PHYTOCHEMISTRY

Volume 3

Marine Sources, Industrial Applications, and Recent Advances

PHYTOCHEMISTRY

Volume 3

Marine Sources, Industrial Applications, and Recent Advances

Edited by

Chukwuebuka Egbuna

Jonathan Chinenye Ifemeje, PhD

Shashank Kumar, PhD

Nadia Sharif, PhD

AAP APPLE ACADEMIC PRESS

Apple Academic Press Inc.
3333 Mistwell Crescent
Oakville, ON L6L 0A2
Canada

Apple Academic Press Inc.
9 Spinnaker Way
Waretown, NJ 08758
USA

First issued in paperback 2021

Exclusive worldwide distribution by CRC Press, a member of Taylor & Francis Group

Phytochemistry, Volume 3: Marine Sources, Industrial Applications, and Recent Advances

ISBN 13: 978-1-77463-523-0 set
ISBN 13: 978-1-77463-434-9 (pbk)
ISBN 13: 978-1-77188-761-8 (hbk)

Phytochemistry, 3-volume set

ISBN 13: 978-1-77188-762-5 (hbk)

Library and Archives Canada Cataloguing in Publication

Phytochemistry / edited by Chukwuebuka Egbuna, Jonathan Chinenye Ifemeje, PhD, Shashank Kumar, PhD, Nadia Sharif, PhD.

Includes bibliographical references and indexes.
Contents: Volume 3. Marine sources, industrial applications, and recent advances.
Issued in print and electronic formats.
ISBN 978-1-77188-761-8 (v. 3 : hardcover).--ISBN 978-1-77188-762-5 (set : hardcover).--
ISBN 978-0-429-42615-5 (v. 3 : PDF).--ISBN 978-0-429-42627-8 (set : PDF)

1. Botanical chemistry. I. Egbuna, Chukwuebuka, editor II. Ifemeje, Jonathan Chinenye, editor
III. Kumar, Shashank, editor IV. Sharif, Nadia, editor

QK861.P65 2019 572'.2 C2018-904824-7 C2018-904875-1

CIP data on file with US Library of Congress

Apple Academic Press also publishes its books in a variety of electronic formats. Some content that appears in print may not be available in electronic format. For information about Apple Academic Press products, visit our website at **www.appleacademicpress.com** and the CRC Press website at **www.crcpress.com**

ABOUT THE EDITORS

Chukwuebuka Egbuna

Chukwuebuka Egbuna is a chartered chemist, a chemical analyst, and an academic researcher. He is a member of the Institute of Chartered Chemists of Nigeria (ICCON), the Nigerian Society of Biochemistry and Molecular Biology (NSBMB), the Royal Society of Chemistry (RSC), United Kingdom, and the Society of Quality Assurance (SQA), USA. He has been engaged in a number of roles at New Divine Favor Pharmaceutical Industry Limited, Akuzor Nkpor, Anambra State, Nigeria, and Chukwuemeka Odumegwu Ojukwu University (COOU), Nigeria. He has attended series of conferences and workshops and has collaboratively worked and published quite a number of research articles in the domain of phytochemistry. He has edited books with top publishers such as Springer Nature and Elsevier. He is a reviewer and an editorial board member for various journals, including serving as a website administrator for the *Tropical Journal of Applied Natural Sciences* (TJANS), a journal of the faculty of Natural Sciences, COOU. His primary research interests are in phytochemistry, food and medicinal chemistry, analytical chemistry, and nutrition and toxicology. He obtained his BSc and MSc degrees in biochemistry at Chukwuemeka Odumegwu Ojukwu University.

Jonathan Chinenye Ifemeje, PhD

Jonathan Chinenye Ifemeje, PhD, is an Associate Professor in the Department of Biochemistry, Faculty of Natural Sciences, Chukwuemeka Odumegwu Ojukwu University, Nigeria. He obtained his PhD in applied biochemistry from Nnamdi Azikiwe University, Awka, Nigeria, and his MSc degree in nutrition and toxicology from the University of Port-Harcourt, Nigeria. He has to his credits over 40 publications in both local and international journals. Dr. Ifemeje is currently the Coordinator, Students Industrial Work Experience Scheme (SIWES), COOU, and has served as an external examiner for various institutions. He is the Managing Editor of the *Tropical Journal of Applied Natural Sciences* and is serving as a reviewer and an editorial board member for various journals. He has worked extensively in the area of phytochemistry, nutrition, and toxicology. He is a member of various institutes, including the Institute of Chartered Chemists of Nigeria

(ICCON), the Nigerian Society of Biochemistry and Molecular Biology (NSBMB), and the Society of Quality Assurance (SQA).

Shashank Kumar, PhD

Shashank Kumar, PhD, is working as Assistant Professor at the Center for Biochemistry and Microbial Sciences, Central University of Punjab, Bathinda, India. He obtained his BSc, MSc, and PhD Biochemistry from the Department of Biochemistry, University of Allahabad, India. He worked as Postdoctoral Fellow at the Department of Biochemistry, King George's Medical University, Lucknow, India. Dr. Kumar has about 60 published scientific papers/reviews/editorial articles/book chapters in various national and international peer-reviewed journals and has been cited more than 1200 times. He has edited several books on topics such as the "concepts in cell signaling," "carbohydrate metabolism: theory and practical approach," and so forth. He has expertise in the areas of free radical biology, cancer biology, characterization of plant natural products, xenobiotic metabolism, and microbiology. He is familiar with many biochemical techniques such as spectrophotometry, enzyme-linked immunosorbent assay, electrophoresis, polymerase chain reaction, real-time polymerase chain reaction, flow cytometry, thin-layer chromatography, high-performance liquid chromatography, liquid chromatography–mass spectrometry, cell culture, and microbiological techniques. He has presented his research findings at more than 25 national/international conferences and attended about 30 workshops at different universities and medical colleges throughout the India. Dr. Kumar is a life time member of Italo-Latin American Society of Ethnomedicine, and the Indian Sciences Congress Association, and member of the Asian Council of Science Editors, Dubai, UAE, and Publication Integrity and Ethics, London. He has been awarded the Junior/Senior and Research Associate Fellowships formulated and funded by various Indian agencies, such as Indian Council of Medical Research, University Grants Commission, Council of Scientific and Industrial Research India. Dr. Kumar laboratory has been funded by the University Grant Commission, India, and the Department of Science and Technology, India, for working on effects of various phytochemicals on cancer cell signaling pathway inhibition.

Nadia Sharif, PhD

Nadia Sharif, PhD, is currently working as a Visiting Lecturer at the Biotechnology Department of Lahore College for Women University, Lahore, Pakistan. She obtained her MSc degree in Zoology from Bahauddin Zakariya

University, Multan, Pakistan, and did her PhD in Biotechnology, Department of Lahore College for Women University, Lahore, Pakistan. She has been awarded the Indigenous and International Fellowship (IRSIP) by the Higher Education Commission, Pakistan. She has visited the Chemical and Biochemical Engineering Department of The Johns Hopkins University, USA, for her PhD research. She has about 20 published scientific papers/reviews/book chapters in various national/international peer-reviewed journals. Dr Nadia Sharif is serving as a reviewer to the *British Microbiology Research Journal, African Journal of Microbiology Research* and *Natural Product Journal*. She has expertise in areas of phycology, industrial biotechnology, microbiology, molecular biology, biostatistics, and biochemistry. She is familiar with many biochemical techniques such as spectrophotometry, electrophoresis, PCR, ASE, TLC, HPLC, GC-MS, cell culture, and microbiological techniques. She has a great interest in working for the sustainable use of natural resources. She has presented her research findings in more than ten national conferences and attended about 30 workshops at the majority of major universities and colleges throughout Pakistan.

CONTENTS

CONTRIBUTORS

Musarat Amina
Department of Pharmacognosy, College of Pharmacy, King Saud University, P. O. Box-2457, Riyadh 11451, Saudi Arabia

Hanan M. Al-Yousef
Department of Pharmacognosy, College of Pharmacy, King Saud University, Riyadh, Saudi Arabia

Syeda Nazish Arshad
Department of Chemistry, Lahore College for Women University, Lahore, Pakistan

Maria Aslam
University Institute of Diet and Nutritional Sciences, Faculty of Allied Health Sciences, University of Lahore, Pakistan

C. S. Chanotiya
Department of Analytical Chemistry, Central Institute of Medicinal and Aromatic Plants, Lucknow, India

Juliana Cotabarren
Centro de Investigación de Proteínas Vegetales (CIPROVE), Departamento de Ciencias Biológicas, Facultad de Ciencias Exactas, Universidad Nacional de La Plata, 47 y 115 s/N, B1900AVW, La Plata, Argentina

Basu Maan Daas
Department of Chemistry, Netaji Subhash Mahavidyalaya, Udaipur, Tripura, India

Hussien M. Daffalla
National Centre for Research, Commission for Biotechnology and Genetic Engineering, Mohamed Nageeb St. No. 61, 11111 Khartoum, Khartoum, Sudan

Chukwuebuka Egbuna
Department of Biochemistry, Faculty of Natural Sciences, Chukwuemeka Odumegwu Ojukwu University, Anambra State 431124, Nigeria

Azza Migdam Elsheikh
National Centre for Research, Commission for Biotechnology and Genetic Engineering, Mohamed Nageeb St. No. 61, 11111 Khartoum, Khartoum, Sudan

Anywar Godwin
Makerere University, Department of Plant Sciences, Microbiology & Biotechnology, P. O. Box 7062, Kampala Uganda

Sechene Stanley Gololo
Department of Biochemistry, School of Science and Technology, Sefako Makgatho Health Sciences University, Ga-Rankuwa, Pretoria, South Africa

Rakesh Kumar Gupta
School of Environment and Earth Science, Environmental Science and Technology, Central University of Punjab, Bathinda, Punjab, 151001, India

Hafsa Kamran
University Institute of Diet and Nutritional Sciences, Faculty of Allied Health Sciences, University of Lahore, Pakistan

Merve Keskin
Department of Chemistry, Faculty of Science, Karadeniz Technical University, Trabzon, Turkey

Şaban Keskin
Department of Chemistry, Faculty of Science and Literature, Bilecik Şeyh Edebali University, Bilecik, Turkey

Sidra Khalid
University Institute of Diet and Nutritional Sciences, Faculty of Allied Health Sciences, University of Lahore, Pakistan

Sevgi Kolaylı
Department of Chemistry, Faculty of Science, Karadeniz Technical University, Trabzon, Turkey

Ramesh Kumar
Department of Biochemistry, University of Allahabad, Allahabad 211002, India

Shashank Kumar
School of Basic and Applied Sciences, Department of Biochemistry and Microbial Sciences, Central University of Punjab, Bathinda, Punjab, 151001, India

Vinesh Kumar
Department of Sciences, Kids' Science Academy, Roorkee, Uttarakhand, India

Prem Prakash Kushwaha
School of Basic and Applied Sciences, Department of Biochemistry and Microbial Sciences, Central University of Punjab, Bathinda, Punjab, 151001, India

Rebati Malik
School of Basic and Applied Sciences, Department of Biochemistry and Microbial Sciences, Central University of Punjab, Bathinda, Punjab, 151001, India

Santosh Kumar Maurya
School of Basic and Applied Sciences, Department of Biochemistry and Microbial Sciences, Central University of Punjab, Bathinda, Punjab, 151001, India

Andrew G. Mtewa
Department of Chemistry, Institute of Technology, Malawi University of Science and Technology, Malawi
Department of Pharmacology and Therapeutics, Mbarara University of Science and Technology, Uganda

Neelma Munir
Department of Biotechnology, Lahore College for Women University, Lahore Pakistan

T. B. Mutsauri
Departamento de Farmacia, Instituto de Farmacia y Alimentos, Universidad de La Habana, Cuba. Calle 222, entre 23 y 29, # 2317, La Coronela, La Lisa, La Habana, Cuba

Sana Nayab
Department of Chemistry, Lahore College for Women University, Lahore, Pakistan

Ashish Kumar Nayak
Department of Microbial Genomics and Diagnostic Laboratory, Regional Plant resource center, Bhubaneshwar, India

Shagufta Naz
Department of Biotechnology, Lahore College for Women University, Lahore Pakistan

Onyeka Kingsley Nwosu
National Biosafety Management Agency (NBMA), Abuja, Nigeria

Walter David Obregón
Centro de Investigación de Proteínas Vegetales (CIPROVE), Departamento de Ciencias Biológicas, Facultad de Ciencias Exactas, Universidad Nacional de La Plata, 47 y 115 s/N, B1900AVW, La Plata, Argentina

David Okechukwu Okeke
Department of Applied Biochemistry, Nnamdi Azikiwe University, Awka, Nigeria

Olumayowa Vincent Oriyomi
Institute of Ecology and Environmental Studies, Obafemi Awolowo University, Ile- Ife, Osun State, Nigeria

Maria Catherine B. Otero
College of Medicine Research Center, Davao Medical School Foundation, Inc., Davao City, Philippines

Abhay K. Pandey
Department of Biochemistry, University of Allahabad, Allahabad 211002, India

Juan Abreu Payrol
Departamento de Farmacia, Instituto de Farmacia y Alimentos, Universidad de La Habana, Cuba. Calle 222, entre 23 y 29, # 2317, La Coronela, La Lisa, La Habana, Cuba

Sergey V. Pospelov
Department of Agriculture & Agrochemistry, Faculty Agrotechnology & Ecology, Poltava State Agrarian Academy, 1/3 Skovorody St., Poltava, 36003, Ukraine

A. Samad
Department of plant pathology, Central Institute of Medicinal and Aromatic Plants, Lucknow India

Arvind Saroj
Department of plant pathology, Central Institute of Medicinal and Aromatic Plants, Lucknow, India

Duncan C. Sesaazi
Department of Pharmacology and Therapeutics, Mbarara University of Science and Technology, Uganda

Hameed Shah
CAS Key Laboratory for Biomedical Effects of Nanomaterials and Nanosafety, National Center for Nanoscience and Technology, Beijing, China
University of Chinese Academy of Science, Beijing 100049, China

Nadia Sharif
Department of Biotechnology, Lahore College for Women University, Lahore Pakistan

Yogita Sharma
Department of Sciences, Kids' Science Academy, Roorkee, Uttarakhand, India

Pushpendra Singh
National Institute of Pathology, New Delhi, India

Atul Kumar Srivastava
Department of plant pathology, Central Institute of Medicinal and Aromatic Plants, Lucknow India

Genevieve D. Tupas
College of Medicine, Department of Pharmacology, Davao Medical School Foundation, Inc., Davao City, Philippines

Inidia Rubio Vargas
Departamento de Farmacia, Instituto de Farmacia y Alimentos, Universidad de La Habana, Cuba. Calle 222, entre 23 y 29, # 2317, La Coronela, La Lisa, La Habana, Cuba

ABBREVIATIONS

4-HC	4-Hydroperoxycyclophosphamide
ACE	Angiotensin-I-converting enzyme
ACGs	Annonaceous acetogenins
AGPs	Arabinogalactan-proteins
ALDH1	Aldehyde dehydrogenase 1
AMPs	Antimicrobial peptides
AP-1	Activator protein 1
ASE	Accelerated solvent extraction
ATP	Adenosine triphosphate
ATRA	All-trans-retinoic acid
Bcl-2	B-cell lymphoma 2
BT	Biotransformation
CAA	Cellular antioxidant activity
CA	Caffeic acid
CE-MS	Capillary electrophoresis coupled with mass spectrometry
CP	Clonal propagation
CSC	Cell suspension culture
CSCs	Cancer stem cells
CS	Chitosan
CVS	Cell volume after sedimentation
DDT	Dichlorodiphenyltrichloroethane
DMAPP	Dimethylallyl pyrophosphate
DW	Dry weight
EGCG	Epigallocatechin-3-gallate
EOs	Essential oils
EPA	Environmental Protection Agency
ESTs	Expressed sequence tags
FD	Freeze drying
FW	Fresh weight
GAGs	Glycosaminoglycans
GC	Gas chromatography
GFC	Gel filtration chromatography
GS	GSH synthetase

GSH	Glutathione
GST	Glutathione S-transferase
hGSH	Homoglutathione
HIV	Human immunodeficiency virus
HMB-PP	(E)-4-Hydroxy-3-methyl-but-2-enyl pyrophosphate
HMG-CoA	3-hydroxy-3-methylglutaryl-CoA
hPC	Homophytochelatins
HPLC-DAD	High-Performance Liquid Chromatography-Diode-Array Detection
HPLC	High-performance liquid chromatography
HUVEC	Human umbilical vein endothelial cell
IAA	Indole-3-acetic acid
IBA	Indole-3-butyric acid
IgE	Immunoglobulin E
IPC	Immobilized plant cells
IPP	Isopentenyl pyrophosphate
LC	Liquid chromatography
MAE	Microwave-assisted extraction
MALDI	Matrix-assisted laser desorption ionization
MALDI-TOF	Matrix-assisted laser desorption/ionization time-of-flight
MAPK	Mitogen-activated protein kinase
MD	Maximum diameter
MDR	Multidrug resistance
MEP	Methylerythritol phosphate
MMP	Metalloproteinase
MP	Micropropagation
MS	Mass spectrometry
MS	MURASHIGE and Skoog
MT	Metallothioneins
MVA	Mevalonic acid
NAA	1-Naphthaleneacetic acid
NADPH	Nicotinamide adenine dinucleotide phosphate
NAFDAC	National Agency for Food and Drug Administration and Control
NBT	Nitroblue tetrazolium
NMR	Nuclear magnetic resonance
NPs	Nanoparticles
NSKE	Neem seed kernel extract

PAL	Phenylalanine ammonia lyase
PCC	Plant cell culture
PCD	programmed cell death
PCS	Phytochelatin synthase
PCs	Phytochelatins
PCV	Packed cell volume
PEF	Pulsed-electric field extraction
PEs	Phorbol esters
PFE	Pressurized liquid extraction
PGE2	Prostaglandin E2
PGRs	Plant growth regulators
PHWE	Pressurized hot water extraction
PLE	Pressurized liquid extraction
PMS	Phenazine methosulphate
PPO	Polyphenol oxidase
PTC	Plant tissue culture
PUFAs	Polyunsaturated fatty acids
QqQ-MS	Triple Quadrupole-Mass Spectrometers
RA	Retinoic acid
RARs	Retinoic acid receptors
ROS	Reactive oxygen species
RP-HPLC	Reversed-phase high-performance liquid chromatography
rpm	Revolutions per minute
RXRs	Retinoid X receptors
SD	Spray drying
SEg	Somatic embryogenesis
SFC	Supercritical fluid chromatography
SFD	SPRAY FD
SFE	Supercritical fluid extraction
SOD	Superoxide dismutase
T-DNA	Transfer DNA
Ti	Tumor-inducing
TRAIL	Tumor necrosis factor-related apoptosis-inducing ligand
UAE	Ultrasound-assisted extraction
UV	Ultraviolet
WIPO	World Intellectual Property Organization
γECS	γ-EC synthetase

FOREWORD

I am pleased to write the foreword for this book, *Phytochemistry, Volume 3: Marine Sources, Industrial Applications, and Recent Advances*. The scope of the volume is multifaceted with deep scientific content. The volume covers trending topics from emerging areas of phytochemistry, including marine phytochemistry, production of phytochemicals through *in vitro* culture, phytochemical biopesticides, and other recent advances. Though there are a few books in this category, the organization of this book particularly makes it exceptional. I commend the editors and the chapter contributors for the good work.

I do believe that everyone with related interest will find this book very useful.

—**Prof. Chukwunenye C. Anene**
Dean Faculty of Natural Sciences,
Former Ag. Vice Chancellor
Chukwuemeka Odumegwu Ojukwu University, Nigeria

PREFACE

This book, *Phytochemistry, Volume 3: Marine Sources, Industrial Applications, and Recent Advances,* is a comprehensive book on phytochemistry written by professionals from key institutions. The contributors are authors of the finest academic traditions. The chapters were drawn carefully and integrated sequentially to aid flow, consistency, and continuity. This book is designed to be useful to researchers, teachers, students, phytochemists, plant biochemists, food and medicinal chemists, marine chemists, nutritionists, analytical chemists, industrialists, and plant biotechnologists.

The chapters were grouped into four parts: Part I: Marine Sources of Secondary Metabolites; Part II: Industrial and Medicinal Applications of Phytochemicals; Part III: Environmental Concerns and Eco-Friendly Control Measures; and Part IV: Recent Advances.

In Part I, Chapter 1, Sharif et al. presents marine phytochemistry and fundamentals. In Chapter 2, Musarat and Hanan discusses marine sponge alkaloids with its potentials as anticancer agents. Chapter 3, by Nwosu and Okeke, presents marine antioxidants and assay methods. In Chapter 4, Sharif et al. details the various extraction and identification protocols.

In Part II, Chapter 5, Shah et al. presents an introduction on the biotechnological approach in the *in vitro* production of phytochemicals. Chapter 6 by Daffalla and Elsheikh provides a comprehensive detail on the *in vitro* production of phytochemicals. Hanan presents the practical steps involved in the production of phytochemicals by plant tissue culture in Chapter 7. In Chapter 8, Kumar and Pandey presents the medicinal and industrial applications of bromelain. Chapter 9 by Payrol et al. is a detailed study on the cysteine proteases from plants and their applications. Keskin et al. presents phytotherapy and encapsulation in Chapter 10. Chapter 11 is a review of the effective processing methods for fruits and vegetables.

In Part III, Chapter 12, Gololo presents the effects of environmental factors on the accumulation of phytochemicals in plants. Kumar and Sharma in Chapter 13 further emphasize the effects of the environmental factors on the chemical constituents and the biological characteristics of some medicinal plants. Chapter 14 by Otero and Tupas is a review of phytochelatins and heavy metal tolerance in plants as regards to phytoremediation. Chapter 15 by Oriyomi details the phytochemical biopesticides. In Chapter 16, Gupta et al. discusses the sustainable approach to integrated pest management. Saroj et al. in Chapter 17 presents the role of essential oils in pest control and disease management. In Chapter 18, Daas presents the potentials of phytochemicals in serving as mild steel eco-friendly corrosion inhibitors.

In Part IV, Chapter 19, Malik et al. presents findings of novel terpenoids as an anticancer stem cell agents. Chapter 20 by Pospelov is a comprehensive study of the phytohemagglutinins activities of Echinacea species in ontogenesis. The author presents novel findings spanning many years of research including a new technique for conducting mass analysis for determining the hemagglutination activity of Echinacea extracts.

As highlighted above, this book contains trending chapters written by professionals. I recommend this book to researchers, students, and everyone with interest in phytochemistry. My sincere appreciation goes to the chapter contributors for their great contributions, patience, and cooperation during the editorial process. I will remain grateful to the volunteer reviewers and my co-editors. A special thanks goes to my family for their support and patience during the editorial process. To the management of Apple Academic Press, I will remain thankful for your guidance and support. To the readers, I appreciate your thoughtfulness and would welcome reviews about the book with an open heart. Thank you.

—Chukwuebuka Egbuna
MNSBMB, MICCON; AMRSC
Department of Biochemistry, Faculty of Natural Sciences,
Chukwuemeka Odumegwu Ojukwu University,
Anambra State- 431,124, Nigeria
E-mail: egbuna.cg@coou.edu.ng

PART I

Marine Sources of Secondary Metabolites

CHAPTER 1

PHYTOCHEMICALS OF MARINE ORIGINS

NADIA SHARIF[1*], SANA NAYAB[2], SYEDA NAZISH ARSHAD[2], NEELMA MUNIR[1], and SHAGUFTA NAZ[1]

[1]*Department of Biotechnology, Lahore College for Women University, Lahore, Pakistan, Tel.: +923237501948*

[2]*Department of Chemistry, Lahore College for Women University, Lahore, Pakistan*

[*]*Corresponding author. E-mail: nadiasharif.s7@gmail.com*
[*]*ORCID: https://orcid.org/0000-0002-8125-9270*

ABSTRACT

Oceans are consecrated with a variety of plants and animals. Marine plants consist of microscopic algae to towering underwater kelp forests and undulating seagrass beds. They possess a stock of several types of natural products as they are developed in a chemically rich environment. These compounds are also biomedically important and are obtained from aquatic life by using sophisticated extraction techniques. Due to their pharmacological activities, these compounds are frequently used in the treatment of lethal diseases such as cancer, arthritis, and acquired immunodeficiency syndrome. This chapter throws light on the recent advances and outcomes in the field of marine phytochemistry.

1.1 INTRODUCTION

The aquatic region has a wide range of temperature underneath freezing temperatures in Antarctic waters to around 350°C in deep hydrothermal vents, wide pressure range, oligotrophic to a eutrophic range of nutrients, and far-reaching photic and non-photic regions. From microorganisms to mammals, this wide-ranging variability has expedited a lot of speciation at all phylogenetic levels. Although the marine biodiversity is far more than terrestrial organisms, looking up in the making for the use of marine herbal products as pharmaceutical marketers is yet in its beginning due to the privation of ethnomedical antiquity and the problems that are related to the assortment of marine organisms (Faulkner, 1992). The progress of new secluded operating machines and new diving techniques has resulted in the collection of marine samples in recent times, from shallow to deep waters from which about 5000 novel compounds have been derived. The marine plants grow within the reach of sunlight for photosynthesis and nearby ice and salt water surface. Algae that are the plentiful type of marine plants are essential for a balanced ecosystem as well as for maintaining food chain (Teagle et al., 2017). Water is the requirement of life. Earlier plants including algae were designed in physiques of saline water that covers the prehistoric Earth. In the Silurian period (about 441–410 million years past), some aquatic plants started to grow on land; however, a lot of plants endured merely water based. The importance of marine plants can be evaluated as they are fundamental organisms to provide the nourishment in the food web and without their existence, it was not possible for the marine animals to evolve or survive (Carpenter, 2014).

Marine plants are comprised of microscopic algae to towering underwater kelp forests and undulating seagrass beds. Regardless of this diversity, the majority of marine plants play an enormous role in marine ecosystems. The very base of the marine food web is formed by tiny algae that are only visible when they multiply into large blooms. Bull kelp and giant kelp like large and multicellular algae in marine environment provide the protection and food to numerous marine species. Many marine animals are harbored by the marine flowering plants or seagrasses, such as eelgrass or surfgrass. Depending on the tolerance to light, air, waves, and predators grazing, different marine plants thrive in different environments. The evolutionary history of the marine plants is traced from the fossils found in the marine sediments formed by algae. The plate tectonics involving changes in ocean shape and continents movement has greatly affected the distribution of marine plants. Marine plants included small unicellular organisms to big convoluted systems. Two major types of marine plants included the algae/seaweeds and seagrasses. Among these, algae/seaweeds are simple forms of plants and are often microscopic, whereas seagrasses represent members of the more complex plants (Rich and Maier, 2015).

As sunlight is required for the manufacturing of food in all marine plants, therefore, they generally grow in nearby water planes. Nutrients are also collected from elements that fluxes wash up from sea floors. Marine plants can acclimatize to a particular state, like inadequate light and the caves underwater. Several are phosphorescent, producing chemical lights. Phytoplanktons are the minutest marine plants. They are single-celled and make the foundation of the marine food chain. Bacillariophyta diatoms are glossy infinitesimal cells which are recurrently associated together in chains. A small number of marine plants (angiosperms); though grow in the tropical coasts, are frequently accrued flowering marine plants. Green algae (Chlorophyta) are the utmost marine plant. Chlorophyll makes these algae to have bright green coloring. As the leaves of algae calcify, the layers are added to ocean deposits. Botanists consider that 200,000 algae species occur, although just 36,000 are known. Red algae (Rhodophyta), supplied with pigment phycoerythrin, are the major type of marine plants and the most diverse. Some red algae stick to corals, hence making reefs. Both green and red algae species favor cold to warm water. Contrary, brown algae (Phaeophyta), tinted with the pigment fucoxanthin, are generally present in temperate or cold water, and also some species living in tropics. On reefs, brown algae commonly are the prevailing organisms. Blue-green bacteria or cyanobacteria are principally microscopic constituents which alter nitrogen from the atmosphere into forms that furthermost marine plants can consume (Morrissey et al., 2016).

Marine biotechnology is the study which includes the procedures to create the partial or full alteration of products, to mend animals or plants, or to advance microorganisms for precise consumptions. Through molecular and biotechnological procedures, humans have been capable to explicate numerous natural means (Jha and Zi-Rong, 2004). The marine environs might comprise 80% of the world's animal and plant species. Currently, various bioactive complexes have been hauling out from many marine animals and marine organisms (Haefner, 2003). The exploration of different metabolites as of marine organisms has occasioned the sequestration of more or less of 10,000 metabolites, several of which are capable of pharmacodynamic activities. Natural products have extensively been supplied as pigments, foods, insecticides, fragrances, medicines, and so forth. Because of their tranquil openness, land plants have aided the key foundation of therapeutically valuable goods, particularly for outmoded or traditional medicine. The ocean provides a diverse living environment for invertebrates as it covers 70% of the earth's surface. In terms of chemicals and biology, the marine environment is rich in diversity. Marine plants are a unique source of chemical compounds that may have potential industrial applications in pharmacy, medicine, agriculture, cosmetics, and research. The reservoir of bioactive natural compounds that are provided by the marine environment is exceptional as a lot of them show the chemical and structural features that are not present in land natural products. Marine organisms have evolved biochemical and physiological contrivances that comprise the bioactive compounds for the applications in communication, predation protection, infection, reproduction, and competition (Halvorson, 1998).

Hence in near future, the marine natural products are going to play a major role in drug discovery. Till now, approximately 7000 natural products of marine origin have been extracted in which algae comprise 25%, sponges 33%, coelenterates 18%, while 24% includes bryozoans, echinoderms, mollusks, and ascidians (Kijjoa and Sawangwong, 2004).

1.2 DISCOVERY OF MARINE PHYTOCHEMICALS

Four steps of drug discovery from marine plants are the identification of drug target, validation of target, identification of lead compounds, and optimization (see Volume 1 and 2 of this book for more information). Completely new therapeutic approaches have been opened up by the marine natural products. Their advantages include the use of marine drug availability, identification, and appreciation of unique biochemical pathways. These have contributed to research tools in biochemistry and molecular cell biology (Grabley and Sattler, 2003).

Saponins, flavonoids, alkaloids, anthraquinones, and volatile oils are the various chemical components of marine organisms. For the identification of phytochemicals, rapid and reproducible analytical techniques have been developed and these techniques include the high-performance liquid chromatography (HPLC) combined with different detectors like diode array detector, refractive index detector, a mass spectrometric detector, and evaporative light scattering detector. A significant step to check or control for crude drugs quality as well as to elucidate their therapeutic mechanism is by analyzing and screening the bioactive compounds. The compounds of marine origin discovered initially were noxious or were not operative in the treatment of pharmaceutical tenacities diseases. Instead, they are beneficial as agrochemicals, cosmetic ingredients, or biological tools (Fenical, 1997).

A lot of drugs are derived from aquatic organisms. One example is a neurotoxin isolated from a snail, with potency 10,000 times more than morphine. For the treatment of herpes virus and cancer, two compounds have been isolated from sponge and also an antibiotic has been derived from fungi. Nevertheless, there are numerous other compounds that are isolated from a marine source and presently are in clinical trials, and it is probable that several additional might progress to the treatment.

The conventional methods employed for extraction, isolation, and identification of phytochemicals were discussed in details in Chapter 4 of this volume.

1.3 UNIQUENESS OF MARINE PHYTOCHEMICALS

The marine vegetation comprises of microflora (cyanobacteria, bacteria, fungi, and Actinobacteria), microalgae, macroalgae (seaweeds), and flowering plants (mangroves and other halophytes). Inhabiting nearly 71% of globally, the sea is opulent in biodiversity, and the microalgae and microflora unaided organize higher than 90% of marine biomass. This huge aquatic floral reserve will compromise a pronounced opportunity for finding the novel medications. It cannot be deprived of that with 3.5 billion years of presence on land and knowledge in biosynthesis; the aquatic microflora lingers environment's greatest cradle of elements. The aquatic entities produce unique compounds to endure risky differences in salinity, pressure, temperature, and so forth, prevalent in their environs, and the compounds formed are inimitable in variety, organizational, and efficient structures (Kathiresan et al., 2008).

The efforts for the extraction of medicines from the ocean came into limelight lately in the 1960s. Nevertheless, the efficient analysis initiated in the mid-1970s, through the period of 1977–1987, brought about 2500 novel metabolites from diverse aquatic organisms. Researchers have noticeably established the aquatic environs as the tremendous basis of unique compounds, not present in land cradles. Until now, more than 10,000 compounds are extracted from aquatic organisms, though much more new complexes are revealed each year. Nearly 300 exclusive rights on bioactive aquatic natural products were acquired amid 1969 and 1999 (Kathiresan et al., 2008). Certain aquatic organisms are demonstrated to be the persuasive foundations of treatments. These are generally invertebrates that comprise sponges, sea fans, sea hares, sea corals, nudibranchs, tunicates, and bryozoans. Currently, it is assumed that contagious floras extant in the invertebrates are liable for the fabrication of curative complexes. The exploration of aquatic faunal and floral species is essentially unheeded. Various complexes derivatives of aquatic entities have anticancer and antioxidant bioactivities yet they are essentially unknown well.

Since ancient times, the aquatic organisms are cast-off for pharmaceutical applications in China, India Europe, and Near East. China and Japanese are utilizing seaweeds for feeding. The seaweeds particularly brown seaweeds are opulent in iodine which results in a minimum occurrence of glandular ailments and goiter. Antiquity divulges that maritime states were using seaweeds as a vermifuge, general anesthetic, and liniment similarly for the treatment of gout, cough, abrasions goiter, venereal illness, and so forth. Sterols and associated complexes existent in seaweeds are able to low plasma blood cholesterol level. Seaweed nutritional filaments accomplish diverse functions like antitumor antioxidant, antimutagenic, and anticoagulant. The seaweeds also impart a significant part in alteration of triglyceride breakdown in the humanoid body. Calcium, sodium, and potassium are accompanying by low mean systolic pressure and low menace of hypertension. All seaweeds propose an amazing level of potassium that is alike with our plasma level. Seaweed extract is remarkably analogous to human blood plasma. Two Japanese investigators applied an inimitable practice of seaweed compounds mixing with water to ancillary entire blood while transfusion and this has been effectively strained in about 100 procedures (Langseth, 1995).

Even though the practice of seaweeds as a source of drugs is not as common as it was previously, seaweed polymer excerpt used in medicine, pharmacy, and biochemistry is well established. Efforts are in process for the introduction of jelly capsules that are made of seaweed alginic acid and secrete insulin so that diabetic patient gets freed from the injection. The lozenge concentrates fortification on the patient's immune system and white blood cells. Seaweed exudates like carrageenan isolated from red seaweed or algin isolated from brown seaweed are opulent sources of soluble fibers (Langseth, 1995).

Numerous aquatic plants are able to produce bioactive materials that exhibit antibacterial, antifungal, antiviral activities, and also antialgal activities (Li and Hu, 2005). The fermentation of an *Eisenia bicyclis* broth with *Candida utilis* YM-1 in the course of 1 day enriched the phenolic content such as dieckol, phlorofucofuroeckol A, eckol, and dioxinodehydroeckol and activity of inhibition against methicillin-resistant *Staphylococcus aureus* and foodborne pathogenic bacteria. Cell wall and storage of green, brown, and red seaweed polysaccharides, together with ulvans, alginates, fucans, laminarin, and carrageenans are able to elicit resistance retorts in plants against pathogens.

1.4 CLASSES OF PHYTOCHEMICALS

Marine organisms are a rich source of biologically active and therapeutically compelling compounds. Polysaccharides and polyphenols are the utmost set of complexes that are valid for biological activities such as anticancer and antioxidant activity. There are above 40,000 diverse species of phytoplankton, 680 species of aquatic algae, including Chlorophyta, Phaeophyta, and Rhodophyta generally known as green, brown, and red seaweeds, respectively, and 71 mangrove plant species recognized globally in the aquatic biotope. They offer amino acids, vital fatty acids, vitamins, bioflavonoids, ionic trace minerals, enzymes, and other compounds.

1.4.1 ALKALOIDS

The term alkaloid was formally suggested by Meissner in 1819 to describe "alkali-like" complexes originated in plants; nevertheless, it was not indeed distinct (Swan, 1967). They include the major collection of secondary chemical components prepared generally of ammonia complexes, consisting essentially of nitrogen bases manufactured from amino acid with numerous radicals substituting one or more of the hydrogen atoms in the peptide ring, utmost encompassing oxygen (see Chapter 2, Volume 1 for more information). The complexes have elementary possessions and are alkaline in response, altering the red litmus paper blue. In actual, one or more nitrogen atoms that are contemporaneous in an alkaloid characteristically has 1, 2, or 3° amines, subsidize to the alkalinity of the alkaloid. The degree of alkalinity of alkaloid differs significantly, contingent on the organization of the molecule, and occurrence and position of the functional groups. The mainstream of alkaloids occurs in solid form like atropine, certain as liquids containing hydrogen, nitrogen, and carbon. Maximum alkaloids are generously solvable in alcohol and yet they are thriftily soluble in water, their salts are generally decipherable. The alkaloids solutions are strongly nasty. These nitrogenous compounds work in the defense of plants against pathogens and herbivores and are broadly oppressed as drugs, amphetamines, tranquilizers, and toxins because of their powerful activities. In natural surroundings, the alkaloids occur in huge quantities in the roots and seeds of plants and frequently in amalgamation with vegetable acids. Alkaloids have drug solicitations as analgesics and central nervous system stimulants (Madziga et al., 2010). Above 12,000 alkaloids are recognized to occur in around 20% of plant species and only a few have been subjugated for therapeutic determinations.

The term alkaloid ends with the suffix –ine and alkaloids of plants origin in clinical use contain the anesthetics morphine and codeine, the muscle relaxant (+)-tubocurarine, the antibiotics berberine and sanguinarine, the vinblastine anticancer agent, the anti-arrhythmic ajmaline, the pupil dilator atropine, and the sedative scopolamine. Other significant plant originated alkaloids include the addictive amphetamines caffeine, ergotamine, nicotine, ephedrine, and cocaine. Amino acids turn as antecedents for the biosynthesis of alkaloids with lysine and ornithine generally utilized as preparatory constituents. As the time passed, the delineation has altered to a compound that has nitrogen atom(s) in a cyclic ring. The term alkaloid includes halogenated cyclic nitrogen-containing elements and various biological amines. The latter is not present in land plants and is particular to aquatic organisms; aquatic algae are included in them. Regarding alkaloids chemistry and its anticancer activities, numerous studies are available in terrestrial plants; however, insufficient data is available in marine plants (Guven et al., 2010). The first alkaloid is morphine that was isolated from a terrestrial plant in 1805, whereas in 1969, hordenine as the first marine alkaloid was extracted. Today, about 2000 alkaloids are recognized. Their occurrence is rare in marine algae and abundant in terrestrial plants.

Among numerous kinds of compounds acquired from plants, conventionally the alkaloids have been of attention because of their pronounced biological activities in humans and animals. Well-known examples of anticancer alkaloids are taxol that is available clinically since 1994 from the western yew, *Taxus brevifolia*, and camptothecin and derivatives of *Camptotheca acuminata* presently are in clinical trials. Marine algae alkaloids are divided into three groups, first are a group of indole and halogenated indole alkaloids, the second group are phenylethylamine alkaloids, and rest alkaloids are included in the third group. In structure, most of the marine algae alkaloids are related to indole and phenylethylamine groups. The phytoconstituents and activities of these alkaloids were not completely examined. In comparison with terrestrial plants, marine plant-derived alkaloids are rare (Gross et al., 2006).

A huge and progressively developing set of secondary metabolites is included in marine indole alkaloids. The biological activities of these varied alkaloids make numerous complexes of this group striking as the starting points for the advancement of pharmaceutical products. Numerous marine-derived indoles remained attractive for different biological activities such as antimicrobial, antioxidant, cytotoxic, and antineoplastic. Furthermore, it acts on human receptors and enzymes. Pyridoacridine also represents a large family of alkaloids possessing inimitable marine nitrogenous composites. Different marine organisms such as sponges (see Chapter 2 and 3 of this volume for details), ascidians, anemones, prosobranch mollusk, and tunicates are evidenced for their presence. A great interest in accordance with pyrido-acridines is raised due to their substantial biological activities. Anticancer activity possessing alkaloids are also extracted from coastal mangroves (Kathiresan and Duraisamy, 2005). Another alkaloid is Rhizophrine, which is a most important component of *Rhizophora mucronata* and *Rhizophora stylosa* leaves. Likewise, the acanthicifolin presence in *Acanthus illicifolius*, brugine, an alkaloid with sulfur, in *Bruguiera sexangula*, and benzoquinones in *Aegiceras corniculatum* and *Kandelia kandel* are reported.

Indole alkaloids are either consequential from direct indole precursor or from tryptophan. In microorganisms and plants, the indole precursor is made from chorismate via anthranilate and indole-3-glycerol-phosphate. The eventual phase of the tryptophan biosynthesis is rescindable and thus free indole can also be made in this catabolic procedure. An anonymous algicolous fungus sampled from the surface of the marine Rhodophyta alga *Gracilaria verrucosa* led to the extraction of Nb-acetyltryptamine. 2-methylsulfinyl-3-methylthio-4,5,6-tribromoindole, 3-methylsulfinyl-2,4,6-tribromoindole, and 4,6-dibromo-2,3-di(methylsulfinyl)indole were extracted from the Formosan red alga *Laurencia brongniartii*. 2,3,4,6-tetrabromo-1-methyl-1H-indole was sequestered from the marine red alga *Laurencia decumbens*. From the marine red alga *Laurencia similis,* 3,5,6-tribromo-1H-indole, 3,5,6-tribromo-1-methyl-1H-indole, 2,3,6-tribromo-1H-indole, 3,5-dibromo-1-methyl-1H-indole, and 2,5-dibromo-1-methyl-1H-indole were extracted (Li et al., 2010).

Granulatamides A and B were sequestered from the soft coral *Eunicella granulate* and it exhibited cytotoxic activity alongside the tumor cell lines DU-145, LNCaP, SK-OV-3, IGROV, IGROV-ET, SK-BR3, SK-MEL-28, HMEC1, A549, K562, PANC1, HT-29, LOVO, LOVO-DOX, HeLa, and HeLa-APL (GI50—concentration which possessions a growth inhibition of 50%—1.7–13.8 μm). N-acetylated aplicyanins B, D, and F are effective antimitotic as well as cytotoxic activities alongside the tumor cell lines HT-29 (GI50 0.39, 0.33, and 0.47 μm, correspondingly), A549 (GI50 0.66, 0.63, and 1.31 μm, correspondingly), and MDA-MB-231 (GI50 0.42, 0.41, and 0.81 μm, correspondingly), while aplicyanin E exhibit merely cytotoxic effects (GI50 values 7.96–8.70 μm) (Reyes et al., 2008).

1.4.2 POLYPHENOLS

The terms phenolics, polyphenolics, phenols, or polyphenol are imparted to extracts that are natural constituents and impart color to plant fruits. Through the action of phenylalanine ammonia lyase (PAL) action, the phenolics are produced from phenylalanine in plants. They are essential for plants and have many roles. They are applied to the rule over human pathogenic permanency as they fight against the herbivores and pathogens via plant defense mechanisms. Their three classes include (a) flavonoids: polyphenols that are comprised catechins, flavones, flavanones, and xanthones, (b) non-flavonoid polyphenolics, and (c) most common phenolic acid of marine plants that is caffeic acid proceeded by chlorogenic acid that is responsible for allergic dermatitis in humans (Kar, 2007). As natural antioxidants, phenolics are used as nutraceuticals, are applied for the treatment of heart ailment, and help fight against cancer and inflammations. Hesperidin, naringin, chlorogenic, rutin, and flavones are examples of some other phenols. Phenolics of marine origin are considered as a significant group of natural antioxidants. Phenolics are made up of one or more aromatic rings and have one or more hydroxyl groups. Chemically, polyphenols classes are coumestans and isoflavones like isoflavonoids, flavones, flavanones, flavanols, flavonols, flavanonols, anthocyanins like flavonoids hydroxycinnamic acids and hydroxybenzoic acids like phenolic acids, tannins and proanthocyanidins like phenolic polymers, lignin, and stilbenes. Structurally, several thousand polyphenolics are reported as the secondary metabolites of marine plants. Their sources include fruits, vegetables, cereals, and leguminous plants. Many factors affect their concentration such as technological, environmental, and genetic factors.

Polyphenols provide protection against pathogens and ultraviolet radiation (Lee and Lip, 2003). Phenols are also involved in plants growth, reproduction, and pigmentation. Phlorotannins group of phenolic compounds are abundant in brown algae and is present in lower quantity in red algae. They constitute the cell wall but are also important for therapeutic properties and secondary ecological functions. They are important against human immunodeficiency virus (HIV), inflammatory, aging, cancer, diabetes, bacterial, and allergic infections. Additionally, to protect against UV radiation, they are involved in protective mechanism against biotic factor and play an integral role in algae reproduction (Frankel, 1998). Because of the health benefits discussed above, this group of compounds is receiving an increasing concern by the food manufacturers and consumers. Antioxidants from natural sources need to be explored further for their great potential. The sustenance of significant omega-3 polyunsaturated fatty acids (PUFAs) like eicosapentaenoic acid (C20:5 n-3) and docosahexaenoic acid (C22:6 n-3) have enormous beneficial effects on human health. Nevertheless, lipid oxidation is the possibility that might affect the seafood having the great quantities of PUFAs (Boyd et al., 1993). Lipid oxidation has a lot of harmful effects and to overcome the possible toxicity and food safety concerns instead of synthetic antioxidants, there is an increase in adaptation for natural antioxidants (Maqsood and Benjakul, 2013). For natural antioxidants, the food industry is focusing more towards the phenolic compounds of the marine source. Different marine phytochemicals including phenolic compounds are reported to retard the oxidation of lipids in a different kind of seafood.

As stated above, the polyphenols of plants are composed of one or more phenolic rings and are formed as a result of plants secondary metabolism. In the terrestrial environment, vegetables, fruits, tea, beer, winc, chocolate, and coffee are made up of phenolic compounds. Moreover, in recent years, they are also extracted and applied to food as colorants and to enhance the shelf life of food. Though the sources from where these compounds are extracted affect their activities, this is credited to the varied factors like the environment in which it grows, its genotype or variety, temperature, light, growth time, environment, type of soil and their dispensation, and postharvest storage. Phenolic contents and antioxidant activities or both and other biological activities and quantity of active compounds are all affected by the listed factors. The antimicrobial, antioxidant, and scavenging activities of polyphenols are comprehensively disseminated in plants (Bors et al., 1990). The high amount of polyphenols like flavonoids, lignin, epicatechin, phenolic acids gallic acid, anthocyanidins, tannins, catechin, and epigallocatechin are observed in seagrass, seaweed, and mangrove like marine plants. The health and nutritional benefits of these polyphenol composites are great like they help act against oxidation, bacteria, cancer, inflammation, viruses, and human platelet aggregation. It is described that the augmented nutritional consumption of natural antioxidants and the abridged coronary heart disease, cancer transience likewise extended life expectancy. Moreover, polyphenols with high antioxidant activity and natural metal chelators inhibit diverse toxic metal ion-induced organ dysfunctions (Xu et al., 2006). The prior research proposes that polyphenols can restore α-tocopherol by reducing the α-tocopheroxyl radical. The association of anticarcinogenic and antioxidant activity is confirmed in a chemically swayed mouse carcinoma system with low-molecular-weight polyphenols (Kakegawa et al., 1985). The aquatic red algae, for example, *Osmundea pinnatifida*, has been widely known for the antileishmanial, antioxidant, antimicrobial, and antifungal activities (Shibata et al., 2002). In addition, scutellarein 4′-methyl ether has antiallergic, anticytotoxic, and anticancer bioactivities in vivo and in vitro (Yuan et al., 2005).

Marine and land polyphenols are comparative in a few regards, however very specific in their compound configurations. Land polyphenols are constructed in light of flavonoids or gallic acids. Marine polyphenols, phlorotannins of algae, are just recognized in brown algae and are restricted to phloroglucinol polymers (Heo et al., 2005). These are usually distributed in plant vegetation and are high molecular weight phenol compounds. Tannins are dissolvable in water and alcohols are originated in the stem, root, bark, and external layers of plant tissue. Tannins have a distinctive highlight to tan, that is, to change over things into leather. They are acidic in response and the acidic response is ascribed to the nearness of phenolics or carboxylic group (Kar, 2007). Tannins are composed of hydrolyzable tannins yet condensed tannins. The hydrolyzable tannins are known as gallotannins and ellagitannins. On heating, they make pyrogallic acid. Co-joint examples concerning hydrolyzable tannins include the aflavins, daidzein, and genistein yet glycitein. In Ayurveda, formulations primarily grounded over tannin-rich flora have been utilized for the remedy concerning ailments like diarrhea, rhinorrhea, and leucorrhoea. Six phlorotannins were identified from the brown seaweeds *E. bicyclis* and *Eclonia kurome* through HPLC analysis, these include phloroglucinol, phloroglucinol tetramer (MW 478), eckol, phlorofucofuroeckol A, dieckol, 8,8′-bieckol. The crude phlorotannins extracts showed inhibitory effects on HAase (Nakamura et al., 1996). As compared to an anti-allergic drug (disodium cromoglycate), half-maximal inhibition (IC50) values of crude phlorotannins of *E. bicyclis* and *E. kurome*, two land polyphenols (catechin, epigallocatechin gallate), prevent four times resiliently (Fukuyama et al., 1989).

Edible seaweeds retain comprehensive potential bioactive constituents: polyphenols and phlorotannins (Zhao et al., 2007). Edible seaweed like *Palmaria palmate* possesses antioxidant activities and inhibits the cancer cell propagation. Brown seaweed *Ecklonia cava* enzyme hydrolysis produces a big quantity of complexes with increased biological activities in comparison to water and organic extract counterparts. Phloroglucinol and its polymers named eckol (a trimer), phlorofucofuroeckol A (a pentamer), dieckol, and 8,8′-bieckol (hexamers) separated from *E. bicyclis* show antioxidant activity. The phlorotannins isolated from *E. kurome* perform as antiplasmin inhibitor; though, additional phlorotannins bioactivities, from the physiological viewpoint of humans, are still obscure (Setty et al., 1976).

1.4.3 SAPONINS

The term saponins is coined from a plant *Saponaria vaccaria* (*Quillaja saponaria*). Two main types of saponins comprise triterpene saponins and steroid saponin. Saponins are harmful and cause a lot of illness, like by causing hemolysis; they are responsible for cattle poisoning and mucous membrane irritation (Kar, 2007). Saponins are also medicinally useful as they possess both anticancer and hypolipidemic activities. The two noteworthy sorts of steroidal saponins are diosgenin and hecogenin. Steroidal saponins are utilized as a part of the commercial production of sex hormones for clinical use. For instance, progesterone is gotten from diosgenin. The most copious beginning material for the production of progesterone is diosgenin secluded from *Dioscorea* species, once provided from Mexico, and now from China. Other steroidal hormones, for example, cortisone and hydrocortisone, can be set up from the starting material hecogenin, which can be detached from sisal leaves discovered broadly in East Africa (Sarker and Nahar, 2007).

The uses of saponins are as natural detergents, well known to primitive people as fish poisons. The intriguing pharmacological properties related to the Chinese medication "giwieng" are viewed as a panacea and other fascinating biological activities, for example, spermicidal (Netz and Opatz, 2015), molluscicidal, antimicrobial, anti-inflammatory, and cytotoxic activities. Pharmacologically significant steroidal saponins such as sapogenisis and sapogenins are produced by *Avicennia officinalis*. Modified terpenes that are Liomonds are known insect antifeedant and growth regulators (Yim et al., 2005).

1.4.4 POLYSACCHARIDES

Throughout the most recent couple of years, restorative and pharmaceutical industries have demonstrated an expanded concern for marine polysaccharides. Polysaccharides or glycans are a group of constituents with the most widely recognized components of monosaccharide like D-glucose, D-fructose, D-galactose, L-galactose, D-mannose, L-arabinose, and D-xylose. Certain monosaccharide byproducts present in polysaccharides incorporate the amino sugars (D-glucosamine and D-galactosamine) and also their products (N-acetylneuraminic corrosive and N-acetylmuramic corrosive) and simple sugar acids (glucuronic and iduronic acids). Carrageenans, agar, and alginate are algae-derived polysaccharides. Agar provides the prime support to algae cell walls; it is an unbranched polysaccharide and it is extracted from the genera *Gelidium* and *Gracilaria*. Galactose sugar molecules are involved in its constitution. Carrageenans are polysaccharides of galactan with rotating 1,3- and 1,4-connected galactose buildups, which fill spaces between the cellulosic plant structures of seaweeds (Matsuda et al., 2003). The active constituents retained in algae polysaccharides are principally sulfated ones. Through the tumoricidal activities of natural killer cells and macrophages, the sulfated polysaccharides are involved in enhancing the innate immune response (Berry et al., 2004). In order to present the antigen to helper T-cells and to produce TNF-alpha and interleukin-1 beta kind of cytokines, the antigen-presenting cells move in and out of tumor tissues. Therefore, T-helper cells advance the action of cytotoxic T-cell, which has a strong cytotoxic impact on tumor cells. Sulfated polysaccharides can improve the versatile invulnerable reaction by advancing such a process. It is also reported that the sulfated polysaccharides diagnose number cell adhesion systems. They augment the proliferative response of T-lymphocytes by binding CD2, CD3, and CD4 in T-lymphocytes (Aisa et al., 2005). A sulfated polysaccharide (B-1) extracted from marine *Pseudomonas* sp. Culture filtrate persuades human leukemic cells apoptosis (Berteau and Mulloy, 2003). PI-88, a sulfated oligosaccharide, persuades pancreatic islet carcinoma apoptosis, whereas sulfated glycosaminoglycans (GAGs) restrict the transcription functionality and consequently persuade the murine melanoma cells apoptosis.

Fucoidan is a derivative of the cell wall of the rhodophytes and it is the sulfated polysaccharides representative (Sadir et al., 2001). Fucoidan imparts human lymphoma HS-Sultan cell lines apoptosis and causes the caspase-3 stimulation and extracellular signal-regulated kinase pathway downregulation (Richard et al., 2006). They are capable of diverse biological activities, going from comparatively unpretentious perfunctory sustenance roles to added convoluted special effects on cellular functions binding proteins like adhesion proteins (Li et al., 2008), growth factors, cytokines (Zemani et al., 2005), and diverse enzymes, comprising coagulation proteases. Consequently, they contribute as GAGs in cell adhesion, proliferation, differentiation, and migration. Fucoidan is involved in modulating clinically pertinent spectacles like angiogenesis, atherosclerosis, and tumor metastasis (Sweeney et al., 2000). For as far back as decade, fucoidans disengaged from various species have been widely contemplated because of their differed biological activities like cell reinforcement, restorative potential in surgery, gastric defensive impacts, blood lipids decreasing, anticomplementary activity against renalpathy, hepatopathy, and uropathy, and its action as antivirus, anticoagulant, antitumor, antithrombotic, and immunomodulatory agent. Contrasted and other sulfated polysaccharides, fucoidans, have been progressively examined lately to build up the medications or food utilitarian. The characteristics of fucoidan, like its sulfation, molecular weight, conformation of its sugar residues, and type are dependent upon the species of seaweed (Matou et al., 2002).

Sulfation is perilous for fucoidan in vivo activity. Particularly, desulfated fucoidan fails to stimulate in vitro angiogenesis or the in vivo induction of immature CD34+ cell mobilization. The protamine presence causes the abolishing of native fucoidan mobilization (Carte, 1996). The principal sulfation configuration consists of a trisulfated disaccharide recurrence analogous to the one present in heparin. Nevertheless, heparin has no influence on in vitro angiogenesis induction through human umbilical vein endothelial cell (HUVEC) and is not involved in immature CD34+ cell mobilization. Moreover, pentosan sulfate, heparan sulfate, and chondroitin sulfate constrain in vitro angiogenesis and show anticoagulant activities. Fucoidan can disturb heparan sulfate development dynamic/cytokine buildings and can be ancillary for cell-surface heparan sulfates in balancing out the development dynamic/development dynamic receptor collaboration. Fucoidan can intercede development factor-initiated endothelial progenitor cell (EPC) separation by connecting with a "receptor" that advances endothelial cell attachment, movement, expansion, and separation, coordinates with a development dynamic receptor and transduces the intracellular signs obligatory to actuate the angiogenic phenotype. Such alleged fucoidan receptor may comprehend a sugar-binding domain that collaborates with the fucoidan starch backbone.

1.4.5 CHLOROPHYLL

Chlorophylls are responsible for the giving the premise to organisms on land, the oxygen in the air, and impart colors to plants. These colors have been streamlined amid advancement for the proficient gathering of daylight and the consequent vitality transduction into great vitality mixes such as adenosine triphosphate (ATP) and Nicotinamide adenine dinucleotide phosphate (NADPH). Synthetically, chlorophylls are cyclic tetrapyrroles (Mochizuki et al., 2010). Chlorophylls have specifically a few chattels that evidently condense them vital for photosynthesis (Grimm et al., 2006). Chlorophylls intensely absorb visible and near-infrared light, which is vital for light harvesting, and they possess long-lived excited states which avert damage to the transitorily stowed energy into heat.

Chlorophyll and its resultants are additionally utilized broadly in pharmacological items. Chlorophyll is stated as to quicken twisted recuperating by over 25% in a few investigations. Subsequently, chlorophyll empowers tissue development, keeps the headway of microscopic organisms, and accelerates the injury recuperating process. Chlorophyll is comparative in substance structure to hemoglobin and, all things considered, is anticipated to animate tissue development in a comparable manner by the help of a fast CO_2 and O_2 interchange (Ma and Dolphin, 1999). Due to this property, chlorophyll is utilized not just in the treatment of ulcers and oral sepsis yet additionally in proctology.

A chronic ulcer is a critical medical issue in the public arena, with extensive phases essential for its cure (Ma and Dolphin, 1999). Chlorophyll's capacity to expand the rate of mending is an achievement for ulcer sufferers. The use of balms comprising chlorophyll derivatives was present to dispose of torment following a few days as well as to enhance the presence of the influenced tissues (Louda et al., 2008). The release from the ulcer and its feature odor additionally enhanced altogether following a couple of days of chlorophyll action (Louda et al., 2008). Analogous assets, which form chlorophyll a key compound in the treatment of ulcers, likewise form its key in the treatment of post-agent wounds from rectal surgery.

1.4.6 AMINES/PEPTIDES

The species and amount of marine bioactive peptides are more than that of land bioactive peptides; though marine life forms are presented to more extraordinary conditions than that terrestrial which influence the marine bioactive peptides to have huge distinctive amino acid conformations and successions from terrestrial bioactive peptides. In addition, marine bioactive peptides can be acquired from different marine plants, animals, and lower life forms. Each is one of a kind as a group; marine bioactive peptides have preferred bioactivity in a few zones over land bioactive peptides thinking about their incredible ordered assorted variety and extraordinary qualities (Wang et al., 2017).

The estimation of cell reinforcement movement is an essential screening strategy. Some compound techniques are utilized, including decreasing force, hydroxyl radical rummaging action, superoxide anion radicals searching action, rummaging responsive oxygen species, and restraint of lipid peroxidation. Notwithstanding the wide utilization of these substance cell antioxidant action tests, none of them consider the bioavailability, take-up, and mechanism of the cancer prevention agent mixes (Liu and Finley, 2005). Lately, cell culture models give a method that is savvy and moderately quick and can clarify metabolic issues (Wolfe and Liu, 2007). One approach is to utilize the cell cellular antioxidant status measured by the methyl thiazolyl tetrazolium test and ensure HepG2 cells against H_2O_2-incited cytotoxicity.

Nonetheless, since the convergence of H_2O_2 is not clear, this technique ought to have a preparatory test. Likewise, cellular antioxidant activity (CAA) is identified with HepG2 cells. The CAA test is deliberated a higher indicator of in vivo activity as compared to in vitro assays since it includes the acquaintance of the antioxidants to the intricacy of biological substrates beneath the physical settings (Frankel and Meyer, 2000). Unquestionably, the best antioxidant agent is applied for animal models and human examinations, though they are not suitable for the preliminary examinations as are time-taking and expensive (Liu and Finley, 2005). As such, despite the fact that there is an extraordinary variety of strategies utilized for antioxidant agent testing, there are no endorsed institutionalized techniques.

Hypertension is a standout amongst the most widely recognized cardiovascular illness around the world (Wilson et al., 2011). Around 75% of hypertensive ailment, 54% of strokes, 25% of other cardiovascular maladies, and 47% of ischemic coronary illness were attributable worldwide to hypertension (Lawes et al., 2008). Among the procedures identified with hypertension and in the control of circulatory blood pressure, the angiotensin-I-converting enzyme (ACE) assumes a vital part. ACE can catalyze the transformation of angiotensin I to angiotensin II, and angiotensin II is an intense vasoconstrictor that builds peripheral vascular protection and subsequently lifts arterial pressure (Skrbic and Igic, 2009).

In this way, in the advancement of medications to control hypertension, ACE inhibitors and angiotensin receptor blockers are currently utilized clinically for the cure of different cardiovascular maladies. Be that as it may, the engineered medications, for example, enalapril, captopril, and lisinopril (Elavarasan et al., 2016), are accepted to have certain symptoms such as angioneurotic edema, skin rash, or loss of taste. Because of these unfavorable symptoms, there is a pattern towards empowering the advancement of normal ACE inhibitors. Lately, normally happening peptides with ACE inhibitory action were acquired from different marine life forms, for example, green algae, sea cucumber (*Acaudina molpadioides*), tuna, sole (*Limanda aspera*), blue mussels (*Mytilus edulis*) (Je et al., 2005), jumbo squid (*Dosidicus gigas*), oysters (*Crassostrea gigas*), and shrimp. The disclosure of the far-reaching dispersion of antimicrobial peptides (AMPs) in the course of recent years has given bits of knowledge into the intrinsic resistance frameworks that allow multicellular life forms (Zasloff, 2002). Advancing through the positive choice, the AMPs are considered as profoundly substantial immune effectors (El-Gamal et al., 2013).

Because of their unique living condition, properties and structure, currently, much consideration has been paid to marine-determined bioactive peptides. The marine plants are in close contact with organisms and give a tremendous source of AMPs. Furthermore, vast seawater harbors have 106 bacterial and 103 fungal cells for each milliliter, and most marine life forms have particular populaces of microorganisms on their surfaces or inside the bounds of their tissues. Researchers have isolated AMPs from Atlantic cod (*Gadus morhua*), mud crab (*Scylla paramamosain*), oyster (*C. gigas*), yellow catfish (*Pelteobagrus fulvidraco*) (Su, 2011), sponge (*Trichoderma* sp.), and marine snail (*Cenchritis muricatus*), and the AMPs from marine life forms are inexpensive, safe, and natural, having high bioactivity. These marine organism-derived peptides showed other bioactivities as well like anticoagulation, immunomodulation, antitumor activity, appetite suppression, calcium binding, cardiovascular protection, neuroprotection, and antidiabetic activity (Cheung et al., 2015).

1.4.7 ESSENTIAL OILS

Essential oils are the volatile and odorous products of numerous animals and plant species. Essential oils keep a potential of evaporation upon air exposure at room temperature and hence also denoted as volatile oils or eerie oils. Essential oils enhance the aroma of some species and contribute the essences or odoriferous constituents of the aromatic plants (Martinez et al., 2008).

Essential oils are stashed unswervingly through the plant protoplasm or by the hydrolysis of several glycosides and structures like the plant structures that are directly allied with the excretion of essential oils such as Lamiaceae, for example, *Lavandula angustifolia* glandular hairs, oil tubes of Apiaceae, for example, *Foeniculum vulgare* and *Pimpinella anisum*, Piperaceae, for example, *Piper nigrum*—black pepper modified parenchymal cells, and pine oil passages of Schizogenous. Different parts of plants like stem, leaves, roots, flowers, and rhizomes are linked to the essential oils. More than 200 different chemical components are associated with flavor and odor of the essential oils, contributed by the trace constituents (Firn, 2010).

Different methods for the preparation of essential oils include direct steam distillation, expression, and extraction via enzymatic hydrolysis. In direct steam distillation process, the plant part is boiled in a distillation flask; it passes the volatile oil and steam through the water condenser and consequently collects the extracted oil in Florentine flask. Selection of the distillation process among direct, steam and water, and water distillation depends upon the source of the extraction material. Extrusion or expression of volatile oils is achieved through the sponge process, scarification, rasping, or by a mechanical method. While using the sponge method, first the washed plant material is cut into two halves and squeezed; oozed volatile oil is collected through the sponge and then squeezed in the vessel and the floating oil is separated. The scarification apparatus is an Ecuelle a Piquer that is a large funnel made of copper and has a tinned inner layer. To penetrate the epidermis, various pointed metal needles are present. In rasping, initially the peel of the plant part is removed and then oil is extracted while pressing through which oil is oozed. Turbid appearance is later on changed and oil separates from the fluid that is further decanted and filtered. Heavy-duty centrifugal devices are used in the mechanical process of essential oil extraction. The yield of oil has now increased remarkably with the advent of modern mechanical devices.

1.5 MARINE SOURCES AS CRADLES OF METABOLITES

Nature has been a cradle of therapeutic agents since a long time and a striking number of contemporary drugs were extracted from plants; several centered on their utilization in traditional treatment (see Volume 2 of this book). Moreover, researchers have also revealed that the plant aids a phytoremediation mediator (Sajn et al., 2005) as a biosorbent for toxic metals (Malik, 2007), for power alcohol and biogas making as a fertilizer and medicinal plants. Similarly, in its traditional form and at the squat invasion, it obliges as fish food, where herbivorous fishes are kept and cultivated combined with other non-predatory species to endorse the fish progression (Ling, 1960).

Numerous reports are available on the antibacterial, antifungal, antiviral, anti-inflammatory, antidiabetic, antioxidant, and cytotoxic activities of seaweeds (Mohammed et al., 2013). The genus *Sargassum* is broadly disseminated in the clement and tropical oceans of the world. They are well known for their biological activities and secondary metabolites (Deepa et al., 2009). The terpenoid components of sargassum are responsible for vasodilatory effects, cell toxicity, acetylcholine-esterase inhibition, and antioxidant activity. Seaweed inhabits in the clear tropical and intertidal zones. Constitutional analysis of marine algae is not done much. Most of the products of the seaweed industry are obtained from one *Gracilaria*/*Gracilariopsis* species, three *Gelidium* species, and two kelps. Additionally, there are economically important seaweeds and their significance is evaluated by assessing their potential for drug development (Carte, 1996). On the other hand, novel cultivation techniques are explored through extensive laboratory researches resulting in new cultivation initiatives. It is confirmed by different studies that *Sphaerococcus coronopifolius* is a good source of antibacterial compounds (Ireland et al., 1993); *Ulva lactuca* shows anti-inflammatory modules; and *Portieria hornemannii* has potential as an anti-tumor agent (Ali et al., 2002). A unique compound sphingosine with antiviral activity is extracted from *Ulva fasciata*. Stypoldione, as a potent cytotoxic metabolite that is involved in the prevention of mitotic spindle formation and microtubule polymerization inhibition, has been sequestered from the tropical brown alga, *Stypopodium zonale* (Xu et al., 2002). *P. hornemannii* is recognized as a unique cradle of cytotoxic penta-halogenated monoterpene, halomon, which showed one of the best differential cytotoxicity airings steered by the National Cancer Institute, USA. Halomon was designated for the development of preclinical treatment; subsequently, it showed toxicity to renal colon brain and tumor cell lines. An inhibitor of adenosine kinase in the form of the iodinated nucleoside is extracted from *Hypnea valitiae*, and it helped to study nucleotide regulation and metabolism other than studying the adenosine receptors (Carte, 1996).

Codium iyengarii algae inhabitant Arabian Sea Karachi coast found rich with two new steroidal glycosides, iyengarosides A and B, and iyengadione that are effective against numerous bacteria (Blunt et al., 2004). Two new bioactive sterols were also isolated from *Sargassum carpophyllum* in the South China Sea. Some of their functions include cytotoxicity against cancer cell lines and morphological abnormalities in plant pathogenic fungus *Pyricularia oryzae*. Stigmast sterol of *Sargassum polycystum* is sampled from North China Sea. Algae among the marine organism are a rich source of components of worth importance. Algae are involved in converting the PUFAs in arachidonic acids that are involved in homeostasis in mammalian systems as well as help coping different diseases like cancer, ulcers, asthma, psoriasis, arteriosclerosis, and heart diseases (Perry et al., 1988).

1.6 MECHANISM OF ACTION OF PHYTOCHEMICALS

Diverse mechanisms of action of phytochemicals have been recommended. They might obstruct microorganisms, affect certain metabolic procedures, or might temper gene expression as well as signal transduction paths. Phytochemicals might moreover be applied as chemopreventive or chemo-therapeutic mediators with chemoprevention denoting to the practice of mediators to constrain, converse, or impede tumorigenesis. As molecular mechanisms may be communal to chemoprevention and cancer therapy, so the chemopreventive phytochemicals are applicable to cancer therapy (for more details, see Volume 1 and 2 of this book). A different mode of actions is exhibited by the essential oils and extracts of plants, like the intrusion of the cell membrane phospholipids that resulted in cellular constituent's loss and increase in permeability. Certain detailed modes of actions are deliberated here.

1.6.1 ANTIOXIDANTS

Reactive oxygen species (singlet oxygen, superoxide, peroxyl radicals, hydroxyl radicals, and peroxynite) cause the oxidative stress that leads to cellular destruction. Antioxidants provide protection to cells against the damaging effects of these reactive oxygen species (Mattson and Cheng, 2006). A number of diseases like atherosclerosis, carcinogenesis, cerebral and cardiac ischemia, diabetic pregnancy, neurodegenerative disorders, aging, rheumatic disorder, and DNA damage are treated with natural antioxidants, and hence, they provide protection and maintenance against degenerative and chronic diseases (Jayasri et al., 2009).

Antioxidants scavenge the "free-oxygen radicals" to give a relatively "stable radical." In the form of metastable chemical species, the free radicals apt to snare electrons from the instantaneous environs molecules. These radicals uncertainty does not scavenge efficiently in time and might harm vital biomolecules such as DNA, mitochondria, lipids, and proteins, comprising all membranes leading to abnormalities and disease conditions (Uddin et al., 2008). Therefore, free radicals convoluted in a lot of diseases like atherosclerosis, tumor inflammation, diabetes, rheumatoid arthritis, gastrointestinal ulcerogenesis, hemorrhagic shock, cystic fibrosis, infertility, asthma, early senescence cardiovascular disorders, parkinsonism, Alzheimer's-like neurodegenerative diseases, and acquired immunodeficiency syndrome. Insufficient amount of antioxidants is produced by the human body which plays an important role in the prevention of oxidative stress. The body has the natural antioxidant mechanisms like catalases and glutathione that remove the free radicals produced in the body (Sen, 1995). Hence, this insufficiency should be fulfilled in the form of new phytochemicals search, finding efficient methods for extraction and determining phytochemicals basic structures and mode of action.

Plants free radicals scavenging molecules with great antioxidant activity include terpenoids, flavonoids, vitamins, and phenols. In the human body, free radicals are scavenged by plants-, vegetables-, and fruits-derived flavonols, phenolics, carotenoid, ascorbic acid, and vitamin E. Substantial antioxidant assets have been detailed in phytochemicals that are essential to decrease the incidence of fetal diseases (Hertog et al., 1993; Anderson et al., 2001). Numerous dietary polyphenolic components derivative of plants are further active antioxidants in vitro as compared to vitamins E or C and therefore may subsidize considerably in in vivo protective effects (Jayasri et al., 2009). Antioxidants are often added to foods to avert the oxidation radical chain reactions; they terminate the reaction or delay the oxidation process through inhibition of initiation and propagation step. Food industries are focusing and are providing funds for the commercialization of natural antioxidants instead of synthetic compounds because of the safety concerns of synthetic compounds. Due to safety concerns of synthetic compounds, food industries have focused on finding natural antioxidants to replace synthetic compounds. Additionally, the consumer concern is providing a spur to explore natural sources of antioxidants.

1.6.2 ANTICARCINOGENESIS

Among diverse phytochemicals, the polyphenols are potent carcinogen inhibitors (Liu, 2004). Phenolic acids usually considerably abate the development of the specific cancer-promoting nitrosamines from the dietary nitrites and nitrates. For the treatment of colon cancer, glucosinolates exert a significant protective support in the metabolism of carcinogens. Isothiocyanates and the indole-3-carbinols interfere emphatically, preventing the procarcinogen activation and thus phase II enzymes are activated. Glutathione S-transferase and NADPH quinone reductase are such enzymes which prevent the change in the structure of nucleic acids by especially detoxifying the electrophilic metabolites. A potent phase II enzyme inducer is sulforaphane. It is responsible for the particular cell-cycle arrest. It also causes the cancer cells apoptosis and the apoptosis of the neoplasm (cancer) cells. A significant inhibitor of breast cancer is d-D-gluconolactone that is produced by sulforaphane. Indole-3-carbinol especially prevents the human papillomavirus that causes uterine cancer. In prostate cancer cells, it downregulates the CDK6 and upregulates p21 and p27; it also blocks the estrogen receptors especially existing in the breast cancer cells. d-D-gluconolactone causes the G1 cell-cycle arrest as well as prostate and breast cancer apoptosis and increases p53 expression in cells that are treated with benzopyrene. The depression of B-cell lymphoma 2 (Bel-2) signaling pathways and Akt, NF-kappaB, and Mitogen-activated protein kinase (MAPK) is caused by d-D-gluconolactone at large extent. Neoplasm development in prostate glands, breast, and colon are blocked by the phytosterols. Though the exact mechanism is yet to be discovered, still it is assumed that in the neoplasm development, the ensuing cell-membrane transfer is caused by them and hence reduces the inflammation expressively.

1.6.3 ANTIMICROBIAL ACTIVITY

Plants primary and secondary metabolites that protect them against protozoa, bacteria, fungi, and pathogenic bacteria are now applied to help human diseases (Nascimento et al., 2000). Phytochemicals like phenolic acids help to lower dental caries and urinary tract infections through minimizing the chances of adherence. Plants can also apply the bactericidal or bacteriostatic activity against microorganisms (Jakhetia et al., 2010). It is noteworthy that results of the antimicrobial action of the similar plant fragment confirmed most of the time mottled from study to study. The probable reason might be the sample type, habitat, extraction, and activity testing protocol. Same plant constituents' concentration varies in different geographical regions, topographical factors differences, plant age, and soil composition. Therefore, the technical procedures must noticeably be recognized and sufficiently applied and stated.

1.6.4 ANTI-ULCER

Marine phytochemicals have been reported as potent antiulcer agents. They constrain the growths of *Helicobacter pylori* in vitro and also its urease activity. The efficacy of various excerpts in a liquid medium and at low pH increases their effectiveness even in the human stomach. They also exert an inhibition effect on the kidney and intestine Na^+/K^+ ATPase activity and on alanine transport in rat jejunum (Jakhetia et al., 2010).

1.6.5 ANTIDIABETIC

A phytoconstituent extract "cinnamaldehyde" displays substantial antihyperglycemic effect that results in lowering the triglyceride and total cholesterol levels, simultaneously, causing an increase in high-density lipoproteins (HDL) cholesterol in streptozotocin (STZ)-induced diabetic rats. Thus, cinnamaldehyde could be used as a natural oral agent, with hypolipidemic and hypoglycemic effects. Currently, it is found that the polyphenols having procyanidin type-A polymers are probable to upsurge the quantity of thrombotic thrombocytopenic purpura, insulin resistance, and glucose transporter-4 in 3T3-L1 adipocytes (Jakhetia et al., 2010).

1.6.6 ANTI-INFLAMMATORY

Essential oils from marine phytochemicals have a tremendous anti-inflammatory action and cytotoxicity against HepG2 (human hepatocellular liver carcinoma cell line) cells. It suppresses the nitric oxide production by lipopolysaccharide-stimulated macrophages (Jakhetia et al., 2010).

1.6.7 MULTIFUNCTIONAL TARGETS

A lot of molecular targets of nutritional phytochemicals are reported from cell growth pathways, cell cycle proteins, pro- and antiapoptotic proteins, protein kinases, cell adhesion molecules, and transcription factors to metastasis. It is possible to overcome cancer drug resistance because of multi-target nature of phytochemicals as the multi-faceted mechanism of action perhaps hampers the cancer cell's aptitude to progress resistance against phytochemicals. Phytochemicals cause the modulation of inflammation, redox signaling of transcription factors, and redox-sensitive transcription factors (Surh, 2003). For example, nitric oxide (NO), a signaling molecule of significance in inflammation, is modulated through plant polyphenols and other botanical extracts (Shanmugam et al., 2008). Several phytochemicals are categorized as phytoestrogens that aid health-promoting properties, signifying phytochemicals as marketed nutraceuticals (Moutsatsou, 2007).

1.7 APPLICATIONS OF MARINE BIOACTIVE COMPOUNDS

Recent trends in useful sustenance and dietary supplements have verified that the bioactive molecules shed a most important therapeutic role between ethnical human sicknesses. Nutritionists and biomedical researchers are cooperating to find new bioactive molecules that have expanded intensity and restorative advantages. A lot of world biota consists of marine life that is providing secondary metabolites and bioactive compounds of wide application. These bioactive molecules are involved in anti-fibrotic, antiviral, anti-inflammatory, antiparasitic, anticancer, and antibiotic activities. Additionally, they may cause the activation and inhibition of certain enzymes, and can also act on transporters and sequestrants as modulating a range of physiological pathways (Suleria et al., 2015).

1.7.1 MEDICINE

Many compounds are available in marine plants that provide protection against various diseases. In addition to classified phytochemicals of marine organisms, some compounds, their activities, and finding related to their medicinal benefit are given below. The marine polyphenols, phlorotannins that are phloroglucinol polymers (1,3,5-trihydroxybenzene), are extracted from Phaeophyceae group of algae. They are different from terrestrial phlorotannins and are derived from phloroglucinol (Sanjeewa et al., 2016). Applications of algal phlorotannins include anti-melanogenic, anti-skin aging, antioxidant, anti-inflammatory, hepatoprotective, and anti-allergic activity. Among brown alga-derived phlorotannins, phloroglucinol, eckol, dieckol (Heo et al., 2009), diphlorethohydroxycarmalol (Kim et al., 2015), and octaphlorethol A were described as effective tyrosinase inhibitors. Phlorotannins of three types such as "phloroglucinol, eckol, and dieckol" were quarantined from *E. cava* by Heo et al. (2009). The anti-melanogenic activity of eckol and dieckol was determined by the inhibition of mushroom tyrosinase and melanin synthesis in B16F10 cells.

The Phaeophyceae algae are opulent cradles of meroterpenoid compounds, which are useful for human health. Particularly, the Sargassum genus is reported for containing a high amount of meroterpenoids. Algal meroterpenoids have anti-inflammatory, antioxidant, antiaging, anti-atherosclerotic, anti-adipogenic, antidiabetic, anticarcinogenic, and neuro-protective activities. Fucoidans, a fucose-rich sulfated polysaccharide, is principally present in aquatic brown algae and echinoderms (Fitton et al., 2015). Fucoidans inhibit the activity of tyrosinase, elastase, and matrix metalloproteases (Senni et al., 2006). Protein hydrolysates of peptides and proteins from marine dispensation wastes exhibit different activities like calcium binding, antimicrobial, HIV inhibition of protease, and suppression of appetite actions. Osteoporosis, dental caries, hypertension, and anemia can be prevented by components which bind and solubilize minerals such as calcium (Korhonen and Pihlanto, 2006).

1.7.2 FOOD INDUSTRY

In the recent years, the consumer interest is increased in the relationship between diet and health. There is presently more acknowledge that when joined with a healthy life, useful sustenance may make a positive imitation of well-being and prosperity. Today, consumers need foods to enhance health, increase life, and/or decrease the danger of disease and then lengthen the threshold of health. In particular, some bioactive of interests are proteinaceous in characteristic (or origin) yet consist of amino acids, proteins, and peptides. Furthermore, as the opulent cradles of protein, some marine organisms are best starting materials for the technology of protein-derived bioactive peptides. The focus on seaweed as much a cause over bioactive nitrogenous complexes has currently been appraised (Harnedy and FitzGerald, 2012). Bioactive peptides are particular fragments of proteins that notwithstanding are wellsprings of amino acids nitrogen having probable biological capacities inside the body; these incorporate opioid, antithrombotic, immunomodulatory, antibacterial, and antihypertension actions. Moreover, certain of these peptides may additionally show multifunctional properties (Meisel, 2004).

KEYWORDS

- **antimicrobial**
- **antioxidant**
- **phytochemicals**
- **ocean**
- **seaweed**

REFERENCES

Aisa, Y.; Miyakawa,Y.; Nakazato, T.; Shibata, H.; Saito, K.; Ikeda, Y.; Kizaki, M. Fucoidan Induces Apoptosis of Human HS Sultan Cells Accompanied by Activation of Caspase 3 and Down Regulation of ERK Pathways. *Am. J. Hematol.* **2005,** *78*(1), 7–14.

Ali, M. S.; Saleem, M.; Yamdagni, R.; Ali, M. A. Steroid and Antibacterial Steroidal Glycosides from Marine Green Alga *Codium iyengarii* Borgesen. *Nat. Prod. Lett.* **2002,** *16*(6), 407–413.

Anderson, K. J.; Teuber, S. S.; Gobeille, A.; Cremin, P.; Waterhouse, A. L.; Steinberg, F. M. Walnut Polyphenolics Inhibit In Vitro Human Plasma and LDL Oxidation. *J. Nutr.* **2001,** *131*(11), 2837–2842.

Berry, D.; Lynn, D. M.; Sasisekharan, R.; Langer, R. Poly (β-Amino Ester)s Promote Cellular Uptake of Heparin and Cancer Cell Death. *Chem. Biol.* **2004,** *11*(4), 487–498.

Berteau, O.; Mulloy, B. Sulfated Fucans, Fresh Perspectives: Structures, Functions, and Biological Properties of Sulfated Fucans and an Overview of Enzymes Active Toward this Class of Polysaccharide. *Glycobiology* **2003,** *13*(6), 29–40.

Blunt, J. W.; Copp, B. R.; Munro, M. H.; Northcote, P. T.; Prinsep, M. R. Marine Natural Products. *Nat. Prod. Rep.* **2004,** *21*(1), 1–49.

Bors, W.; Heller, W.; Michel, C.; Saran, M. Flavonoids as Antioxidants: Determination of Radical-Scavenging Efficiencies. *Methods Enzymol.* **1990,** *186,* 343–355.

Boyd, L.; Green, D.; Giesbrecht, F.; King, M. Inhibition of Oxidative Rancidity in Frozen Cooked Fish Flakes by Tert Butylhydroquinone and Rosemary Extract. *J. Sci. Food. Agric.* **1993,** *61*(1), 87–93.

Carpenter, N. E. *Chemistry of Sustainable Energy*, 1st ed.; CRC Press: Florida, USA, 2014; p 446.

Carte, B. K. Biomedical Potential of Marine Natural Products. *Bioscience* **1996,** *46*(4), 271–286.

Cheung, R. C.; Ng, T. B.; Wong, J. H. Marine Peptides: Bioactivities and Applications. *Mar. Drugs* **2015,** *13*(7), 4006–4043.

Deepa, M.; Usha, P.; Nair, C.; Prasanna, K. Antipyretic Activity of Seeds from *Nelumbo nucifera* in Albino Rat. *Vet. World* **2009,** *2,* 213–214.

El-Gamal, M. I.; Abdel-Maksoud, M. S.; Oh, C. H. Recent Advances in the Research and Development of Marine Antimicrobial Peptides. *Curr. Top. Med. Chem.* **2013,** *13*(16), 2026–2033.

Elavarasan, K.; Shamasundar, B. A.; Badii, F.; Howell, N. Angiotensin I-Converting Enzyme (ACE) Inhibitory Activity and Structural Properties of Oven- and Freeze-Dried Protein Hydrolysate from Fresh Water Fish (*Cirrhinus mrigala*). *Food Chem.* **2016,** *206,* 210–216.

Faulkner, D. J. Biomedical Uses for Natural Marine Chemicals. *Oceanus* **1992,** *35*(1), 29–35.

Fenical, W. New Pharmaceuticals from Marine Organisms. *Trends Biotechnol.* **1997,** *15*(9), 339–341.

Firn, R. *Nature's Chemicals: the Natural Products that Shaped Our World*, 1st ed.; Oxford University Press: UK, 2010; p 264.

Fitton, J.; Dell'Acqua, G.; Gardiner, V.-A.; Karpiniec, S.; Stringer, D.; Davis, E. Topical Benefits of Two Fucoidan-Rich Extracts from Marine Macroalgae. *Cosmetics* **2015,** *2*(2), 66.

Frankel, E. *Lipid Oxidation*, 2nd ed.; Oily Press: Scotland, 1998; p 488.

Frankel, E. N.; Meyer, A. S. The Problems of Using One Dimensional Methods to Evaluate Multifunctional Food and Biological Antioxidants. *J. Sci. Food. Agric.* **2000,** *80*(13), 1925–1941.

Fukuyama, Y.; Kodama, M.; Miura, I.; Kinzyo, Z.; Kido, M.; Mori, H.; Nakayama, Y.; Takahashi, M. Structure of an Anti-Plasmin Inhibitor, Eckol, Isolated from the Brown Alga *Ecklonia kurome* Okamura and Inhibitory Activities of its Derivatives on Plasma Plasmin Inhibitors. *Chem. Pharm. Bull.* **1989,** *37*(2), 349–353.

Grabley, S.; Sattler, I. Natural Products for Lead Identification: Nature is a Valuable Resource for Providing Tools. *Mod. Methods Drug Discovery* **2003,** *93,* 87–107.

Grimm, B.; Porra, R.; Rüdiger, W.; Scheer, H.; Eds. *Advances in Photosynthesis and Respiration, Chlorophylls and Bacteriochlorophylls: Biochemistry, Biophysics, Functions and Applications;* Springer: Dordrecht, The Netherlands, 2006; Vol. 25.

Gross, H.; Goeger, D. E.; Hills, P.; Mooberry, S. L.; Ballantine, D. L.; Murray, T. F.; Valeriote, F. A.; Gerwick, W. H. Lophocladines, Bioactive Alkaloids from the Red Alga *Lophocladia* sp. *J. Nat. Prod.* **2006,** *69*(4), 640–644.

Guven, K. C.; Percot, A.; Sezik, E. Alkaloids in Marine Algae. *Mar. Drugs* **2010,** *8*(2), 269–284.

Haefner, B. Drugs from the Deep: Marine Natural Products as Drug Candidates. *Drug Discovery Today* **2003,** *8*(12), 536–544.

Halvorson, H. Aquaculture, Marine Sciences and Oceanography: A Confluence. *N. Engl. J. Higher. Educ. Econ. Dev.* **1998,** *13*(1), 38–40.

Harnedy, P. A.; FitzGerald, R. J. Bioactive Peptides from Marine Processing Waste and Shellfish: A Review. *J. Funct. Foods* **2012,** *4*(1), 6–24.

Heo, S.-J.; Park, P.-J.; Park, E.-J.; Kim, S.-K.; Jeon, Y.-J. Antioxidant Activity of Enzymatic Extracts from a Brown Seaweed *Ecklonia cava* by Electron Spin Resonance Spectrometry and Comet Assay. *Eur. Food Res. Technol.* **2005,** *221*(1–2), 41–47.

Heo, S.-J.; Ko, S.-C.; Cha, S.-H.; Kang, D.-H.; Park, H.-S.; Choi, Y.-U.; Kim, D.; Jung, W.-K.; Jeon, Y.-J. Effect of Phlorotannins Isolated from *Ecklonia cava* on Melanogenesis and their Protective Effect Against Photo-Oxidative Stress Induced by UV-B Radiation. *Toxicol. In Vitro* **2009,** *23*(6), 1123–1130.

Hertog, M. G.; Feskens, E. J.; Kromhout, D.; Hollman, P.; Katan, M. Dietary Antioxidant Flavonoids and Risk of Coronary Heart Disease: the Zutphen Elderly Study. *Lancet* **1993,** *342*(8878), 1007–1011.

Ireland, C.; Copp, B.; Foster, M.; McDonald, L.; Radisky, D.; Swersey, J. Biomedical Potential of Marine Natural Products. In *Marine Biotechnology;* Attaway D, Zeborsky O., Eds.; Plenum Press: New York, 1993; pp 1–43.

Jakhetia, V.; Patel, R.; Khatri, P.; Pahuja, N.; Garg, S.; Pandey, A.; Sharma, S. Cinnamon: A Pharmacological Review. *J. Adv. Sci. Res.* **2010,** *1*(2), 19–23.

Jayasri, M.; Lazar, M.; Radha, A. A Report on the Antioxidant Activity of Leaves and Rhizomes of *Costus pictus* D. Don. *Int. J. Integr. Biol.* **2009,** *5*(1), 20–26.

Je, J. Y.; Park, P. J.; Byun, H. G.; Jung, W. K.; Kim, S. K. Angiotensin I Converting Enzyme (ACE) Inhibitory Peptide Derived from the Sauce of Fermented Blue Mussel, *Mytilus edulis*. *Bioresour. Technol.* **2005,** *96*(14), 1624–1629.

Jha, R. K.; Zi-Rong, X. Biomedical Compounds from Marine Organisms. *Mar. Drug* **2004,** *2*(3), 123–146.

Kakegawa, H.; Matsumoto, H.; Satoh, T. Activation of Hyaluronidase by Metallic Salts and Compound 48/80, and Inhibitory Effect of Anti-Allergic Agents on Hyaluronidase. *Chem. Pharm. Bull.* **1985,** *33*(2), 642–646.

Kar, A. *Pharmacognosy and Pharmacobiotechnology,* Revised-Expanded 2nd ed.; New Age International Publishers: New Delhi, 2007; pp 332–600.

Kathiresan, K.; Duraisamy, A. Current Issue of Microbiology. *ENVIS. Cent. Newsl.* **2005,** *4,* 3–5.

Kathiresan, K.; Nabeel, M. A.; Manivannan, S. Bioprospecting of Marine Organisms for Novel Bioactive Compounds. *Sci.Trans. Environ. Technov.* **2008,** *1,* 107–120.

Kijjoa, A.; Sawangwong, P. Drugs and Cosmetics from the Sea. *Mar. Drugs*, **2004,** *2*(2), 73.

Kim, K.-N.; Yang, H.-M.; Kang, S.-M.; Ahn, G. N.; Roh, S. W.; Lee, W.; Kim, D. K.; Jeon, Y.-J. Whitening Effect of Octaphlorethol a Isolated from Ishige Foliacea in an In Vivo Zebrafish Model. *J. Microbiol. Biotechnol.* **2015,** *25*(4), 448–451.

Korhonen, H.; Pihlanto, A. Bioactive Peptides: Production and Functionality. *Int. Dairy J.* **2006,** *16*(9), 945–960.

Langseth, L. *Oxidants, Antioxidants, and Disease Prevention;* ILSI Europe: Brussels, **1995**; p 1–32.
Lawes, C. M.; Vander Hoorn, S.; Rodgers, A. Global Burden of Blood-Pressure-Related Disease, 2001. *Lancet* **2008,** *371*(9623), 1513–1518.
Lee, K.; Lip, G. The Role of Omega-3 Fatty Acids in the Secondary Prevention of Cardiovascular Disease. *QJM* **2003,** *96*(7), 465–480.
Li, F.-M.; Hu, H.-Y. Isolation and Characterization of a Novel Antialgal Allelochemical from *Phragmites communis*. *Appl. Environ. Microbiol.* **2005,** *71*(11), 6545–6553.
Li, B.; Lu, F.; Wei, X.; Zhao, R. Fucoidan: Structure and Bioactivity. *Molecules* **2008,** *13*(8), 1671–1695.
Li, C.-S.; Li, X.-M.; Cui, C.-M.; Wang, B.-G. Brominated Metabolites from the Marine Red Alga *Laurencia similis*. *Zeitschrift. Fur. Naturfors.* **2010,** *65b,* 87–89.
Ling, S. Control of Aquatic Vegetation. *Int. Inland. Fish. Train. Cent. Indon* **1960,** *1,* 12
Liu, R. H. Potential Synergy of Phytochemicals in Cancer Prevention: Mechanism of Action. *J. Nutr.* **2004,** *134*(12), 3479S–3485S.
Liu, R. H.; Finley, J. Potential Cell Culture Models for Antioxidant Research. *J. Agric. Food Chem.* **2005,** *53*(10), 4311–4314.
Louda, J.; Neto, R.; Magalhaes, A.; Schneider, V. Pigment Alterations in the Brown Mussel *Perna perna*. *Comp. Biochem. Physiol. B Biochem. Mol. Biol.* **2008,** *150*(4), 385–394.
Ma, L.; Dolphin, D. The Metabolites of Dietary Chlorophylls. *Phytochemistry* **1999,** *50*(2), 195–202.
Madziga, H.; Sanni, S.; Sandabe, U. K. Phytochemical and Elemental Analysis of *Acalypha wilkesiana* Leaf. *J. Am. Sci.* **2010,** *6*(11), 510–514.
Malik, A. Environmental Challenge vis a vis Opportunity: The Case of Water Hyacinth. *Environ. Int.* **2007,** *33,* 122–138.
Maqsood, S.; Benjakul, S. Effect of Kiam (*Cotylelobium lanceolatum* Craib) Wood Extract on the Haemoglobin-Mediated Lipid Oxidation of Washed Asian Sea Bass Mince. *Food Bioprocess Technol.* **2013,** *6*(1), 61–72.
Martinez, M. J. A.; Lazaro, R. M.; Del Olmo, L. M. B.; Benito, P. B. Anti-Infectious Activity in the Anthemideae Tribe. *Stud. Nat. Prod. Chem.* **2008,** *35,* 445–516.
Matou, S.; Helley, D.; Chabut, D.; Bros, A.; Fischer, A.-M. Effect of Fucoidan on Fibroblast Growth Factor-2-Induced Angiogenesis In Vitro. *Thromb. Res.* **2002,** *106*(4), 213–221.
Matsuda, M.; Yamori, T.; Naitoh, M.; Okutani, K. Structural Revision of Sulfated Polysaccharide B-1 Isolated from a Marine Pseudomonas Species and its Cytotoxic Activity Against Human Cancer Cell Lines. *Mar. Biotechnol.* **2003,** *5*(1) 13–19.
Mattson, M. P.; Cheng, A. Neurohormetic Phytochemicals: Low-Dose Toxins that Induce Adaptive Neuronal Stress Responses. *Trends Neurosci.* **2006,** *29*(11), 632–639.
Meisel, H. Multifunctional Peptides Encrypted in Milk Proteins. *Biofactors* **2004,** *21*(1–4), 55–61.
Mochizuki, N.; Tanaka, R.; Grimm, B.; Masuda, T.; Moulin, M.; Smith, A. G.; Tanaka, A.; Terry, M. J. The Cell Biology of Tetrapyrroles: A Life and Death Struggle. *Trends Plant Sci.* **2010,** *15*(9), 488–498.
Mohammed, H. A.; Uka, U. N.; Yauri, Y. A. B. Evaluation of Nutritional Composition of Water Lily (*Nymphaea lotus* Linn.) from Tatabu Flood Plain, North-Central, Nigeria. *J. Fish. Aquat. Sci.* **2013,** *8*(1), 261.
Morrissey, J. F.; Sumich, J. L.; Pinkard-Meier, D. R. *Introduction to the Biology of Marine Life*, 10th ed.; Jones & Bartlett Learning: USA, 2016; p 396.

Moutsatsou, P. The Spectrum of Phytoestrogens in Nature: Our Knowledge is Expanding. *Hormones* **2007,** *6*(3), 173.

Nakamura, T.; Nagayama, K.; Uchida, K.; Tanaka, R. Antioxidant Activity of Phlorotannins Isolated from the Brown Alga *Eisenia bicyclis*. *Fish. Sci.* **1996,** *62*(6), 923–926.

Nascimento, G. G.; Locatelli, J.; Freitas, P. C.; Silva, G. L. Antibacterial Activity of Plant Extracts and Phytochemicals on Antibiotic-Resistant Bacteria. *Braz. J. Microbiol.* **2000,** *31*(4), 247–256.

Netz, N.; Opatz, T. Marine Indole Alkaloids. *Mar. Drugs*, **2015,** *13*(8), 4814–4914.

Perry, N. B.; Blunt, J. W.; Munro, M. H. G.; Pannell, L. K. Mycalamide A, an Antiviral Compound from a New Zealand Sponge of the Genus Mycale. *J. Am. Chem. Soc.* **1988,** *110*(14), 4850–4851.

Reyes, F.; Fernández, R.; Rodríguez, A.; Francesch, A.; Taboada, S.; Ávila, C.; Cuevas, C. Aplicyanins A–F, New Cytotoxic Bromoindole Derivatives from the Marine Tunicate *Aplidium cyaneum*. *Tetrahedron* **2008,** *64*(22), 5119–5123.

Rich, V. I.; Maier, R. M. *Aquatic Environments*, 3rd ed.; Elsevier: USA, 2015; pp 111–138.

Richard, B.; Bouton, M. C.; Loyau, S.; Lavigne, D.; Letourneur, D.; Jandrot-Perrus, M.; Arocas, V. Modulation of Protease Nexin-1 Activity by Polysaccharides. *Thromb. Haemostasis* **2006,** *95*(2), 229.

Sadir, R.; Baleux, F.; Grosdidier, A.; Imberty, A.; Lortat-Jacob, H. Characterization of the Stromal Cell-Derived Factor-1α-Heparin Complex. *J. Biol. Chem.* **2001,** *276*(11), 8288–8296.

Sajn, S. A.; Bulc, T.; Vrhovsek, D. Comparison of Nutrient Cycling in a Surface-Flow Constructed Wetland and in a Facultative Pond Treating Secondary Effluent. *Water Sci. Technol.* **2005,** *51,* 291–298.

Sanjeewa, K. K. A.; Kim, E. A.; Son, K. T.; Jeon, Y. J. Bioactive Properties and Potentials Cosmeceutical Applications of Phlorotannins Isolated from Brown Seaweeds: A Review. *J. Photochem. Photobiol. B* **2016,** *162,* 100–105.

Sarker, S.; Nahar, L. *Chemistry for Pharmacy Students: General, Organic and Natural Product Chemistry,* 1st ed.; John Wiley & Sons: New Jersey, 2007; p 396.

Sen, C. K. Oxygen Toxicity and Antioxidants: State of the Art. *Indian J. Physiol. Pharmacol.* **1995,** *39*(3), 177–196.

Senni, K.; Gueniche, F.; Foucault-Bertaud, A.; Igondjo-Tchen, S.; Fioretti, F.; Colliec-Jouault, S.; Durand, P.; Guezennec, J.; Godeau, G.; Letourneur, D. Fucoidan a Sulfated Polysaccharide from Brown Algae is a Potent Modulator of Connective Tissue Proteolysis. *Arch. Biochem. Biophys.* **2006,** *445*(1), 56–64.

Setty, B. S.; Kamboj, V. P.; Garg, H. S.; Khanna, N. M. Spermicidal Potential of Saponins Isolated from Indian Medicinal Plants. *Contraception* **1976,** *14*(5), 571–578.

Shanmugam, K.; Holmquist, L.; Steele, M.; Stuchbury, G.; Berbaum, K.; Schulz, O.; Benavente García, O.; Castillo, J.; Burnell, J.; Garcia Rivas, V. Plants Derived Polyphenols Attenuate Lipopolysaccharides Induced Nitric Oxide and Tumour Necrosis Factor Production in Murine Microglia and Macrophages. *Mol. Nutr. Food. Res.* **2008,** *52*(4), 427–438.

Shibata, T.; Fujimoto, K.; Nagayama, K.; Yamaguchi, K.; Nakamura, T. Inhibitory Activity of Brown Algal Phlorotannins Against Hyaluronidase. *Int. J. Food Sci. Technol.* **2002,** *37*(6), 703–709.

Skrbic, R.; Igic, R. Seven Decades of Angiotensin (1939–2009). *Peptides* **2009,** *30*(10), 1945–1950.

Su, Y. Isolation and Identification of Pelteobagrin, a Novel Antimicrobial Peptide from the Skin Mucus of Yellow Catfish (*Pelteobagrus fulvidraco*). *Comp. Biochem. Physiol. B. Biochem. Mol. Biol.* **2011,** *158*(2), 149–154.

Suleria, H. A. R.; Osborne, S.; Masci, P.; Gobe, G. Marine-Based Nutraceuticals: An Innovative Trend in the Food and Supplement Industries. *Mar. Drug* **2015,** *13*(10), 6336–6351.

Surh, Y.-J. Cancer Chemoprevention with Dietary Phytochemicals. *Nat. Rev. Cancer* **2003,** *3*(10), 768–780.

Swan, G. A. *An Introduction to the Alkaloids;* Blackwell Scientific: Oxford, UK, 1967.

Sweeney, E. A.; Priestley, G. V.; Nakamoto, B.; Collins, R. G.; Beaudet, A. L.; Papayannopoulou, T. Mobilization of Stem/Progenitor Cells by Sulfated Polysaccharides Does Not Require Selectin Presence. *Proc. Natl. Acad. Sci. U.S.A.* **2000,** *97*(12), 6544–6549.

Teagle, H.; Hawkins, S. J.; Moore, P. J.; Smale, D. A. The Role of Kelp Species as Biogenic Habitat Formers in Coastal Marine Ecosystems. *J. Exp. Mar. Biol. Ecol.* **2017,** *492,* 81–98.

Uddin, S. N.; Akond, M.; Mubassara, S.; Yesmin, M. N. Antioxidant and Antibacterial Activities of Trema Cannabina. *Middle-East J. Sci. Res.* **2008,** *3*(2), 105–108.

Wang, X.; Yu, H.; Xing, R.; Li, P. Characterization, Preparation, and Purification of Marine Bioactive Peptides. *BioMed Res. Int.* **2017,** *2017,* 16.

Wilson, J.; Hayes, M.; Carney, B. Angiotensin-I-Converting Enzyme and Prolyl Endopeptidase Inhibitory Peptides from Natural Sources with a Focus on Marine Processing By-Products. *Food Chem.* **2011,** *129*(2), 235–244.

Wolfe, K. L.; Liu, R. H. Cellular Antioxidant Activity (CAA) Assay for Assessing Antioxidants, Foods, and Dietary Supplements. *J. Agric. Food. Chem.* **2007,** *55*(22), 8896–8907.

Xu, S.; Ding, L.; Wang, M.; Peng, S.; Liao, X. Studies on the Chemical Constituents of the Algae *Sargassum polycystcum*. *Chin. J. Org. Chem.* **2002,** *22*(2), 138–140.

Xu, S.; Luo, L.; Zhu, L.-Q.; Li, Z.; Qiu, L.-L.; Chen, Q.; Xu, C.-F. Reversal Effect of 4′-Methylether-Scutellarein on Multidrug Resistance of Human Choriocarcinoma JAR/VP16 Cell Line. *Prog. Biochem. Biophys.* **2006,** *33*(11), 1061–1073.

Yim, J. H.; Son, E.; Pyo, S.; Lee, H. K. Novel Sulfated Polysaccharide Derived from Red-Tide Microalga *Gyrodinium impudicum* Strain KG03 with Immunostimulating Activity In Vivo. *Mar. Biotechnol.* **2005,** *7*(4), 331–338.

Yuan, Y. V.; Carrington, M. F.; Walsh, N. A. Extracts from Dulse (*Palmaria palmata*) are Effective Antioxidants and Inhibitors of Cell Proliferation In Vitro. *Food Chem. Toxicol.* **2005,** *43*(7), 1073–1081.

Zasloff, M. Antimicrobial Peptides of Multicellular Organisms. *Nature* **2002,** *415*(6870), 389–395.

Zemani, F.; Benisvy, D.; Galy-Fauroux, I.; Lokajczyk, A.; Colliec-Jouault, S.; Uzan, G.; Fischer, A. M.; Boisson-Vidal, C. Low-Molecular-Weight Fucoidan Enhances the Proangiogenic Phenotype of Endothelial Progenitor Cells. *Biochem. Pharmacol.* **2005,** *70*(8), 1167–1175.

Zhao, M.; Yang, B.; Wang, J.; Liu, Y.; Yu, L.; Jiang, Y. Immunomodulatory and Anticancer Activities of Flavonoids Extracted from Iitchi (*Litchi chinensis* Sonn) Pericarp. *Int. Immunopharmacol.* **2007,** *7*(2), 162–166.

CHAPTER 2

MARINE SPONGE ALKALOIDS: A SOURCE OF NOVEL ANTICANCER AGENTS

MUSARAT AMINA* and HANAN M. AL-YOUSEF

Department of Pharmacognosy, College of Pharmacy, King Saud University, Riyadh, Saudi Arabia. Tel.: 011-805320

**Corresponding author. E-mail: musarat.org@gmail.com.*
**ORCID: https://orcid.org/0000-0003-4545-253X.*

ABSTRACT

The marine environment has always been a source of novel classes of biologically active compounds. Primitive organisms are the source of a vast range of secondary metabolites which enable them to flourish in a harsh marine environment, and in particular huge wealth of unique and rare novel classes of metabolites produced by marine sponges has continuously attracted the attention of researchers who are trying to develop new drugs. The present chapter describes the research on novel anticancer alkaloids obtained from marine sponges. More than 110 isolated novel antitumor cytotoxic compounds confirmed activity in vitro cancer cell lines bioassay and are of current interest to national cancer institutes for further in vivo evaluation. This chapter describes the structure, origin cytotoxic, and anticancer evaluation of sponge-derived alkaloids.

2.1 INTRODUCTION

The search for natural bioactive compounds from primitive marine organisms is still an emerging field in comparison to long traditional terrestrial pharmacognosy. However, in the last two or three decades, isolation of fascinating array of unique metabolites with pronounced biological activities has attracted the tremendous attention of scientists (Newman and Cragg, 2007). Most of the pharmacologically active compounds, predominantly alkaloids and terpenoids were obtained from marine sponges and are considered as an important producer of novel diverse marine metabolites. Around 5300 different new and natural compounds have been reported from sponges every year with promising biological activities associated with them which include anticancer, antiviral, antibacterial, antimalarial, antifungal, immunosuppressive, anthelminthic, anti-inflammatory, and muscle relaxants activities (Molinski et al., 2009). In addition, uncommon nucleosides, marine sponges also produce other classes of alkaloids, sterols, terpenes, amino acid derivatives including cyclic peptides, fatty acids, peroxides, and so forth. Several sponge-derived constituents are already in preclinical and clinical trials as agents against cancer, microbial infections, inflammation, and other diseases (Newman and Cragg, 2004). However, in many cases, development of drug is severely hampered due to a limited supply of the respective compounds as they are often present only in little amounts in the sponge tissue.

The word cancer is burdened globally and about 8.8 million victims of malignant tumors are claimed per year, which is causing one in six deaths worldwide (WHO, online available). Current two major issues with anticancer therapy are safety and low efficacy. Therefore, the need for identification of new anticancer strategies with a better pharmacotoxicological profile, to be used individually or in combination with conventional chemotherapy, is required. Natural constituents in this context could play a vital role as they are less toxic in comparison to conventional chemotherapy drugs, more effective, easily available, and inexpensive (Amin et al., 2009). Natural compounds are usually considered better and safe profile drugs than traditional anticancer agents and their ability to prevent cancer formation and development is through interaction with multiple cell signaling pathways (Amin et al., 2009).

In this chapter, we describe the novel anticancer alkaloids isolated from marine sponges. The structures, origin, and pharmacological activities associated with an isolated marine sponge are reviewed (Fig. 2.1), with the main emphasis on the anticancer potential of poised isolated constituents: imidazole, indoles, pyridines, pyrrolesquinolones, isoquinolines, guanidines, and other structural families.

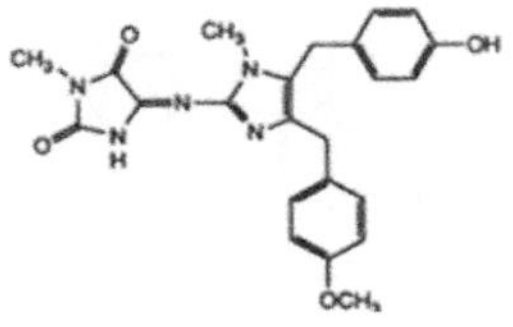

(1) Naamidines

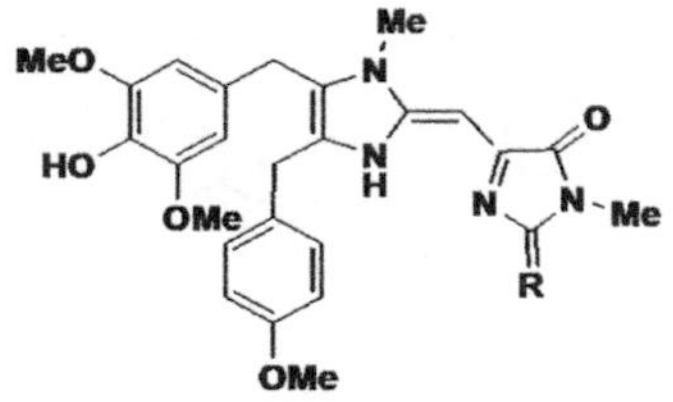

(2) Naamidines H R= O
(3) Naamidines I R = NMe

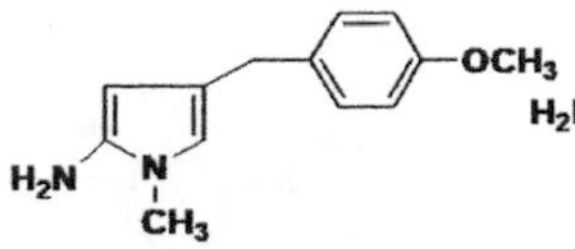

(4) Methyldorimidazole

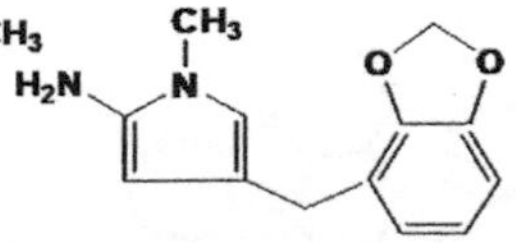

(5) Preclathridine B

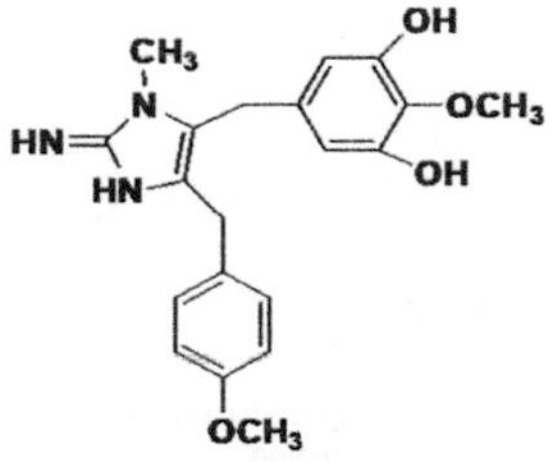

(6) Naamine E

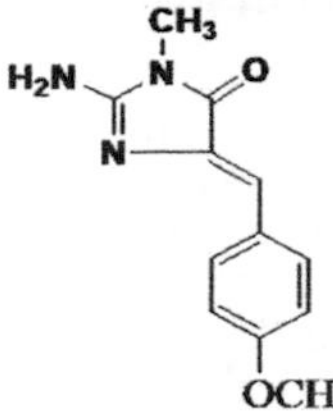

(7) Leucettamine C

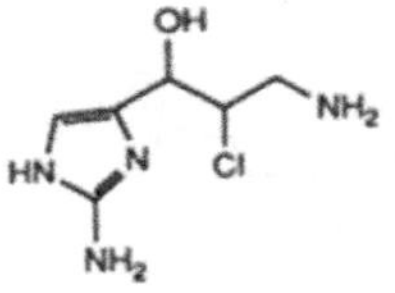

(8) Girolline

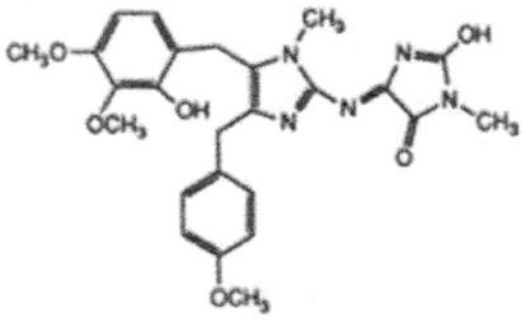

(9) Pyronaamide

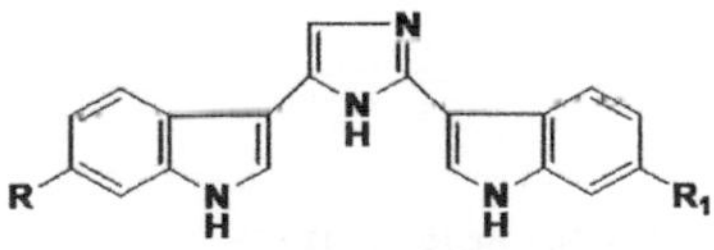

(10) Nortopsentins A R =R_1= Br
(11) Nortopsentins B R =Br, R_1= H
(12) Nortopsentins C R =H, R_1= Br

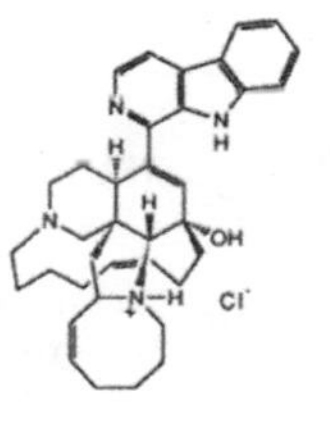

(13) Manzamine A

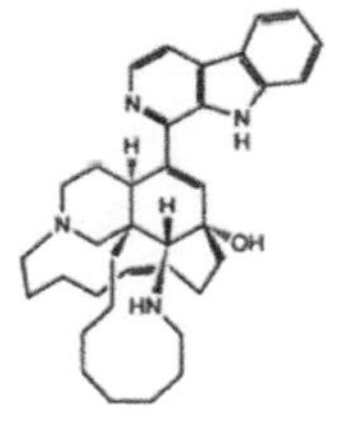

(14) Manzamine B

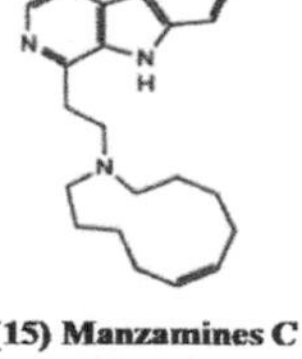

(15) Manzamines C

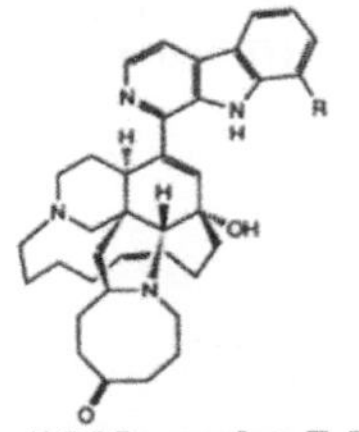

(16) Manzamines E, R= H,
(17) Manzamines F, R= OH

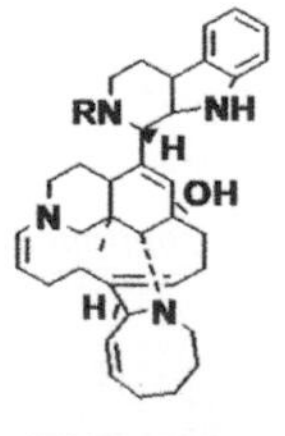

(18) N-Methyl-epi-manzamine D
(19) epi-Manzamine D

FIGURE 2.1 Alkaloids isolated from marine sponges.

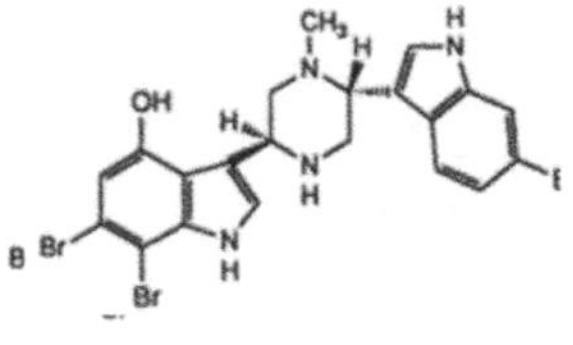

(20) Dragmacidin

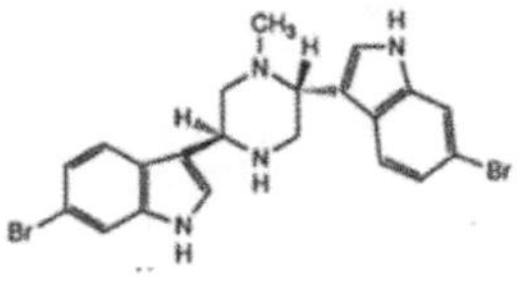

(21) Dragmacidon A

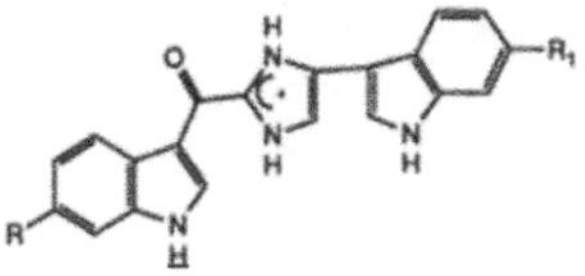

(22) Topsentins A, R =R,1= H
(23) Topsentins B1, R = OH, R_1= H
(24) Topsentins B2, R = OH, R_1 = Br

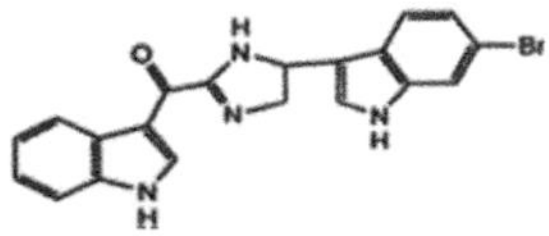

(25) dihydrodeoxybromo topsentin

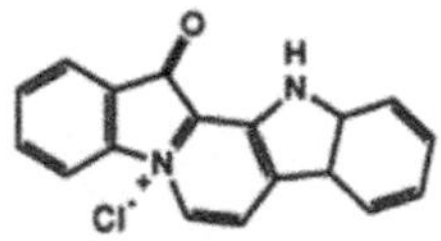

(26) Fascaplysin

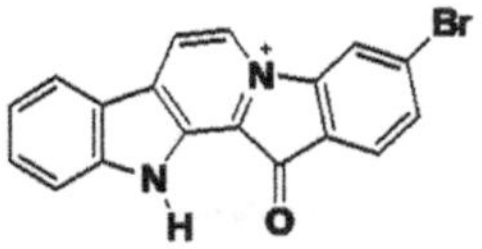

(27) 3-Bromofascaplysin

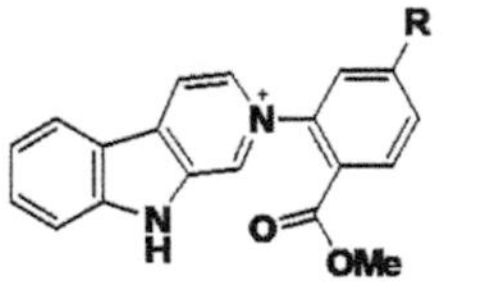

(28) 14-bromoreticulatine, R Br

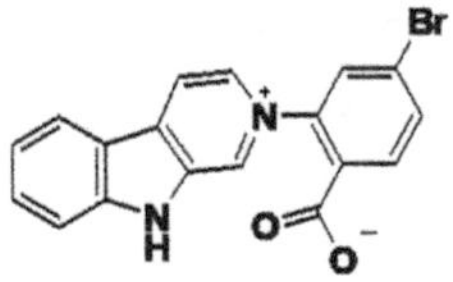

(29) 14-bromoreticulatate, R = Br

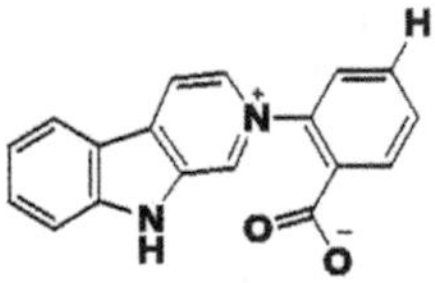

(30) Reticulatate, R = H

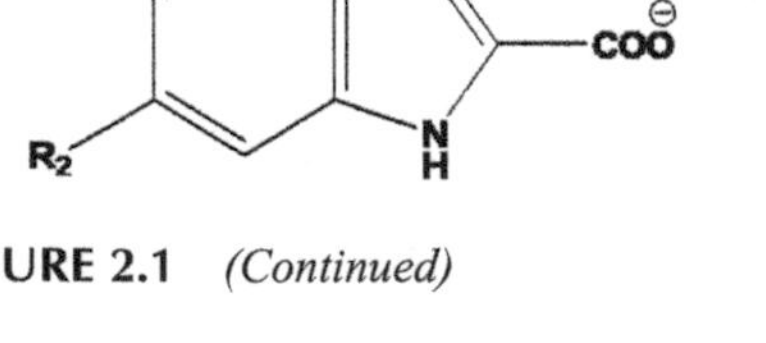

(31) Trachycladinole A, R_1 = Br, $R_{2,3,4}$ = H
(32) Trachycladinole B, R_1 = Br, $R_{2,3}$ =H, R_4 =Me
(33) Trachycladinole C, R_1 = Br, R_2 = OH, $R_{3,4}$ =H
(34) Trachycladinole D, R_1 = Br, R_2 =OH, R_3 = Me, R_4 =H
(35) Trachycladinole E, R_1 = Br, R_2 = H, R_3 = Me, R_4 = OH
(36) Trachycladinole F, R_1 = Br, $R_{2,4}$ = OH, R_3 = Me
(37) Trachycladinole G, $R_{1,2,3,4}$ = H

FIGURE 2.1 *(Continued)*

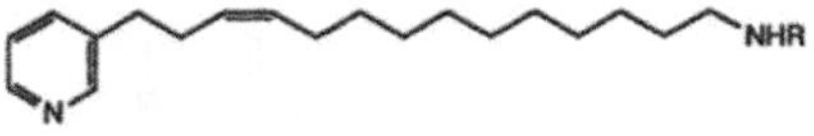

(38) TheonelladinsA, R = H
(39) TheonelladinsA, R = CH_3

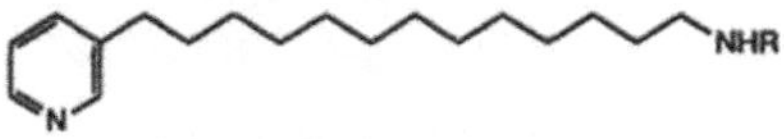

(40) TheonelladinsA, R = H
(41) TheonelladinsA, R = CH_3

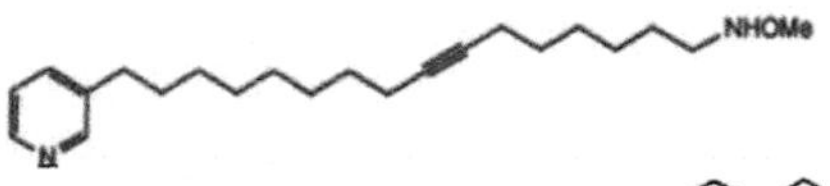

(42) Niphatynes A

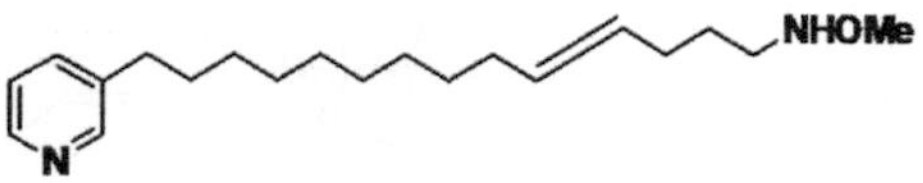

(43) Niphatynes B

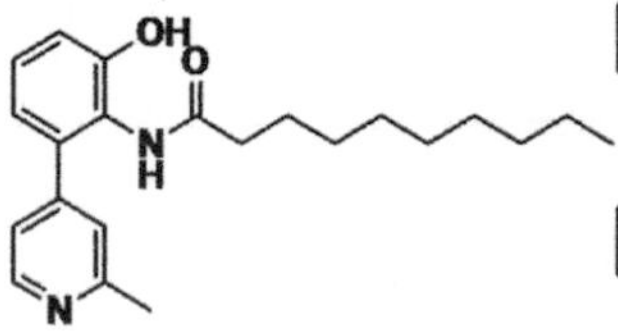

(44) Echinoclathrines A

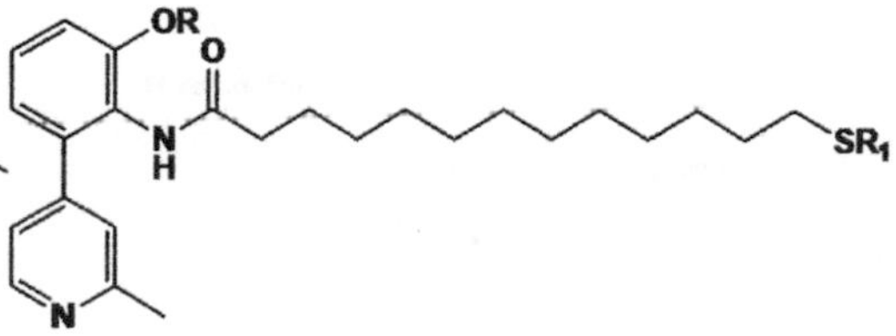

(45) Echinoclathrine B, R = H, R_1 = Ac
(46) Echinoclathrine C, R = R_1 = H

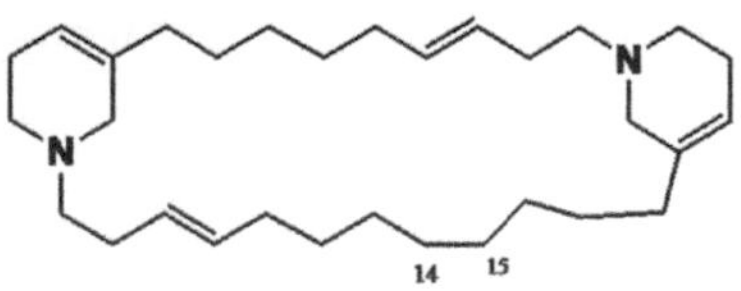

(47) Haliclamines A
(48) Haliclamines B14

FIGURE 2.1 *(Continued)*

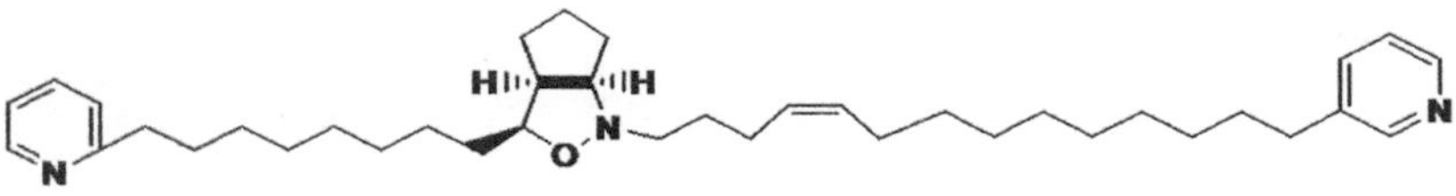

(49) Pyrinodemins A

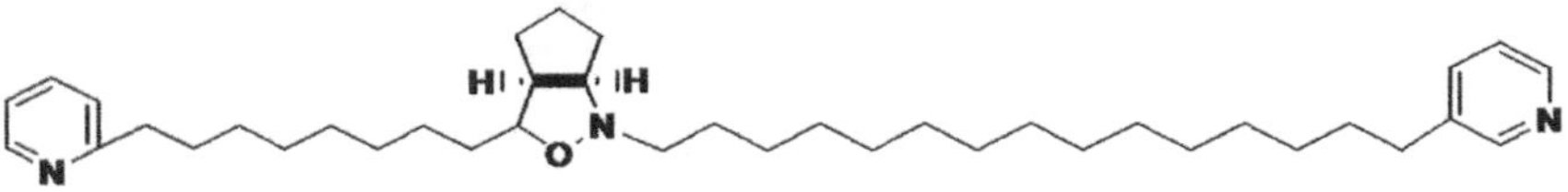

(50) Pyrinodemins B

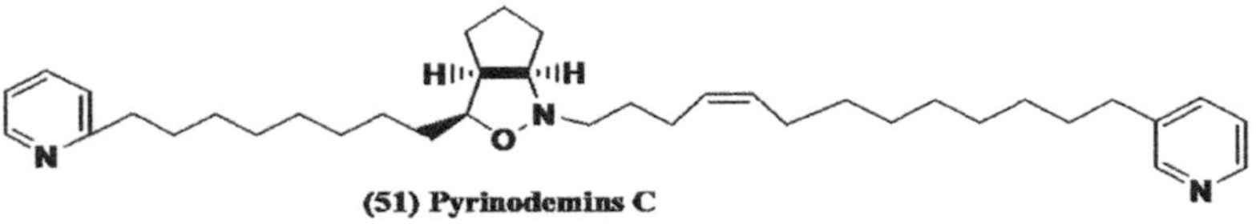

(51) Pyrinodemins C

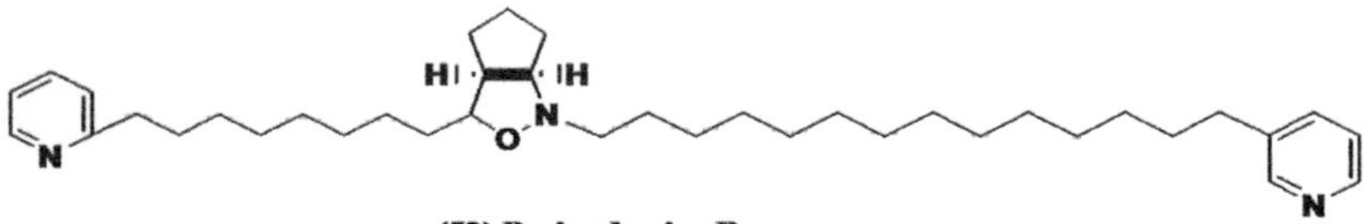

(52) Pyrinodemins B

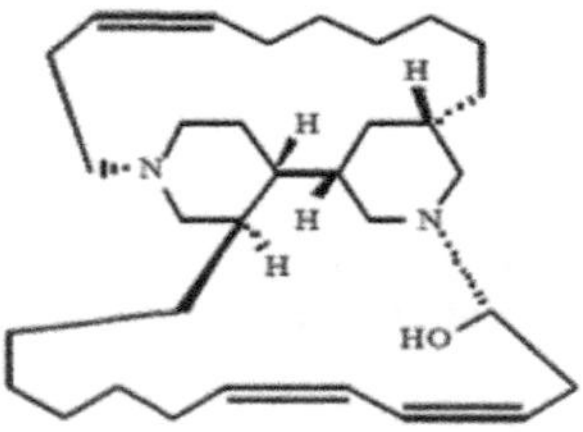

(53) Arenosclerins A

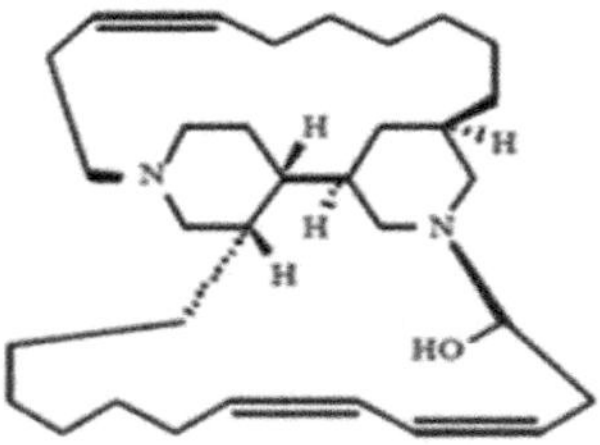

(54) Arenosclerins A

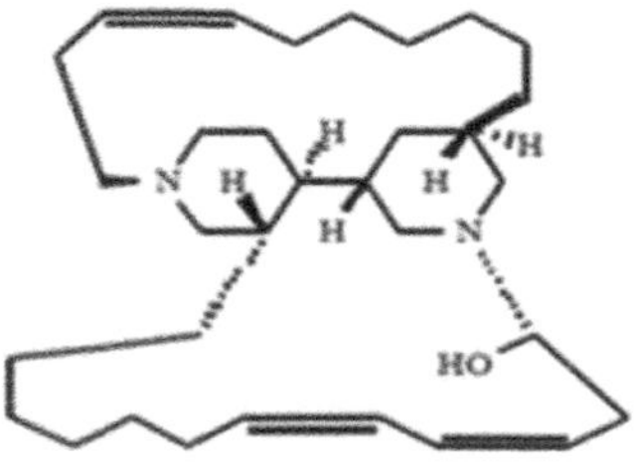

(55) Arenosclerins A

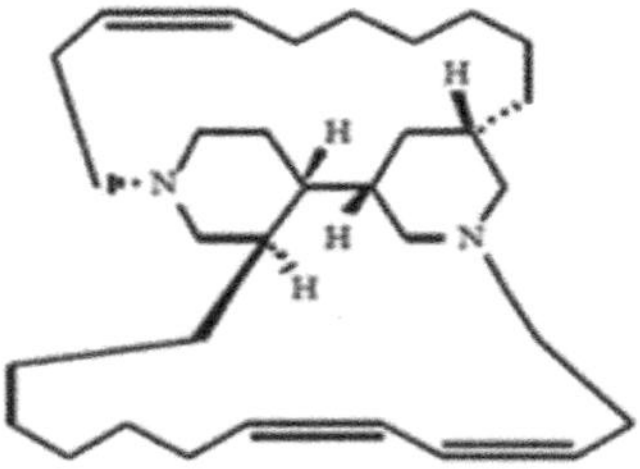

(56) Haliclonacyclamie E

FIGURE 2.1 *(Continued)*

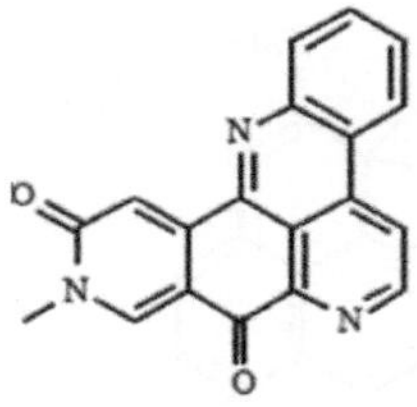

(57) Amphimedine

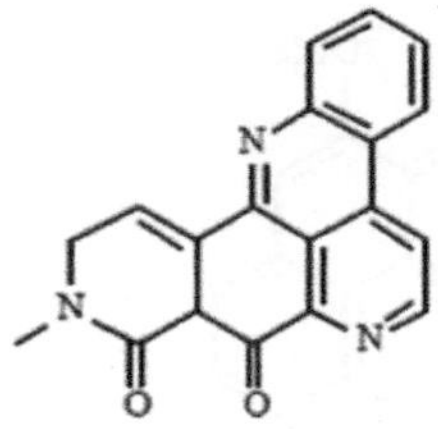

(58) Neoamphimedine

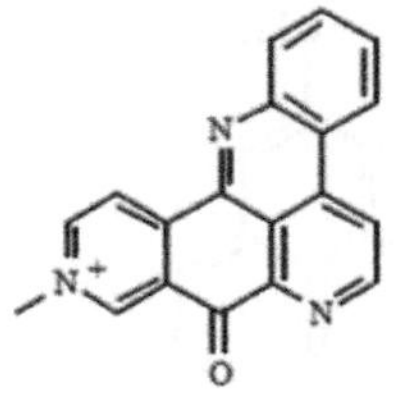

(59)Deoxyamphimedine

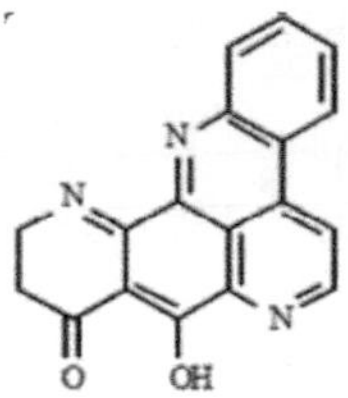

(60) Labuanine A

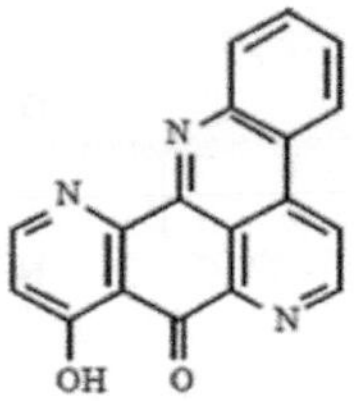

(61) 9-aminobenzo[b] pyrido[4,3,2-de] [1,10] phenanthrolin-8(8H)-one

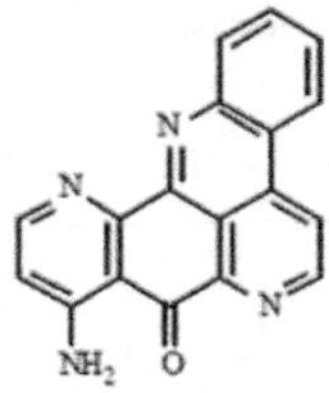

(62) 9-hydroxybenzo[b] pyrido[4,3,2-de] [1,10]phenanthrolin-8(8H)-one

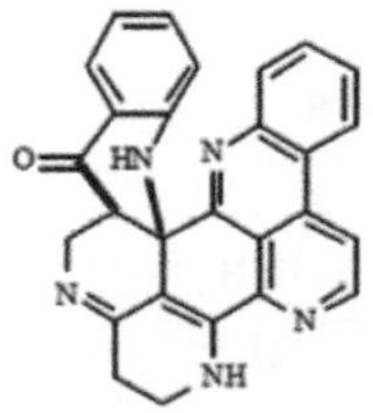

(63) Biemnadin

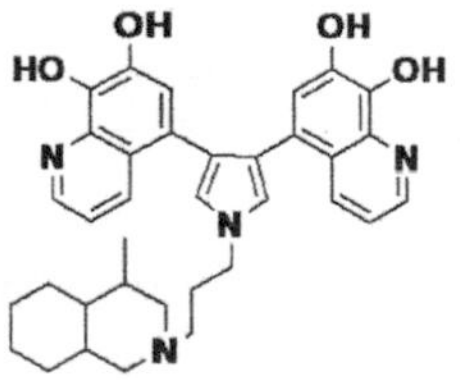

(64) Halitulin

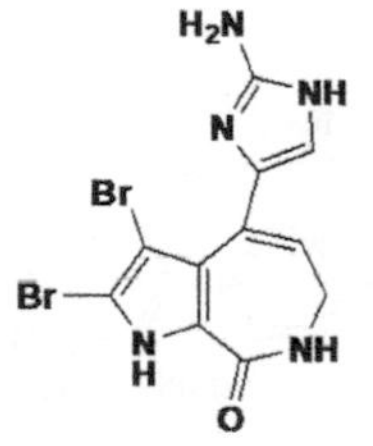

(65) Imidazolylpyrroloazepines

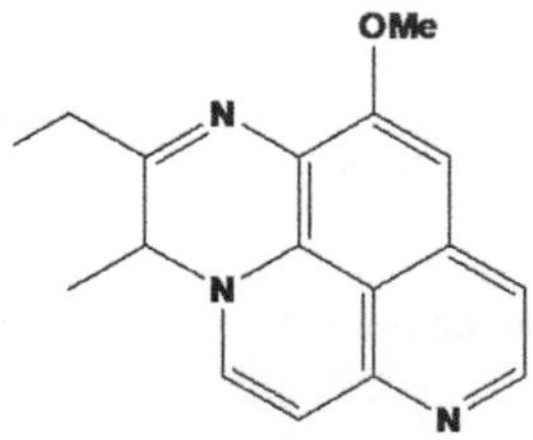

(66) 8,9,9-Trimethoxy-9H-benzo[de] [1,6]naphthyridine

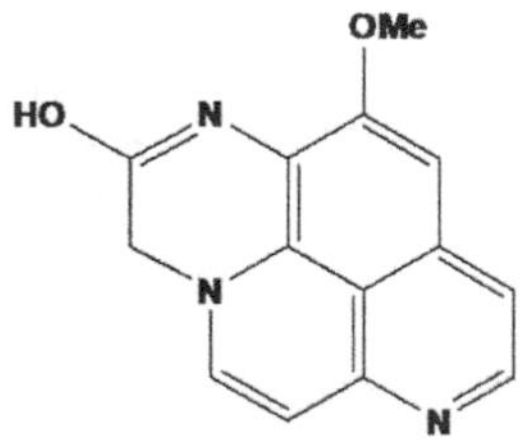

(67)

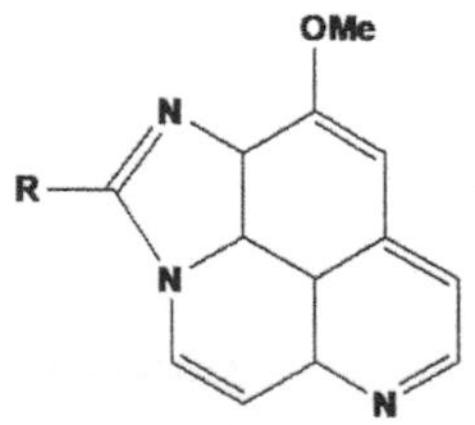

(68) R = CH-(Me)2
(69) R = H

FIGURE 2.1 *(Continued)*

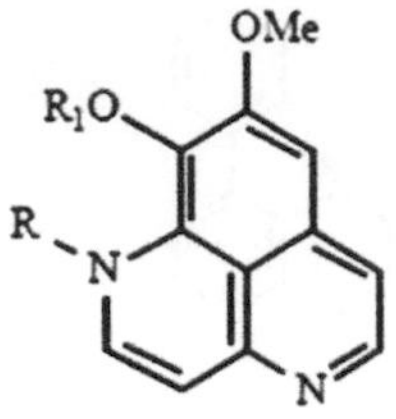

(70) Aaptamine R= H, R1= Me
(71) Isoaaptamine R=Me, R1=H

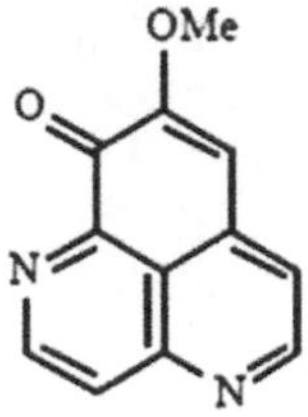

(72) Demethyl(oxy)aaptamine

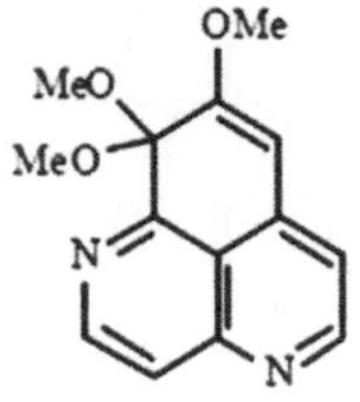

(73) Dimethylketal

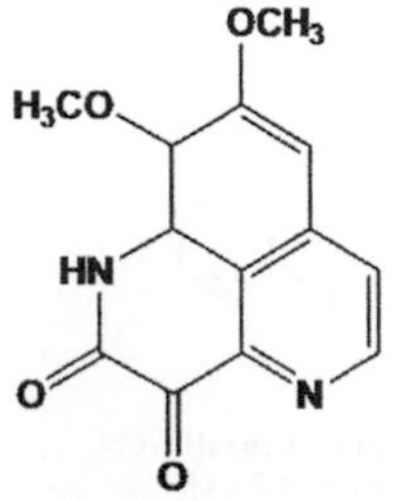

(74) 2,3-dihydro-2,3-dioxoaaptamine

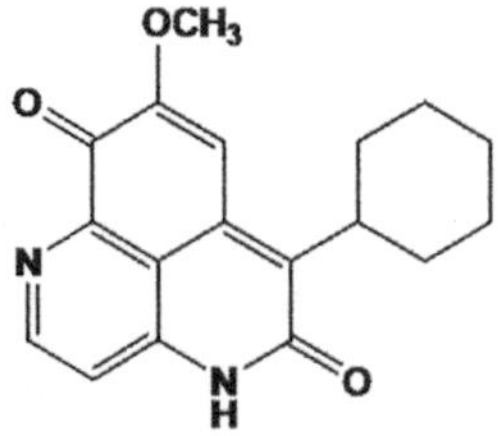

(75) 6-(N-morpholinyl)-4,5-dihydro-5-oxodemethyl(oxy)aaptamine

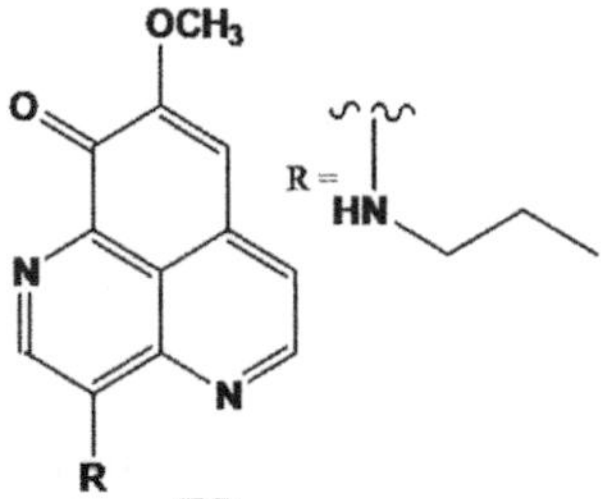

(76)

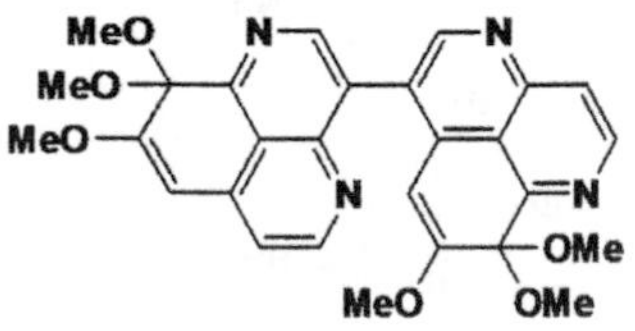

(77) Suberitine A

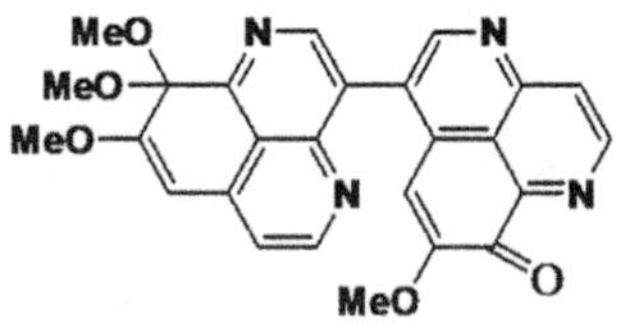

(78) Suberitine B

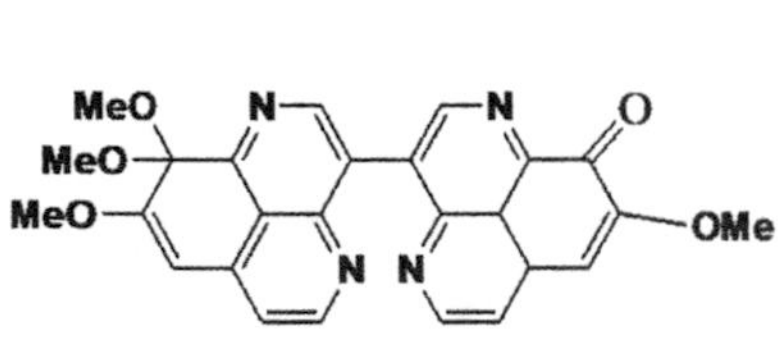

(79) Suberitine C

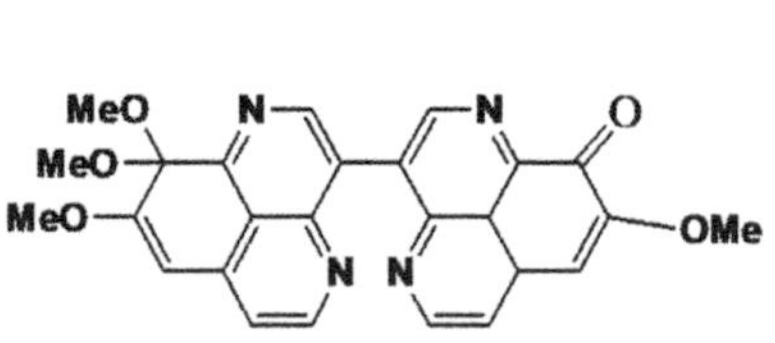

(80) Suberitine D

FIGURE 2.1 *(Continued)*

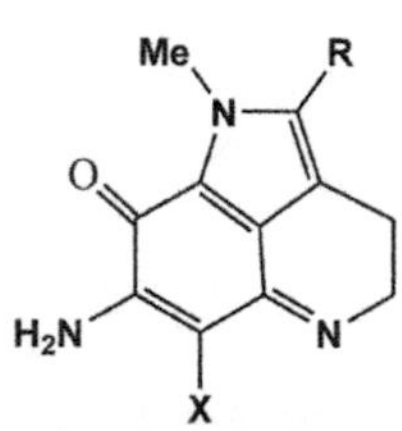

(81) Isobatzelline A, R = SMe, X = Cl
(82) Isobatzelline B, R = SMe, X = H
(83) Isobatzelline C, R = H, X = Cl

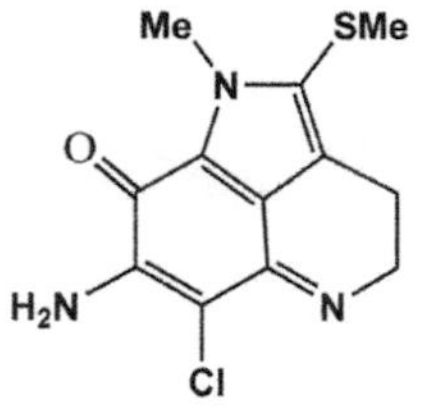

(84) Isobatzelline D

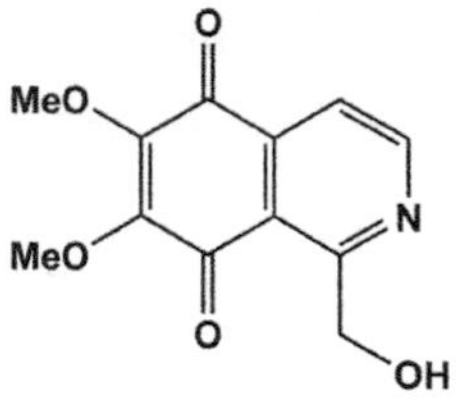

(85) Renierol

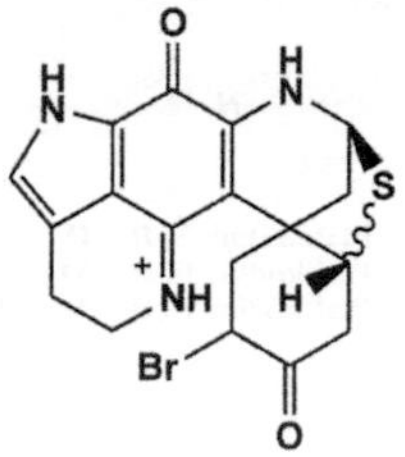

(86) Discorhabdins A

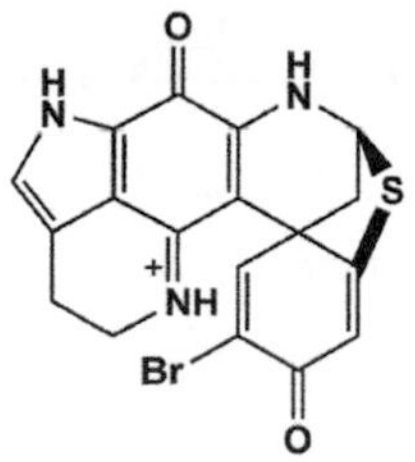

(87) Discorhabdins B

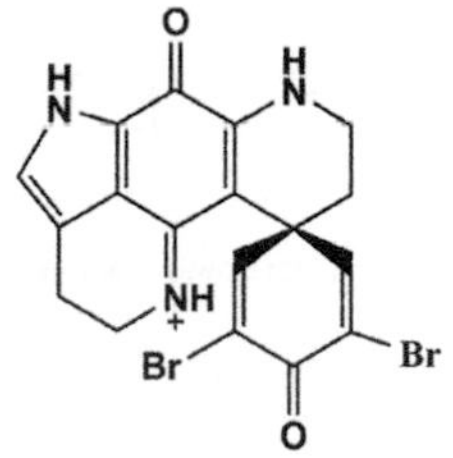

(88) Discorhabdins C

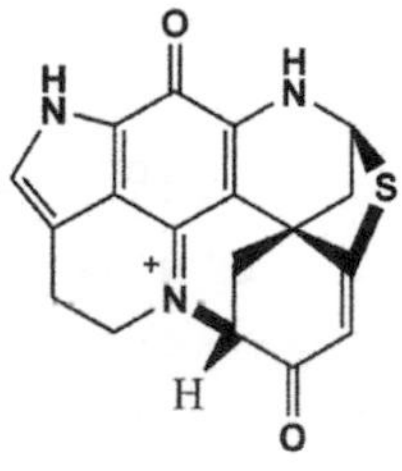

(89) Discorhabdins D

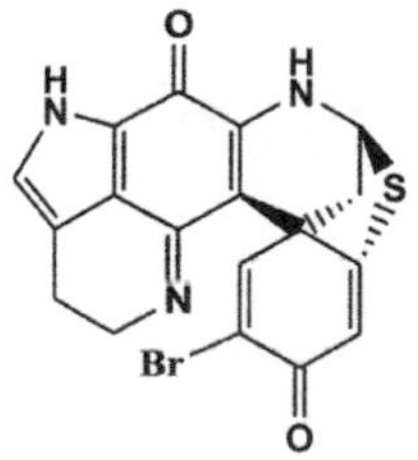

(90) Prianosin A

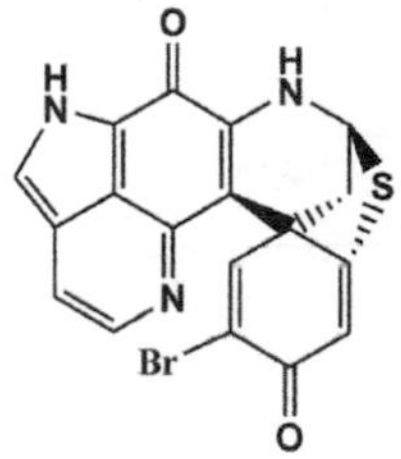

(91) Prianosin B

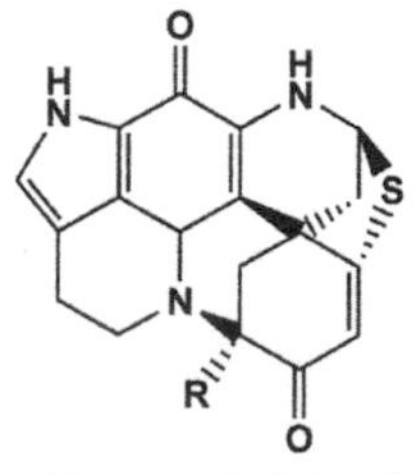

(92) Prianosin C, R = OH
(93) Prianosin D, R = H

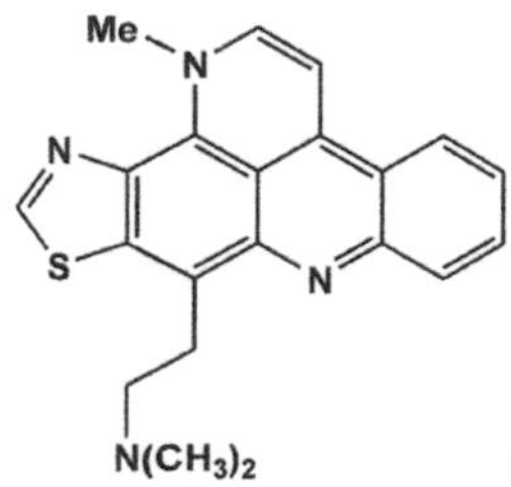

(94) Dercitin

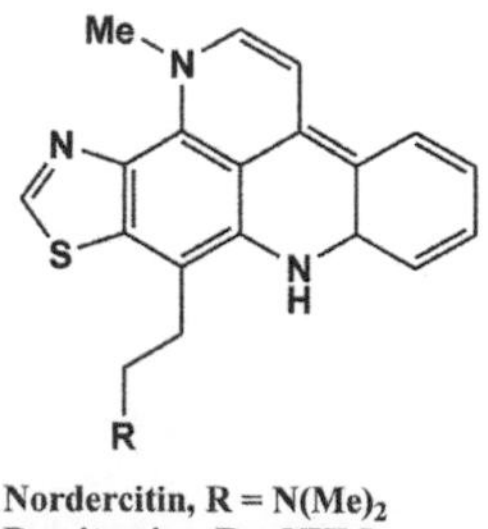

(95) Nordercitin, R = N(Me)$_2$
(96) Dercitamine, R = NHMe
(97) Dercitamine, R = NHCOCH$_2$CH$_3$

FIGURE 2.1 *(Continued)*

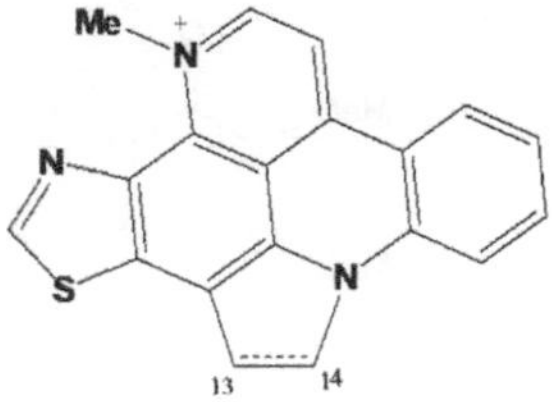

(98) Cyclodercitin (13, 14 dihydro)
(99) Cyclodercitin

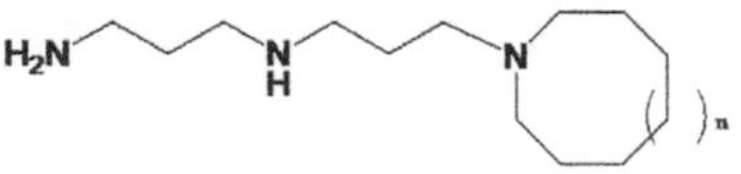

(100) Motuporamine A, n = 6
(101) Motuporamine B, n = 7

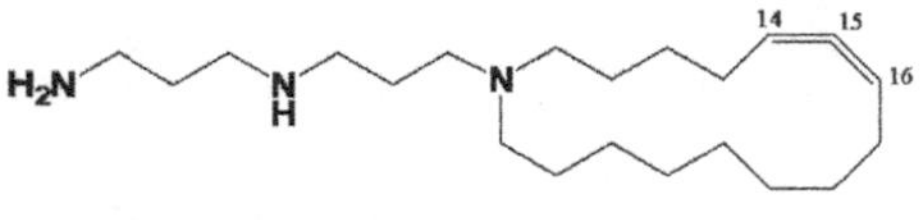

(102) Motuporamine C, = 14, 15 or 15, 16

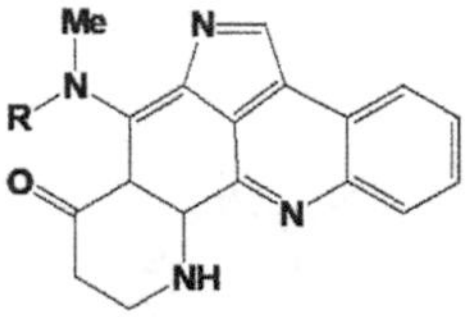

(103) Plakinidine A, R = H
(104) Plakinidine B, R = Me
(105) Plakinidine C, R = Me-Me

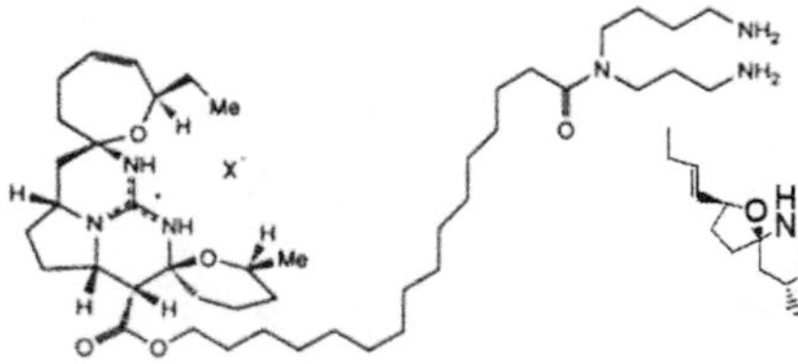

(106) Ptilomycalin A

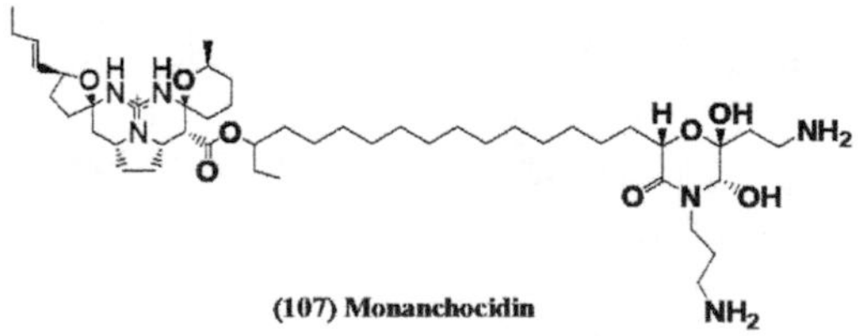

(107) Monanchocidin

FIGURE 2.1 *(Continued)*

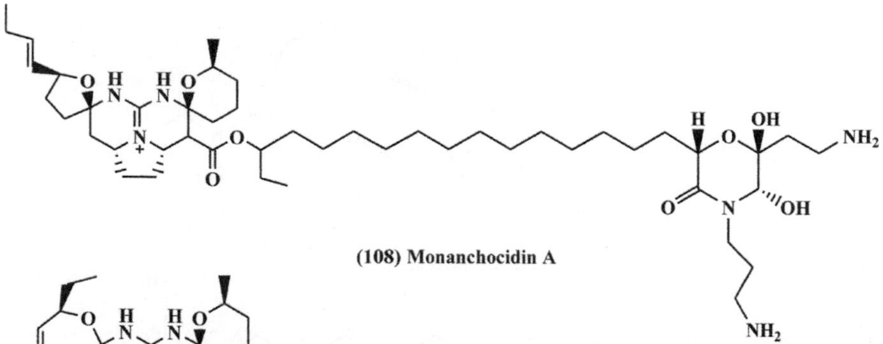

(108) Monanchocidin A

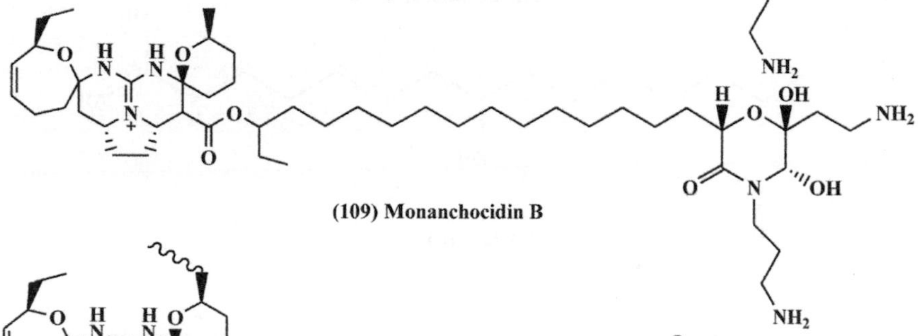

(109) Monanchocidin B

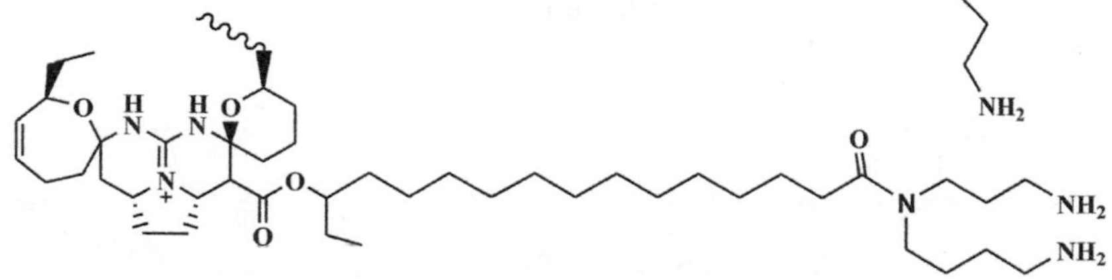

(110) Monanchomycalin C

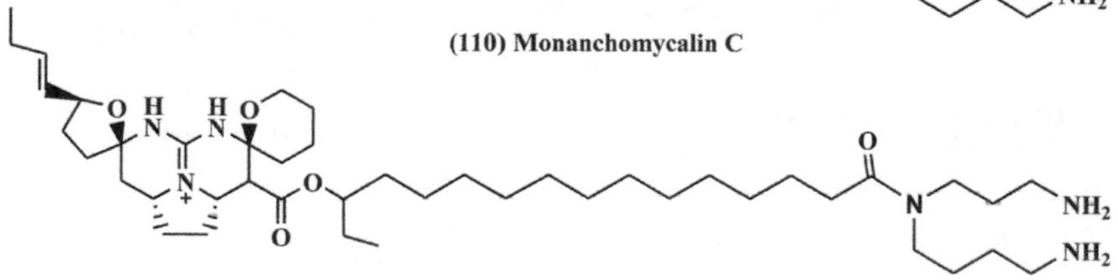

(111) Monanchomycalin B

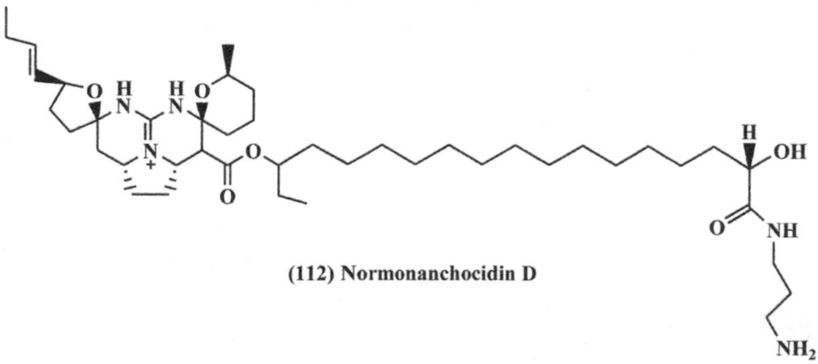

(112) Normonanchocidin D

FIGURE 2.1 *(Continued)*

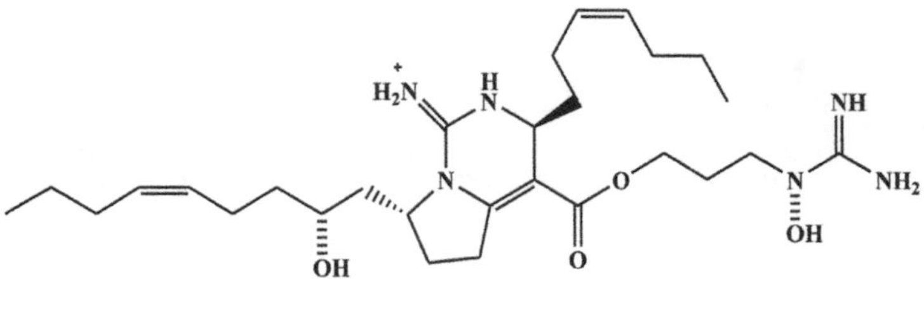

(113) Urupocidin A

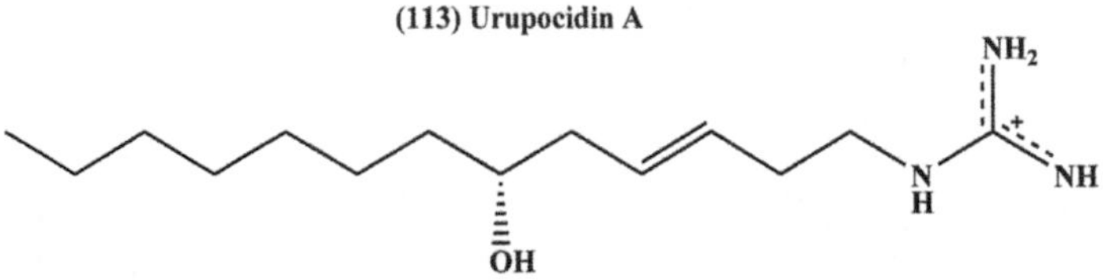

(114) Pulchranin A

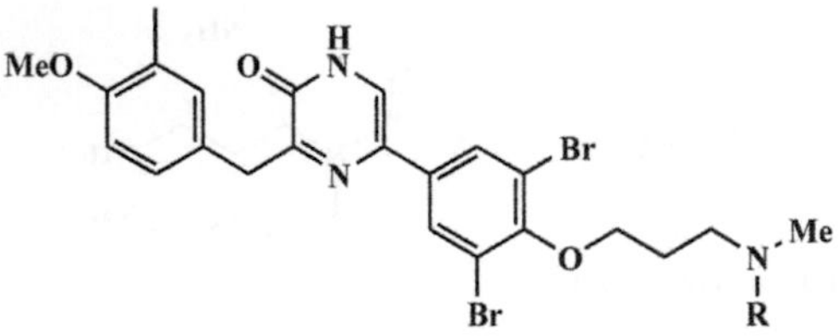

(115) Ma'damine A, R = Me
(116) Ma'damine B, R = H

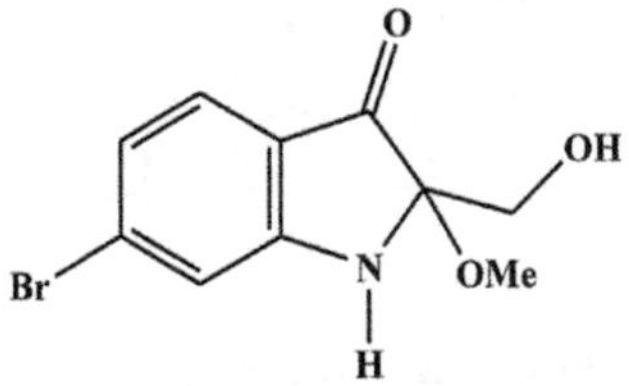

(117) Matemone

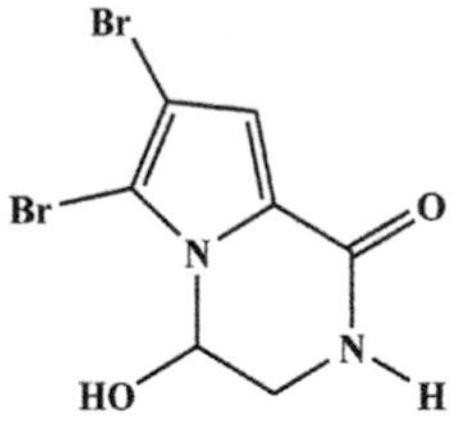

(118) Longamide

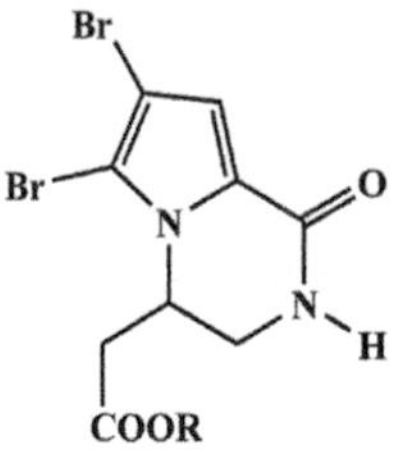

(119) Longamide B, Me , R = Me
(119) LongamideB, R = H
(120) Hanishin R= Et

FIGURE 2.1 *(Continued)*

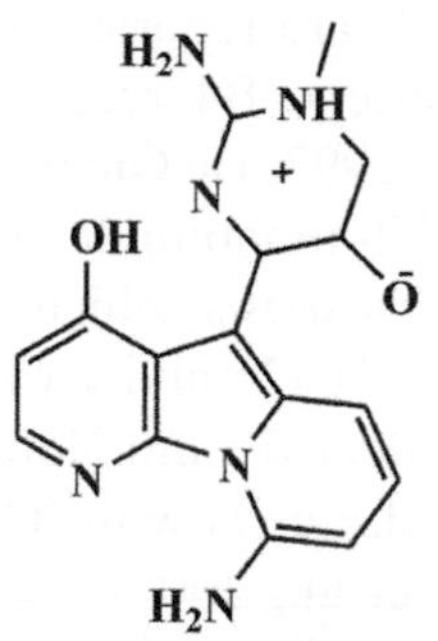

(121) Variolin A

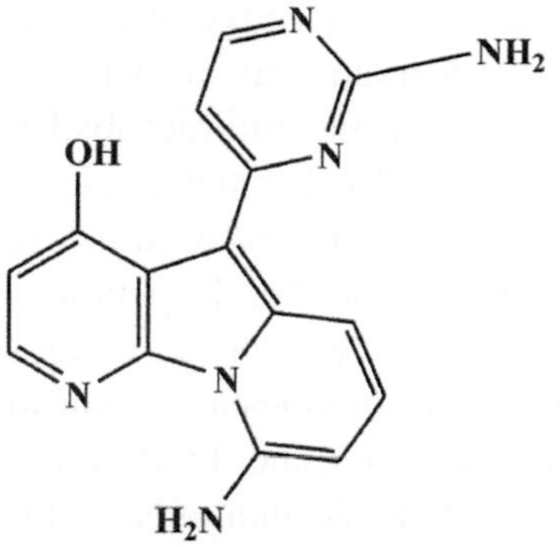

(122) Variolin B

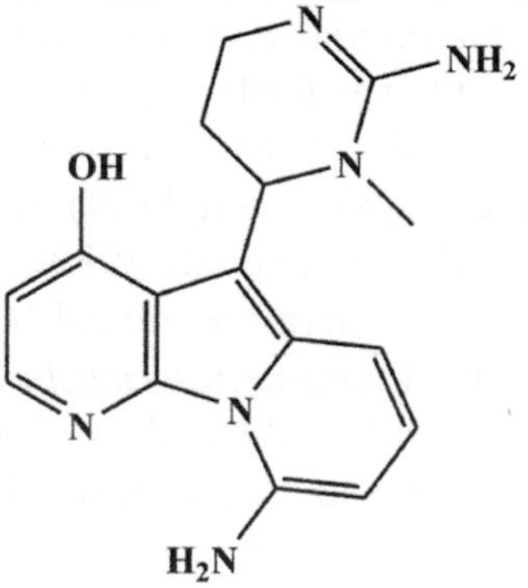

(123) Variolin C

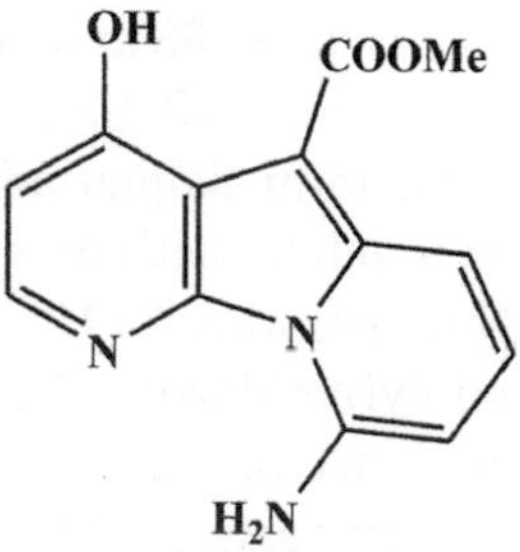

(124) Variolin D

FIGURE 2.1 *(Continued)*

2.2 MARINE SPONGE ALKALOIDS AND THEIR ANTICANCER POTENTIALS

2.2.1 CYTOTOXIC IMIDAZOLES ALKALOIDS

Naamidines are the biologically active imidazole alkaloids, commonly found in *Leucetta, Clathrina,* and *Leucosolenia* genera of the marine sponges (Carmely et al. 1989; Ciminiello et al., 1990; Ralifo et al., 2007). Structurally, they are comprised of central imidazole ring to which one or two modified benzyl groups are attached at the N-3 or C-4, C-5 positions, and most of the alkaloids belonging to this group contain a hydantoin or hydantoin derivative at the N-6 position. These alkaloids are reported for various biological properties such as cytotoxic, leukotriene B4 receptor antagonist, and antimicrobial activities (Plubrukarn et al., 1997; De Guzman et al., 1999). Carmel et al. (1989) reported a series of 2-aminoimidazole alkaloids called naamidines (e.g., **1**) from *Leucetta chagosensis* which is a marine sponge. Two imidazole alkaloids, naamidines H (**2**) and I (**3**), were extracted from *L. chagosensis* (marine sponge) collected from North Sulawesi, Indonesia and showed cytotoxicity against HeLa cells with IC_{50} values of 5.6 and 15 μg/mL, respectively (Tsukamoto et al., 2007). Two new imidazole alkaloids, methyldorimidazole (**4**), preclathridine B (**5**) along with known compounds naamine E (**6**) and leucettamine C (**7**) were isolated by *L. chagosensis* (Hassan et al., 2009). The isolated compounds showed cytotoxicity against P388 at 2–10 μg/mL (Y. Kashman, personal communication). Girolline (**8**), obtained from *Pseudaxinyssa cantharella,* was found active against P388 at 0.001–1 μg/mL and the activity was further confirmed in vivo in mice (P388 at 1 mg/kg doses (Ahond et al., 1988). The sponge *Leucetta* from Saipan and Guam was the source of pyronaamide (**9**) and found to inhibit activities of KB cells (MIC 5 μg/mL) (Akee et al., 1990).

Nortopsentins A (**10**), B (**11**), and C (**12**), having a characteristic 2,4-bis (3-indolyl)imidazole skeleton were obtained from *Spongsorites ruetzleri*, a deepwater marine sponge. Nortopsentins A, B, and C showed in vitro cytotoxicity against P388 cell: IC_{50} (mg/mL) 7.6, 7.8 and 1.7, respectively (Sakemi and Sun, 1991; Sun et al., 1991; Kawasaki et al., 1996).

2.2.2 ANTITUMOR INDOLE ALKALOIDS FROM MARINE SPONGES

Manzamines are one of the most complex alkaloidal structures. Manzamine A (**13**) is found in the *Haliclona* sp., *Pellina* sp., *Xestospongia* sp., and *Pachypellina* sp. from marine sponges and reported to possess various biological properties such as antimicrobial, anti-inflammatory, and anticancer activities (Radwan et al., 2012). Manzamine A (**13**) was extracted from a *Haliclona* sp. of sponge from Okinawa as its hydrochloride salt with an IC_{50} of 0.07 μg/mL against P388 cells in vitro (Sakai et al., 1986) and enhanced the sensitivity to tumor necrosis factor-related apoptosis-inducing ligand (TRAIL)-apoptosis inducers in human adenocarcinoma pancreatic cells (Guzman et al., 2011). The same sponge resulted in the disclosure of manzamines B (**14**) and C (**15**) (Sakai et al., 1987), while as manzamines E (**16**) and F (**17**) were later isolated from genus *Xestospongia* (Ichiba et al., 1988). Manzamines A–F showed cytotoxicity against P388 cells in vitro: IC_{50} (μg/mL) 0.07, 0.06, 0.03, 0.05, and 0.05, respectively. A marine sponge crude extract designated PAL93-055 collected from Palau resulted in the isolation of two new isomeric manzamines, namely *N*-Methyl-*epi*-manzamine D (**18**) and *epi*-manzamine D (**19**). These two isolated isomers (**18, 19**) showed cytotoxic effects against B16F10 and HeLa cell lines with highest potency (IC_{50}: 0.1 mg/mL) for N-methyl-*epi*-manzamine D (**18**) for B16F10 cell line and were consistent with previously reported manzamine alkaloids (Zhou et al., 2000).

Dragmacidin (**20**), obtained from deepwater sponge, was found to be toxic to P388 cells (IC_{50}: 15 μg/mL) as well as to KCT-8 human colon, A549 human lung, and MD-AMB human mammary cells, all with IC_{50} of 1–10 μg/mL (Kohmoto et al., 1988). Another closely related compound dragmacidon A (**21**) was later reported by Morris and Andersen (1989), which exhibited cytotoxicity against Ll210 cells with ED_{50}, 10 μg/mL similar to dragmacidin.

Topsentins, bisindole alkaloids were discovered almost at the same time by two different groups. Bartik et al. (1987) in Belgium were the first to report topsentins A (**22**), B1 (**23**), and B2 (**24**) from *Topsentia genitrix* sponge and their toxicity effects to fish at 15–20 mg/L (Braekman et al., 1987). Subsequently, Tsujii and Rinehart (1988) also isolated topsentins A (designated deoxytopsentin), B1 (designated, topsentin), and B2 (designated, bromotopsentin) along with a new metabolite dihydrodeoxybromo topsentin (**25**) from family Halichondriidae, a deepwater sponge. Also, in vitro and very weak in vivo activities against P388 (IC_{50}: 12.0, 2.0, 7.0, 4.0 μg/mL) and tumor-initiating cell, TIC132 at 75 mg/kg, TIC126 at 75 mg/kg, respectively were reported.

Fascaplysin (**26**) is an unusual pentacyclic-fused planar alkaloid isolated from *Fascaplysinopsis bergquist* sp. sponge (Roll et al., 1988). Recently, three new members of fascaplysin, namely 3-bromofascaplysin (**27**), 14-bromoreticulatine (**28**), 14-bromoreticulatate (**29**) along with reticulatate (**30**), were isolated from the sponge *Fascaplysinopsis reticulate* and two collections of the tunicate *Didemnum* sp. (Segraves et al., 2003). These isolates (**26–30**) were tested for in vitro solid tumor selectivity against a panel of human and murine tumor cells. Among all tested compounds, fascaplysin (**26**) exhibited murine solid tumor selectivity and was found to be most cytotoxic. Beside this, fascaplysin (**26**) possesses a vast range of biological activities including antimicrobial, p56 tyrosine kinase, HIV-1-RT, antimalarial, potency to various cancer cell lines (Hörmann et al., 2001; Kirsch et al., 2000; Schmidt and Faulkner, 1996; Jimenez et al., 1991a and 1991b). It induces apoptosis, cell-cycle arrest, and reactive oxygen specie generation (Hamilton, 2014). Moreover, fascaplysin also exhibited synergistic cytotoxicity with the topoisomerase I inhibitors in competent to camptothecin, 10-hydroxycamptothecin, and topotecan on chemoresistant NCI-H417 small cell lung cancer, but the mechanism of action is still unknown (Hamilton, 2014).

Trachycladindoles A-G (**31–37**), a 2-amino-4, 5-dihydroimidazole bearing alkaloids have been isolated from *Trachycladus laevispirulifer* (Southern Australian marine sponge). They displayed a substitution-dependent pattern cytotoxicity against human cancer cell lines A549, MDA-MB-231, and HT-29 (Capon et al., 2008).

2.2.3 CYTOTOXIC PYRIDINES ALKALOIDS FROM MARINE SPONGES

Theonelladins are the pyridine skeleton alkaloids. Theonelladins A (**38**), B (**39**), C (**40**) and D (**41**) were isolated from the *Theonella swinhoe* in addition to swinholide macrolides (Kobayashi et al., 1989). Theonelladins A–D exhibited in vitro cytotoxicity against L1210 cells: IC_{50} (μg/mL) 4.7, 1.0, 3.6, and 1.6, respectively, and KB cells: ED_{50} (μg/mL) 10.0, 3.6, 10, and 5.26, respectively. Also, the theonelladins are reported to be 20 times more efficient in causing the release of Ca^{2+} from sarcoplasmic reticulum than caffeine. Other pyridine-related alkaloids niphatynes A (**42**) and B (**43**) have been isolated from *Niphates* sp. collected from Fiji, which were cytotoxic against P388 cells: IC_{50} (μg/mL) 0.5 (Quinoa and Crews, 1987).

Echinoclathrines A–C (**44–46**), the new class of pyridine alkaloids possessing 4-aryl-2-methylpyridine moiety as the main structure element, were isolated from *Echinoclathria* sp. from an Okinawan sponge. All these compounds (**44–46**) were tested for cytotoxic properties and results showed that compound **44** was cytotoxic against A-549, HT-29, and P388 cells with IC_{50} value of 10 μg/mL. Also, compounds **44** and **45** demonstrated weak immunosuppressive activity in a mixed lymphocyte reaction assay with IC_{50} of 7.9 and 9.7 μg/mL, respectively (Kitamura et al., 1999).

The macrocyclic alkaloids haliclamines A (**47**) and B (**48**) extracted from a sponge belonging to genus *Haliclona* were reported to be active against various cell assays: P388 cells—IC_{50} (μg/mL) 0.75, 0.36; L1210 cells: IC_{50} (μg/mL) 1.5, 0.9; inhibition of cell division of eggs of sea urchin *Hemicentrotus pulcherrimus*: IC_{50} (μg/mL) 5, 10, respectively (Fusetani et al., 1989). Biogenetically, these alkaloids are closely related to halitoxin (Schmitz et al., 1978).

The unique *bis*-3-alkylpyridine alkaloids containing *cis*-cyclopent[*c*] isoxazolidine moiety, pyrinodemins A-D (**49–52**) and related -alkyl pyridine alkaloids have been isolated from *Amphimedon* sp. from the Okinawan marine sponge (Hirano et al., 2000a). Cytotoxicity evaluation revealed pyrinodemin (A–D [**49–52**]). Compounds **50** and **51** demonstrated significant cytotoxicity against KB epidermoid carcinoma cells (IC_{50}: 0.5 mg/mL, each) and murine leukemia L1210 (IC_{50}: 0.07, 0.06, and 0.08 mg/mL, respectively) in vitro comparable to pyrinodemin A (Hirano et al., 2000a). Novel tetracyclic alkylpiperidine alkaloids, arenosclerins A (**53**), B (**54**), and C (**55**) along with haliclonacyclamie E (**56**) have been isolated from *Arenosclera brasiliensis*, a marine sponge (Torres et al., 2002). All these compounds were tested for cytotoxicity and showed an almost similar range of cytotoxicity, irrespective of the cancer cell line tested.

Marine sponge *Amphimedon* sp. collected from Okinawan resulted in the isolation of two bis-3-alkylpyridine alkaloids, pyrinodemin G, and pyrinodemin H. The structures of pyrinodemins G and H are composed of N-methoxy amide moiety and an α,β-unsaturated 3,5-disubstituted δ-lactone moiety at a junction of two 3-alkylpyridines, respectively. There is a possibility of multiple structures for pyrinodemins G and H. Furthermore, pyrinodemins G and pyrinodemin H showed significant antitumor activity against P388 murine leukemia cells with IC_{50} values of 9.6 and 2.5 mg/mL (Williams et al., 1998).

The pyridoacridines constitute an interesting class of secondary metabolites from a marine source and many compounds of this series are reported to possess potent cytotoxic activity (Molinski, 1993; Ding et al., 1999). Amphimedine (**57**) was the first pyridoacridine alkaloid isolated from marine organism *Amphimedon* sp. in 1983 (Schmitz et al., 1983). A few years later, De Guzman et al. reported the isolation of neoamphimedine (**58**) and deoxyamphimedine (**59**), two structurally related compounds, from two tropical Xestospongia sponges (Tasdemir et al., 2001). Neoamphimedine (**58**) showed significant antineoplastic activity tumors in athymic mice. The results showed that neoamphimedine was as effective as 9-aminocamptothecinin in HCT-116 tumors-bearing mice and as effective asetoposide in KB tumors-bearing mice. However, amphimedine (**57**) neither showed any potent antineoplastic activity nor induced any catenation or DNA aggregation in vitro. Therefore, the results suggested that neoamphimedine (**58**) possesses two-mediated mechanism of anticancer and cytotoxicity potential (Marshalla et al., 2003). Pyridoacridine alkaloids, labuanine A (**60**), (9-aminobenzo[b] pyrido[4,3,2-de] [1,10] phenanthrolin-8(8H)-one (**61**)), (9-hydroxybenzo[b] pyrido[4,3,2-de] [1,10]phenanthrolin-8(8H)-one) (**62**) and biemnadin (**63**), were extracted from *Biemna fortis* from an Indonesian marine sponge (Aoki et al., 1969). The isolated pyridoacridine alkaloids induced multipolar neuritogenesis in more than 50% of cells at 0.03–3 μM concentration. Compound

(**60**), exhibited the strongest neuritogenic activity and induced increase in acetylcholinesterase, arrested cell cycle at the G2/M phase and a neuronal marker in Neuro 2A. Whereas compounds (**61**), (**62**), and (**63**) induced neurite outgrowth in more than 50% of cells at 1–3 μM concentration. The huge difference in neuritogenic activity between compounds (**61**) and (**62**) is due to the presence of amino group at C-9 (Fuente et al., 2001).

2.2.4 CYTOTOXIC PYRROLES ALKALOIDS FROM MARINE SPONGES

A novel bisquinolinylpyrrole named as halitulin (**64**) has been isolated from the *Haliclona tulearensis,* a marine sponge, and has shown potent cytotoxicity against panel of cell lines, such as murine leukemia P388 (IC_{50}: 0.025 mg/mL), human colon carcinoma HT-29 (IC_{50}: 0.012 mg/mL), human melanoma MEL-28 (IC_{50}: 0.025 mg/mL), and human lung carcinoma A-549 (IC_{50}: 0.012 mg/mL) (Kashman et al., 1999). Wright and Thompson in 1987 reported imidazolyl pyrroloazepines alkaloid (**65**) from *Teichaxinella morchella* and *Ptilocaulis walpersi* sponges and showed mild cytotoxicity against L1210 cells (IC_{50}: 10.0 μg/mL).

2.2.5 ANTITUMOR QUINOLINES AND ISOQUINOLINES ALKALOIDS

An unidentified species from Indonesian marine sponge of genus *Xestospongia* sp. has resulted in isolation of four new novel (**66–69**) alkaloidal compounds from aaptamine class in addition to known aaptamine (**70**), isoaaptamine (**71**), demethyl(oxy)aaptamine (**72**) and its dimethylketal (**73**) (Calcul et al., 2003; Shen et al., 1999). These compounds were screened for antitumor against KB cells and all the tested compounds (**70–73**) showed significant cytotoxic activity on KB cells (ID_{50} mg/mL, 3.7, 0.5, 1.8, 3.5, new four compounds **66–69**=>10). In another study, antitumor activity screening of compound (isoaaptamine, demethyl(oxy)aaptamine) against Ehrlich ascites tumors in mice showed 95% of inhibition in mice pretreated with compounds (**71**) and (**72**) at 25 μg/mL (Fedoreev et al., 1988). These compounds were also reported from genus *Suberites* of the marine sponges. Compounds (**71**) and (**72**) were also reported from the *Aaptos aaptos* sponge and showed toxic effects on HeLa cells with ED_{50}: 2 and 0.87 μg/mL, respectively (Nakamura et al. 1987). Shubina et al. (2010) reported

2,3-dihydro-2,3-dioxoaaptamine (**74**), 6-(*N*-morpholinyl)-4,5-dihydro-5-oxodemethyl(oxy)aaptamine (**75**), and 3-(methylamino)demethyl(oxy) aaptamine (**76**) from the Vietnamese sponge *Aaptos* sp. All the isolated compounds were tested for apoptosis-inducing activity and compound (**76**) showed promising apoptosis-inducing activity (40% of early and 56% of late apoptosis at 208 μM concentration).

Four new dimeric aaptamine alkaloids, suberitines A (**77**), B (**78**), C (**79**), and D (**80**) together with two known monomers have been isolated from marine sponge *Aaptossu beritoids*, collected from Xisha Island in South China. Cytotoxic evaluation of suberitine A–D (**77–80**) against P388, K565, and HeLa cell lines, suberitines B and D showed potent cytotoxicites against selected P388 cell lines with IC_{50} values of 1.8 and 3.5 μM, respectively (Liu et al., 2012).

Isobatzellines A–D (**81–84**) are the pyrroloquinoline alkaloids that were reported to be obtained from *Batzella* sp. of the Caribbean sponge (Sun et al., 1990). Significant cytotoxicity has been reported for these isolated Isobatzellines A–D; in addition to antifungal activity against *Candida albicans*. Renierol (**85**) isolated from the *Xestospongia caycedoia* Fijian sponge and inhibited the growth of L1210 cell with IC_{50} value 3 μg/mL (McKee and Ireland, 1987).

2.2.6 CYTOTOXICDISCORHABDINS/PRIANOSINSALKALOIDS

Discorhabdins and prianosins are unusual but closely related fused pyrrolophenanthroline sulfur-containing alkaloids, which were independently reported by two groups of researchers. These natural discorhabdin alkaloids possess a unique structure with core tetracyclic pyrroloiminoquinone skeleton bound to spirocyclohexanone at the C-6 position and few contain sulfur-containing substituents at the carbon-6 position (Hu et al., 2011). The first reported compound was discorhabdin C (**88**) by Perry et al. in 1986. Few years later, the same group reported remaining discorhabdins, that is, discorhabdins A (**86**), B (**87**), D (**89**) (Perry et al., 1988a and 1988b). The other sources for these discorhabdins reported were *Latrunculia brevis, Prianos* sp., and *Haplosclerida.* Cytotoxicity results for this class of compounds showed that compounds (**86**), (**87**), and (**88**) were inactive in vivo P388 cell lines (TIC < 12%, toxic dose 2 mg/kg), while discorhabdin D (**89**) was found active in vivo against P388 cell lines (TIC132% at 20 mg/kg dose). Thus, the results showed that only discorhabdin D showed modest in vivo activity against P388 cell line: TIC at 20 mg/kg. Kobayashi et al. in 1987 isolated prianosin A (**90**) from *Prianos melanos,* an Okinawan sponge. Structurally prianosin A is a non-protonated form of discorhabdin A. Other prianosins B–D (**91–93**) were reported by Cheng et al. in 1988. Cytotoxicity screening of prianosins A–D (**91–93**) against Ll210, L5178Y cell lines and results showed that only prianosin D (**93**), induced Ca^{2+} release from sarcoplasmic reticulum with a potency 10 times that of caffeine.

2.2.7 POLYCYCLIC AROMATIC ALKALOIDS: ACRIDINE ALKALOIDS

During the last few years, polycyclic aromatic alkaloid obtained from sponges and ascidians, containing a tetracyclic moiety in common, includes the acridine ring system. Amphimedine was the first described compound of this series and has been isolated from *Amphimedon* sp. from a gum sponge. Amphimedine showed in vitro activity against P388 cells with ED_{50} value of 0.4 μg/mL but proved inactive in vivo (Schmitz et al., 1983).

Dercitin (**94**), obtained from various species of *Dercitus*, a deepwater sponge, which was found active against P388 in vitro with an IC_{50} value of 0.54 μg/mL as well as in vivo with TIC 170 at 5 mg/kg and against human cancer cell lines HCT-8, A-549, and T47D in vitro with an IC_{50} value of 1.0 μg/mL. Mechanism of action studies revealed that dercitin disrupts the DNA, RNA, and protein synthesis in the P388 system by binding to DNA and inhibiting nucleic acid synthesis. It is an effective inhibitor of DNA Nick translation at concentrations that disrupt the superhelical density of DNA. It relaxes covalently closed supercoiled ΦX174DNA, indicating intercalation as the mode of binding (Burres et al., 1989). Dercitin was slightly active against B16 tumors in mice in vivo (TIC125 at 1.25 mg/kg). In addition, dercitin is reported to possess immunosuppressive and antiviral activity. The remaining members of dercitin family, namely nordercitin (**95**), dercitamine (**96**), dercitamide (**97**), and cyclodercitin (**98**) have been isolated from two species of family Pachastrellidae, a deepwater sponge (Gunawardana et al., 1989; see Gunawardana et al., 1992). These compounds (nordercitin, dercitamine, dercitamide, and cyclodercitin) showed cytotoxic activity against P388 cells with IC_{50} (μM) 4.79, 26.7, 12.0, and 1.9, respectively, in addition to immunosuppressive activity.

Cyclodercitin (**98**) easily undergoes oxidation on exposure to air to give cyclodercitin (Δ^{13}) (**99**), which is also cytotoxic. Cytotoxic motuporamines A–C (**100–102**) are the first example of macrocyclic alkaloids reported from the *Xestospongia exigua,* a marine sponge (Williams et al., 1998). *X. exigua* are extracted by bioassay-guided fractionation resulted in isolation of mixture of motuporamines A (**100**), B (**101**), and C (**102**) along with known members of 3-alkyl piperidine alkaloidal series xestospongin/araguspongine and petrosin. The motuporamines having spermidine-like substructure represent a new class of cytotoxic alkaloids derived from sponge which are biogenetically formed of basic building blocks, that is, ammonia, acrolein, and a long-chain dialdehyde involving a pathway of 3-alkylpiperidine alkaloids isolated from marine sponges in the order Haplosclerida. The underivatized mixture of motuporamines demonstrated modes of cytotoxicity against a panel of human solid tumor cancer cell lines in vitro with an IC_{50} value of 0.6 mg/mL (Baldwin and Whitehead., 1992; Andersen et al., 1996). Thorectandramine, a novel quaternary hexacyclic alkaloid, has been isolated from genus *Thorectandra* from a Palauan sponge (Charan et al., 2002). The compound showed in vitro cytotoxicity against MALME-3M (melanoma), OVCAR-3 (ovarian), MCF-7 (breast), and A549 (non-small lung cell cancer) four human tumor cell lines (Charan et al., 2002).

Plakinidines are acridine alkaloids with slight variation in the acridine moiety from the Fiji sponge and a *Plakortis* sp. assayed using an antiparasite bioassay, which led to the isolation of plakinidines A (**103**) and B (**104**) (Inman et al., 1990). Subsequently, plakinidine A was reported to inhibit reverse transcriptase activity at 1 μg/mL. In the same year West et al. (1990) described the isolation of plakinidines A (**103**), in addition to plakinidines B (**104**) and C (**105**) from the same source and reported cytotoxicity against L1210 cells with IC_{50} values of 0.7, 0.1, and 0.3 μg/mL respectively.

2.2.8 CYTOTOXIC GUANIDINES ALKALOIDS

Ptilomycalin A (**106**), a novel guanidine polycyclic alkaloid, obtained from the Caribbean sponge from *Ptilocaulis spiculifer* (Kashman et al., 1989) and *Hemimycale* sp. from a Red Sea sponge, which showed toxic effects on P388 cells (IC_{50}: 0.1 μg/mL) as well as antifungal activity against *C. albicans* and antiviral activity against herpes simplex virus (HSV) at 0.2 μg/mL.

Guzii et al. (2010) reported a novel polycyclic guanidine alkaloid monanchocidin (**107**) from marine sponge *Monanhora pulchra* that induced cell death in human leukemia THP-1, human cervix epitheloid carcinoma HeLa, and mouse epidermal JB6C141 cells with IC_{50} value of (μM) 5.1, 11.8, and 12.3, respectively. Monanchocidin also induces 60% of early apoptosis in THP-1 cells at 3.0 μM. Urupocidins A and B, bisguanidine alkaloids with an unprecedented skeleton derived from polyketide precursors and having N-alkyl-N-hydroxylguanidine moiety, were obtained from the same sponge, that is, *M. pulchra* by Makarieva et al. (2014) and urupocidin A showed the increase in the production of nitric oxide in murine macrophages through inducing inducible nitric oxide synthase expression. Recently, eight new rare guanidine alkaloids, namely monanchocidin A (**108**), monanchocidin B (**109**), monanchomycalin C (**110**), ptilomycalin A (**106**), monanchomycalin B (**111**), normonanchocidin D (**112**), urupocidin A (**113**), and pulchranin A (**114**) have been isolated from *M. pulchra.* All of these constituents showed cytotoxic properties and are able to prevent epidermal growth factor-induced neoplastic transformation of JB6 P+ Cl4 1 cells in vitro. Moreover, the current study suggests that these marine guanidine alkaloids hold potential to eliminate human cancer cells and prevent cancer cell formation and spreading (Dyshlovoy et al., 2016).

2.2.9 BROMINE CONTAINING ALKALOIDS

Ma'edamines A–B (**115–116**) are the bromotyrosine alkaloids, possessing unique 2(1H) pyrazinone moiety sandwich between two bromotyrosine units and were extracted from *Suberea* sp. from the Okinawan marine sponge. Biogenetically, ma'edamines A and B may be originated by 11, 12-dehydro form of aplysamine-2 or purpuramine H through formation of a six-membered ring and dehydroxylation. Cytotoxic screening of ma'edamines A (**115**) and B (**116**) showed cytotoxicity against L1210 murine leukemia cells (IC_{50}: 4.3 and 3.9 mg/mL, respectively), and KB epidermoid carcinoma cells (IC_{50}: 5.2 and 4.5 mg/mL, respectively) in vitro. Furthermore, compound (**115**) exhibited in vitro inhibitory activity against c-erbB-2 kinase (IC_{50}: 6.7 mg/mL), whereas compound (**116**) proved to be inactive (IC_{50} > 10 mg/mL) (Hirano et al., 2000b).

Matemone (**117**), a bromine-containing oxindole alkaloid along with known 6-bromoindole-3-carbaldehyde was isolated from *Iotrochota purpurea* sponge collected from the Indian Ocean, exhibited mild cytotoxicity against growth of three cell lines: pancreatic cancer MIA PaCa-2 cell line, lung cancer NSCLC-N6 L16 strain18, and prostate cancer DU145 cell line with IC50 (mg/mL) 24, 30, and 27 respectively (Carletti et al., 2000).

A bromopyrrole longamide (**118**) was obtained originally from *Agelas longissima* from a Caribbean sponge and later was also isolated from Japanese marine sponge from *Homaxinella* sp. (Umeyama et al., 1998). The compound showed cytotoxicity against lymphocytic leukemia P388 cells, in addition to antibacterial activity (MIC 60 mg/mL). Longamide B methyl ester in racemic form was isolated from isolated from as *Homaxinella* sp. and showed weak in vitro cytotoxic activity against lymphocytic leukemia P388 cells (30 mg/mL) (Umeyama et al., 1998). The corresponding longamide B (**119**) acid in racemic form has been isolated from the *Agelas dispar* from the Caribbean marine sponge showed modest antibiotic activity against several strains of Gram-positive bacteria (MIC 50 mg/mL). Hanishin (**120**), the ethyl ester of longamide B has been isolated from highly polymorphic extracts of *Acanthella carteri* sponge and showed cytotoxicity toward human non-small lung carcinoma NSCLC-N6 cells (9.7 mg/mL) (Mancini et al., 1997).

2.2.10 CYTOTOXIC PYRIMIDINE ALKALOIDS

Variolins A–D (**121–124**) is a group of heterocyclic alkaloidal compounds obtained from *Kirkpatrickia variolosa,* an Antarctic marine sponge, and are composed of tricyclic skeleton, which has no precedents in either terrestrial or marine natural products, a pyrido[3′, 2′:4, 5]pyrrolo[1,2-*c*] pyrimidine, substituted at position 5. Biological screening of these compounds exhibited interesting antiviral and antitumor activity against murine leukemia P388 cells (Perry et al., 1994; Trimurtulu et al., 1994). Variolin B showed potent cytotoxic and cytostatic effects against various human leukemia K-562, U-937, MOLT-4 cell lines and Jurkatt, human ovarian carcinoma OVCAR-3, SKOV-3 cell lines, and human intestinal carcinoma LoVo cell line. Variolin B was equally effective against LoVo carcinoma and its multidrug resistant variant LoVo/Dx overexpressing Pgp. The concentration of variolin B in the nM range for 1 h cause G1 cell arrest and a decrease in progression rate of S-phase cells to G2, while as concentrations in mM range for a little time induced blockade in G2 phase. Studies revealed that variolin B is a strong activator of apoptosis assessed by biochemical and morphological methods (Erba et al., 2002).

2.2.11 ALKALOIDS DERIVED FROM SPONGES IN CLINICAL/PRECLINICAL TRIAL

Sponges have proven to be an interesting source of a large array of bioactive alkaloids, and few of them reported in the literature can potentially compete with anticancer alkaloids isolated from terrestrial plants, and are in clinical or preclinical trials. Soni et al. (2000) discovered the new potential use of fascaplysin, a marine sponge-derived natural product. While investigating for inhibitors of cyclin-dependent protein kinases and key enzymes involved in the mammalian cell cycle, they observed that fascaplysin selectively inhibited Cdk4 kinase in vitro with an IC_{50} 0.35 μM. Molecular modeling studies showed that fascaplysin binds to the ATP binding pocket of Cdk4 by interacting through a bidentate hydrogen bond/acceptor pair (Soni et al., 2000). The fact that fascaplysin caused G1 arrest not only in normal human fibroblasts but also in both human colon carcinoma and osteogenic sarcoma cell lines make this marine chemical an interesting candidate for the further study of cellular processes regulated by Cdk4 kinase in mammalian cells.

Manzamine is another series of sponge which was studied by Zhou et al. (2000) in novel antiangiogenesis, while Hirano et al. (2000b) showed that ma'edamine A had inhibitory activity against the c-erbB-2 kinase in vitro. All these compounds were tested in cytotoxicity assays that most commonly consisted of panels of either human or murine tumor cell lines. In a few reports, cytotoxicity studies were very extensive and included the National Cancer Institute 60-tumor cell line screen (Calcabrini et al., 2017). These novel compounds exhibited potent cytotoxic activity, defined as an IC_{50} of 4.0 g/mL, and would appear as possible candidates for studying mechanism of action. This would help to determine if the reported cytotoxicity was the result of a pharmacologic rather than a toxic effect on the tumor cell used for the reported investigation.

2.3 CONCLUSION

Marine sponges have been clearly established as a source of novel alkaloids possessing promising anticancer and cytotoxic properties that can be used for selecting hits in various pharmacotherapeutic areas. At least three leads are already in clinical trials or appear to be destined for such testing. These attained leads and the promise of uncovering new biochemical techniques that may be crucial for studying disease mechanisms provide a continuing impetus for further exploration of marine sponges as a potential source of anticancer drugs.

KEYWORDS

- **sponge**
- **marine environment**
- **alkaloids**
- **anticancer**
- **secondary metabolites**

REFERENCES

Ahond, A.; Zurita, M. B.; Collin, M.; Fizames, C.; Laboute, P.; Lavelle, F.; Laurent, D.; Poupat, C.; Pusset, J.; Pusset, M.; Thoison, O.; Potier, P. Girolline, a New Antitumoral Compound Extracted from the Sponge, *Pseudaxinyssa cantharella* sp. (Axinellidae). C. *R. Acad. Sci. Paris.* **1988,** *307,* 145–148.

Akee, R. K.; Carroll, T. R.; Yoshida, W. Y.; Scheuer, P. J.; Stout, T. J.; Clardy, J. Two Imidazole Alkaloids from a Sponge. *J. Org. Chem.* **1990,** *55*(6), 1944–1946.

Aoki, S.; Wei, H.; Matsui, K.; Rachmat, R.; Kobayashia, M. *Bioorg. Med. Chem.* **2003,** *11,* 1969.

Amin, A. R.; Kucuk, O.; Khuri, F. R.; Shin, D. M. Perspectives for Cancer Prevention with Natural Compounds. *J. Clin. Oncol.* **2009,** *27,* 2712–2725.

Andersen, R. J.; Van Soest, R. W. M.; Kong, F. 3-Alkylpiperidine Alkaloids Isolated from Marine Sponges in the Order Haplosclerida. In *Alkaloids, Chemical and Biological Perspectives;* Pelletier, S. W., Ed.; Pergamon: New York, 1996; pp 301–355.

Bartik, K.; Braekman, J. C.; Daloze, D.; Stoller, C.; Huysecom, J.; Vandevyver, G.; Ottinger, R. Topsentins, New Toxic Bis-Indole Alkaloids from the Marine Sponge *Topsentia genitrix. Can. J. Chem.* **1987,** *65,* 2118–2121.

Braekman, J. C.; Daloze, D.; Stoller, C. Synthesis of Topsentin-A, a Bisindole Alkaloid of the Marine Sponge *Topsentia genetrix. Bull. Soc. Chim. Belg.* **1987,** *96*(10), 809–812.

Burres, N. S.; Sazesh, S.; Gunawardana, G. P.; Clement, J. J. Antitumor Activity and Nucleicacid Binding Properties of Dercitin, a New Acridine Alkaloid Isolated from a Marine *Dercitus* species Sponge. *Cancer Res.* **1989,** *49*(19), 5267–5274.

Baldwin, J. E.; Whitehead, R. C. On the Biosynthesis of Manzamines. *Tetrahedron Lett.* **1992,** *33,* 2059–2062.

Carmely, S.; Dan, M.; Kashman, Y. 2-Arnino Imidazole Alkaloids from the Marine Sponge *Leucetta chagosensis*. *Tetrahedron* **1989,** *45*(7), 2193–2200.

Ciminiello, P.; Fattorusso, E.; Mangoni, A.; Benedetto, D. B.; Pavone, V. Structure of Clathridine Zn-Complex, a Metabolite of the Marine Sponge *Clathrina clathrus*. *Tetrahedron* **1990,** *46,* 4387–4392.

Calcul, L.; Longeon, A.; Mourabit, A. A.; Guyot, M.; Bourguet-Kondracki, M.-L. Novel Alkaloids of the Aaptamine Class from an Indonesian Marine Sponge of the Genus *Xestospongia*. *Tetrahedron* **2003,** *59,* 6539–6544.

Cheng, J.; Ohizumi, Y.; Walchli, M. R.; Nakamura, H.; Hirata, Y.; Sasaki, T.; Kobayashi, J. Prianosins B, C, and D, Novel Sulfur-Containing Alkaloids with Potent Antineoplastic Activity from the Okinawan Marine Sponge *Prianos melanos*. *J. Org. Chem.* 1**988,** *53*(19), 4621–4624.

Charan, R. D.; McKee, T. C.; Gustafson, K. R.; Pannell, L. K.; Boyd, M. R. Thorectandramine, a Novelβ-Carboline Alkaloid from the Marine Sponge *Thorectandra* sp. *Tetrahedron Lett.* **2002,** *43,* 5201–5204.

Carletti, I.; Banaigs, B.; Amade, P. Matemone, a New Bioactive Bromine-Containing Oxindole Alkaloid from the Indian Ocean Sponge *Iotrochota purpurea*. *J. Nat. Prod.* **2000,** *63,* 981–983.

Capon, R. J.; Peng, C.; Dooms, C. Trachycladindloes A-G: Cytotoxic Heterocycles from an Australian Sponge *Trachycladus laevispirulifer*. *Org. Biomol. Chem.* **2008,** *6,* 2765–2771.

Calcabrini, C.; Catanzaro, E.; Bishayee, A.; Turrini, E.; Fimognari, C. Marine Sponge Natural Products with Anticancer Potential: An Updated Review. *Mar. Drugs.* **2017,** *15,* 310.

De Guzman, F. S.; Carte, B.; Troupe, N.; Faulkner, D. J.; Harper, M. K.; Concepcion, G. P.; Mangalindan, G. C.; Matsumoto, S. S.; Barrows, L. R.; Ireland, C. M. Neoamphimedine: A New Pyridoacridine Topoisomerase II Inhibitor Which Catenates DNA. *J. Org. Chem.* **1999,** *64,* 1400–1402.

Ding, Q.; Chichak, K.; Lown, J. W. Pyrroloquinoline and Pyridoacridine Alkaloids from Marine Sources. *Curr. Med. Chem.* **1999,** *6,* 1–27.

Dyshlovoy, S. A.; Tabakmakher, K. M.; Hauschild, J. Shchekaleva, R. K.; Otte, K.; Guzii, A. G.; Makarieva, T. N.; Kudryashova, E. K.; Fedorov, S. N.; Shubina, L. K.; Bokemeyer, C.; Honecker, F.; Stonik, V. A.; Amsberg, G. V. Guanidine Alkaloids from the Marine Sponge *Monanchora pulchra* Show Cytotoxic Properties and Prevent EGF-Induced Neoplastic Transformation in Vitro. *Mar. Drugs.* **2016,** *14,* 133.

Erba, E.; Tognon, G.; Jimeno, J.; Faircloth, G. T.; D'lncalci. M. Novel Antitumor Agents: Marine Sponge Alkaloids, Their Synthetic Analogs and Derivatives. *Eur. J. Cancer* **2002,** *38*(7), S33.

Fusetani, N.; Yasumuro, K.; Matsunaga, S.; Hirota, H. Haliclamines A and B, Cytotoxicmacrocyclic Alkaloids from a Sponge of the Genus *Haliclona. Tetrahedron Lett.* **1989,** *30*(49), 6891–6894.

Fuente, J. A.; Martin, M. J.; Blanco, M. M.; Pascual-Alfonso, E.; Avendano, C.; Menendez, J. C. *Bioorg. Med. Chem.* **2001,** *9,* 1807.

Fedoreev, S. A.; Prokofeva, N. G.; Denisenko, V. A.; Rebachuk, N. M. Cytotoxic Activity of Aaptamines Derived from *Suberitidae* Sponges. *Khim. Farm. Zh.* **1988,** *22*(8), 943–946.

Guzman, E. A.; Johnson, J. D.; Linley, P. A.; Gunasekera, S. E.; Wright, A. E. A Novel Activity from an Old Compound: Manzamine a Reduces the Metastatic Potential of AsPC-1 Pancreatic Cancer Cells and Sensitizes them to TRAIL-Induced Apoptosis. *Invest. New Drugs* **2011,** *29,* 777–785.

Gunawardana, G. P.; Kohmoto, S.; Burres, N. S. New Cytotoxic Acridine Alkaloids from Two Deep Water Marine Sponges of the Family Pachastrellidae. *Tetrahedron Lett.* **1989,** *30*(33), 4359–4362.

Gunawardana, G. P.; Koehn, F. E.; Lee, A. Y.; Clardy, J.; He, H.; Faulkner, D. J. Pyridoacridine Alkaloids from Deep-Water Marine Sponges of the Family Pachastrellidae: Structure Revision of Dercitin and Related Compounds and Correlation with the Kuanoiamines. *J. Org. Chem.* **1992,** *57,* 1523–1526.

Guzii, A. G.; Makarieva, T. N.; Denisenko, V. A.; Dmitrenok, P. S.; Kuzmich, A. S.; Dyshlovoy, S. A.; Krasokhin, V. B.; Stonik, V. A. Monanchocidin: A New Apoptosis-Including Polycyclic Alkaloid from the Marine Sponge *Monanchora pulchra. Organic Lett.* **2010,** *12*(19), 4292–4295.

Hörmann, A.; Chaudhuri, B.; Fretz, H. DNA Binding Properties of the Marine Sponge Pigment Fascaplysin. *Bioorg. Med. Chem.* **2001,** *9,* 917–921.

Hamilton, G. Cytotoxic Effects of Fascaplysin Against Small Cell Lung Cancer Cell Lines. *Mar. Drugs* **2014,** *12,* 1377–1389.

Hu, J.-F.; Fan, H.; Xiong, J.; Wu, S.-B. Discorhabdins and Pyrroloiminoquinone-Related Alkaloids. *Chem. Rev.* **2011,** *111*(9), 5465–5491.

Hirano, K.; Kubota, T.; Tsuda, M.; Mikami, Y.; Kobayashi, J. Pyrinodemins B.-D. Potent Cytotoxic Bis-Pyridine Alkaloids from Marine Sponge *Amphimedon* sp. *Chem. Pharm. Bull.* **2000a,** *48,* 974–977.

Hirano, K.; Kubota, T.; Tsuda, M.; Watanabe, K.; Fromont, J.; Kobayashi, J. Ma'edamines A and B, Cytotoxic Bromotyrosine Alkaloids with a Unique 2 (1H) Pyrazinone Ring from Sponge *Suberea* sp. *Tetrahedron* **2000b,** *56,* 8107–8110.

Hassan, W. H. B.; Al-Taweel, A. M.; Proksch, P. Two New Imidazole Alkaloids from *Leucetta chagosensis* Sponge. *Saudi J. Pharm. Chem.* **2009,** *17,* 295–289.

Ichiba, T.; Sakai, R.; Kohmoto, S.; Saucy, G.; Higa, T. New Manzamine Alkaloids from a Sponge of the Genus *Xestospongia*. *Tetrahedron Lett.* **1988,** *29*(25), 3083–3086.

Inman, W. D.; O'Neill-Johnson, M.; Crews, P. Novel Marine Sponge Alkaloids: Plakinidine A and B, Anthelmintic Active Alkaloids from a *Plakortis* Sponge. *J. Am. Chem. Soc.* **1990,** *112*(1), 1–4.

Jimenez, C.; Quinoa, E.; Adamczeski, M.; Hunter, L. M.; Crews, P. Tryptophan-Derived Pigments and Accompanying Sesterterpenes from *Fascaplysinopis reticulata. J. Org. Chem.* **1991a,** *56,* 3403–3410.

Jimenez, C.; Quinoa, E.; Crews, P. Novel Marine Sponge Alkaloids 3. ß-Carbolinium Salts from *Fascaplysinopsis reticulate. Tetrahedron Lett.* **1991b,** *32,* 1843–1846.

Kashman, Y.; Koren-Goldshlager, G.; Gravalos, M. D.; Schleyer, M. Halitulin, a New Cytotoxic Alkaloid from the Marine Sponge *Haliclona tulearensis*. *Tetrahedron Lett.* **1999,** *40,* 997–1000.

Kawasaki, I.; Yamashita, M.; Ohta, S. Total Synthesis of Nortopsentins A-D. Marine Alkaloids. *Chem. Pharm. Bull.*, **1996,** *44,* 1831–1839.

Kohmoto, S.; Kashman, Y.; McConnell, O. J.; Rinehart, K. L.; Wright, A.; Koehn, F.; Dragmacidin, a New Cytotoxic Bis (Indole) Alkaloid from a Deep Water Marine Sponge, *Dragmacidon* sp. *J. Org. Chem.* **1988,** *53*(13), 3116–3118.

Kirsch, G.; König, G. M.; Wright, A. D.; Kaminsky, R. A New Bioactive Sesterterpene and Antiplasmodial Alkaloids from the Marine Sponge *Hyrtios* cf. *erecta*. *J. Nat. Prod.* **2000,** *63,* 825–829.

Kitamura, A.; Tanaka, J.; Ohtani, I. I.; Higa, T. Echinoclathrines A–C: A New Class of Pyridine Alkaloids from an Okinawan Sponge, *Echinoclathria* sp. *Tetrahedron* **1999,** *55,* 2487–2492.

Kobayashi, J.; Cheng, J. F.; Ishibashi, M.; Nakamura, H.; Ohizumi, Y. I.; Hirata, Y.; Sasaki, T.; Lu, H.; Clardy, J.; Prianosin, A. A Novel Antileukemic Alkaloid from the Okinawan Marine Sponge *Prianosmelanos. Tetrahedron Lett.* **1987,** *28*(43), 4939–4942.

Kobayashi, J.; Murayama, T.; Ohizumi, Y.; Sasaki, T.; Ohta, T.; Nozoe, S. Theonelladins A-D, Novel Antineoplastic Pyridine Alkaloids from the Okinawan Marine Sponge *Theonella swinhoei. Tetrahedron Lett.* **1989,** *30*(36), 4833–4836.

Liu, C.; Tang, X.; Li, P.; Li, G. Suberitine A–D, Four New Cytotoxic Dimeric Aaptamine Alkaloids from the Marine Sponge *Aaptos suberitoides. Org. Lett.* **2012,** *14*(8), 1994–1997

Marshalla, K. M.; Matsumotoa, S. S.; Holdenb, J. A.; Concepciond, G. P.; Tasdemirc, D.; Irelandc, C. M.; Barrows, L. R. The Anti-Neoplastic and Novel Topoisomerase II-Mediated Cytotoxicity of Neoamphimedine, a Marine Pyridoacridine. *Biochem. Pharmacol.* **2003,** *66,* 447–458.

Makarieva, T. N.; Ogurtsova, E. K.; Denisenko, V. A.; Dmitrenok, P. S.; Guzii, T. A. G.; Pislyagin, E. A.; Eskov, A. A.; Kozhemyako, D. L.; Wang, A. Y.-M.; Stonik, V. A. Urupocidin A: A New, Including iNOS Expression Bicyclic Guanidine Alkaloid from the Marine Sponge *Monanchora pulchra. Organ. Lett.* **2014,** *16*(16), 4292–4295.

Mancini, I.; Guella, G.; Amade, P.; Roussakis, C.; Pietra, F. Hanishin, a Semiracemic, Bioactive C_9 Alkaloid of the Axinellid Sponge *Acanthella carteri* from the Hanish Islands. *Tetrahedron Lett.* **1997,** *38,* 6271.

McKee, T. C.; Ireland, C. M. Cytotoxic and Antimicrobial Alkaloids from the Fijian Sponge *Xestospongia caycedo. J. Nat. Prod.* **1987,** *50*(4), 754–756.

Molinski, T. F. *Chem. Rev*. **1993,** *93,* 1825.

Molinski, T. F.; Dalisay, D. S.; Lievens, S. L.; Saludes, J. P. Drug Development From Marine Natural Products. *Nat. Rev.* **2009,** *8,* 69–83.

Morris, S.; Andersen, R. J. Brominated Bis (Indole) Alkaloids from the Marine Sponge *Hexadella* sp. *Tetrahedron* **1989,** *46*(3), 715–720.

Nakamura, H.; Kobayashi, J.; Ohizumi, Y.; Hirata, Y. Aaptamines, Novel Benzo[De][1,6] Naphthyridines from the Okinawan Marine Sponge *Aaptos aaptos. Chem. Soc. Perkin Trans. 1.* **1987,** *1,* 173–176.

Newman, D. J.; Cragg, G. M. Marine Natural Products and Related Compounds in Clinical and Advanced Preclinical Trials. *J. Nat. Prod.* **2004,** *67,* 1216–1238.

Newman, D. J.; Cragg, G. M. Natural Products as Sources of New Drugs Over the Last 25 Years. *J. Nat. Prod.* **2007**, *70*, 461–477.

Perry, N. B.; Blunt, J. W.; McCombs, J. D.; Munro, M. H. G. Discorhabdin C, a Highly Cytotoxic Pigment from a Sponge of the Genus *Latrunculia. J. Org. Chem.* **1986,** *51*(26), 5476–5478.

Perry, N. B.; Blunt, J. W.; Munro, M. H. G. Cytotoxic Pigments from New Zealand Sponges of the Genus *Latrunculia:* Discorhabdins A, B, and C. *Tetrahedron* **1988a,** *44*(6), 1727–1734.

Perry, N. B.; Blunt, J. W.; Munro, M. H. G.; Higa, T.; Sakai, R. Discorhabdin D, an Antitumor Alkaloid from the Sponges *Latrunculia brevis* and *Piranos* sp. *J. Org. Chem.* **1988b,** *53*(17), 4127–4128.

Perry, N. B.; Ettouati, L.; Litaudon, M.; Blunt, J. W.; Munro, M. H. G.; Parkin, S.; Hope, H. Antiviral and Antitumor Agents from a New Zealand Sponge, *Mycale* sp. *Tetrahedron* **1994,** *50,* 3987–4000.

Plubrukarn, A.; Smith, D. W.; Cramer, R. E.; Davidson, B. S. (2E,9E)-Pyronaamidine 9-(N-Methylimine), a New Imidazole Alkaloid from the Northern Mariana Islands Sponge *Leucetta* sp. cf. *chagosensis*. *J. Nat. Prod.* **1997,** *60*, 712–715.

Quinoa, E.; Crews, P. Niphatynes, Methoxylamine Pyridines from the Marine Sponge *Niphates* sp. *Tetrahedron Lett.* **1987,** *28*(22), 2467–2468.

Radwan, M.; Hanora, A.; Khalifa, S.; Abou-El-Ela, S. H. Manzamines: A Potential for Novel Cures. *Cell Cycle* **2012,** *11,* 1765–1772.

Ralifo, P.; Tenney, K.; Valeriote, F. A.; Crews. P. A Distinctive Structural Twist in the Aminoimidazole Alkaloids from a Calcareous Marine Sponge: Isolation and Characterization of Leucosolenamines A and B. *J. Nat. Prod.* **2007,** *70,* 33–38.

Roll, D. M.; Ireland, C. M.; Lu, H. S. M.; Clardy, J. Fascaplysin, an Unusual Antimicrobial Pigment from the Marine Sponge *Fascaplysinopsis* sp. *J. Org. Chem.* **1988,** *53*(14), 3276–3278.

Sakemi, S.; Sun, H. H. Biological Activities of Nortopsentin A-C (1–3), IC50 Againist P388 (pg/mL): 1, 7.6; 2, 7.8; 3, 1.7. *J. Org. Chem.* **1991,** *56,* 4304–4307.

Sakai, R.; Higa, T.; Jefford, C. W.; Bernardinelli, G. Manzamine A, a Novel Antitumor Alkaloid from a Sponge. *J. Am. Chem. Soc.* **1986,** *108*(20), 6404–6405.

Sakai, R.; Kohmoto, S.; Higa, T.; Jefford, C. W.; Bernardinelli, G. Manzarnines Band C, Two Novel Alkaloids from the Sponge *Haliclona* sp. *Tetrahedron Lett.* **1987,** *28*(45), 5493–5496.

Segraves, N. L.; Lopez, S.; Johnson, T. A.; Said, S. A.; Fu, X.; Schmitz, F. J.; Pietraszkiewicz, H.; Valeriote, F. A.; Crews, P. Structures and Cytotoxicities of Fascaplysin and Related Alkaloids from Two Marinephyla—*Fascaplysinopsis* Sponges and Didemnum Tunicates. *Tetrahedron Lett.* **2003,** *44,* 3471–3475.

Schmidt, E. W.; Faulkner, D. J. Palauolol, a New Anti-Inflammatory Sesterterpene from the Sponge *Fascaplysinopsis* sp. from Palau. *Tetrahedron Lett.* **1996,** *37,* 3951–3954.
Schmitz, F. J.; Hollenbeak, K. H.; Campbell, D. C. Marine Natural Products: Halitoxin, Toxic Complex of Several Marine Sponges of the Genus *Haliclona. J. Org. Chem.* **1978,** *43,* 3916–3922.
Schmitz, F. J.; Agarwal, S. K.; Gunasekera, S. P. Amphimedine, New Aromatic Alkaloid from Pacific Sponge, *Amphimedon* sp. Carbon Connectivity Determination from Natural Abundance Carbon-13-Carbon-13 Coupling Constants. *J. Am. Chem. Soc.* **1983,** *105,* 4835–4836.
Shen, Y.-C.; Lin, T.-T.; Sheu, J.-H.; Duh, C.-Y. Structures and Cytotoxicity Relationship of Isoaaptamine and Aaptamine Derivatives. *J. Nat. Prod.* **1999,** *62,* 1264–1247.
Shubina, L. K.; Makarieva, T. N.; Dyshlovoy, S. A.; Fedorov, S. N.; Dmitrenok, P. S.; Stonik, V. A. Three New Aaptamines from the Marine Sponge *Aaptos* sp. and Their Proapoptotic Properties. *Nat. Prod. Res.* **2010,** *5,* 1881–1884.
Sun, H. H.; Sakemi, S.; Burres, N.; McCarthy, P. Isobatzellines A, B, C, and D. Cytotoxic and Antifungal Pyrroloquinoline Alkaloids from the Marine Sponge *Batzella* sp. *J. Am. Chem. Soc.* **1990,** *55,* 4964–4966.
Sun, H. H.; Sakemi, S.; Gunasekera, S.; Kashman, Y.; Lui, M.; Burres, N.; McCarthy, P. Bis-Indole Imidazole Compounds Which are Useful Anticancer and Antimicrobial Agents. U. S. Patent 4,970,226, *Chem. Abstr.* **1991,** *115,* 35701z.
Soni, R.; Muller, L.; Furet, P.; Schoepfer, J.; Stephan, C.; Zumstenin-Mecker, S.; Fretz, H.; Chaudhuri, B. Inhibition of Cyclin-Dependent Kinase 4 (cdk4) by Fascaplysin, a Marine Natural Product. *Biochem. Biophys. Res. Coummun.* **2000,** *275*(3), 877–884.
Tsujii, S.; Rinehart, K. L. Topsentin, Bromotopsentin, and Dihydrodeoxytopsentin: New Antiviral and Antitumor Bis (Indolyl) Imidazoles from Caribbean Deep Sea Sponges of the Family Halichondriidae. Structural and Synthetic Studies. *J. Org. Chem.* **1988,** *53*(23), 5446–5453.
Torres, Y. R.; Berlinck, R. G. S.; Nascimento, G. G. F.; Fortier, S. C.; Pessoa, C.; de Moraes, M. O. Antibacterial Activity Against Resistant Bacteria and Cytotoxicity of Four Alkaloid Toxins Isolated from the Marine Sponge *Arenosclera brasiliensis. Toxicon* **2002,** *40,* 885–891.
Tasdemir, D.; Marshall, K. M.; Mangalindan, G. C.; Concepcion, G. P.; Barrows, L. R.; Harper, M. K.; Ireland, C. M. Deoxyamphimedine, a New Pyridoacridine Alkaloid from Two Tropical *Xestospongia* Sponges. *J. Org. Chem.* **2001,** *66,* 3246–3248.
Trimurtulu, G.; Faulkner, D. J.; Perry, N. B.; Ettouati, L.; Litaudon, M.; Blunt, J. W.; Munro, M. H. G.; Jameson, G. B. Alkaloids from the Antarctic Sponge *Kirkpatrickia varialosa*. Part 2 Variolin-A and *N*(3′)-Methyl Tetrahydrovariolin-B. *Tetrahedron* **1994,** 50, 3993–4000.
Tsukamoto, S.; Kawabata, T.; Kato, H.; Ohta, T.; Rotinsulu, H.; Mangindaan, R. E. P.; Soest, R. W. M. V.; Ukai, K.; Kobayashi, H.; Namikoshi, M. Naamidines H and I, Cytotoxic Imidazole Alkaloids from the Indonesian Marine Sponge *Leucetta chagosensis. J. Nat. Prod.* **2007,** *70,* 1658–1660
Umeyama, A.; Ito, S.; Yuasa, E.; Arihara, S.; Yamada, T. A New Bromopyrrole Alkaloid and the Optical Resolution of the Racemate from the Marine Sponge *Homaxinella* Sp. *J. Nat. Prod.* **1998,** *61,* 1433–1434.
Williams, D. E.; Lassota, P.; Andersen, R. J. Motuporamines A–C, Cytotoxic Alkaloids Isolated from the Marine Sponge *Xestospongia exigua* (Kirkpatrick) *J. Org. Chem.* **1998,** *63,* 4838–4841.

Wright, A. E.; Thompson, W. C. Antitumor Compositions Containing Imidazolylpyrroloazepines (WO 8707274 A2), *Chem. Abstr.* **1987,** *110*(17), 147852c.

West, R. R.; Mayne, C. L.; Ireland, C. M.; Brinen, L. S.; Clardy, J. Plakinidines: Cytotoxicalkaloid Pigments from the Fijian sponge *Plakortis* sp. *Tetrahedron Lett.* **1990,** *31*(23), 3271–3274.

World Health Organization. http://who.int/mediacentre/factsheets/fs297/en/ (accessed July 6, 2017).

Zhou, B.-N.; Slebodnick, C.; Johnson, R. K.; Mattern, M. R.; Kingston, D. G. I. New Cytotoxic Manzamine Alkaloids from a Palaunsponge. *Tetrahedron* **2000,** *56,* 5781–5784.

CHAPTER 3

MARINE ANTIOXIDANTS AND ASSAY METHODS

ONYEKA KINGSLEY NWOSU[1,*] and DAVID OKECHUKWU OKEKE[2]

[1]*National Biosafety Management Agency (NBMA), Abuja, Nigeria, Tel.: +2348065002754*

[2]*Department of Applied Biochemistry, Nnamdi Azikiwe University, Awka, Nigeria*

[*]*Corresponding author. E-mail: nwosuonyeka6@gmail.com*
[*]*ORCID: https://orcid.org/0000-0003-1197-6810*

ABSTRACT

The marine organisms are now an emphasis of natural products drug discovery research because of its relatively unexplored biodiversity compared to terrestrial environment. Research has been developed using many biotechnological tools to harness and to produce new marine essential compounds with the aim of increasing the availability and chemical diversity of marine organisms' essential constituents. Indeed the bioprospecting marine organisms for secondary metabolite production are a promising area in marine biotechnology. Most of these marine organisms are great sources of natural antioxidants and nutritional compounds. This chapter examines the concepts of marine organisms, the antioxidants of the marine organisms (algae and sponges), and determination of antioxidant activities.

3.1 INTRODUCTION

The marine environment is a good source of chemical and biological active compounds. The organisms that occupy the marine environment are said to be potential sources of interesting compounds for uses towards economic development like the food industry, neutraceuticals, pharmaceutical industry, cosmetic industry, and so many other industrially important compounds (Marine Biotechnology, 2003). There are enormous marine-based products within the marine environment which can increasingly promote the exploitation of the vast diversity of the marine life. The marine ecosystem still remains an untapped reservoir of biologically active compounds which have considerable capabilities to provide chemical constituents towards the development of new conventional and ethnopharmacological drugs and as well as supply food ingredients towards the progress of new functional foods and nutraceuticals. However, production of ample amount of persistent quality and inexpensive marine products has been the foremost impediment for marine biotechnologists, notwithstanding the boundless potential of marine organisms (Slevan et al., 2012).

Research has been developed using many biotechnological tools to harness and to produce new marine essential compounds with the aim of increasing the incessant availability and chemical diversity of marine organisms' essential constituents. Certainly, the hunting of marine organisms for the production of secondary metabolite is an auspicious area in marine biotechnology. Most of these marine organisms are the richest sources of natural antioxidants and nutritional compounds (Balakrishan et al., 2014). The antioxidants usually produced by the marine environment include flavonoids, benzoic acid, gallic acid, and cinnamic acid (Al-Saif et al., 2014). Marine environment can thereby be considered as producers of substances that are useful for the treatment of human diseases since antioxidants application serves as an efficient method in avoiding or minimizing or reducing the formation of toxic oxidation products, lipid peroxidation in food products, and maintaining nutritional quality. Among the demerits of the marine environment as benefits to human health is that secondary metabolites from their ecosystem are often produced only in trace amounts in such that large quantity of sources must be collected to be able to attain adequate amounts of the target compound.

3.2 MARINE ORGANISMS

The marine environment contains more than 200,000 described species of invertebrates and algae, however, it is estimated that this number is but a small percentage of the entire number of species that have yet to be discovered and described. Conservatives estimates suggest that marine environment subsurface bacteria could constitute as much as 10% of the total living biomass carbon in the biosphere. However, thousands of chemical compounds have been isolated from a relatively small number of these species that have been studied to date.

Marine plants, animals, and microbes produce compounds that have potential as pharmaceuticals due to the secondary metabolites they contain. The marine organisms became a focus of natural products drug discovery research due to its relatively unexplored biodiversity when compared to terrestrial environment. The thought of marine organisms as the basis of natural products for pharmaceuticals and therapeutics was introduced by the first work of Bergmann in the 1950s (Bergmann and Feeney, 1951) which led to the only two marine-derived pharmaceuticals that are clinically available today; anticancer drug, Ara-C and antiviral drug, Ara-A. Among the vast array of marine organisms with exclusive biological properties, the most studied and characterized are algae (seaweeds) and sponges.

3.2.1 ALGAE

Marine algae are chlorophyll-containing organisms made up of a cell or grouped together in colonies or as organisms with many cells, occasionally interacting together as simple tissues (Lordan et al., 2011). The marine algae, therefore, would be classified as unicellular or multicellular vegetative organisms that do not have true roots or stems and greatly vary in morphology and size up to 70 m long, 3 - 10 μm in length and growing up to 50 cm/day (El Gamal, 2010). Marine algae are a heterogeneous group of plants with long fossil history which can be classified into two main groups according to their size. They are:

i) Macroalgae: They occupy the littoral zone, which included green algae, brown algae, and red algae. They are mainly considered by biologists as the seaweeds. They possess several characteristics that are used to categorize them including the nature of their chlorophyll, the presence, and absence of flagella and their cell wall chemistry.
ii) Microalgae: They are known as phytoplankton and dominate in both benthic and littoral habitats and also throughout the ocean waters. The phytoplankton comprises organisms such as diatoms (bacillariophyta), dinoflagellates (dinophyta), blue-green algae (cyanophyta), yellow-brown and green flagellates (chlorophyta, prasinophyta, prymnesiophyta, chrysophyta, cryptophyta, and rhaphidiophyta). As

photosynthetic organisms, this group plays a key role in the productivity of oceans and constitutes the basis of the marine food chain (Bold and Wyne, 1985).

3.2.1.1 MACROALGAE (SEAWEEDS)

Macroalgae or seaweeds are a source of biologically active phytochemicals, which comprise of fatty acids, polysaccharides, carotenoids, phycobilins, vitamins, sterols, phycocyanins, and tocopherol among others (Lordan et al., 2011). The nutritional and chemical composition of the macroalgae depends on many factors which include species, water temperature, geographical origin, seasonal, environmental, and physiological variations, and processing methods (Mabeau and Fleurence, 1993). The high antioxidant content is one of the major nutritive features of macroalgae. Seaweeds are well known for containing reactive antioxidant molecules such as glutathione (GSH) when fresh, as well as secondary metabolites like carotenoids (ά- and β-carotene, fucoxanthin, astaxanthin), catechins, and tocopherols (Yuan et al., 2005). Among macroalgae, natural antioxidants, terpenoids, phlorotannins, polyphenols, phenolic acids, anthocyanins, hydroxycinnamic acid derivatives, and flavonoids are important (Bandoniene and Murkovic, 2002). Flavonoids have effective antiviral, anti-allergic, and have free radical scavenging abilities and also offer protection against cardiovascular mortality. Table 3.1 shows some algae proven to possess some antioxidants.

TABLE 3.1 Algae Sources of Nutritional Antioxidants

Antioxdants	Specie of algae	References
Vitamin C	*Ulva* sp., *Monostroma undulatum, Undaria pinnatifida, Ascophyllum nodosum, Laminaria digitata, Porphyra umbilicalis, Palmaria palmata, Thalassiosira pseudonana, Chaetoceros muelleri, Gracilaria changgi*	MacArtain et al. (2007), Bocanegra et al. (2009), Brown et al. (1997)
Vitamin E	*Ulva rigida, A. nodosum, Dunaliella tertiolecta, U. pinnatifida, L. digitata, P. umbilicalis, P. palmata*	Taboada et al. (2010), MacArtain et al. (2007), Carballo-Cárdenas et al. (2003)
Carotenoids	*Porphyridium cruentum*	Rebolloso-Fuentes et al. (2000)

TABLE 3.1 *(Continued)*

Antioxdants	Specie of algae	References
α-carotene	*Chlorella pyrenoidosa, Dunaliella salina*	Inbaraj et al. (2006), Hu et al. (2008)
β-carotene	*A. nodosum, C. pyrenoidosa, Chlorella vulgaris, Chlorococcum, D. salina, Fucus serratus, Fucus vesiculosus, G. changgi, Haematococcus pluvialis, L. digitata, Laminaria saccharina, Pelvetia canaliculata, Phormidium* sp., *Porphyra tenera, Synechocystis* sp.	Inbaraj et al. (2006), Cha et al. (2010), Yuan et al. (2002), Hu et al. (2008), Okai et al. (1996), Plaza et al. (2010)
Antheraxan-thin	*D. salina, L. digitata, L. saccharina*	Yokthongwattana et al. (2005)
Lutein	*C. pyrenoidosa, C. vulgaris, Chlorella zofingiensis, Chlorococcum, D. salina, H. pluvialis, Muriellopsis* sp., *Phormidium* sp., *P. tenera, Scenedesmus almeriensis.*	Del Campo et al. (2007), Inbaraj et al. (2006), Cha et al. (2010), Yuan et al. (2002), Hu et al. (2008), Okai et al. (1996), Rodri-guez-meizoso et al. (2008)
Zeaxanthin	*L. saccharina, P. canaliculata, Phormidium* sp., *A. nodosum, C. pyrenoidosa, D. salina, F. serratus, F. vesiculosus, H. pluvialis, Himanthalia elongata, L. digitata, L. saccharina, P. canaliculata, Synechocystis* sp.	Inbaraj et al. (2006), Hu et al. (2008), Plaza et al. (2010), Rodriguez-meizoso et al. (2008)
α-tocopherol	*P. cruentum, Laminaria ochroleuca, Saccorhiza polychides, Himanthalia elongate*	Durmaz et al. (2007), Sánchez-Machado et al. (2002)
γ-tocopherol	*Tetraselmis suecica, P. cruentum*	Carballo-Cárdenas et al. (2003), Durmaz et al. (2007)
Pheophytin a	*C. vulgaris, P. cruentum*	Cha et al. (2010), Rebolloso-Fuentes et al. (2000)
Pheophytin b	*C. vulgaris, P. cruentum*	Cha et al. (2010), Rebolloso-Fuentes et al. (2000)
Polyphenols	*Fucus* sp., *H. pluvialis, Laminaria* sp., *Porphyra* sp., *Spongiochloris spongiosa, Undaria* sp.	Bocanegra et al. (2009), Klejdus et al. (2009), Bocanegra et al. (2009)
Astaxanthin	*C. vulgaris, Chlorococcum* sp.	Mendes et al. (1995), Li and Chen (2001)

Source: Adapted from ref Lordan et al. (2011). https://creativecommons.org/licenses/by/3.0/

3.2.1.2 MICROALGAE

There are over 50,000 different species of microalgae of which only a few have been characterized (Bhakuni and Rawat, 2005). This group of microorganisms is exceptionally diverse and represents a major unexploited resource of valued bioactive compounds and biochemicals such as pigments, antioxidants, fatty acids, and vitamins (Mata et al., 2010). Microalgal production of carotenoids, such as β-carotene and astaxanthin, has been an attractive area of research as they are valuable bioactive ingredients that can present at relatively high concentrations in algal cells. Moreover, larger quantities of carotenoids can be produced when cultivated algae are induced by controlling certain environmental growth conditions. The strains of microalgae that are recently being studied for use as natural producers of commercial carotenoids include *Dunaliella salina, Sarcina maxima, Chlorella protothecoides, Chlorella vulgaris,* and *Haematococcus pluvialis*.

D. salina has been found to be the most appropriate organism for the mass production of β-carotene as it can produce β-carotene in the range of 14% of its dry weight (Metting, 1996). β-carotene has strong antioxidant properties which help to mediate the harmful effects of free radicals implicated in numerous life-threatening diseases, including many forms of coronary heart disease, premature aging, cancer, and arthritis. The antioxidant qualities of β-carotene can also assist the body in suppressing the effects of premature aging caused by ultraviolet (UV) rays (Dembitsky and Maoka, 2007). Momentous amounts of xanthophylls, especially zeaxanthin, which possesses distinctive biological properties with potential for disease prevention can be accumulated by *D. salina* (Yokthongwattana et al., 2005). β-carotene derived from microalgae is more biologically active than synthetically produced β-carotene and can be marked as a "natural" food additive (Rasmussen and Morrissey, 2007). Natural β-carotene also contains numerous carotenoids and essential nutrients that are not present in the synthetic form and can be consumed in greater quantities as the body tissues regulate its use (Olson and Krinsky, 1995).

Carotenoids and chlorophylls are also antioxidants that can be produced in both closed and open-culture systems by another unicellular alga known as "*Haematococcus*" (Rasmussen and Morrissey, 2007). *H. pluvialis* has the capacity to accumulate large quantities (1.5–3% of dry weight) of the high-value carotenoid, astaxanthin. *H. pluvialis* has been considered as a dietary supplement in the United States and it has also been approved in several European countries for human consumption (Mata et al., 2010). With up to 10 times antioxidant activity stronger than other carotenoids, astaxanthin provides defensive activity against inflammation, cancer, and UV light. The health benefits of astaxanthin alongside with its strong coloring characteristics make it a prospective ingredient for use in the cosmetics, nutraceutical, and food and feed industries.

Antioxidants vitamins A, C, E, biotin, and folic acid are also found to be in high concentrations in many microalgae and are largely rich in chlorophylls (Spolaore et al., 2006). Microalgae are rich sources of nutritious and biologically active compounds, however, not only is it their huge variety that marks these microorganisms fascinating but also the likelihood of growing them in diverse conditions and using them as natural reactors, results in an enhancement of certain bioactive compounds. Though, prior to this, the algal material must be analyzed for the presence of toxic compounds.

3.2.2 SPONGES

Sponges are among the first classes of marine invertebrates to be studied by natural products chemists. Sponges are multicellular, undifferentiated organisms equipped with an adept water-filtration system. Although technically considered animals, physiologically sponges are among the simplest metazoans. Possessing no differentiated tissue to form digestive, nervous, and circulatory systems, they are composed primarily of a porous network of channels and chambers through which water moves. Following phagocytosis through apertures at the inhalant surface (ostia), food particles are filtered through progressively smaller sieve-like channels into the mesohyl for metabolism. The sieves are designed because indiscrete intake of water and particles by non-selective filter feeders result in ingestion of many particles which are of no biochemical value to the sponge. In order to retain sufficient nutrients for metabolism while simultaneously keeping waste levels from overwhelming the filtering system, the sponge must constantly excrete particles from its aqueous environment. Materials that cannot be used for energy are eliminated through apertures (oscules) in the exhalant surface. The entire sponge biomass is involved primarily in maintaining its low-pressure water-pumping system (Bergquist, 1978).

There have been misconceptions about sponges among taxonomists by lack of consistent defining characteristics of sponge morphology. Amorphous shapes, color variability within a species, and both flexibility in size and pigment intensity depending on the degree of light exposure create classification challenges. However, advancements in biochemical and histological tests aid classification of collected sponges, and other researchers have begun exploring the interesting technique of chemotaxonomy—identification by differential metabolite production. Chemotaxonomy has been used to distinguish sponges down to the genera, but cannot be used to determine classification at the species level (Verpoorte, 1998). There are three classes of sponges:

i) Demospongiae: This class includes 95% of identified species and spans a wide range of habitats from intertidal depths to marine trenches in fresh or brackish water.
ii) Hexactinellida: This class is characterized by six-membered hexactine siliceous spicules. This rather unusual class lacks a mesohyl matrix and is morphologically the most distinct from other poriferan classes.
iii) Calcarea: This class is composed of calcium carbonate-based skeletal materials. Crystalline calciferous spicules may grow individually or as one mass.

3.2.2.1 ANTIOXIDANTS FROM SPONGES

Sponges produce bioactive metabolites as part of their defensive system and they rarely develop a synergistic relationship with both algae and microorganisms. The symbionts to an extent are the true source of secondary metabolites found in sponges. Biotic factors such as epifaunal diversity and morphology alongside abiotic factors like pH, salinity, temperature, and so forth which are influenced by seasonal changes are responsible for the biosynthesis of secondary metabolites. Even though many bioactives have been found in sponges, only a few of these compounds have been commercialized. Therefore, the study of the chemical ecology of secondary metabolites is a hopeful value. Interestingly, these secondary metabolites are promises for developing potent drugs (Bell, 2008). Among these bioactive compounds, antioxidants are of special interest due to the functions of free radicals in many ailments including cancer, aging, and atherosclerosis. Marine sponge extracts from unused by-products such as head and viscera of salmon have been heavily investigated as cheap sources of natural antioxidants (Wu and Bechtel, 2008). However, few works have been carried out to investigate antioxidant properties of marine natural products isolated from sponges.

Extracts of *Fascaplysinopsis reticulate, Callyspongia siphonella, Niphates furcate, Callyspongia* sp., *Callyspongia clavata*, and *Pseudosaberities clavatus* collected from a coral island of Kish was found to possess high hydroxyl and DPPH (2,2-diphenyl-1-picrylhydrazyl) radical scavenging activity (Seradj et al., 2012). *Rhabdastrella globostella* and *Spirastrella inconstans* var. digitata (Dendy) extracts were found to elevate above the control basal values of the specific activity of almost all the antioxidant-related enzymes including glutathione peroxidase, glutathione reductase, catalase, and superoxide dismutase (SOD) in the extract-treated rats (Chairman et al., 2012). Also, *Aurora globostellata* was found to possess high-DPPH radical scavenging activity exhibiting a good antioxidant activity (Sugappriya and Sudarsanam, 2016). These sponges are said to possess antioxidant activities due to its possession of high-phenolic and aromatic compounds.

Several studies have demonstrated that numerous bioactive metabolites originally extracted from sponges, were in fact synthesized or transformed by bacterial strains. Hence, the sponge-associated bacteria could make up a renewable source of biomedical agents. As accumulated evidence suggests, it offers the likelihood to use the sponge-associated bacteria for the production of biologically active substances instead of the sponge itself. Because bacteria quickly produce excess amounts of biomass, biologically active secondary products can simply be produced in huge amounts on a biotechnological scale without the necessity to harvest or cultivate the sponge (Donia and Hamman, 2003).

3.3 DETERMINATION OF ANTIOXIDANT ACTIVITY

The interpretation of results obtained from in vitro measurement of the antioxidant activity of a marine organism or of a crude plant extract should be handled with caution. The selection of the appropriate assay to be used ought to be based on the intended applications of the antioxidant. The methods to examine the antioxidant activity of a sample can be divided in principle into major categories:

1. Measuring its capability to donate an electron or hydrogen atom to a specific ROS or to an electron acceptor.
2. Testing its ability to remove any source of oxidative initiation, for example, inhibition of enzymes, absorption of UV radiation, and chelation of transition metal. Free radicals can also be reduced by other mechanisms like:
   i. Metal chelation by complexing with transition metal ions, thereby hindering metal-catalyzed initiation and decomposition of lipid hydroperoxides.
   ii. Reducing the rate at the initiation of new radicals.
3. The other mechanisms include oxygen scavenging, singlet oxygen quenching, and blocking of peroxidant effects by binding certain proteins containing catalytic metal sites.

Enzymatic and nonenzymatic methods can be used to determine and or measure the antioxidant activities of marine organisms.

3.3.1 ESTIMATION OF ENZYMATIC ANTIOXIDANTS

The enzymatic antioxidants normally analyzed in the parts marine organism sample are SOD, catalase, peroxidase, glutathione S-transferases (GSTs) and polyphenol oxidase (PPO).

3.3.1.1 ESTIMATION OF SUPEROXIDE DISMUTASE

Principle: SOD assay is based on the inhibition of the formation of NADH-phenazine methosulphate (PMS)-nitroblue tetrazolium (NBT) formazon. The color formed at the end of the reaction can be sampled into butanol and measured at 560 nm.

Reagents: Sodium pyrophosphate buffer (0.025 M, pH 8.3); PMS (186 μM); NBT (300 μM); NADH (780 μM); glacial acetic acid; n-butanol; potassium phosphate buffer (50 mM, pH 6.4).

Preparation of enzyme sample: The sample (0.5 g) should be ground with 3.0 mL of potassium phosphate buffer, centrifuged at 2000 g for 10 min, and the supernatants should be used for the assay.

Assay: The assay mixture should contain 1.2 mL of sodium pyrophosphate buffer, 0.1 mL of PMS, 0.3 mL of NBT, 0.2 mL of the enzyme preparation, and water in a total volume of 2.8 mL. The reaction should be initiated by the addition of 0.2 mL of NADH. The mixture should be incubated at 300°C for 90 s and arrested by the addition of 1.0 mL of glacial acetic acid. The reaction mixture should then be shaken with 4.0 mL of n-butanol, allowed to stand for 10 min and centrifuged. In the butanol layer, the intensity of the chromogen should be measured at 560 nm in a spectrophotometer.

One unit of enzyme activity is defined as the amount of enzyme that gave 50% inhibition of NBT reduction in 1 min.

3.3.1.2 ESTIMATION OF CATALASE

Principle: At 240 nm, the UV absorption of hydrogen peroxide can be measured. This absorbance decreases when degraded by the enzyme catalase. The enzyme activity can be calculated from the decrease in absorbance.

Reagents: Phosphate buffer: 0.067 M (pH 7.0); hydrogen peroxide (2 mM) in phosphate buffer.

Preparation of enzyme sample: A 20% homogenate of the sample should be prepared in phosphate buffer. The homogenate should be centrifuged and the supernatant should be used for the enzyme assay.

Assay: H_2O_2-phosphate buffer (3.0 mL) should be taken in an experimental cuvette, followed by the quick addition of 40 μL of enzyme sample and mixed thoroughly. Using a spectrophotometer, the time required for a decrease in absorbance by 0.05 units should be recorded at 240 nm. The enzyme solution containing H_2O_2-free phosphate buffer should serve as the control.

One enzyme unit should be calculated as the amount of enzyme required to decrease the absorbance at 240 nm by 0.05 units.

3.3.1.3 ESTIMATION OF PEROXIDASE

Principle: In the presence of the hydrogen donor pyrogallol or dianisidine, peroxidase converts H_2O_2 to H_2O and O_2. Spectrophotometrically, the oxidation of pyrogallol or dianisidine to a colored product called purpurogalli can be followed at 430 nm.

Reagents: Pyrogallol—0.05 M in 0.1 M phosphate buffer (pH 6.5); H_2O_2—1% in 0.1 M phosphate buffer (pH 6.5).

Preparation of enzyme sample: A 20% homogenate should be prepared in 0.1 M phosphate buffer (pH 6.5) from the sample, clarified by centrifugation and the supernatant should be used for the assay.

Assay: To 3.0 mL of pyrogallol solution, 0.1 mL of the enzyme sample should be added and the spectrophotometer should be adjusted to read zero at 430 nm. To the test cuvette, 0.5 mL of H_2O_2 should be added and mixed. In the spectrophotometer, the change in absorbance should be recorded every 30 s for up to 3 min. One unit of peroxidase is defined as the change in absorbance/minute at 430 nm.

3.3.1.4 ESTIMATION OF GLUTATHIONE S-TRANSFERASE

Principle: The principle of GST assay is based by its ability to conjugate Glutathione (GSH) and 1-chloro-2, 4-dinitrobenzene (CDNB), the extent of conjugation causing a proportionate change in the absorbance at 340 nm.

Reagents: Glutathione (1 mM); 1-chloro-2,4-dinitrobenzene (CDNB) (1 mM in ethanol); phosphate buffer (0.1 M, pH 6.5).

Preparation of enzyme sample: The sample (0.5 g) should be homogenized with 5.0 mL of phosphate buffer. For the assay, the homogenates should be centrifuged at 5000 rpm for 10 min and the supernatants should be used.

Assay: The activity of the enzyme should be determined by observing the change in absorbance at 340 nm. The reaction mixture contained 0.1 mL of GSH, 0.1 mL of CDNB and phosphate buffer in a total volume of 2.9 mL. The reaction should be initiated by the addition of 0.1 mL of the enzyme sample. The readings were recorded every 15 s at 340 nm against distilled water blank for a minimum of 3 min in a spectrophotometer. The assay mixture without the sample should serve as the control to monitor nonspecific binding of the substrates.

GST activity should be calculated using the extinction coefficient of the product formed (9.6 mM^{-1} cm^{-1}) and should be expressed as nanomoles of CDNB conjugated/minute.

3.3.1.5 ESTIMATION OF POLYPHENOL OXIDASE

Principle: Phenol oxidases are copper-comprising proteins that catalyze the aerobic oxidation of phenolic substrates to quinines, which are autooxidized to dark brown pigments known as melanin. These can be estimated spectrophotometrically at 495 nm.

Reagents: Tris-HCl (50 mM, pH 7.2) containing sorbitol (0.4 M) and NaCl (10 mM); phosphate buffer (0.1 M, pH 6.5); catechol solution (0.01 M).

Preparation of enzyme sample: The enzyme sample should be prepared by homogenizing 0.5 g of sample tissue in 2.0 mL of the sample on medium containing tris HCl, sorbitol, and NaCl. At 2000 g the homogenate should be centrifuged for 10 min and the resultant supernatant should be used for the assay.

Assay: Phosphate buffer (2.5 mL) and 0.3 mL of catechol solution should be added in the cuvette and the spectrophotometer should be set at 495 nm. The enzyme sample (0.2 mL) should be added and the change observed in the absorbance should be recorded for every 30 s up to 5 min in a spectrophotometer.

One unit of catechol oxidase or laccase is defined as the amount of enzyme that transforms 1 μmol of dihydrophenol to 1 μmol of quinone per min.

The activity of PPO can be calculated using the formula:

Enzyme units in the sample = K × (μA/minute),

where, K for catechol oxidase = 0.272; K for laccase = 0.242.

3.3.2 ESTIMATION OF NONENZYMATIC ANTIOXIDANTS

The nonenzymatic antioxidants normally analyzed in samples are ascorbic acid, α-tocopherol, total carotenoids, lycopene, reduced glutathione, total phenols, flavonoids, and chlorophyll.

3.3.2.1 ESTIMATION OF ASCORBIC ACID

Principle: Treatment with activated charcoal converts ascorbate into dehydroascorbate which reacts with 2,4-dinitrophenylhydrazine to form osazones. When osazone is dissolved in sulfuric acid, it produces an orange-colored solution, whose absorbance can be measured spectrophotometrically at 540 nm.

Reagents: TCA (4%); 2,4-dinitrophenyl hydrazine reagent (2%) in 9N H_2SO_4; thiourea (10%); sulfuric acid (85%); standard ascorbic acid solution: 100 µg/mL in 4% TCA.

Preparation of sample: Ascorbate should be prepared from 1 g of the sample using 4% TCA and the volume should be made up to 10 mL with the same. The supernatant obtained after centrifugation at 2000 rpm for 10 min should be treated with a pinch of activated charcoal, shaken vigorously using a cyclomixer, and kept for 5 min. By centrifugation, charcoal particles should be removed and aliquots should be used for the estimation.

Procedure: Standard ascorbate ranging between 0.2mL - 1.0mL and the aliquot of the treated supernatant ranging between 0.5mL - 1.0mL should be taken. The volume should be made up to 2.0 mL with 4% TCA. DNPH reagent (0.5 mL) should be added to all the tubes, followed by two drops of 10% thiourea solution. The contents should be mixed and incubated at 370°C for 3 h resulting in the formation of osazone crystals. The crystals should be dissolved in 2.5 mL of 85% sulfuric acid, in cold. To the blank alone, DNPH reagent and thiourea should be added after the addition of sulfuric acid. The tubes should be cooled in ice and the absorbance should be taken at 540 nm in a spectrophotometer.

A standard graph should be constructed using an electronic calculator set to the linear regression model. The concentration of ascorbate in the samples should be calculated and expressed in terms of mg/g of sample.

3.3.2.2 ESTIMATION OF TOCOPHEROL

Principle: The Emmerie–Engel reaction is based on the reduction of ferric to ferrous ions by tocopherols, which, with 2,2′-dipyridyl, forms a red color.

Tocopherols and carotenes are first sampled with xylene and read at 460 nm to measure carotenes. A correction is made for this after adding ferric chloride and read at 520 nm.

Reagents: Absolute alcohol; xylene; 2,2′-dipyridyl (1.2 g/L in n-propanol); ferric chloride solution (1.2 g/L in ethanol); standard solution (D, L-α-tocopherol, 10 mg/L in absolute alcohol); sulfuric acid (0.1 N).

Preparation of sample: The sample (2.5 g) should be homogenized in 50 mL of 0.1 N sulfuric acid and allowed to stand overnight. The contents of the flask should be shaken vigorously and filtered through Whatman No.1 filter paper. Aliquots of the filtrate should be used for the estimation.

Procedure: In three stoppered centrifuge tubes, 1.5 mL of the sample, 1.5 mL of the standard, and 1.5 mL of water should be pipetted out separately. To all the tubes, 1.5 mL of ethanol and 1.5 mL of xylene should be added, mixed well, and centrifuged. Xylene (1.0 mL) layer should be transferred into another stoppered tube. To each tube, 1.0 mL of dipyridyl reagent should be added and mixed well. The mixture (1.5 mL) should be pipetted out into a cuvette and the absorbance is taken at 460 nm. Ferric chloride solution (0.33 mL) should be added to all the tubes and mixed well. The red color developed should be read exactly after 15 min at 520 nm in a spectrophotometer.

The concentration of tocopherol in the sample should be calculated using the formula:

$$Tocopherols\ (\mu g) = \frac{Sample\ Abs\,520 - Abs\,460 \times 0.29 \times 0.15}{Standard\ Abs\,520}.$$

3.3.2.3 ESTIMATION OF TOTAL CAROTENOIDS AND LYCOPENE

Principle: Total carotenoids and lycopene can be estimated in a sample using petroleum ether and estimated at 450 nm and 503 nm, respectively.

Reagents: Petroleum ether (40–60°C); anhydrous sodium sulfate; calcium carbonate; alcoholic potassium hydroxide (12%).

Procedure: The experiment is done in the dark to avoid photolysis of carotenoids once the saponification is complete. The sample (0.5 g) should be homogenized and saponified with 2.5 mL of 12% alcoholic potassium hydroxide in a water bath at 60°C for 30 min. The saponified sample should be transferred to a separating funnel containing 10–15 mL of petroleum ether and mixed well. The lower aqueous layer should then be transferred to another separating funnel and the upper petroleum ether layer containing the carotenoids should be collected. The procedure should be repeated until the aqueous layer become colorless. A small amount of anhydrous sodium sulfate should be added to the petroleum ether sample to remove excess moisture. The final volume of the petroleum ether sample should be noted. The absorbance of the yellow color should be read in a spectrophotometer at 450 nm and 503 nm using petroleum ether as blank. The amount of total carotenoids and lycopene should be calculated using the formulae:

$$Amount\ of\ total\ carotenoids = \frac{Abs\,450 \times Volume\ of\ sample \times 100 \times 4}{Weight\ of\ the\ sample}$$

$$Amount\ of\ lycopene = \frac{3.12 \times Abs\,503 \times Volume\ of\ the\ sample \times 100}{Weight\ of\ the\ sample}.$$

The total carotenoids and lycopene are expressed as mg/g of the sample.

3.3.2.4 *ESTIMATION OF REDUCED GLUTATHIONE*

Principle: Reduced glutathione in reaction with DTNB (5,5′-dithiobis nitrobenzoic acid) produces a yellow colored product that absorbs at 412 nm.

Reagents: TCA (5%); phosphate buffer (0.2 M, pH 8.0); DTNB (0.6 mM in 0.2 M phosphate buffer); standard GSH (10 nmol/mL of 5% TCA)

Preparation of sample: A homogenate should be prepared with 0.5 g of the sample with 2.5 mL of 5% TCA. The precipitated protein should be centrifuged at 1000 rpm for 10 min. The supernatant (0.1 mL) should be used for the estimation of GSH.

Procedure: The supernatant (0.1 mL) should be made up to 1.0 mL with 0.2 M sodium phosphate buffer (pH 8.0). Standard GSH corresponding to concentrations ranging between 2 and 10 nmol should also be prepared. About 2 mL of freshly prepared DTNB solution should be added and the intensity of the yellow color developed should be measured in a spectrophotometer at 412 nm after 10 min.

The values are expressed as nanomoles GSH/g sample.

3.3.2.5 *ESTIMATION OF TOTAL PHENOLS*

Principle: Phenols react with the phosphomolybdic acid in Folin–Ciocalteau reagent to produce a blue-colored complex in alkaline medium, which can be estimated spectrophotometrically at 650 nm.

Reagents: Ethanol (80%); Folin–Ciocalteau reagent (1 N); sodium carbonate (20%); standard catechol solution (100 μg/mL in water).

Procedure: The sample (0.5 g) should be homogenized in 10X volume of 80% ethanol. The homogenate should be centrifuged at 10,000 rpm for 20 min. The procedure should be repeated with 80% ethanol. The supernatants should be pooled and evaporated to dryness. The residue is then dissolved in a known volume of distilled water. Different aliquots should pipette out and the volume in each tube should be made up to 3.0 mL with distilled water. Folin–Ciocalteau reagent (0.5 mL) should be added and the tubes must be placed in a boiling water bath for exactly 1 min. The tubes should be cooled and the absorbance is taken at 650 nm in a spectrophotometer against a reagent blank. Standard catechol solutions (0.2–1 mL) corresponding to 2.0–10 μg concentrations should also be treated as above.

The concentration of phenols is expressed as mg/g tissue.

3.3.2.6 ESTIMATION OF FLAVONOIDS

Principle: Flavonoids react with vanillin to produce a colored product, which can be measured spectrophotometrically.

Reagents: Vanillin reagent (1% in 70% sulfuric acid); catechin standard (110 μg/mL).

Preparation of sample: The samples (0.5 g) should first be prepared with methanol:water mixture (2:1) and secondly with the same mixture in the ratio 1:1. The samples should be shaken well and allowed to stand overnight. The supernatants should be pooled and the volume should also be measured. This supernatant should be concentrated and then used for the assay.

Procedure: A known volume of the sample should be pipetted out and evaporated to dryness. Vanillin reagent (4.0 mL) should be added and the tubes should be heated in a boiling water bath for 15 min. Varying concentrations of the standard can also be treated in the same manner.

The optical density should be read in a spectrophotometer at 340 nm. A standard curve is constructed and the concentration of flavonoids in each sample is well calculated. The values of flavonoids are expressed as mg/g sample.

3.3.2.7 ESTIMATION OF CHLOROPHYLL

Principle: Chlorophyll is prepared in 80% acetone and the absorbance is measured at 645 and 663 nm. The amount of chlorophyll is calculated using the absorption coefficient.

Reagent: Acetone (80%, prechilled).

Procedure: Chlorophyll should be prepared from 1 g of the sample using 20 mL of 80% acetone. The supernatant should be transferred to a volumetric flask after centrifugation at 5000 rpm for 5 min. The solution should be repeated until the residue become colorless. The volume in the flask should be made up to 100 mL with 80% acetone. The absorbance of the sample should be taken in a spectrophotometer at 645 and 663 nm against 80% acetone blank. The amount of total chlorophyll in the sample should be calculated using the formula:

$$Total\ Chlorophyll = \frac{20.2\,(Abs\,645) + 8.02\,(Abs\,663) \times V}{1000 \times W},$$

where V = final volume of the sample; W = fresh weight of the leaves. The values are expressed as mg chlorophyll/g sample.

3.3.3 EVALUATION OF THE RADICAL SCAVENGING EFFECTS

The scavenging effects of samples are usually evaluated against 2,2-diphenyl-2-picrylhydrazyl (DPPH), 2,2-azino-bis (3-ethylbenzothiazoline-6-sulphonic acid) (ABTS), hydrogen peroxide, superoxide, nitric oxide, and hydroxyl radicals.

3.3.3.1 DPPH RADICAL SCAVENGING EFFECTS

The ability of samples to scavenge the DPPH radical are usually tested in a rapid dot-plot screening and quantified using a spectrophotometric assay.

Principle: DPPH radical reacts with an antioxidant compound that can donate hydrogen, and gets reduced. DPPH, when acted upon by an antioxidant, is converted into diphenyl picryl hydrazine. This can be identified by the conversion of purple to light yellow color.

a) Dot-plot rapid assay

Reagents: TLC plates (silica gel 60 F254-Merck); DPPH (0.4 mM) in methanol.

Procedure: Aliquots of the sample should be spotted carefully on TLC plates and dried for 3 min. The sheets bearing the dry spots should be placed upside down for 10 s in a 0.4 mM DPPH solution and should be layer-dried. The stained silica layer should reveal a purple background with yellow spots, which should show radical scavenging capacity.

b) DPPH spectrophotometric assay

Reagents: DPPH—2,2-diphenyl-2-picrylhydrazyl hydrate (0.3 mM in methanol); methanol.

Procedure: The marine sample (20 μL) should be added to 0.5 mL of methanolic solution of DPPH and 0.48 mL of methanol. The mixture should be allowed to react at room temperature for 30 min. Methanol should serve as the blank and DPPH in methanol without the sample should serve as the positive control. After 30 min of incubation, the discoloration of the purple color should be measured at 518 nm in a spectrophotometer. The radical scavenging activity should be calculated as follows:

$$\%\ \text{Antioxidant activity} = \frac{(\text{Absorbance of control} - \text{Absorbance of sample})}{(\text{Absorbance of control})} \times 100.$$

3.3.3.2 ABTS SCAVENGING EFFECTS

The antioxidant effect of the marine sample can be studied using ABTS (2,2′-azino-bis-3-ethylbenzthiazoline-6-sulphonic acid) radical cation decolorization assay.

Reagent: ABTS solution (7 mM with 2.45 mM ammonium persulfate).

Procedure: ABTS radical cations (ABTS+) are produced by reacting ABTS solution (7 mM) with 2.45 mM ammonium persulphate. The mixture should be allowed to stand in the dark at room temperature for 12–16 h before use. Aliquots (0.5 mL) of the three different samples should be added to 0.3 mL of ABTS solution and the final volume made up to 1 mL with ethanol. The absorbance should be taken at 745 nm in a spectrophotometer and the percent inhibition was calculated using the formula.

$$Inhibition\,(\%) = \frac{(Control - Test) \times 100}{Control}.$$

3.3.3.3 HYDROGEN PEROXIDE SCAVENGING EFFECTS

Reagents: Phosphate buffer (0.1 M, pH 7.4); H_2O_2 (40 mM) in phosphate buffer.

Procedure: A solution of H_2O_2 (40 mM) should be prepared in phosphate buffer. Marine samples at the concentration of 10 mg/μL should be added to the H_2O_2 solution (0.6 mL) and the total volume made up to 3 mL. The absorbance of the reaction mixture should be recorded at 230 nm in a spectrophotometer. A blank solution containing phosphate buffer, without H_2O_2 should be prepared. The extent of H_2O_2 scavenging of the sample should be calculated as:

$$\%\ Scavenging\ of\ Hydrogen\ Peroxide = \frac{((Abs\ of\ Blank - Abs\ of\ sample 230) \times 100)}{Abs\ of\ Blank}.$$

3.3.3.4 MEASUREMENT OF SUPEROXIDE SCAVENGING ACTIVITY

Principle: This assay is based on the inhibition of the production of NBT formazon of the superoxide ion by the sample and is measured spectrophotometrically at 560 nm.

Reagents: EDTA (0.1 M containing 1.5 mg of NaCN); NBT (1.5 mM); riboflavin (0.12 mM); phosphate buffer (0.067 M, pH 7.6).

Procedure: Superoxide anions should be generated in samples that should contain in 3.0 mL, 0.02 mL of the marine samples (20 mg), 0.2 mL of EDTA, 0.1 mL of NBT, 0.05 mL of riboflavin, and 2.64 mL of phosphate buffer. The control tubes should also be set up where dimethyl sulfoxide (DMSO) should be added instead of the sample. All the tubes should be vortexed and the initial optical density measured at 560 nm in a spectrophotometer. The tubes should be illuminated using a fluorescent lamp for 30 min. The absorbance should be measured again at 560 nm. The difference in absorbance before and after illumination is indicative of superoxide anion scavenging activity.

3.3.3.5 MEASUREMENT OF NITRIC OXIDE SCAVENGING ACTIVITY

Principle: Sodium nitroprusside in aqueous solution, at physiological pH, spontaneously generates nitric oxide, which interacts with oxygen to produce nitrite ions that are estimated spectrophotometrically at 546 nm.

Reagents: Sodium nitroprusside (100 mM); phosphate buffered saline (pH 7.4); Griess reagent (1% sulphanilamide, 2% H_3PO_4 and 0.1% naphthylethylenediamine dihydrochloride)

Procedure: The reaction should be initiated by adding 2.0 mL of sodium nitroprusside, 0.5 mL of PBS, 0.5 mL of the sample (50 mg), and incubated at 25°C for 30 min. Griess reagent (0.5 mL) should be added and incubated for another 30 min. Control tubes should be prepared without the samples. The absorbance should be taken at 546 nm against the reagent blank, in a spectrophotometer.

3.3.3.6 MEASUREMENT OF HYDROXYL RADICAL SCAVENGING ACTIVITY

The extent of hydroxyl radical scavenging from Fenton reaction is quantified using 2′-deoxyribose oxidative degradation.

Principle: The principle of the assay is the quantification of 2′-deoxyribose degradation product, malondialdehyde, by its condensation with thiobarbituric acid.

Reagents: Deoxyribose (2.8 mM); ferric chloride (0.1 mM); EDTA (0.1 mM); H_2O_2 (1 mM); ascorbate (0.1 mM); KH_2PO4-KOH buffer (20 mM, pH 7.4); thiobarbituric acid (1%)

Procedure: The reaction mixture contained 0.1 mL of deoxyribose, 0.1 mL of $FeCl_3$, 0.1 mL of EDTA, 0.1 mL of H_2O_2, 0.1 mL of ascorbate, 0.1 mL of KH_2PO4-KOH buffer and 20 μL of the sample in a final volume of 1.0 mL. The mixture should be incubated at 37°C for 1 h. At the end of the incubation period, 1.0 mL of TBA should be added and heated at 95°C for 20 min to develop the color. After cooling, the Thiobarbituric acid reactive substances (TBARS) formation should be measured spectrophotometrically at 532 nm against an appropriate blank. The hydroxyl radical scavenging activity should be determined by comparing the absorbance of the control with that of the sample. The percent TBARS production for positive control (H_2O_2) should be fixed at 100% and the relative percent TBARS should be calculated for the sample treated groups.

KEYWORDS

- **antioxidants**
- **marine antioxidants**
- **sponge**
- **DPPH**
- **radical scavenging**

REFERENCES

Al-Saif, S. S.; Abdel-Raouf, N.; El-Wazanani, H. A.; Aref, L. A. Antibacterial Substances from Marine Algae Isolated from Jeddah Coast of Red Sea, Saudi Arabia. *Saudi J. Biol. Sci.* **2014,** *21,* 54–64.

Balakrishan, D.; Kandasamy, D.; Nithyanand, P. A Review on Antioxidant Activity of Marine Organisms. *Int. J. ChemTech. Res.* **2014,** *6*(7), 3431–3436.

Bandoniene, D.; Murkovic, M. On-line HPLC-DPPH Screening Method for Evaluation of Radical Scavenging Phenols Extracted from Apples (*Malusdomestica L.*). *J. Agric. Food Chem.* **2002,** *50,* 2482–2487.

Bell, J. J. The Functional Roles of Marine Sponges. *Estuarine Coastal Shelf Sci.* **2008,** *79,* 341–353.

Bergmann, W.; Feeney, R. J. Contribution to the Study of Marine Products, XXXII. The Nucleosides of Sponges. *J. Org. Chem.* **1951,** *16,* 981–987.

Bergquist, P. R. *Sponges*, 2nd ed.; University of California Press: Berkeley, 1978.

Bhakuni, D. S.; Rawat, D. S. *Bioactive Marine Natural Products*, 1st ed.; Anamaya Publishers: New Delhi, 2005.

Bocanegra, A.; Bastida, S.; Benedí, J.; Ródenas, S.; Sánchez-Muniz, F. J. Characteristics and Nutritional and Cardiovascular-Health Properties of Seaweeds. *J. Med. Food* **2009,** *12,* 236–258.

Bold, H. C.; Wynne, M. J. *Introduction of the Algae Structure and Reproduction*, 2nd ed.; Prentice-Hall Inc, Englewood Cliffs: New Jersey, 1985; pp 1–33.

Brown, M. R; Jeffrey, S. W.; Volkman, J. K.; Dunstan, G. A. Nutritional Properties of Microalgae for Mariculture. *Aquaculture* **1997,** *151,* 315–331.

Carballo-Cárdenas, E. C.; Tuan, P. M.; Janssen, M.; Wijffels, R. H. Vitamin E (α-tocopherol) Production by the Marine Microalgae *Dunaliella tertiolecta* and *Tetraselmis suecica* in Batch Cultivation. *Biomol. Eng.* **2003,** *20,* 139–147.

Cha, K. H.; Kang, S. W.; Kim, C. Y.; Um, B. H.; Na, Y. R.; Pan, C. H. Effect of Pressurized Liquids on Extraction of Antioxidants from *Chlorella vulgaris*. *J. Agric. Food Chem.* **2010,** *58,* 4756–4761.

Chairman, K.; Singh, R.; Alagumuthu, G. Cytotoxic and Antioxidant Activity of Selected Marine Sponges. *Asian Pac. J. Trop. Dis.* **2012,** *1,* 234–238.

Del Campo, J. A.; García-González, M.; Guerrero, M. G. Outdoor Cultivation of Microalgae for Carotenoid Production: Current State and Perspectives. *Appl. Microbiol. Biotechnol.* **2007,** *74,* 1163–1174.

Dembitsky,V. M.; Maoka, T. Allenic and Cumulenic Lipids. *Prog. Lipid Res.* **2007,** *46,* 328–375.

Donia, M.; Hamman, M. T. Marine Natural Products and their Potential Application as Anti-Infective Agents. *Lancet Infect. Dis.* **2003,** *3,* 338–348.

Durmaz, Y.; Monteiro, M.; Bandarra, N.; Gokpinar, S.; Isik, O. The Effect of Low Temperature on Fatty Acid Composition and Tocopherols of the Red Microalga, *Porphyridium cruentum*. *J. Appl. Phycol.* **2007,** *19,* 223–227.

El Gamal, A. A. Biological Importance of Marine Algae. *Saudi Pharm. J.* **2010,** *18,* 1–25.

Hu, C. C.; Lin, J. T.; Lu, F. J.; Chou, F. P.; Yang, D. J. Determination of Carotenoids in *Dunaliella salina* Cultivated in Taiwan and Antioxidant Capacity of the Algal Carotenoid Extract. *Food Chem.* **2008,** *109,* 439–446.

Inbaraj, B. S.; Chien, J. T.; Chen, B. H. Improved High Performance Liquid Chromatographic Method for Detersmination of Carotenoids in the Microalga *Chlorella pyrenoidosa*. *J. Chromatogr.* **2006,** *1102,* 193–199.

Klejdus, B.; Kopecký, J.; Benesová, L.; Vacek, J. Solid-Phase/ Supercritical-Fluid Extraction for Liquid Chromatography of Phenolic Compounds in Freshwater Microalgae and Selected. *Cyanobacterial Species*. *J. Chromatogr.* **2009,** *1216,* 763–771.

Li, H.-B.; Chen, F. Preparative Isolation and Purification of Astaxanthin from the *Microalga Chlorococcum* Sp. by High-Speed Counter-Current Chromatography. *J. Chromatogr.* **2001,** *925,* 133–137.

Lordan, S.; Ross, P.; Stanton, C. Marine Bioactives as Functional Food Ingredients: Potential to Reduce the Incidence of Chronic Diseases. *Mar. Drugs* **2011,** *9,* 1056–1100.

Mabeau, S.; Fleurence, J. Seaweeds in Food Products: Biochemical and Nutritional Aspects. *Trends Food Sci. Technol.* **1993,** *4,* 103–107.

MacArtain, P.; Gill, C. I. R.; Brooks, M.; Campbell, R.; Rowland, I. R. Nutritional Value of Edible Seaweeds. *Nutr. Rev.* **2007,** *65,* 535–543.

Marine Biotechnology. Basis sand Applications: Abstracts of an International Symposium; Spain, February 25-March 1, 2003. *Biomol. Engr.* **2003**, 20, 37–82.

Mata, T. M.; Martins, A. A.; Caetano, N. S. Microalgae for Biodiesel Production and other Applications: A Review. *Renewable Sustainable Energy Rev.* **2010,** *14,* 217–232.

Mendes, R. L.; Fernandes, H. L.; Coelho, J. P.; Reis, E. C.; Cabral, J. M.; Novais, J. M.; Palavra, A. F. Supercritical CO_2 Extraction of Carotenoids and other Lipids from *Chlorella vulgaris*. *Food Chem.* **1995,** *53,* 99–103.

Metting, F. B. Biodiversity and Application of Microalgae. *J. Ind. Microbiol.* **1996,** *17,* 477–489.

Okai, Y.; Higashi-Okai, K.; Yano, Y.; Otani, S. Identification of Antimutagenic Substances in an Extract of Edible Red Alga, *Porphyra tenera (asadusa-nori)*. *Cancer Lett.* **1996,** *100,* 235–240.

Olson, J. A.; Krinsky, N. I. Introduction: The Colourful, Fascinating World of the Carotenoids: Important Physiologic Modulators. *FASEB J.* **1995,** *9,* 1547–1550.

Plaza, M.; Santoyo, S.; Jaime, L.; García-Blairsy Reina, G.; Herrero, M.; Señoráns, F. J.; Ibáñez, E. Screening for Bioactive Compounds from Algae. *J. Pharm. Biomed. Anal.* **2010,** *51,* 450–455.

Sánchez-Machado, D.; López-Hernández, J.; Paseiro-Losada, P. High-Performance Liquid Chromatographic Determination of [alpha]-Tocopherol in Macroalgae. *J. Chromatogr.* **2002,** *97,* 277–284.

Seradj, H.; Moein, M.; Eskandari, M.; Maaref, F. Antioxidant Activity of Six Marine Sponges Collected from the Persian Gulf. *Iran. J. Pharm. Sci.* **2012,** *8*(4), 249–255.

Slevan, G. P.; Rawikumar, S.; Ramu, A.; Neelakandan, P. Antagonistic Activity of Marine Sponge Associated *Streptomyces* sp. against Isolated Fish Pathogens. *Asian Pac. J. Trop. Dis.* **2012,** *2,* S724–S728.

Spolaore, P.; Joannis-Cassan, C.; Duran, E.; Isambert, A. Commercial Applications of Microalgae. *J. Biosci. Bioeng.* **2006,** *101,* 87–96.

Sugappriya, M.; Sudarsanam, D. Free Radical Screening Activity of Marine Sponge Auwora Globostellata. *Asian J. Pharm. Clin. Res.* **2016,** *9*(4), 210–212.

Rasmussen, R. S.; Morrissey, M. T. Marine Biotechnology for Production of Food Ingredients. *Adv. Food Nutr. Res.* **2007,** *52,* 237–292.

Rebolloso Fuentes, M. M.; Acién Fernández, G.; Sánchez Pérez, J.; Guil Guerrero. Biomass Nutrient Profiles of the Microalga *Porphyridium cruentum*. *Food Chem.* **2000,** *70,* 345–353.

Rodríguez-Meizoso, I.; Jaime, L.; Santoyo, S.; Cifuentes, A.; Garcia-Blairsy Reina, G.; Señoráns, F.; Ibáñez, E. Pressurized Fluid Extraction of Bioactive Compounds from *Phormidium* Species. *J. Agric. Food Chem.* **2008,** *56,* 3517–3523.

Taboada, C.; Millán, R.; Míguez, I. Composition, Nutritional Aspects and Effect on Serum Parameters of Marine Algae *Ulva rigida*. *J. Sci. Food Agric.* **2010,** *90,* 445–449.

Verpoorte, R. Exploration of Nature Chemodiversity: The Role of Secondary Metabolites as Leads in Drugs Development. *Drug Discovery Today*, **1998,** *3,* 232–238.

Wu, T. H.; Bechtel, P. J. Salmon By-Products Storage and Oil Extraction. *Food Chem.* **2008,** *111*(4), 868–871.

Yokthongwattana, K.; Savchenko, T.; Polle, J. E. W.; Melis, A. Isolation and Characterization of a Xanthophyll-rich Fraction from the Thylakoid Membrane of *Dunaliella salina* (green algae). *Photochem. Photobiol. Sci.* **2005,** *4,* 1028–1034.

Yuan, J. P.; Chen, F., Liu, X.; Li, X. Z. Carotenoid Composition in the Green *Microalga Chlorococcum. Food Chem.* **2002,** *76,* 319–325.

Yuan, Y. V.; Bone, D. E.; Carrington, M. F. Antioxidant Activity of Dulse (*Palmaria palmata*) Extract Evaluated in Vitro. *Food Chem.* **2005,** *91,* 485–494.

References and Further Readings on Measurement of Antioxidant Activity

Bayfield, R. F.; Cole, E. R. Colorimetric Estimation of Vitamin A with Trichloroacetic Acid. *Methods Enzymol.* **1980,** *67,* 189–195.

Kakkar, A. K. Colorimetric Assay of SOD. *Anal. Biochem.***1984,** *47*(2), 389–394.

Luck, H. Catalase. In *Methods of Enzymatic Analysis;* Bergmeyer, H-U., ed.; Academic Press: New York, 1974; Vol. II, pp 885–890.

Reddy, K. P.; Subhani, S. M.; Khan, P. A.; Kumar, K. B. Effect of Light and Benzyl Adenine and Dark Treated Graving Rice (*Oryza sativa*) Leaves Changes in Gluthione Peroxidases Activity. *Plant Cell Physiol.* **1995,** *26,* 987–994.

Roe, J. H.; Kuether, C. A. The Determination of Ascorbic Acid in Whole Blood and Urine through the 2,4-dinitrophenylhydrazine Derivative of Dehydroascorbic Acid. *J. Biol. Chem.* **1943,** *147,* 399.

Rosenberg, H. R. *Chemistry and Physiology of the Vitamins;* Interscience Publisher: New York, 1992; pp 452–453.

CHAPTER 4

EXTRACTION OF MARINE PHYTOCHEMICALS: METHODS AND TECHNIQUES

NADIA SHARIF[1,*], NEELMA MUNIR[1], and SHAGUFTA NAZ[1]

[1]*Department of Biotechnology, Lahore College for Women University, Lahore 54000, Pakistan, Tel.: +92 3237501948*

Corresponding author. E-mail: nadiasharif.s7@gmail.com

ORCID: https://orcid.org/0000-0002-8125-9270

ABSTRACT

It is imperative to document proper, specific, practical, and eco-friendly supportive extraction systems for marine phytochemicals. These procedures should fulfill the necessities in regard to the extraction and isolation of the bioactive of interests. Conventional extraction systems are comparatively time-taking, requiring high solvent volumes and are extensively laborious. These methods regularly deliver low selectivity and extraction of bioactive compounds from marine plants. The utilization of new best-in-class extraction methods, for example, pressurized liquid extraction, supercritical fluid extraction, ultrasound-assisted extraction, accelerated solvent extraction (ASE®), and microwave-assisted extraction systems have proven a successful contrasting option to the issues experienced with the utilization of conventional extraction techniques.

4.1 INTRODUCTION

Considering the immense biodiversity of marine organisms, the utilization of proper approaches that are able to quickly screen diverse marine metabolites are of remarkable importance. To outline the isolation technique, a lot of factors need to be considered. These factors comprise dissolvability, atomic weight, and heat resistance. At first, a reasonable extraction method ought to be chosen. The utilization of naturally clean propelled extraction methods is important for the proper extraction of a bioactive. After extraction, the bioactive properties of the extract are accessed through the various in vitro and in vivo assays such as antihypertensive, antimicrobial and antioxidants. After confirming the biological activities and functional categorization, the next step is the chemical categorization. Structural confirmation is possible through analytical techniques that are dependent on temperature, pH, and solubility (Tejesvi et al., 2008; Grosso et al., 2015).

The extraction of bioactive components from the marine plant is a pragmatic workout at different conditions with different solvents. The failure or success of the extraction method relies on the condition of extraction. The partition of the crude extracts or chromatographic techniques to fractionate the extract grounded on the acid property, polarity, or atomic size is the next step. Recrystallization, distillation or sublimation methods are applied to offer appropriate wholesome structural exploration (Grosso et al., 2015). The polarity of the compound of interest is of importance for the solvent choice. Other factors such as molecular affinity between solute and solvent, cosolvent use, mass transfer, human toxicity, financial feasibility and environmental safety must likewise be considered in deciding the solvent for the extraction of bioactive compounds (Cowan, 1999). More details can be obtained from *Volume 1* of this book.

4.2 CONVENTIONAL EXTRACTION TECHNIQUES

The extraction of bioactive compounds from marine plant samples can be achieved by numerous conventional extraction techniques. Mostly, these techniques rely on the application of mixing/heat and extracting the power of different solvents. The bioactive yield can be influenced by the technique for molding and extraction. Different solvents can be utilized to separate distinctive phytoconstituents (Wong and Kitts, 2006). Acid hydrolysis is a significant chemical modification that is able to bring a significant change in structural and functional properties (Lee and Jeffries, 2011). It is a preferred method over other pretreatments due to its effectiveness and low cost (Loow et al., 2016). Commonly used dilute acids include H_2SO_4, HNO_3, HCl, H_3PO_4, and other acids. On the other hand, alkali hydrolysis of different plant samples is also tried in different experiments but a lot of times it results in reduced functionality and is of little benefit (Kristinsson and Rasco, 2000).

Enzymatic hydrolysis from animal and plant cradles has been deliberated extensively and by numerous authors over the past 60 years, and it is still the most commonly used method for adding value to the target organism. The preferred commercial enzymes are of bacterial origin, including Alcalase, Neutrase, and Flavourzyme, as well as from animals and plants, including trypsin, pepsin, papain, bromelain (see Chapter 8 of this volume), and subtilisin. The conventional techniques for the extraction of bioactive compounds from diverse plants are Soxhlet extraction, maceration, and hydrodistillation. Soxhlet extractor was first suggested by German chemist Franz Ritter Von Soxhlet (1879). The Soxhlet extraction has extensively been utilized for extracting valued bioactive compounds from numerous natural cradles. It is recognized as a model for the comparison of novel extraction substitutes.

4.2.1 MACERATION

Maceration was utilized as a part of homemade tonic for quite a while. It turned into a famous and modest approach to get fundamental oils and bioactive mixes. For small-scale extraction, maceration forms the most part comprising of a few stages. Right off the bat, pounding of plant materials into little molecules is utilized to expand the surface zone for legitimate blending with the dissolvable. Also, in maceration process, fitting a dissolvable named as menstruum is included in a shut vessel. Thirdly, the fluid is stressed off however, the marc which is the strong deposit of this extraction procedure is squeezed to recuperate a huge measure of blocked arrangements. The material gets stressed and the press out fluid is blended and isolated and separated by filtration. Periodic shaking in maceration encourages extraction in two ways; (a) enhanced dissemination, (b) expel concentrated arrangement from the example surface for conveying the new dissolvable to the menstruum for more extraction yield (Azmir et al., 2013).

4.2.2 HYDRODISTILLATION

Hydrodistillation is performed before dehydration of plant materials without solvents. Steam distillation, direct steam distillation and water distillation are three different hydrodistillation methods (Vankar, 2004). In hydrodistillation, to start with, the plant materials are pressed into a still compartment; second, water is included and after that conveyed to boil. On the other hand, coordinate steam is infused into the plant material. Boiling water and steam go about as the fundamental compelling components to free bioactive mixes of plant tissue. Circuitous cooling by water gathers the vapor blend of water and oil. Consolidated blend flows from the condenser to a separator, where oil and bioactive mixes isolated from the water (Silva et al., 2005). Hydrodistillation includes three principles in physicochemical procedures; decomposition by heat, hydro-diffusion, and hydrolysis. At a high extraction temperature, some volatile components might be lost. This disadvantage restrains its utilization for thermolabile compound extraction.

4.3 NONCONVENTIONAL EXTRACTION TECHNIQUES

Though different extraction systems exist, some are known as conventional and some as nonconventional that are available for the isolation and characterization of marine plant materials. The nonconventional extraction system seems more natural to me because of diminished utilization of manufactured and natural chemicals, decreased operational time, and better yield and nature of concentrate that has been produced in the recent 50 years (Grosso et al., 2015). To overcome the limitations of conventional extraction methods and the demand for new extraction systems to augment the inclusive yield and discernment of bioactive constituents from plant materials has resulted in advanced extraction techniques introducing techniques such as enzyme digestion, microwave heating, supercritical fluids and accelerated solvents extraction systems (Troy et al., 2017). The benefits of nonconventional extraction methods are reduced consumption of organic solvent, automation and reduced extraction time. Some of the most promising nonconventional extraction techniques are ultrasound-assisted extraction, enzyme-assisted extraction, microwave-assisted extraction (MAE), pulsed-electric field-assisted extraction, supercritical fluid extraction (SFE) and pressurized liquid extraction (PLE) (Selvamuthukumaran and Shi, 2017).

4.3.1 ULTRASOUND-ASSISTED EXTRACTION

Ultrasound-assisted extraction (UAE) works by increasing the porousness of the cell wall of the sample. It causes fast extraction as UAE considerably decreases the time of extraction and raises the yield of extraction, as it produces cavitation bubbles in the solvent during the expansion phase (Zou et al., 2013). The local tensile strength of the liquid exceeds because of the negative pressure exerted by the expansion cycle (Wang, 2011).

Unconstrained arrangement rises in the fluid below its boiling point, that is, cavitation impact, because of dynamic focusing and increment in the mechanical pushing, that is, inner contact of the cells (Mukherjee, 2002). The UAE relies on many components: (a) force, (b) time, (c) dissolvable, (d) temperature, (e) throb, (f) network (Lavoie and Stevanovic, 2007).

The utilization of ultrasound can be partitioned into two unmistakable classes: low intensity–high recurrence (100 kHz–1 MHz) and high intensity–low recurrence (in the vicinity of 20 and 100 kHz) ultrasound, the latter being the main case that prompts the interruption of cell dividers and films (Kong et al., 2014).

4.3.2 PULSED-ELECTRIC FIELD EXTRACTION

Pulsed-electric field extraction (PEF) technique is utilized to enhance mass transfer practices, it disrupts cell membranes. The sample lattice is put between two anodes in a group or a consistent stream treatment chamber and presented to repetitive electric frequencies (Hz–kHz) with an extreme (0.1–80 kV/cm) electric field for brief periods (from a few nanoseconds to a few milliseconds). A restrained PEF treatment is determined by the application of 100–10,000 μs treatment times with field strength of 0.5–1.0 kV/cm in the range of 1–10 kV/cm and short times (5–100 μs). The utilization of electric pulses causes the arrangement of reversible or irreversible pores in the cell films, characterized as electroporation or electro-permeabilization, which thus helps the fast dissemination of the solvents and the improvement of the mass exchange of intracellular mixes (Zbinden et al., 2013; Poojary et al., 2016). The particular analyte's extraction can be accomplished by regulating the pore arrangement, which is reliant on the force of the treatment connected (electric field quality, single pulse length, repetition frequency of the external electric pulses, duration, intensity and amplitude of particular energy input) and the cell attributes (i.e., shape, size, direction of introduction in the electric field). Depending on different factors, either reversible or irreversible pores are generated in the membranes. Irreversible pores formation is of great significance for abstraction of bioactive compounds from marine microorganisms (Zbinden et al., 2013; Raso et al., 2016).

4.3.3 MICROWAVE-ASSISTED EXTRACTION

In the last decade, MAE has been effectively utilized for the extraction of numerous biologically active compounds from a variety of natural cradles

(Navarro et al., 2007; Perino-Issartier et al., 2011). This technique has been reported to enhance the extraction yield of bioactive compounds from various matrices compared to traditional solid-liquid extraction (Kaufmann and Christen, 2002). MAE involves the extraction of high-value composites from natural cradles such as functional food ingredients, phytonutrients, pharmaceutical, and nutraceutical actives from biomass. MAE is an effective technique that proceeds with irradiation of microwave to hasten the removal of diverse compounds of natural cradles. It involves the use of electromagnetic waves with a frequency range of 300 MHz–1000 GHz (Patil and Shettigar, 2010).

MAE acts upon the quick and discerning centralized heating of moisture in the sample by microwaves. In general, the mechanism of MAE is through inter- and intramolecular friction, together with collision and movement of a very large number of charged ions, triggering quick heating of the reaction system and the subsequent breakdown of cell walls and membranes (Grosso et al., 2015). Because of centralized heating and maintenance of pressure within the sample cells, a fast exchange of extracted compounds from cells to the extracting solvent takes place. In MAE, both mass and heat incline slog in a similar direction, whereas it works in opposite directions in conventional heating. Therefore, a direct heating to the surface matrix of sample exists in conventional heating and it is subsequently followed by surface to the core heating through conduction (Choi et al., 2006).

Though the usage of MAE may vitiate bioactive carbohydrates because of localized high temperature (Routray and Orsat, 2012), numerous studies have reported the significant use of MAE for the extraction of bioactive materials from marine organisms. Several investigators have applied MAE for fish tissues (Reyes et al., 2009), oysters (Bhattacharya et al., 2015), and shrimp (Tsiaka et al., 2015). Acid hydrolysis of proteins for peptide mass mapping and tandem mass spectrometric analysis of peptides through MAE has also been reported (Zhong et al., 2005). Furthermore, MAE apposite the degradation of special organisms such as algae, have cells that are enclosed by a vibrant, intricate, and carbohydrate-rich cell wall that requires the breakdown of cell walls principally significant (Popper et al., 2011). Some investigators have deliberated the antioxidant activity of sulfated polysaccharides from Brown Seaweed (Yuan and Macquarrie, 2015) under different algae/water ratios, extraction times and pressures. These researches indicated that MAE is an effective technology.

4.3.4 PRESSURIZED LIQUID EXTRACTION

Pressurized liquid extraction (PLE) is also recognized as pressurized fluid extraction (PFE), accelerated solvent extraction (ASE), high-pressure solvent extraction or enhanced solvent extraction (Nieto et al., 2010), and was introduced in 1996 (Richter et al., 1996). PLE involves the application of pressure at temperatures higher than the normal boiling point of liquids. Combined high pressures and temperatures are used that utilize a small amount of solvent and provide faster extraction. When high temperature is applied, it increases the solubility of the analyte with high mass transfer rate, decreases the surface tension and viscosity of the solvent, hence improving extraction yield (Herrero et al., 2006a; Mendiola et al., 2007).

The PLE instrumentation is quite simple; it has a solvent reservoir that is coupled to a high-pressure pump through which solvent is introduced in the system. An oven where the extraction cell is placed, a valve is also present to maintain the pressure inside the system. For the collection of extract, a vial is placed at the end of the extraction system. Moreover, the framework could outfit with a condenser gadget for fast cooling of the resultant concentrate. The extraction time is variable as indicated by the example to be tested (Nieto et al., 2010). Ever since the early advent of PLE, there has been a great deal of exertion centered on getting bioactive mixes from marine sources. Presumably, the fundamental explanation behind the critical improvement of PLE-based systems is the likelihood of its robotization alongside the lessened extraction time and solvents required, as specified beforehand. PLE has been used, for example, to think carotenoids from *Dunaliella salina* microalgae. The best yields were obtained with ethanol and no essential extraction temperature and time (160°C and 17.5 min). The examination of compound depiction by tiptop liquid chromatography (LC) joined with diode display revelation (High-Performance Liquid Chromatography-Diode-Array Detection (HPLC-DAD) raised that the concentrates contained, other than all-trans-b—carotene and isomers, a couple of different minor carotenoids that seemed to contribute earnestly to the cancer prevention agent action of concentrates (Breithaupt, 2004; Herrero et al., 2006b).

PLE has been used, for example, to isolate carotenoids from brown macroalgae, *Himanthalia elongata*, *Eisenia bicyclis* and *Cystoseira abies-marina.* It was noted that ethanol at high temperatures yields higher fucoxanthin than other oxygenated carotenoids. Based on the selected solvent, PLE is reported as an idyllic system for the separation of bioactive phenolic complexes from marine algae (*Porphyra tenera*-nori, *Stypocaulon scoparium* and *Undaria pinnatifida*-wakame (Wang et al., 2010; Lopez et al., 2011).

4.3.5 SUPERCRITICAL FLUID EXTRACTION

SFE is an alternative extraction method which was introduced by Hannay and Hogarth in 1879. A significant attribute of SFE is the exceedingly diminished (frequently to zero) work of lethal natural solvents. CO_2 is the dissolvable most regularly used to remove bioactive mixes from common sources utilizing SFE. In fact, CO_2 has a progression of properties for bioactive extraction: it is fetched effective, its basic conditions are feasible (30.9°C and 73.8 bar), and it is an ecologically well-disposed dissolvable that is generally recognized as safe for use in the nutrition industry (Ibanez et al., 2012).

An interesting application of SFE is the screening of phenols, flavonoids such as phenolic compounds from marine cradles. An innovative hyphenated practice was advanced for the extraction and fortitude isoflavones from marine macroalgae (*Halopytis incurvus*, *Chondrus crispus*, *Sargassum vulgare*, *Hypnea spinella*, *Porphyra* sp., *U. pinnatifida*, and *Sargassum muticum*), *Spongiochloris spongiosa* freshwater algae, and *Scenedesmus* and *Nostoc* like cyanobacteria (Klejdus et al., 2010). Moreover, SC–CO_2 extraction use was reported to get the flavonoid antioxidants from *Chlorella vulgaris*. Authors compared SC–CO_2 extraction at 50°C, 310 bars, utilizing 50% aqueous ethanol as a modifier, with ultrasonic extraction with 50% aqueous ethanol. It was found that flavonoid contents gained under SFE conditions were considerably high as compared to UAE. It leads to a high antioxidant activity but correspondingly improved lung cancer metastasis inhibition (Wang et al., 2010).

4.3.6 PRESSURIZED HOT WATER EXTRACTION

Pressurized hot water extraction (PHWE), also known as superheated water extraction, pressurized low polarity water extraction or subcritical water extraction is a particular use of PLE with H_2O as extracting solvent. PHWE is built on using H_2O at temperatures above its atmospheric boiling point but keeping it as a liquid through pressure. In static PHWE, a batch process occurs in one or many extraction cycles while the solvent is replaced in between. In dynamic PHWE, it involves continuous flow and pumping of solvent at a selected flow rate by the extraction vessel that contains the sample. So it requires a somewhat more sophisticated HPLC pump in order to control the water flow rate and a pressure restrictor or a micrometering valve instead of static open/close valve (Herrero et al., 2006a; Mendiola et al., 2007).

HPLC-DAD, HPLC-Triple Quadrupole-Mass Spectrometers (QqQ-MS), and gas chromatography (GC)–MS were used to determine the chemical composition. Short-chain fatty acids turned out to be accountable for the antimicrobial activity, whereas the antioxidant activity is correlated with vitamin E, together with simple phenols, carmelization produces, and neoformed antioxidants isolated while the extraction at high temperatures (Plaza et al., 2010). The current research stated that PHWE at high temperatures is involved in extracting new antioxidant compounds as was done for microalga *Haematococcus pluvialis*. Different microalgae (*C. vulgaris*), macroalgae (*S. vulgare*, *Porphyra* spp., *C. abies*-marina, *S. muticum*, *U. pinnatifida*, and *Halopitys incurvus*), and plants (rosemary, thyme, and verbena) were studied for extraction via PLE (Plaza et al., 2010). Phycobiliproteins from the *Spirulina platensis* cyanobacteria were extracted through PLE. Capillary electrophoresis coupled with mass spectrometry (CE-MS) was applied to monitor and optimize the PLE of proteins from *S. platensis*. The combinational application of PLE and CE-MS permitted the achievement of extracts rich in phycobiliproteins in short extraction times (Herrero et al., 2006a).

4.4 ISOLATION AND PURIFICATION TECHNIQUES

In a characteristic technique to discover the marine bioactive, the compounds primarily extracted from the aquatic organisms, the excerpt is vetted for a special bioactivity, fractionated, and finally filtered to yield a single bioactive molecule. In addition, for an effectual process, it is necessary to clearly research methods such as membrane filtration systems, gel or size exclusion chromatography, ion-exchange column chromatography, and reversed-phase high-performance liquid chromatography (RP-HPLC) (Patil and Shettigar, 2010).

4.4.1 MEMBRANE FILTRATION

Membrane filtration can be used at different levels. Ultrafiltration with a high molecular weight cut-off can be used for the separation of non-hydrolyzed compounds. Membrane filtration can be operated at normal temperature, and there are no chemical reactions during the process. Membrane filtration can provide a high amount of separation compared to other chromatographic separation, and then, this technology always shows applications for the separation and recovery of bioactive compounds from diverse raw matrices (Li et al., 2012).

In recent years, many researchers have used membrane filtration as the first purification step. An example is the use of cross-flow microfiltration to make the galacturonic acid content of pectin increase from 68.0–72.2%. The membrane filtration technology has demonstrated a potential application in the separation of bioactive products.

4.4.2 GEL FILTRATION

The partially purified extract could be subjected to gel filtration chromatography (GFC) and ion-exchange chromatography, with reversed-phase C_{18} HPLC for the final purification step (Nazeer and Kumar, 2011; Zhang et al., 2012). GFC, likewise called size exclusion chromatography, has been utilized for more than 40 years for the isolation, desalting, and estimation of the atomic weight of certain molecules. GFC is the least difficult and mildest of the majority of the chromatography systems and isolates particles based on sizes. Its partition system is to channel atoms as per their sizes; some littler particles enter the pores of the gel and undergo a more drawn out separation, while bigger atoms indicate considerably shorter maintenance times. Thus, a critical favorable position of GFC is that elution conditions can be shifted to suit the sort of test and also the necessities for advanced cleaning, investigation or capacity without changing the division (Wang et al., 2017).

Trypsin inhibitor was purified from Yellowfin Tuna (*Thunnus albacores*) roe, followed by column chromatography on Sephacryl S-200, Sephadex G-50, and diethylaminoethyl-cellulose, and it was finally found to have an apparent molecular weight of 7×104 Da. (Wu et al., 2014). Sephadex is recommended for rapid group separation such as desalting and buffer exchange and it is widely used in the marine organism purification field (Bougatef et al., 2010; Hsu, 2010). Thus, GFC is cumbersome, time-consuming, and costly, its high selectivity and high resolution make this technology applicable to various separation and purification fields.

4.4.3 LIQUID CHROMATOGRAPHY (LC)

4.4.3.1 HIGH-PERFORMANCE LC

HPLC is an extensively applied method for the separation, identification, and purification of bioactive compounds (Singh et al., 2014). Analysis involving

HPLC could fully reflect the information of the sample and does not require the collection of fractions; preparative HPLC needs to consider the purity, production, production cycle, and operating cost. Furthermore, RP-HPLC is applied to fractionate samples based on their different assets, particularly when analyzing the structural and configurational assets of compounds (So et al., 2016; Song et al., 2016). The main advantages of this technology include the ease of operation, high resolution, and sensitivity, and it always uses a short time to get the elution spectra compared to the GFC and IEX, which each time is essentially about20–30 h long.

In recent years, HPLC is usually combined with qualitative equipment such as mass spectrometry (MS) and LC followed by tandem mass spectrometric recognition, a standard method for the characterization bioactive molecules (Vijaykrishnaraj and Prabhasankar, 2015), which has revealed a new era in the physical explication of compounds (Careri and Mangia, 2003); even though this technique is very particular and stout, it is exclusive and time-consuming (Mann and Jensen, 2003). Electrospray ionization and matrix-assisted laser desorption ionization (MALDI) have been identified as imperative tools for bioactive compounds detection and categorization (Leonil et al., 2000); matrix-assisted laser desorption/ionization time-of-flight (MALDI-TOF) mass spectrometric analysis is the backbone analysis for various hydrolysates or semipurified fractions (Singh et al., 2014) of marine microorganisms and so forth.

4.4.3.2 LIQUID CHROMATOGRAPHY-NUCLEAR MAGNETIC RESONANCE

The combination of chromatographic separation technique with nuclear magnetic resonance (NMR) spectroscopy is one of the powerful and time-saving approaches for the separation and structural interpretation of unidentified composite and mixes, particularly for the structure analysis of oxygen and light-sensitive materials. The online liquid chromatography-NMR (LC-NMR) practice permits the incessant recording of time changes as they appear in the chromatographic run, automated data procurement, and LC-NMR advances in speed and sensitivity of detection (Daffre et al., 2008). The recent introduction of pulsed field gradient technique in high-resolution NMR as well as three-dimensional technique improves the application in structure elucidation and molecular weight information. These new hyphenated techniques are helpful in the areas of pharmacokinetics, toxicity elucidations, drug metabolism, and drug discovery progression.

4.4.4 GAS CHROMATOGRAPHY

Coupling capillary column GC with Fourier-transform infrared spectrometer provides an effective resource for separating and recognizing the components of various mixtures. GC-MS technique can be directly interfaced with rapid scan mass spectrometer of different forms. The flow rate from a capillary column is normally kept low enough that the column output can be served directly into the ionization chamber of MS. The simplest mass detector in GC is the ion trap detector. In this technique, ions are created from the eluted sample by electron effect or chemical ionization and stowed in a radio frequency field; the ensnared ions are then evicted from the area of storage to an electron multiplier detector. The discharge is meticulous so that scanning on the basis of the mass-to-charge ratio is probable. The ions ploy detector is remarkably dense and less affluent than quadruple instruments. GC-MS instruments have been used for documentation of hundreds of constituents that are present in the natural and biological system (Daffre et al., 2008; Nagani et al., 2012).

4.4.5 SUPERCRITICAL FLUID CHROMATOGRAPHY

Supercritical fluid chromatography (SFC), the most technologically advanced extraction system, is a hybrid of gas, usually CO_2 and liquid chromatography that combines some of the best features of each. The liquid is impelled via a cylinder that holds the material needed to be extracted. Furthermore, the extract-laden liquid is driven into a parting chamber where the extract is parted from the gas and the gas is mended for reuse. This technique is an essential third kind of column chromatography that is starting to find application in numerous industrial, administrative and research laboratories. Coupled SFE-SFC and coupled SFE-GC and SFE-LC systems are available for a critical analysis.

KEYWORDS

- **bioactive compounds**
- **conventional extraction**
- **enzymatic hydrolysis**
- **marine phytochemicals**
- **membrane filtration**

REFERENCES

Azmir, J.; Zaidul, I.; Rahman, M.; Sharif, K.; Mohamed, A.; Sahena, F.; Jahurul, M.; Ghafoor, K.; Norulaini, N.; Omar, A. Techniques for Extraction of Bioactive Compounds from Plant Materials: A Review. *J. Food. Eng.* **2013,** *117,* 4, 426–436.

Bhattacharya, M.; Srivastav, P. P.; Mishra, H. N. Thin-Layer Modeling Of Convective And Microwave-Convective Drying of Oyster Mushroom (Pleurotus Ostreatus). *J. Food. Sci. Technol.* **2015,** *52*(4), 2013–2022.

Bougatef, A.; Nedjar-Arroume, N.; Manni, L.; Ravallec, R.; Barkia, A.; Guillochon, D.; Nasri, M. Purification and Identification of Novel Antioxidant Peptides from Enzymatic Hydrolysates of Sardinelle (Sardinellaaurita) by-Products Proteins. *Food. Chem.* **2010,** *118*(3), 559–565.

Breithaupt, D. E. Simultaneous HPLC Determination of Carotenoids used as Food Coloring Additives: Applicability of Accelerated Solvent Extraction. *Food. Chem.* **2004,** *86*(3), 449–456.

Careri, M.; Mangia, A. Analysis of Food Proteins and Peptides by Chromatography and Mass Spectrometry. *J. Chrom. A*, **2003,** *1000*(1), 609–635.

Choi, I.; Choi, S. J.; Chun, J. K.; Moon, T. W. Extraction Yield of Soluble Protein and Microstructure of Soybean Affected by Microwave Heating. *J. Food. Process. Pres.* **2006,** *30*(4), 407–419.

Cowan, M. M. Plant products as antimicrobial agents. *Clin. Microbiol. Rev*, **1999**, *12(4),* 564–582.

Daffre, S.; Bulet, P.; Spisni, A.; Ehret-Sabatier, L.; Rodrigues, E. G.; Travassos, L. R. Bioactive Natural Peptides. *Stud. Nat. Prod. Chem.* **2008,** *35*, 597–691.

Grosso, C.; Valentão, P.; Ferreres, F.; Andrade, P. B. Alternative and Efficient Extraction Methods for Marine-Derived Compounds. *Mar. Drug.* **2015,** *13*(5), 3182–3230.

Herrero, M.; Cifuentes, A.; Ibañez, E. Sub-and Supercritical Fluid Extraction of Functional Ingredients from Different Natural Sources: Plants, Food-By-Products, Algae And Microalgae: A Review. *Food. Chem.* **2006a,** *98*(1), 136–148.

Herrero, M.; Jaime, L.; Martín-Álvarez, P. J.; Cifuentes, A.; Ibáñez, E. Optimization of the Extraction of Antioxidants from Dunaliella Salina Microalga by Pressurized Liquids. *J. Agricul Food. Chem.* **2006b,** *54*(15), 5597–5603.

Hsu, K-C. Purification of Antioxidative Peptides Prepared from Enzymatic Hydrolysates of Tuna Dark Muscle by-Product. *Food. Chem.* **2010,** *122*(1), 42–48.

Ibanez, E.; Herrero, M.; Mendiola, J. A.; Castro-Puyana, M. Extraction and Characterization of Bioactive Compounds with Health Benefits from Marine Resources: Macro and Micro Algae, Cyanobacteria, and Invertebrates. In: *Marine BioactiveCompounds;* Maria, H., Ed.; Springer: Boston, 2012; pp 55–98.

Kaufmann, B.; Christen, P. Recent Extraction Techniques for Natural Products: Microwave-Assisted Extraction And Pressurised Solvent Extraction. *Phytochem. Anal.* **2002,** *13*(2), 105–113.

Klejdus, B.; Lojková, L.; Plaza, M.; Snoblova, M.; Sterbova, D. Hyphenated Technique for the Extraction and Determination of Isoflavones in Algae: Ultrasound-Assisted Supercritical Fluid Extraction Followed by Fast Chromatography with Tandem Mass Spectrometry. *J.Chrom. A.* **2010,** *1217*(51), 7956–7965.

Kong, W.; Liu, N.; Zhang, J.; Yang, Q.; Hua, S.; Song, H.; Xia, C. Optimization of Ultrasound-Assisted Extraction Parameters of Chlorophyll from Chlorella Vulgaris Residue after Lipid

Separation using Response Surface Methodology. *J. Food. Sci. Technol.* **2014,** *51*(9), 2006–2013.

Kristinsson, H. G.; Rasco, B. A. Fish Protein Hydrolysates: Production, Biochemical, and Functional Properties. *Cri. Rev. Food. Sci. Nut.* **2000,** *40*(1), 43–81.

Lavoie, J. M.; Stevanovic, T. Selective Ultrasound-Assisted Extractions of Lipophilic Constituents from Betula Alleghaniensis and B. Papyrifera Wood at Low Temperatures. *Phytochem. Analysis.* **2007,** *18*(4), 291–299.

Lee, J-W.; Jeffries, T. W. Efficiencies of Acid Catalysts in the Hydrolysis of Lignocellulosic Biomass Over A Range of Combined Severity Factors. *Bioresour. Technol.* **2011,** *102*(10), 5884–5890.

Leonil, J.; Gagnaire, V.; Mollé, D.; Pezennec, S.; Bouhallab, S. Application of Chromatography and Mass Spectrometry to the Characterization of Food Proteins and Derived Peptides. *J. Chrom. A.* **2000,** *881*(1), 1–21.

Li, K.; Xing, R.; Liu, S.; Li, R.; Qin, Y.; Meng, X.; Li, P. Separation of Chito-Oligomers with Several Degrees of Polymerization and Study of Their Antioxidant Activity. *Carbohydr. Polym.* **2012,** *88*(3), 896–903.

Loow, Y-L.; Wu, T. Y.; Jahim, J. M.; Mohammad, A. W.; Teoh, W. H. Typical Conversion of Lignocellulosic Biomass into Reducing Sugars Using Dilute Acid Hydrolysis and Alkaline Pretreatment. *Cellulose.* **2016,** *23*(3), 1491–1520.

Lopez, A.; Rico, M.; Rivero, A.; de Tangil, M. S. The Effects of Solvents on the Phenolic Contents and Antioxidant Activity of Stypocaulon Scoparium Algae Extracts. *Food. Chem.* **2011,** *125*(3), 1104–1109.

Mann, M.; Jensen, O. N. Proteomic Analysis of Post-Translational Modifications. *Nature Biotechnol.* **2003,** *21*(3), 255–261.

Mendiola, J. A.; Herrero, M.; Cifuentes, A.; Ibañez, E. Use of Compressed Fluids for Sample Preparation: Food Applications. *J. Chrom. A.* **2007,** 1152(1), 234–246.

Mukherjee, P. K. *Quality Control of Herbal Drugs: An Approach Ro Evaluation of Botanicals*; 1st ed. Vol 2; Business Horizons Publication:New Delhi, 2002; pp 379–447.

Nagani, K.; Kaneria, M.; Chanda, S. Pharmacognostic Studies on the Leaves of Manilkara Zapota L.(Sapotaceae). *Pharmacog. J.* **2012,** *4*(27), 38–41.

Navarro, D. A.; Flores, M. L.; Stortz, C. A. Microwave-Assisted Desulfation of Sulfated Polysaccharides. *Carbohydr. Polym.* **2007,** *69*(4), 742–747.

Nazeer, R.; Kumar, N. S. Purification and Identification of Antioxidant Peptide from Black Pomfret, Parastromateus Niger (Bloch, 1975) Viscera Protein Hydrolysate. *Food. Sci. Biotechnol.* **2011,** *20*(4), 1087.

Nieto, A.; Borrull, F.; Pocurull, E.; Marcé, R. M. Pressurized Liquid Extraction: A Useful Technique to Extract Pharmaceuticals and Personal-Care Products from Sewage Sludge. *Trend. Anal. Chem.* **2010,** *29*(7), 752–764.

Patil, P.; Shettigar, R. An Advancement of Analytical Techniques in Herbal Research. *J. Adv. Sci. Res.* **2010,** *1*(1), 8–14.

Perino-Issartier, S.; Zill-e-Huma.; Abert-Vian, M.; Chemat, F. Solvent Free Microwave-Assisted Extraction of Antioxidants from Sea Buckthorn (Hippophae rhamnoides) Food by-Products. *Food. Bioproc. Technol.* **2011,** *4*(6), 1020–1028.

Plaza, M.; Amigo-Benavent, M.; Del Castillo, M. D.; Ibáñez, E.; Herrero, M. Facts About the Formation of New Antioxidants in Natural Samples After Subcritical Water Extraction. *Food. Res. Int.* **2010,** *43*(10), 2341–2348.

Poojary, M. M.; Roohinejad, S.; Barba, F. J.; Koubaa, M.; Puértolas, E.; Jambrak, A. R.; Greiner, R.; Oey, I., Application of Pulsed Electric Field Treatment for Food Waste

Recovery Operations. In: *Handbook of Electroporation*; Miklavcic D (ed)Springer, Switzerland, 2016; pp 1–18.

Popper, Z. A.; Michel, G.; Hervé, C.; Domozych, D. S.; Willats, W. G.; Tuohy, M. G.; Kloareg, B.; Stengel, D. B. Evolution and Diversity of Plant Cell Walls: from Algae to Flowering Plants. *Annual. Rev. Plant. Biol.* **2011,** *62*, 567–590.

Raso, J.; Frey, W.; Ferrari, G.; Pataro, G.; Knorr, D.; Teissie, J.; Miklavčič, D. Recommendations Guidelines on the Key Information to be Reported in Studies of Application of Pef Technology in Food and Biotechnological Processes. *Innov. Food. Sci. Emerg. Technol.* **2016,** *37*, 312–321.

Reyes, L. H.; Mar, J. L. G.; Rahman, G. M.; Seybert, B.; Fahrenholz, T.; Kingston, H. S. Simultaneous Determination of Arsenic and Selenium Species in Fish Tissues Using Microwave-Assisted Enzymatic Extraction and Ion Chromatography–Inductively Coupled Plasma Mass Spectrometry. *Talanta.* **2009,** *78*(3), 983–990.

Richter, B. E.; Jones, B. A.; Ezzell, J. L.; Porter, N. L.; Avdalovic, N.; Pohl, C. Accelerated Solvent Extraction: A Technique for Sample Preparation. *Anal. Chem.* **1996,** *68(6),* 1033–1039.

Routray, W.; Orsat, V. Microwave-Assisted Extraction of Flavonoids: A Review. *Food. Biopro. Technol*, **2012,** 5(2), 409–424.

Selvamuthukumaran, M.; Shi, J. Recent Advances in Extraction of Antioxidants from Plant by-Products Processing Industries. *Food. Qual. Saf.* **2017,** 1(1), 61–81.

Silva, L.; Nelson, D.; Drummond, M.; Dufossé, L.; Glória, M. Comparison of Hydrodistillation Methods for the Deodorization of Turmeric. *Food. Res. Int.* **2005,** *38*(8), 1087–1096.

Singh, B. P.; Vij, S.; Hati, S. Functional Significance of Bioactive Peptides Derived from Soybean. *Peptides.* **2014,** *54*, 171–179.

So, P. B.; Rubio, P.; Lirio, S.; Macabeo, A. P.; Huang, H-Y.; Corpuz, M. J.; Villaflores, O. B. In Vitro Angiotensin I Converting Enzyme Inhibition by A Peptide Isolated from Chiropsalmus Quadrigatus Haeckel (Box Jellyfish) Venom Hydrolysate. *Toxicon.* **2016,** *119*, 77–83.

Song, R.; Zhang, K-Q.; Wei, R-B. In Vitro Antioxidative Activities of Squid (Ommastrephes Bartrami) Viscera Autolysates and Identification of Active Peptides. *Process. Biochem.* **2016,** *51*(10), 1674–1682.

Tejesvi, M. V.; Kini, K. R.; Prakash, H. S.; Subbiah, V.; Shetty, H. S. Antioxidant, Antihypertensive, and Antibacterial Properties of Endophytic Pestalotiopsis Species from Medicinal Plants. *Canadian. J. Microbiol.* **2008,** *54*(9), 769–780.

Troy, D.; Tiwari, B.; Hayes, M.; Ross, P.; Stanton, C.; Johnson, M.; Stengel, D.; O'Doherty, J.; FitzGerald, R.; McSorley, E. *Marine Functional Foods Research Initiative (NutraMara);* Marine Institute; 2017.

Tsiaka, T.; Zoumpoulakis, P.; Sinanoglou, V. J.; Makris, C.; Heropoulos, G. A.; Calokerinos, A. C. Response Surface Methodology Toward the Optimization of High-Energy Carotenoid Extraction from Aristeus Antennatus Shrimp. *Analyt. Chim. Acta.* **2015,** *877*, 100–110.

Vankar, P. S. Essential Oils and Fragrances from Natural Sources. *Resonan*, **2004,** *9*(4), 30–41.

Vijaykrishnaraj, M.; Prabhasankar, P. Marine Protein Hydrolysates: Their Present and Future Perspectives in Food Chemistry–A Review. *RSC. Advan.* **2015,** *5*(44), 34864-34877.

Wang, H-M.; Pan, J-L.; Chen, C-Y.; Chiu, C-C.; Yang, M-H.; Chang, H-W.; Chang, J-S. Identification of Anti-Lung Cancer Extract from Chlorella Vulgaris CC by Antioxidant Property Using Supercritical Carbon Dioxide Extraction. *Process. Biochem.* **2010,** *45*(12), 1865–1872.

Wang, L. Advances in Extraction of Plant Products in Nutraceutical Processing. *Handb. Nutraceuticals* **2011,** *2,* 15–52.

Wang, X.; Yu, H.; Xing, R.; Li, P. Characterization, Preparation, and Purification of Marine Bioactive Peptides. *BioMed. Res. Int.* **2017,** 2017.

Wong, P. Y. Y.; Kitts, D. D. Studies on the Dual Antioxidant and Antibacterial Properties of Parsley (Petroselinum Crispum) and Cilantro (Coriandrum Sativum) Extracts. *Food. Chem.* **2006,** *97*(3), 505–515.

Wu, J-L.; Ge, S-Y.; Cai, Z-X.; Liu, H.; Liu, Y-X.; Wang, J-H.; Zhang, Q-Q. Purification and Characterization of a Gelatinolytic Matrix Metalloproteinase from the Skeletal Muscle of Grass Carp (Ctenopharyngodon Idellus). *Food. Chem.* **2014,** *145*, 632–638.

Yuan, Y.; Macquarrie, D. Microwave Assisted Extraction of Sulfated Polysaccharides (Fucoidan) from Ascophyllum Nodosum and its Antioxidant Activity. *Carbohydr. Polym.* **2015,** *129,* 101–107.

Zbinden, M. D.; Sturm, B. S.; Nord, R. D.; Carey, W. J.; Moore, D.; Shinogle, H.; Stagg-Williams, S. M. Pulsed Electric Field (PEF) as an Intensification Pretreatment for Greener Solvent Lipid Extraction from Microalgae. *Biotechnol. Bioeng.* **2013,** *110*(6), 1605–1615.

Zhang, Y.; Duan, X.; Zhuang, Y. Purification and Characterization of Novel Antioxidant Peptides from Enzymatic Hydrolysates of Tilapia (Oreochromis Niloticus) Skin Gelatin. *Peptides*. **2012,** *38*(1), 13–21.

Zhong, H.; Marcus, S. L.; Li, L. Microwave-Assisted Acid Hydrolysis of Proteins Combined with Liquid Chromatography Maldi Ms/Ms for Protein Identification. *J. Am. Soc. Mass. Spectrom.* **2005,** *16*(4), 471–481.

Zou, T-B.; Jia, Q.; Li, H-W.; Wang, C-X.; Wu, H-F. Response Surface Methodology for Ultrasound-Assisted Extraction of Astaxanthin from Haematococcus Pluvialis. *Marin. Drug* **2013,** *11*(5), 1644–1655.

PART II

Industrial and Medicinal Applications of Phytochemicals

CHAPTER 5

BIOTECHNOLOGY APPROACH TO THE PRODUCTION OF PHYTOCHEMICALS: AN INTRODUCTION

HAMEED SHAH[1,2], ANDREW G. MTEWA[3,4], CHUKWUEBUKA EGBUNA[5,*], ANYWAR GODWIN[6], and DUNCAN C. SESAAZI[4]

[1]*CAS Key Laboratory for Biomedical Effects of Nanomaterials and Nanosafety, National Center for Nanoscience and Technology, Beijing, China*

[2]*University of Chinese Academy of Science, Beijing 100049, China*

[3]*Department of Chemistry, Institute of Technology, Malawi University of Science and Technology, Malawi*

[4]*Department of Pharmacology and Therapeutics, Mbarara University of Science and Technology, Uganda*

[5]*Department of Biochemistry, Faculty of Natural Sciences, Chukwuemeka Odumegwu Ojukwu University, Anambra State 431124, Nigeria. Tel.: +2347039618485*

[6]*Department of Plant Sciences, Microbiology and Biotechnology, Makerere University, P. O. Box 7062, Kampala, Uganda*

**Corresponding author. E-mail: egbuna.cg@coou.edu.ng; egbunachukwuebuka@gmail.com*

**ORCID: https://orcid.org/0000-0001-8382-0693*

ABSTRACT

This chapter details the biotechnological approach to the production of phytochemicals. The production of phytochemicals is usually known to be natural in plants. Recently, the propagation techniques have taken newer paths involving the preservation of plant species that saw the advantage of further manipulation of the growth environment of the plants to suit better growth patterns. Researchers understood that similar methods can be used to enhance the production of specific phytochemicals for potential drug leads, food additives, and fragrances. This first worked with the use of plant parts being grown on other plants, then in laboratory bioreactor setups and in modern days, the use of plant cell cultures. Plant cell culturing techniques have an advantage in that they are clean and allow flexibility in the attainment of the exact phytochemicals so desired. This technique is the best so far for propagation. However, it is an expensive venture that requires huge financial investments.

5.1 INTRODUCTION

The dependence of human beings on plants is an open secret which dates back to time immemorial, and still, human beings are constantly dependent on plants, for their curiosity of novel drugs isolation to treat different diseases and their use as fuels in certain parts of the world. The phytochemists are well aware of the fact that drugs isolation is a tedious job, which is more cynical in terms of natural products quality and yield, primarily due to environmental changes either accidentally in the form of acid rains, storms, and floods, or natural in the shape of latitude and altitude change of the same species in different locations of the world, and in some cases with effects from plants disease and so forth. These problems along with the advancement of knowledge in terms of understanding the plant pathways lead to the synthesis of different compounds. The effects of different nutritional and environmental factors on the plants make the scientists able to develop some artificial techniques to overcome their desire for obtaining some specific molecules or plants as a whole which could be better utilized for the welfare of human beings. In order to deal properly with these issues, there emerge a need to applying the technique of cell and tissue culture, which involve the in vitro cultivation of a desired plant in a controlled environment by providing all the requisites in an artificial environment such as the nutrition's required for its normal growth, including organic and inorganic salts, obligatory vitamins, plant growth hormones and amino acids and so forth. A well-established laboratory with the accomplished medium for growth is in the ominous need for this process to complete. The process makes researchers able to obtain the desired drugs in a time-independent manner from the natural environmental cycles. They also obtain the required product in more yield and without the internal changes of decomposition or other structural changes due to many factors involved with the growth of the plant in the natural environment and through the natural cycles. The technique is also valuable in terms of obtaining the desired drugs without leading to the deforestation of the plants.

Plant cell and tissue culture is an important area of phytochemistry which although being nascent, is highly important due to some aspects such as the source of obtaining different cost-effective phytochemicals, obtaining the desired products with better quality and quantity under a controlled and properly observed system, preserving the plant species, minimizing cost and labor effects and so forth.

Since the beginning of the 20th century, scientists have returned to nature as a source of potential drugs in pharmaceutical development (Georgiev, 2013; Pant, 2014). Plants constitute the largest part of the natural source of known natural products (over 80%) including pharmaceuticals in drug discovery (Smetanska, 2008). Many drugs in the market today came from the information and materials of indigenous knowledge of plants and their traditional uses (Pant, 2014). Already, over 25% of modern medicines are derived indirectly or directly from plants, especially with 60% in cancer therapy and 75% in infectious diseases, but also for drugs used in immunosuppression therapy and metabolic syndrome-related diseases' treatment (Georgiev, 2014). The most common and typical way of obtaining phytochemicals and other such important natural product compounds is through extraction from the source plants (Ochoa-Villarreal et al., 2016). In the course of the years, population increase and demand for plant products (medicines, clothing, and shelter), infrastructural development, and social gratification (illegal trade, religion, and pleasure) have contributed to the exploitation and depletion of plants including medicinal plants (De Luca et al., 2012; Chattopadhyay et al., 2004). Many plant species are still at a threat of depletion from their natural habitats in regard to the projected population growth of about a third by 2050 (FAO, 2009) which will have increased social demand for more plant use and exploitation. With the need for phytochemicals for continuous drug discovery and development, nutritional, and social needs, techniques of plant cell culture are providing alternatives for production and harvesting of bioactive compounds from plants without contributing to plant species' depletion. The culturing of plant cells is a latent source of important phytochemicals which can be used as pharmaceuticals, nutraceuticals, and food additives among which are colorants, flavors, and fragrances (Smetanska, 2008; Zhong, 2001). Plant cell culture has been practiced as early as the

1930s with the first patent for phytochemical production from cell culture filed in 1956 by Pfizer Inc., (Ratledge and Sasson, 1992). As reported by Smetanska (2008), the progression of the techniques in 1989, saw a phytochemical, Shikonin, being for the first time produced on an industrial scale by Mitsui Petrochemical Industries Ltd. Plant cell culture has established its place in commercial applications as well as in biochemistry, genetics, pharmaceutical, and cell biology research. To date, there are not less than 28,000 patents related to plant cell culture products in various fields of natural products applications (Ochoa-Villarreal et al., 2016) and this still remains a cutting age next-generation technology in phytochemical use and allied natural product compounds.

5.2 HISTORICAL BACKGROUND OF PLANT CELL/TISSUE CULTURE

The theoretical base for plant tissue culture is provided by the cell theory put forward by Schleiden in 1838 and Schwann in 1839. Thus, it is the regenerative ability of plant cells, which is readily expressed by plant cells and tissue culture, through the help of suitable chemical and environmental stimuli, soon after its separation from parent plant followed by in vitro culture. An auxiliary step was taken by the German Scientist, Gottlieb Haberlandt, whom in his address to the German Academy of Sciences in 1902 while discussing his experiments on cell culture growth, proposed that in future such studies will bring interesting information about cells in terms of their properties and potentialities. Unfortunately, he did not get any satisfactory results from his own culturing experiments, yet he is the pioneer in establishing the concept of totipotency and hence is known as the father of plant tissue culture. Soon after Gottlieb Haberlandt experiments and concept of plant tissue culture, much emphasis was given on this burgeoning field by scientists. In 1904, Hanning succeeded in culturing coniferous embryo that was successfully followed by Brown in 1906 with the culturing of Barley embryos. In 1922, the isolated root tips were cultivated by Kotte which successfully leads to tomato root tip culturing in 1934 by White. Laibach successfully rescued embryos from nonavailable seeds of a cross between Linum perenne × L. austriacum. Full embryo development in the ripening seeds of some species was achieved by Tukey in 1934. LaRue in 1936, also succeeded to develop the phenomena of precocious germination, followed by his attempts for ovary culturing in 1942, and first endospermic tissue culturing of immature maize in 1949. Loo in 1945 and Ball in 1946 likewise cultured the buds successfully. This effective achievement encouraged the scientists to further optimize the conditions for plant cell tissue culture. In 1962, Kanta reported the in vitro pollination and fertilization of plants, primarily based on the earlier achievements of Tuleke, who reported the culturing of cell colonies from Ginko pollen grains in 1953, successfully followed in 1969 by Street for his reports on the culture effected in the presence of organized and disorganized media and which make him able to study virus under the effects of these root media as well as to study plant physiologically under the effects of culture media. In other words, the scientists were aware regarding the role of media and different nutrient agents present in the media, thus having much elaborative potential on the applications effects of plant tissue culture.

5.3 NEED FOR PLANT CELL CULTURE

Different extraction methods are used to avail phytochemicals from the plant matrices sourced from the whole plant, or parts of it. This method avails phytochemicals that were naturally produced by the plants over some time in the past. Some of the challenges with relying on natural source plant produced phytochemicals are as follows:

5.3.1 TYPICAL LOW YIELDS

Active compounds of interest are typically in low concentrations from the source plant-derived matrices (Ochoa-Villarreal et al., 2016), an undertaking which usually proves to be economically costly. For example, a 2-kg sample may yield concentrations in the order of nanograms of a particular compound of interest, and there is no control to that.

5.3.2 SLOW GROWTH RATES OF SOURCE PLANTS

The natural slow growth of some plants have a reducing effect on the production potential of phytochemicals. This means the plant may take years to grow only to produce very low concentrations of desired compounds.

Synthesis of desired phytochemicals provides an alternative route of availing these compounds for use, especially for simpler structured molecules. However, multiple chiral centers for many natural compounds including phytochemicals make total synthesis difficult particularly where they are region- and/or stereo-specific.

5.4 ADVANTAGES OF CELL CULTURING

There are several advantages of producing and ultimately harvesting phytochemicals from plants using plant cell cultures over conventional methods of extraction from plant parts or whole plants. This section highlights some of the advantages which are worth noting and investing for.

5.4.1 CONSERVATION OF PLANT SPECIES

Owing to the depletion of most plant species, the laboratory scientist should be the last to endanger them more and to contribute to the damage. Undertaking plant cell cultures ensure that the actual plant is left alive to blossom whilst science of metabolite harvesting is as well flourishing. The cells can be multiplied and at the same time is kept alive as viable cell lines for further studies.

5.4.2 CONTAMINATION FREE

With the detailed care invested in the biotechnology and the bioprocess, yields are free from insects and microbes (Hussain et al., 2012). It is largely very difficult to ensure microbe-free phytochemical yields from the conventional plant part or tissue extraction technology which is to some extent, likely to affect biochemical analyses due to metabolic activities of the microbes.

5.4.3 HIGH YIELDS AT A REDUCED LABOR COST

Since the cell growth bioprocess is controlled and automated, there will be no need for laborious activities once the set up is done apart from regular monitoring.

High acceptability: Consumer acceptability for plant cell culture products is higher as consumers get to have surety that the products are no-GMO (Murthy et al., 2015).

5.4.4 FREE FROM CLIMATIC AND SOIL CONDITIONS INFLUENCES

Naturally, some phytochemicals may not favorably develop in particular climatic conditions and soil profiles in which the plant is growing. Cell culture phytochemical production can be designed to develop any particular type of metabolites of interest under controlled conditions to or toward targeted desired yields. This means, cells from any type of plant despite where they are traditionally found can be grown at any placc but in controlled conditions to produce the desired phytochemicals in vitro (Hussain et al., 2012).

5.4.5 ENSURE A STABLE SUPPLY CHAIN

Harvesting phytochemicals and other natural compounds from plant cell culturing technology act more as a renewable source of plant compounds with an add-on that one may wish to control production depending on need, thereby establishing a robust chain of supply for various compounds (Ochoa-Villarreal et al., 2016).

Pros of plant tissue culture

The use of plant tissue culture offers several benefits, which include the following:

1. It enables the rapid production of mature plants, in large quantities, which do not require much space or large vessels for storages (Grout, 2017).
2. Tissue culture greatly enhances the production of plants from recalcitrant seeds or seeds with very low germination rates.
3. One can significantly shorten the time required for harvesting since it is no longer necessary to wait for the entire life cycle of seed development, especially for plants that take longer to mature and side (Sharma, 2015).
4. Plant tissue culture is an indispensable tool for producing disease-free plant material.
5. Tissue culture is ideal for the production of facsimile or exact copies of plants with particularly desirable characteristics; for example, in this case, is plants which produce standard quantities of particular compounds of interest

6. It is useful in the mass production of planting material, especially for commercial purposes.
7. Through plant tissue culture, it is possible to have a continuous supply of young planting material throughout the year, irrespective of the season, once an ideal plant tissue culture line is established (George, 2008; Sharma 2015).
8. Plant tissue culture is an ingenious method of plant propagation while bypassing the availability of seeds or even the natural pollinators of the plants. It is also useful for plants that are sterile or do not produce viable seeds.
9. Because plant tissue culture does not require the use or harvesting of a whole plant or large parts of it, it is ideal for cloning of critically endangered plants since the mother plant is virtually left intact.
10. With tissue culture through micropropagation, one usually produces more robust plants. This results in faster growth in comparison to similar plants produced by conventional methods such as seeds or cuttings (Sharma, 2015).
11. Plant material needs little attention between subcultures and there is no labor or materials required for watering, weeding, spraying, and so forth,; micropropagation is most advantageous when it costs less than traditional methods of multiplication (George and Debergh, 2008).

Cons of plant tissue culture

Much as plant tissue culture comes with all these advantages, and benefits, it comes with some challenges. Key among them is the facilities:

1. The resources: Tissue culture requires a highly specialized laboratory for it to be carried out. These laboratories are expensive to set up and run. They require specialized equipment and reagents.
2. The personnel: Tissue culture requires highly trained and skilled personnel to run the laboratories. This staff requires a lot in terms of resources need for training them.
3. Once the parent stock is infected, sick, or susceptible to disease, all the resultant material will possess this undesirable characteristic.
4. Plant tissue culture can result in reduced genetic diversity. This can come about if the current plant stock has a similar genetic makeup. Reduced or low genetic diversity reduces the chances of the plants resisting diseases and pathogens that may attack the plant in future.

5. Not all plants can be successfully cultured by this method because of lack of knowledge on the right medium or because of the secondary metabolites produced by some plants, which inhibit the growth of the explant (an excised portion of a plant from which plant tissue culture is initiated). There are no a one-size fits all as different plant species require differences in their protocols such as the type of nutrient medium among others. As a result, protocols need to be developed for individual plant species, and this is often a tedious process of trial and error.
6. It is a highly laborious and technical exercise and if not well conducted, it can result in contamination of the entire stock.

5.5 BIOTECHNOLOGY APPROACH TO PHYTOCHEMICAL PRODUCTION

The in vitro biotechnology of plant cell culturing involves engineering of metabolic pathways and conditions and is vital for today's and next-generation production of phytochemicals. These activities are conducted on plant cells outside (detached from) the plant as opposed to in vivo activities that are conducted on cells that are well within or surrounded by other plant cells in a plant. Plant cell secondary metabolism engineering mainly aims at lowering levels of undesirable compounds, increasing desired phytochemical content and introducing the production of novel compounds into specific plants (Kirakosyan et al., 2009).

Considerations to invest in an aseptic laboratory environment and apparatus with qualified personnel are required. The first step is to obtain a callus from any part of the whole plant containing cells that are dividing and is known to be highly productive. The knowledge of portions of high productivity helps to maximize the availability of, particularly desired compounds. The callus' friable portions are transferred into a premade liquid medium, made as homogenous as possible, and is then stored under suitable environmental conditions (agitation, air, temperature, light, and others) (Chattopadhyay et al., 2004). The following section outlines details in the techniques used in getting good phytochemical yields from plant cell culturing.

Naturally, plants produce tiny organic molecules involved directly in metabolic processes of development and growth, called primary metabolites. However, they also produce secondary metabolites, which are relatively more abundant in higher plants for chemical defense against insects, microorganisms, and higher predators and for attracting pollinators and seed dispersers (Bhojwani and Dantu, 2013). Among these secondary metabolites is an overwhelming range of phytochemicals that man has used and is still using in medicine, nutrition, cosmetics, and neuro-manipulation among other areas. Science has developed strategies to obtain phytochemicals from these plant materials.

5.6 ENHANCING PHYTOCHEMICAL PRODUCTION

Plant cell culturing and component harvesting and plant cell biotechnology, in general, is made more convenient and attractive through the application of system biology and functional genomics (Kirakosyan et al., 2009). Productivity in a bioreactor can be enhanced by a proper strategy of cultivation, timely feeding of appropriate metabolic precursors, and extraction of any undesired intracellular metabolites (Chattopadhyay et al., 2004).

5.6.1 DELIBERATE ISOLATION OF HIGH YIELDING CELL LINES

The best choice of the parent plant, known to have high levels of the product desired for the induction of callus is always a good starting point. This gives a guarantee of getting best yielding cell lines. This process is systematic and involves actual screening of the wide range of cell clones, among those that are capable of producing highly. The identification and selection of these cell lines can be achieved well if the desired product is pigmented. Selection can be done visually, or by using analytical techniques.

5.6.2 MUTATION STRATEGIES

The involvement of mutation strategies has also been used to get high yielding cell lines. Here, a large cell population is exposed to a toxic inhibitor or environmental stress. Cells that are capable of resisting this procedure are the ones that will grow.

5.6.3 STRESS MODIFICATION

Phytochemical production can also be enhanced by a deliberate manipulation of the culture environment. Many secondary metabolite pathways' expressions can easily be modified by external factors such as stress factors, nutrient levels, growth regulators, and light. Many of the constituents of plant cell culture media are important determinants of growth and yielding of phytochemicals (Misawa, 1985).

5.6.4 CULTURE ENVIRONMENT OPTIMIZATION

The environment in which cultures are grown has proven to be one of the most effective factors in determining the yield of phytochemicals. Temperature is required to be checked, controlled, and specified for each and every species. For example, lowering the temperature at the cultivation stage increases total fatty acid content in each cell, dry weight (Toivonen et al., 1992). Kreis and Reinhard (1992) reported that upon maintaining the temperature at 19°C, digitoxin was transformed to digoxin most favorably, but at 32°C, the yielding of purpurea glycoside was favored more in *Digitalis lanata* cell cultures.

Light application strongly stimulated anthocyanin accumulation in cell cultures of *Vitis hybrids* and *Dausus carota* (Seitz and Hinderer, 1988). This process was also found to affect sesquiterpenes' composition in *Matricaria chamomilla* callus cultures (Mulder-Krieger et al., 1988). It is not only the application of light that positively affects phytochemical yields, light withdrawal also positively contributes to yields as was the case with callus cultures of *Citrus limon* that prompted monoterpenes accumulation (Mulder-Krieger et al., 1988).

5.6.5 pH OF THE MEDIUM

The pH of the culture medium before autoclaving is usually between 5 and 6 and extremes pHs are avoided. As the culture grows hydrogen power in the cells changes. *Chenopodium rubrum* cell culture suspension indicated that an increase in the medium pH from 4.5 to 6.3 enhanced the cytosolic pH of the cells by 3.0 units and their vacuolar pH by about 1.3 units (Husemann et al., 1992).

5.7 TYPES OF PLANT CELL CULTURE

Cell culturing basically consists of three main types: primary cell culture, semicontinuous cell cultures, and continuous cell cultures.

1. Primary cell culture: Cell culturing which involve the direct culturing of cells separated from the parent plant tissue is called primary cell culture. Cell culturing basically starts with biopsy of the tissue isolated from the source (~1 cm^3) through dissection from tissue or organ of the parent organism. Following the dissection, the next step involves the isolation of single cell suspension which is carried out by the removal of cell basal membrane or cell basal connections. The techniques may involve physical interferences, such as cutting with the help of surgical knives, or chemical digestion methods such as using certain chemicals or may involve biological digestion methods such as using enzymes trypsin or collagenase and so forth. In the next steps, these obtained cell suspensions are further purified through different methods, including the serial dilutions along with centrifugations, adherence, antibody coupling to a fluorescent dye, microdissection, and so forth. After the maximum purification, these culturing cells are finally transferred to the cell culture vessels, where the cells being freed from the cellular connections are able to stick to the culture vessel surface while the nonsticky cells and their residuals are removed from the cell culture vessels by centrifugation and so forth, as mentioned in the above lines, which lead to the completion of this initial step in the cell culturing. Primary cell culturing is a tedious job, and could be maintained for a limited time because the cell media is consumed along with the filling up of the space provided for cell growth. It is very important to note that apart from a lot of efforts to isolate and culture pure cells in culture vessels, still there are some other cellular organelles or cells on the cell culture vessels, such as fibroblasts, and toxins and so forth. In other words, it is not completely possible to culture pure cell on the culture vessels during this primary culture, yet, it is still noticeable that this primary culture grown still greatly resembles the tissue culture obtained from the parent organism biopsy, and the complete purification involve further steps, after which the pure cell culture is usually obtained in the secondary culturing by passaging. Thus, this step has drawbacks of not pure cell culture and having limited cell growth and proliferation ability. Then their need further measures to overcome these shortcomings. In the next step, the propagation of the undesired cells could be stopped by different techniques such as through the introduction of medium suitable only for the growth of the required cell culture which may lead to the death of the undesired cells. In the next steps,

providing new cell media for the plant growth could also provide more nutrition and space for the plant cell culture growth.

2. Semicontinuous cell culture: This cell culture is basically dependent on the primary cell culture and involves the further growth of the primary cell culture in a different environment. In semicontinuous cell culture, the medium is continuously changed for 24 h and the cells are also usually diluted, thus making room for the culture growth. However, after a certain point, it becomes unsuitable to continue the culture due to the building up of increasing number of competitors, predators, contaminants, and metabolites. Fibroblasts are still present here, yet the ratio of toxins is almost negligible.

   This culture has the advantage of obtaining more cells with more specificity because here we can introduce some new space and new rich nutrition medium per the specificity of the cell line we are desired in the cell culture, as a result of which we get the specific cells more suitable for their application. The cells in this culture retain the actual number of chromosome pairs and are thus diploid. These are clones cell lines and thus even a single cell is capable to give rise to subsequent generations. Their passaging ability is between 60 and 100 times, and hence considered more suitable in virology. These cultures are used primarily in human chickenpox virus and poliomyelitis virus production.
3. Continuous cell culture: As the name confirms, in these cultures, the cells are grown in a medium where the nutrition is continuously supplied and the grown cell culture is removed simultaneously. In practice, a volume of fresh culture medium is added automatically at a rate proportional to the growth rate of the algae, as for example, while an equal volume of culture is removed, thus maintaining the culture at a maximum growth rate. The process involves the growth of the culture in a medium with a hole, in which after the addition of the fresh media, the old media flow out automatically. The culture has the ability to be well suspended with a maximum concentration of O_2 and CO_2. These cell cultures are also known as immortal, or transformed lines, and are heteroploid with an abnormal number of chromosomes usually not present in pairs. These cell lines are capable to pass through thousands of passages. These cells are obtained by the engineered or spontaneous transformations of the cells in vitro or by the culturing of tumor cells such as HeLa cells or

RD cell lines. Its early development involves the microbial generation for industrial and research purpose.

5.8 BASIC REQUIREMENTS OF PLANT CELL/TISSUE CULTURING

Cell culture is basically an art of keeping live the cells of organisms in an artificial environment by providing all the basic requirements for their normal growth in terms of their food supplementation along with the required hormones and so forth. The cell culturing has covered the areas of vaccine formation, monoclonal antibody, enzyme production, growth factor preparation, hormone production, and interleukin production. The development of regenerative medicine concept is another area of application of cell culture. These all methods involve the transformation/differentiation of the cell from the initial stage of the selective product which mainly depends on the internal cellular program and the outside environmental factors.

As mentioned in the above lines, special working conditions are necessary for cell culturing involving the handling of the cell by sophisticated instruments in the well-equipped labs with sterile conditions and proper planning for the safe contamination of the waste. Cell culturing is achieved only when proper conditions are maintained for the safety of the laboratory. An environment suitable for the reproduction of the cells in the desired direction involves factors such as free space and nutrition support. After the initial growth cell passaging is the desired action which can be achieved keeping in mind the factors such as cell concentration, pH of the new environment, and the time interval between the two passaging actions and so forth. Below are given a short summary of the requirements for maintaining a cell culture and the lab in proper conditions.

5.8.1 LAB SAFETY

Lab safety could be categorized as problems related to the working environment and working material. The working environment involves the flow of air along with the passage of water and so forth, that is, the environment of the lab and definitely some surrounding area, which need to be properly maintained to achieve the best health conditions for the working scientists as well as for the cultured cells and other materials such as chemicals and so forth. In the second category of working materials, there include equipment's, solvents, and other reagents. Chemicals are to be considered as the most erudite and important part of the lab in terms of their inactivity by mishandling along with their corrosive, toxic, mutagenic, and inflammable properties. On the other hand, the proper handling of the instruments is also an important factor in lab safety perspective as it could lead to serious accidents. Different infections are the major safety concerns of the related materials, as the plant cell cultures may contain different viruses, bacteria, and so forth, which may cause the workers to spread different infections in their body per their originating organism from which they had been isolated and they may have these pathogens at the time of handling them. Problems in the cell culture laboratory could harm the human health and the environment. Legal regulations should be firmly followed along with work and security protocols, thoroughly analyzed and procedure well as per the requirements of the location environment and lab conditions. The staff should also be well educated in terms of handling the objects inside the lab and following the rules and regulations. Some important procedures prepared by National Institutes of Health, World Health Organization, and so forth.

5.8.2 CONSTITUENTS OF MEDIA

Media is an important component of the normal cell growth during plant culturing. It should have to provide all the components of the cell culture, which mimics the natural environment that is provided by soil. For example, it should be able to provide 17 essential elements of carbon (C), oxygen (O), hydrogen (H), nitrogen (N), potassium (K), calcium (Ca), phosphorus (P), magnesium (Mg), sulfur (S), iron (Fe), nickel (Ni), chlorine (Cl), manganese (Mn), zinc (Zn), boron (B), copper (Cu), and molybdenum (Mo). Some species growth also requires the presence of more elements of aluminum (Al), cobalt (Co), iodine (I), and sodium (Na). Each plant strain shows a different tendency in growth toward a specific media. Hence, it is very important to maintain specific conditions for the growth of a cell culture in a media.

5.8.3 MACRONUTRIENTS

These are the constituents required in a concentration of more than 0.5 mM/L. The main chemical present in high concentration is the sucrose, one of the main source of C, O, and H for the plant growth. In common mediums, it is used in the concentration range of 20,000–30,000 mg/mL. It acts as a full house for the cell growth along with its role in metabolite signaling. As per the nature of media, other sources of energy such as glucose, sorbitol, raffinose, and so forth may also be used in the medium. Other micronutrients include salts such as $Ca_3 (PO_4)_2$, $Ca (NO_3)_2$, KNO_3, $MgSO_4.7H_2O$, $NaNO_3$, $NH_4H_2PO_4$, NH_4NO_3, NaH_2PO_4. H_2O, $(NH_4)_2SO_4$, $CaCl_2.2H_2O$, $CaCl_2$, KCl, KH_2PO_4, K_2SO_4, and so forth, the concentration of which varies per medium.

5.8.4 MICRONUTRIENTS

These are the constituents required in a concentration less than 0.05 mg/L, and include mainly the metals of iron, molybdenum, copper, zinc, manganese, and boron. These micronutrients are extremely important for the plant growth, although being in very small quantities. Usually, these elements are also introduced as salts in the medium, but in case of iron, usually chelating agents such as EDTA and so forth, which make iron able to be absorbed in low pH.

5.8.5 VITAMINS

These are the organic supplements added to the plant's cultures required for their metabolism, with their role as metabolic cofactors or enzyme cofactors. For example, thiamine is an important cofactor for carbohydrates metabolism and is added in a concentration of 0.1–5 mg/L to the medium. The other commonly used vitamins are pantothenic acid (B5), pyridoxine (B6), nicotinic acid (B3), and myoinositol.

5.8.6 pH

Different types of cells favor different conditions for their growth in terms of pH effect. Mostly, the cell cultures favor the normal growth at basic pH between 7.4 and 7.8. However, some cultures, for instance, the epidermal cells can be grown at acidic media with a pH 5.5; yet, it has not been universally adopted. Phenol red is commonly used as an indicator of pH change. At pH 7.4, it embarks red color, while with a decrease in pH to 7.0, it becomes orange, with a little more decrease to pH 6.5, it then becomes yellow, pink at basic 7.6, while purple at 7.8.

5.8.7 PLANT HORMONES

These supplementary materials are added frequently to the serum-free media and are usually not expressed in the general constituents for any media. The hormones are usually supplemented to the media as organic complex material such as orange juice, tomato juice, coconut water, casein hydrolysate, yeast extract, and so forth.

5.8.8 PLANT GROWTH REGULATORS

Determine the development pathway of plant cells and tissues in the culture medium. The auxins, cytokinins, and gibberellins are most commonly used plant growth regulators. These stimulate cell division and regulate the growth and differentiation of shoots and roots on explants and embryos in liquid or semisolid liquid cultures. Skoog and Miller studied the effects of two plant hormones as growth regulators first and found that high concentration of cytokinin in comparison to auxin lead to better shoots production, while a reverse lead to better roots production. The organic complex material added to the media usually act as a source of plant hormones and as the source of plant growth regulator.

5.9 APPLICATIONS OF PLANT CELL CULTURE

Cell culturing could be applied in different directions if is grown by a proper procedure and maintained under appropriate conditions. Perhaps the big advantage of this technique is that new reshaped cells are obtained in a selective environment, which can be further engineered per our requirements.

5.9.1 AGRICULTURE

Food is the cradle of energy which is primarily obtained from plants. Owing to ecological pollution, along with the political instability in some regions and the low economic and instrumental strength of farmers in some regions, the quality and quantity of food are affecting greatly. Moreover, bad weathers, the soil infertility, annual nature of plants, and the natural low production ability of certain plants along with the increasing population are some extra contributing factors in making the situation worse. In this scenario, the plant cell culturing is a greater hope to overcome these issues because the better quantity and quality could be achieved by applying the artificial environmental, nutritional and genetic modifications in the cells culturing of the plants. For instance, the annual plants could be and have been produced throughout the year for their food and other purposes by providing the artificial environment. Moreover, through genetic engineering, the genes which are causing diseases in plants have been changed with the healthy ones in their seeds. Similarly, the genes involved in the high production of food could be transferred from one plant species to another through genetic engineering, and then their planting could lead to better food. In the scientifically approved environment, the food production is much better than the plants grown by farmers in their traditional manners.

5.9.2 INDUSTRY

Plant cell tissue culture is also actively contributing to the industry. Even in the form of agricultural applications, it is contributing a good asset to the market. Plant tissue culture is being grown both in the developed and developing countries. The plant cell cultures are established and marketed to the laboratories to be available to a scientist for their ongoing research. The plants cultured through plant cell culturing are sold locally and internationally, and a good financial reward is collected from them. The plants culturing for the financial purpose include plants for ornamental purposes, plants culturing in area with high species rate and then their sale to areas or countries of low or not available species, plants growth for specific microbes collection and then those microbes sale at national or international level, plants culturing for specific metabolites production by pharmaceutical industry are some of the applications of plant cell culturing in the industry.

5.9.3 MEDICINAL

Secondary metabolites of medicinal importance are produced through this technique. The production of bioactive metabolites through biotechnological approaches, specifically plant tissue culture is regarded to be on the same side with the industrial agricultural production for secondary metabolites.

5.9.3.1 ANTICANCER DRUGS

Taxol is a common anticancerous drug isolated from the inner bark of several *Taxus* species. The procedure is very costly and laborious, yet the final yield is also very low. Moreover, a high proportion of the plants are destroyed for taxol isolation. Although related procedures, such as total synthesis, or semisynthetic precursors has also been applied, yet the problems of cost and the laborious extraction are the issues. To overcome this diseases of cancer by taxol, plant cell tissue culturing is considered to be the best option. The preliminary studies carried out during the optimization of the culture favors the increased production of taxol and related toxoids from the *Taxus* sp.; however, still there is need to study factors such as gene involvement, biosynthetic pathways, their regulation and so forth, and after all finalization, the technique could be applied commercially.

5.9.3.2 ANTIDIABETIC

Diabetes is a disease increasing day by day, both in the developed and non-developed world. Basically consisting of two types, the type 1 is totally insulin dependent while the type 2 involves primarily usage of some drugs. Both the insulin and the drugs or secondary metabolites such as quercetin used in the diabetes treatment are widely cultured. It is also interesting, that the insulin produced through recombinant deoxyribonucleic acid technology, involving the use of *Escherichia coli* and yeast is safer than the one reported from porcine because the human-derived insulin may contain disease of the parent organisms. On the other hand, secondary metabolites such as quercetin and so forth which have anti-diabetic efficiency is been synthesized by plant cell culture.

5.10 APPLICATIONS OF PLANT TISSUE CULTURE

Plant tissue culture applications involve the aseptic culture of cells, tissues, organs, and their components under specified chemical and physical conditions in vitro. These applications cut across several fields in the plant sciences including conservation biology, agriculture, forestry, plant biotechnology, and horticulture among others (Bhatia and Dahiya, 2015). They include:

1. Providing a useful research tool in phytoremediation studies. Results from plant tissues culture research on phytoremediation can be used to predict the responses of plants to environmental pollutants. This can lead to remodeling of phytoremediation designs and subsequently lower of the conventional whole phytoremediation experiments (Doran, 2009).
2. The conservation of endangered plant species that faced with extinction. The risk is eminent in plants with a complex reproductive biology and threatened by loss of habitat, small population sizes, and their long life cycle (Loyola-Vargas and Vázquez-Flota, 2006).
3. Germplasm storage: The ability to store germplasm for prolonged periods of time especially for plants that are propagated by vegetative means or have recalcitrant seeds is limited when using conventional or traditional means. The use of plant tissue culture overcomes this barrier when applied to other complementary techniques such as cryopreservation under liquid nitrogen at −196°C, which allows for the preservation for decades (Grout, 2017).
4. Production of secondary metabolites: When subjected to the right conditions, the growth and division of cells from an explant can give rise to a mass of undifferentiated cells known as callus. This can be maintained on a semisolid medium as or grown as a suspension of cells in liquid medium. The growing cells of different plant species can yield many valuable secondary metabolites including elite compounds such as pharmaceuticals and cosmetics. Cells can also be grown in a batch culture or grown over longer periods with a limited, continual harvest (Loyola-Vargas and Vázquez-Flota, 2006; Grout, 2017).
5. The production of disease or pathogen-free seeds or plants especially where traditional propagation methods such as the use of cuttings have fueled the spread of diseases in crops. Bacterial pathogens will typically infest the vascular tissues that provide transport to the shoot and root. Viral particles and phytoplasmas, however, are significantly limited by the absence of vascular tissue in the terminal tissues of the meristematic dome (Grout, 2017).
6. Large-scale commercial production of plants used for example in the flower industry and landscaping among others. The regeneration of in vitro plantlets is the supports production en masse of clonal

populations of field or glass-house established plants. This is of particular value when dealing with crops that are, conventionally, vegetatively propagated, for example, fruits, ornamentals and forest trees (Grout, 2017).

7. Plant tissue culture contributes to crop selection and improvement by providing a non-seasonal multiplication system for elite and rare, material. It also provides a selection system that can be used to screen for potentially valuable crop characteristics. In addition, it also facilitates the production of genetically modified plants (Grout, 2017).
8. Research for screening plant cells instead of whole plants for specific purposes such as yield or production of certain compounds, herbicide resistance tolerance among others.
9. Chromosome doubling and induction of polyploidy. These include doubled haploid, tetraploids, and other forms of polyploids. Haploids in plant breeding programs are a useful way of shortening the time required to complete backcross programs. This facilitates the retention of the character under transfer and stabilizes the transferred genetic materials in a homozygous form. The production of dihaploid plants from haploid cultures shortens the time taken to achieve uniform homozygous lines and varieties. The use of haploids in breeding programs makes it possible to isolate individual genomes irrespective of whether they are dominant or recessive (Kumar and Loh, 2012).
10. It can be used to cross distantly related species by protoplast fusion and generation of the novel hybrids (Sharma, 2015).

5.11 LARGE SCALE APPLICATIONS OF PLANT CELL CULTURING

Bioreactors are critical for successful yielding of phytochemicals in an industrial setting (Bhojwani and Dantu, 2013). Care must be taken in the selection of suitable bioreactors to avoid affecting metabolic pathways. In this regard, aggregation of cells, aeration, proper mixing, and shear sensitivity should be taken into account (Chattopadhyay et al., 2004).

It should be noted that plant root and tissue cultures have great genetic stability and at times, better metabolic performances than cell line cultures but their operating techniques and bioreactor development are highly laborious and require huge investments (Flores and Curtis, 1992). Despite that, plant cell cultures have a higher industrial application potential than plant organ and tissue cultures because of closely related know-how invested in microbial cultures over the years. This does not mean the two methods are entirely the same, the differences in the growth type and nature of the cells require the plant cell line to be further developed beyond the microbial cell culture (Payne et al., 1987).

5.12 CONCLUSION AND FUTURE PERSPECTIVES

It is evident that plant cell culturing is involved in our daily life from research to the most dependent things of food and medicine. We are taking help from this technique by enhancing every area of our life related to the plants. It helps us to grow more plants and trees, both as source of medicine as well as for our domestic uses of ornamental or other daily uses, it also helps us to grow more food from plants, along with its support for complicated medicines from plants for the notorious diseases such as cancer and so forth, plant cell cultures have already had a unique and important role in bioproduction, bioconversion, or biotransformation, and biosynthetic studies. From future perspective, it may help in transgenic plant studies, through which it may help to accelerate the conventional multiplication rate of crops related plants, which is important to strive drought in some regions of the world, where the crops are wiped out by diseases, while all the currently employed techniques will definitely improve both methodologically and technically, which will bring more future to human life.

Although phytochemical production through in vivo plant culturing is viable in the laboratory, the feasibility of the bioprocesses and recurrent low yields of compounds of interest from original materials limit its applications in industries (Kirakosyan et al., 2009). The other challenge with cell culture phytochemical production is that the process requires huge capital expenditure and running costs. It is not easy for low-cost production units to have these technologies in place.

See Chapter 6 and 7 for more details.

ACKNOWLEDGMENT

Hameed Shah acknowledges financial support from University of Chinese Academy of Sciences, and The World Academy of Sciences under the CAS-TWAS President's fellowship program.

KEYWORDS

- **plant cell culture**
- **plant tissue culture**
- **secondary metabolites**
- **phytochemicals**
- **plant biotechnology**

REFERENCES

Bhatia, S.; Dahiya, R. Concepts and Techniques of Plant Tissue Culture Science. In *Modern Applications of Plant Biotechnology in Pharmaceutical Sciences*. Bhatia, S.; Sharma, K.; Dahiya, R.; Bera, T. (Eds.; Academic Press: Boston, 2015; pp 121–156.

Bhojwani, S. S.; Dantu, P. K., Production of Industrial Phytochemicals. In *Plant Tissue Culture: An Introductory Text*. Bhojwani, S.S.; Dantu, P.K., Eds.; Springer: New Delhi, 2013; pp 275–286.

Chattopadhyay, S.; Srivastava, A. K.; Bisaria, V. S., Production of Phytochemicals in Plant Cell Bioreactors. In *Plant Biotechn. Mol. Markers;* Srivastava, P. S., Narula, A., Srivastava, S., Eds.; Anamaya Publishers: New Delhi, 2004; pp 117–128.

De Luca, V.; Salim, V.; Atsumi, S. M.; Yu, F. Mining the Biodiversity of Plants: A Revolution in the Making. *Science* **2012,** *336,* 658–1661.

Doran, P. M. Application of Plant Tissue Cultures in Phytoremediation Research: Incentives and Limitations. *Biotechnol. Bioeng.* **2009,** *103*(1), 60–76. DOI: 10.1002/bit.22280.

FAO. How to feed the world. Paper presented at the High-level expert forum, Rome (2009). www.fao.org/fileadmin/templates/wsfs/docs/Issues_papers/HLEF2050_Global_Agriculture.pdf (accessed Jan 18, 2018).

Flores, H. E.; Curtis, W. R. Approaches to Understanding and Manipulating the Biosynthetic Potential of Plant Roots. *Ann. N. Y. Acad. Sci.* **1992,** *665,* 188–209.

George, E. F. Plant Tissue Culture Procedure – Background. In *Plant Propagation by Tissue Culture, 3rd Ed.;* George, E. F., Hall, M. A., De Klerk, G. J., Eds.; Springer: Netherlands, 2008; pp 1–28.

George, E. F.; Debergh, P. C. Micropropagation: Uses and Methods In *Plant Propagation by Tissue Culture,* 3rd Ed.; George, E. F., Hall, M, A., De Klerk, G. J., Eds.; Springer, Netherlands. 2008. Pp. 29-64.

Georgiev, I. M. Editorial (Hot Topic: Coming Back to Nature: Plants as a Vital Source of Pharmaceutically Important Metabolites–Part II A). *Curr. Med. Chem.* **2013,** *20,* 851–851.

Georgiev, I. M. Natural Products Utilization. *Phytochem. Rev.* **2014,** *13*(2), 339–341.

Grout, B. General Principles of Tissue Culture. In *Encyclopedia of Applied Plant Sciences,* 2nd Ed.; Murray, B. G., Murphy, D. J., Eds.; Academic Press: Oxford, 2017; pp. 437–443.

Husemann, W.; Callies, R.; Leibfritz, D. External pH Modifies the Intracellular Ph and the Mode of Photosynthetic Co_2-Assimilation in Photoautotrophic Cell Suspension Cultures of *Chenopodium rubrum* L. *Bot. Acta.* **1992,** *105,* 116.

Hussain, S.; Fareed, S.; Ansari, S.; Rahman, A.; Ahmad, I. Z.; Saeed, M. Current Approaches Toward Production of Secondary Plant Metabolites. *J. Pharm. Bioallied Sci.* **2012,** *4*(1), 10-20.

Kirakosyan, A.; Cseke, L. J.; Kaufman, P. B. The Use of Plant Cell Biotechnology for the Production of Phytochemicals. *Recent Adv. Plant Biotechnol.* **2009,** 15–33.

Kreis, W.; Reinhard, E. 12B-Hydroxylation of Digitoxin by Suspension Cultured Digitalis Lanata Cells: Production of Digoxin in 20 L and 300 L Airlift Reactors. *J. Biotechnol.* **1992,** *26,* 257–273.

Kumar, P. P.; Loh, C. S. Plant Tissue Culture for Biotechnology. In *Plant Biotechnology and Agriculture;* Hasegawa, P. M. Ed.; Academic Press: San Diego, 2012; pp 131–138.

Loyola-Vargas, V. M.; Vazquez-Flota, F. An Introduction to Plant Cell Culture: Back to the Future. *Methods Mol. Biol.* **2006,** *318,* 3–8. DOI: 10.1385/1–59259–959–1:003.

Misawa, M. Production of Useful Plant Metabolites. In *Adv Biochem Eng Biotechnol.* Fiechter, A., Ed., Springer-Verlag: Berlin, 1985; pp 59–88.

Mulder-Krieger, T.; Verpoorte, R.; Svendse, A.; Scheffer, J. Production of Essential Oils and Flavours in Plant Cell and Tissue Cultures, a Review. *Plant Cell, Tissue Organ Cult.* **1988,** *13,* 85–114.

Murthy, H. N.; Georgiev, M. I.; Park, S. Y.; Dandin, V. S.; Paek, K. Y. The Safety Assessment of Food Ingredients Derived from Plant Cell, Tissue and Organ Cultures: A Review. *Food Chem.* **2015,** *176,* 426–432. DOI: 10.1016/j.foodchem.2014.12.075.

Ochoa-Villarreal, M.; Howat, S.; Hong, S. M.; Jang, M. O.; Jin, Y. W.; Lee, E. K.; Loake, G. J. Plant Cell Culture Strategies for the Production of Natural Products. *BMB Rep.* **2016,** *49*(3), 149–158. DOI: 10.5483/BMBRep.2016.49.3.264.

Pant, B. Application of Plant Cell and Tissue Culture for the Production of Phytochemicals in Medicinal Plants. *Adv. Exp. Med. Biol.* **2014,** *808,* 25–39. DOI: 10.1007/978–81–322–1774–9_3.

Payne, G. F.; Shuler, M. L.; Brodelius, P., Plant cell culture. In *Large Scale Cell Culture Technology;* Lydensen, B. K., Ed., Hanser Publishers: New York, 1987; pp 193-229.

Ratledge, C.; Sasson, A. *Production of Useful Biochemicals by Higher-Plant Cell Cultures;* Cambridge University Press: Cambridge, 1992;

Seitz, H. U.; Hinderer, W. Anthocyanins. In *Cell culture and somatic cell genetics of plants;* Constabel, F. Vasil, I. Eds.; Academic Press: San Diego, 1988; Vol. 5, pp 49–76.

Sharma, G. K.; Jagetiya, S.; Dashora, R. *General Techniques of Plant Tissue Culture;* Lulu Press Inc: Raleigh, North Carolina, United States, 2015.

Smetanska, I. *Production of Secondary Metabolites Using Plant Cell Cultures;* Springer-Verlag: Berlin, 2008; Vol. 111.

Toivonen, L.; Laakso, S.; Rosenqvist, H. The Effect of Temperature on Hairy Root Cultures of Catharanthus Roseus: Growth, Indole Alkaloid Accumulation and Membrane Lipid Composition. *Plant Cell Rep.* **1992,** *11,* 395–399.

Zhong, J. J. Biochemical Engineering of the Production of Plant-Specific Secondary Metabolites by Cell Suspension Cultures. In *Plant Cells. Advances in Biochemical Engineering/ Biotechnology;* Zhong, J. J., et al., Eds.; Springer: Berlin, Heidelberg, 2001, Vol. 72, pp 2–24.

CHAPTER 6

SECONDARY METABOLITES ACCUMULATION AND PRODUCTION THROUGH *IN VITRO* CULTURES

HUSSIEN M. DAFFALLA* and AZZA MIGDAM ELSHEIKH

National Centre for Research, Commission for Biotechnology and Genetic Engineering, Mohamed Nageeb St. No. 61, 11111 Khartoum, Sudan

**Corresponding author. E-mail: hdaffalla@yahoo.com; Mob.: +49918349142*

**ORCID: https://orcid.org/0000-0002-7786-8380*

ABSTRACT

In vitro plant culture comprises three distinct types, namely cell, tissue, and organ cultures. Each type of this culture involves three components, namely plant material, medium and culture conditions. In turn, each of these components has various characteristics, for example, concentrations, size, and practices. The utilization of in vitro cultures for the production of secondary metabolites was comprehensively studied to date. Production of many pharmaceuticals, nutraceuticals, food additives, and agrochemicals was successfully realized. However, most of these compounds were still commercially produced directly from intact plants. The high cost is the main restraint for in vitro production of phytochemicals. Therefore, reducing the costs below conventional methods must be the core intention. Cost reduction has been managed mainly by increasing biomass growth and/or biomaterials accumulation. These can be performed through the optimization of the three components of each culture type by manipulating their characteristics. This chapter addressed various achievements in phytochemicals production by in vitro cultures.

6.1 INTRODUCTION

Plant secondary metabolites are derived biosynthetics from the primary metabolites present at a much lower concentration (less than 1% dry weight) and depend mainly on the physiological and developmental stages of plants (Crozier et al., 2009; Nandani et al., 2013). Although they have a slight role in photosynthesis, respiration or growth and development, they are efficiently used for survival and diversification, hence generated during a specific developmental period of the plant (Collin, 2001; Crozier et al., 2009; Nandani et al., 2013). While secondary metabolites have no physio-biochemical functions, they play major biological roles such as pollination attractants, recruiting seed dispersers, environmental adaptations, or protective agents against climatic stress, microorganisms, other plants, and predators (Alfermann et al., 2003). Various types of secondary metabolites were accumulated by arid and semiarid plants to tolerate the harsh abiotic stress, especially water deficiency (Meena and Patni, 2008). During senescence, leaves show beautiful color which is formed to protect the leaf cells from photooxidative damage and for effectiveness in nutrient recovery (Winkel-Shirley, 2002). A further view is that the secondary compounds may be an expedient storage, in which the stored carbon and nitrogen are recycled back into the primary metabolism when there is a demand (Collin, 2001). According to their function, human beings utilized these natural products for centuries to meet their needs for health, food, agricultural, and daily necessities. In particular, plant-derived chemicals are valuable sources for a variety of pharmaceuticals, flavors, aromas, pigments, food additives, dyes, oils, resins, bio-based fuels, plastics, enzymes, preservatives, fragrances, cosmetics, and agrochemicals (Zhong, 2001; Rao and Ravishanker 2002; Alfermann et al., 2003). Plants remain the main exclusive source for many medications. In recent years, there has been an increasing interest in plant antioxidants that are used as an unmodified form of natural food preservatives to replace synthetic substances (Nandani et al., 2013). The WHO reported that medicinal plants are used by around 80% of the world population for treating some diseases as intact plants or their extracts (Smetanska, 2008).

Although secondary plant products are very common, this does not imply that every plant can produce every product. The bioactive compounds are of more limited occurrence. Many of these commercially valuable phytochemicals are secondary metabolites not essential for plant growth, produced in trace amounts, and often accumulate in specialized tissues (Kim et al., 2002; Alfermann et al., 2003). Some secondary metabolites are found only in certain species of families, showing the individuality of species or specific growth condition (Zhong, 2001; Nandani et al., 2013). Similarly, the bioactivities of plants are inimitable to specific plant species or groups as the mixture of secondary products in a particular plant is taxonomically distinct (Meena and Patni, 2008). Also, certain plant organs or just one type of cell could contain only specific secondary compounds (Kim et al., 2002; Rao and Ravishanker, 2002). This particular organ called the medicinal part in pharmacognosy is liable for the accumulation or secretion of those compounds. For instance, flavonoids acting as ultraviolet (UV) protectants are specifically accumulated in epidermal cells (Liu et al., 2008). The expression of the genes responsible for the formation of secondary metabolites is extremely high in the tissue where those metabolites are primarily accumulated. Moreover, only 10% of medicinal plant species are cultivated (Julsing et al., 2007) and the rest are still collected from the wild. The chemical structure of secondary plant products is more complex than that of primary products (James et al., 2008). Slow plant growth rates and ineffective purification procedures have an additional prohibition role in obtaining less sufficient amounts of active compounds (Kim et al., 2002). Efforts to produce large quantities of physiologically active secondary compounds by organic synthesis are ongoing. However, nearly all active secondary compounds are structurally complex, and in many cases, are impossible to synthesize or the yields are too low (Materska, 2008; Nandani et al., 2013). To overcome these difficulties, plant tissue culture techniques have been developed for rapid, large-scale production of cells and their secondary compounds (Rao and Ravishanker, 2002; James et al., 2008). The advantage of this method is providing an uninterrupted and reliable supply of secondary metabolites capable to accumulate a higher concentration of compounds compared to the whole plants. For example, a 750 L bioreactor containing 600 L suspension culture of *Lithospermum erythrorhizon* would yield 1.2 kg of shikonin within 2 weeks, while the plants covering a whole 1 ha would yield about 9 kg shikonin after 4 years (Alamgir, 2017). By calculation, the production of 8 bioreactors in 2 weeks was equal to 4 years of a 1 ha field of shikonin yields. However, few such successful examples on in vitro production of biomaterials were reported. Yet, in vitro plant culture represents a prospective alternative for industrial secondary metabolites production, but there are a number of obstructions in the way that can be classified as physiological such as slow growth rate, heterogeneity, genetic instability, low metabolite content, product secretion, and operational such as the requirement for illumination, mixing, sterilization, and result from biomass growth as shear sensitivity and wall adhesion (Zhong, 2001). Optimization of operational and instrumentation systems to a corresponding advanced technology used in animal and microbial production is compulsory for retrofit existing bioreactor (Smith, 1995). This chapter summarized the works on the production of phytochemicals from the three distinct types of in vitro cultures, namely cell, tissue, and organ cultures in a bioreactor, liquid, and solid systems. The focus will be on providing examples of cultural systems of each culture type as useful guidelines.

6.2 ADVANTAGES OF IN VITRO PLANT CULTURES

In vitro plant culture is the main biotechnology technique that has the potentiality to produce valuable and natural next generation products safe for human use in medical, food and agricultural applications. Various alkaloids, saponins, anthraquinones, polyphenols, and terpenes have been obtained from in vitro cultures of various plant species. Numerous advantages of utilizing in vitro cultures for synthesis of bioactive secondary metabolites, have been listed by many authors (Collin, 2001; Chattopadhyay et al., 2002; Rao and Ravishanker, 2002; Alfermann et al., 2003; Vanisree and Tsay, 2004; James et al., 2008; Smetanska, 2008; Tan et al., 2010; Kuo et al., 2011; Gaosheng and Jingming, 2012; Yildiz, 2012). Below is the summary of the advantages:

1. In vitro propagation of a large number of genetically uniform and pathogen-free clones of a high phytochemical accumulation in a limited time and space.
2. Completely running under controlled environment autonomously from the effects of the abiotic or biotic factors.
3. It is possible to select cultivars with a higher phytochemical productivity.
4. Automation of main culturing steps such as cell growth and hence, regulation of metabolic processes can decrease costs and, simultaneously, increase yield.
5. As cells have a higher rate of metabolism and shorter biosynthetic cycles than intact plants, they can accumulate phytochemicals in higher concentration per dry weight compared to the whole plants.
6. Extraction from the in vitro tissues is much easier than extraction from the complex structure of the entire plant tissues.
7. Biotransformation of the exogenously supplied substrates into valuable products.
8. Production of novel compounds that are not produced or not been detected in intact plants.
9. No herbicide and insecticide required during culturing.

6.3 PRODUCTION OF SECONDARY METABOLITES THROUGH TISSUE CULTURE

Plant cell culture techniques include ordinary undifferentiated cultures (callus, cell suspension, and protoplast), organ (shoot and root cultures), and special cultures (hairy root and immobilized cells). The production of secondary metabolites in plant in vitro cultures is contingent on the degree of cell proliferation and differentiation (George, 2008). Careful selection of productive cells and cultural conditions resulted in an accumulation of several products in higher levels in cultured cells. Notably, every type of culture has its appropriate external cultural conditions such as temperature, gas exchange and light as well as medium conditions like pH, nutrients, and plant growth regulators (PGRs) concentration, which favors cells growth and accumulation of secondary metabolites. For instance, the production of tryptophol in the cell culture of *Ipomoea purpurea* becomes double at pH 6.3 and is inhibited at pH 4.8 (Alamgir, 2017). The endogenous hormones content interact with the exogenous supplement of PGRs not only to induce growth of cells but also the formation of the secondary compounds. Each explant type shows diverse responses, in terms of biomass and phytochemical accretion, to external and internal factors. Praveen et al. (2010) studied the distribution of withanolide-A in eight organs of *Withania somnifera*, and found that the quantity of withanolide-A gradually decreased from young leaves to the root.

To date, many plant species are under commercial utilization to produce natural products using in vitro culture (Table 6.1). Some include *Panax ginseng* (ginsenoside; 27% of dry weight in 20,000 L), *L. erythrorhizon* (shikonin; 20% of dry weight), *Coleus blumei* (rosmarinic acid; 15% of dry weight), *Taxus* spp. (paclitaxel; in 75,000 L), *Coptis japonica* and *Thalictrum minus* (protoberberines; 13.2% of dry weight in 4000 L), and *Morinda citrifolia* (anthraquinones; 18% of dry weight) (Smith, 1995; Collin, 2001; Gaosheng and Jingming, 2012; Alamgir, 2017). On the other hand, several products other than pharmaceuticals have been commercially released. Recently, protecting cosmetic supplements from the cell culture of *Saponaria pumila,* and dietary supplements consisting of the freeze-dried biomass of *Theobroma cacao* cell suspension were trademarked (Georgiev, 2015). The commercial production of natural plant-based insecticides mainly pyrethrum (*Chrysanthemum cinerariaefolium*), nicotine (*Nicotiana* spp.), rotenone (*Lonchocarpus utilis*), and azadirachtin (*Azadirachta indica*) has been gradually increased (George, 2000). Veterinary vaccines were also produced through in vitro cultures with the first vaccine against

TABLE 6.1 Examples of Secondary Metabolites Production from Cell Culture.

Plant species	Medium + PGRs (mg/L)	Explant used	Light regime	Culture period (d)	Products	Yield	References
Arnebia euchroma	M9	Leaf	Dark	10	Naphthoquinone	637.15 mg/L	Kumar et al. (2011)
Artemisia annua	MS + 0.5 BAP + 0.5 1-Naphthaleneacetic acid (NAA)	Leaf	Continuous	12	Artemisinin	0.06%	Lo et al. (2012)
Astragalus missouriensis	MS + NAA 1 + Kin 2	Mesocotyl	Continuous	14	Isoquercitrin, Quercitrin	5.3 mg/g, 8.1 mg/g DW	Ionkova (2009)
Azadirachta indica	MS+ nd	Seed kernel	Dark	12	Azadirachtin	2.98 mg/g	Prakash and Srivastava (2005)
Barringtonia racemosa	B5+2.0 2,4-Dichlorophenoxyacetic acid (2,4-D)	Leaf	16 h	10	Lycopene	0.69 mg/g DW	Behbahani et al. (2011)
Centella asiatica	MS + 2 2,4-D	Leaf	16 h	26	Quercetin, Luteolin, kaempferol	0.146 mg/g, 0.141 mg/g, 0.056 mg/g DW	Tan et al. (2010)
C. asiatica	MS + 3 2,4-D + 1 kin	Leaf	16 h	12	Luteolin	390 µg/g DW	Tan et al. (2013)
Cinchona ledgeriana	WPM + 15 µM Pic*, 0.5 µM BA	Leaf	12 h	49	Quinine	11% DW	Ratnadewi et al. (2013)
Crocus sativus	B5+2 NAA + 2 Indole-3-acetic acid (IAA) + 0.5 BA	Corm	Dark	21	Crocin	1.74 mg/g	Chen et al. (2003)
Ficus deltoidea	MS + 10.74 µM NAA/4.65 µM Kin	Leaf	16 h	21	Rutin, quercetin,	39.13 mg/g, 3.92 mg/g, 8.65 mg/g DW	Ong et al. (2011)

TABLE 6.1 *(Continued)*

Plant species	Medium + PGRs (mg/L)	Explant used	Light regime	Culture period (d)	Products	Yield	References
Morinda citrifolia	B5+2,4-D 5 μmol/L	Nd	Dark	14	Anthraquinones	40 μmol/g FW	Stalman et al. (2003)
Spilanthes acmella	MS + 15 μM BA + 5 μM 2,4-D.	Leaf	16 h	28	Scopoletin	35.63 μg/g DW	Abyari et al. (2016)
Glehnia littoralis	B5 + NAA 1 + kin 0.01	Petiole	dark	20	Anthocyanins	14% DW	Miura et al. (1998)
Papaver bracteatum	MS+ 1 2,4-D + 0.1 kin	Hypocotyl–cotyledon	16 h	16	Thebaine	10.76 μg/g DW	Farjaminezhad et al. (2013)
Psoralea corylifolia	MS+ 1 2,4-D + 0.5 NAA + 1.5 BAP	Leaf	16 h	16	Psoralen	9850 μg/g DW	Ahmed and Baig (2014)
Lavandula vera	LS + 0.2 2,4-D	Nd	dark	11	Rosmarinic acid	3348 mg/L	Georgiev et al. (2007)
Scrophularia striata	MS + NAA 0.5 + BA 2.0	Leaf	dark	17	Acteoside	14.25 μg/g	Khanpour-Ardestani et al. (2015)
Solanum hainanense	MS +1.0 2,4-D + 0.1 BAP	Stem	10 h	28	Solasodine	220.5 mg/g	Loc et al. (2014)
M. citrifolia	MS+ NAA (2.5 μM) +0.5 μM BAP	Root	16 h	45	Anthraquinone	16.99 mg/g DW	Sreeranjini and Siril (2013)
Vitis vinifera	MS + 0.1 BA	Leaf	16 h	14	Phenolics, Resveratrol	71.91 mg/g, 277.89 μg/g DW	Sae-Lee et al. (2014)
Eriobotrya japonica	MS + 2.5 BA + 1 NAA	Leaf	Dark	30	Triterpene	151.54 mg/g	Ho et al. (2018)

TABLE 6.1 *(Continued)*

Plant species	Medium + PGRs (mg/L)	Explant used	Light regime	Culture period (d)	Products	Yield	References
E. japonica	MS+ NAA 0.5	Immature embryo	10	nd	Tormentic acid	63.1 mg/g DW	Li et al. (2017)
S. striata	MS+ 0.5 NAA + 2.0 BA	Stem	Dark	29	Acteoside	14.25 μg/g FW	Khanpour-Ardestani et al. (2015)
Salvia officinalis	MS+ 0.1 NAA+ 0.2 BA + 0.5 2, 4-D	Hypocotyl	Continuous	238	Carnosol, Rosmarinic acid	0.05 mg/g, 18.57 mg/g DW	Grzegorczyk et al. (2005)

PGRs: plant growth regulators, M9: Fujita et al. (1981), MS: Murashige and Skoog (1962), Pic: picloram, B5: Gamborg et al. (1968), WPM: Lloyd and McCown (1980), LS: Linsmaier and Skoog (1965), Nd: not determined.

Newcastle disease virus developed using tobacco BY-2 cells but not released commercially (Georgiev, 2015). Sweeteners used to replace sugar such as glycyrrhizin, stevioside and thaumatin were produced from cell cultures of *Glycyrrhiza glabra*, *Stevia rebaudiana,* and *Thaumatococcus daniellii*, respectively (Rodríguez-Sahagún et al., 2012). The approval for plant cell-based recombinant therapeutic protein for human use was utilizing genetically engineered carrot and tobacco cell cultures patently protected (Georgiev, 2015).

6.3.1 SECONDARY METABOLITES PRODUCTION FROM UNDIFFERENTIATED CULTURES

Undifferentiated culture is the culture of cells in solid medium (callus), in liquid medium (cell suspension) or both in liquid or semisolid medium (protoplasts). Undifferentiated plant cells are genetically heterogeneous that make it promising to select cell strains with superior metabolites production.

6.3.1.1 CALLUS CULTURE

6.3.1.1.1 Initiation of Callus

Callus is an amorphous and undifferentiated mass of thin-walled parenchyma cells frequently growing and dividing. Callus culture involves induction of cell aggregates from proliferating cells, tissues or organ explants on solid or semisolid media commonly containing auxin alone or high auxin/cytokinin ratio. Callusing is normally considered as a response of explants to wounds and appeasers in the form of tissue dedifferentiation. Theoretically, a single living cell is capable of developing into a whole plant and this phenomenon is called cellular totipotency. Gautheret and Nobecourt were the first to induce callus culture from carrot (*Daucus carota* L.) root tissues with the aid of indole-3-acetic acid (IAA) in 1939 (Varshney and Anis, 2014). For the production of a particular compound, it is advantageous to initiate the callus from the plant part that is known to be a high or a specific producer for a compound. The age and physiological status of the mother plant could affect the formation of callus. Callus is mostly classified, according to morphology and texture, into *compact* or *friable*. Compact callus consists of densely aggregated cells. Friable callus consists of loosely associated cells which can easily detach. Compact calli are preferred for initiation of organogenesis or embryogenesis cultures, while the friable calli are used to generate cell suspension cultures. The auxin/cytokinin ratios are the main controllers in determining the type of callus. Generally, the chosen appropriate explant should be fundamentally healthy with vigorous growth. The type of auxin and cytokinin and the ratio between the two are important for callus formation (Lee et al., 2011). The size and the shape of the initial explant are not critical, although proliferation might not occur with explants below a critical size. In general, fairly large pieces of tissues were favored because of the large numbers of cells present increased the chance of obtaining a viable culture. On the other hand, the endogenous content of nutrients and hormones are higher according to the size of the tissue (Yildiz, 2012). Therefore, a high surface area/volume ratio was desirable for maximum growth. The type of explants also affects the nature of cells induced. A single cell or a uniform group of cells produced *homogeneous callus*, while explants excised from an organ consist of many cell types, that is, leaf, root, which produced *heterogeneous callus*.

Callus culture protocol from explant to proliferation usually contains three developmental stages namely, induction, division, and differentiation.

1. Induction stage is where cells prepare to divide and metabolism is activated.
2. Division stage is characterized by a rapid cell division and an increase in metabolic activity, cells become dedifferentiated as meristem materialized, and the cell size reduces due to cell division.
3. Differentiation stage starts with the maturation of some cells, therefore, leading to the expression of certain metabolic pathways that lead to the formation of secondary products. The duration of each stage is dependent on the physiological status of cells and cultural conditions. The metabolite biosynthesis varies accordingly.

6.3.1.1.2 Maintenance of Callus Culture

Callus produces an undifferentiated mass of cells, which are aggregate of heterogeneous or homogenous dedifferentiated cells. Cultures of callus must be optimized for long-term maintenance of high growth rate, biomass gain, and secondary metabolites production. The initial cells induced on the explant are actively growing mass of cells called *primary* callus. The callus can be subcultured or subdivided for one of three reasons, biomass production, the establishment of cell suspension, or to regenerate organs/whole plants with each requiring an appropriate hormonal balance. When primary callus is separated from the remaining explants tissues and subcultured into a same or different media for biomass growth, the newly formed callus is called the *secondary* callus. The biomass enlargement of callus is dependent on the composition of the subsequent medium, mainly on the concentration of auxins and cytokinins. The types and the combination ratios of auxin and cytokinin are imperative for increasing the callus rate of production and growth (Lee et al., 2011). Both percentage induction and growth of callus are important in determining the final dry weight produced by an explant. The higher growth rate is an indicator of biomass gain in a shorter culture period which is important to diminish the production cost. Moreover, higher final dry weight is correlated, in some cases, to high accumulation of secondary products. Maximum stimulation of flavonoids is associated with good biomass growth achieved (Ionkova, 2009). The establishment of callus growth curve, therefore, is essential to verify the point (time) of stationary phase which is the suitable time for subculture process. Scheduled subculture into a fresh medium with the same compositions is imperative for long-term maintenance of the callus nature (friable or compact) and to avoid browning, or for the harvesting of calli with a higher fresh/dry weight or by-product yields. The growth of callus might show a general growth pattern of a sigmoid (S-shaped) curve when growth is plotted against time. Callus curve commonly contains three phases namely: (1) a lag phase with adaptation and initial slow growth, (2) log phase which is the main period for rapid and maximum growth, and (3) the stationary phase where growth is sluggish and lastly, stops. When callus is about to reach the stationary phase, it must be subdivided and subcultured. Callus induced on *Grewia asiatica* explants was stimulated and growth increased when subcultured periodically (Sharma and Patni, 2013).

The PGRs concentration, cell-to-cell contact, type and age of explant, and any early differentiation which is present seem to favor the biosynthesis of secondary products (Parr, 1989). Callus culture was reported to be utilized for phytochemicals production, commonly flavonoids (Filová, 2014). For example, callus culture of *Maackia amurensis* accumulated elevated concentrations of isoflavones and pterocarpans approximately four times higher than the content of the heartwood of intact plants (Fedoreyev et al., 2004). Other phytochemicals also, for example, ginseng was produced by callus culture of Ginsenoside, *Panax ginseng,* which was six times higher than the whole plant (Alamgir, 2017). Callus tissues of *Zataria multiflora* produced a very high level of rosmarinic acid (158.26 mg/g) compared to (12.28 mg/g) that produced by the propagated shoots (Françoise et al., 2007). Matkowski

(2004) compared the production of four isoflavonoid compounds in the calli of *Pueraria lobate* from different explant sources (root, leaf, and stem) (Table 6.2). The results reveal that the kind of explant affected both the total amount of isoflavonoids and the quantity of each compound. It was also found that the age of explant source affected the isoflavonoids content.

Callus culture has several advantages that makes it useful for secondary metabolites production: (1) Can be induced from a wide range of explant sources compared to other cultural types (Table 6.2). (2) It has the possibility to be maintained for longer cultural periods compared to organ cultures. (3) When established, it is easier to use for the initiation of a distinct type of culture, from a single cell to the whole plant. (4) Photosynthesis is inconsequential; can grow under dark condition.

6.3.1.2 CELL SUSPENSION CULTURE

6.3.1.2.1 Initiation of Cell Suspension Culture

Cell suspension culture is induced by suspending an undifferentiated friable callus into liquid media containing PGR. The callus then separates into cells which are uniformly bathed in liquid medium under continuous agitation on horizontal reciprocating or gyratory shakers which favor cells growing in a disorganized form. However, an organ such as leaf was reportedly used for direct induction of cells in liquid media bypassing the callus induction stage. For instance, a rapid growth and mass of cells are released into suspension as leaf sections of *Chenopodium rubrum* are kept floated on Murashige and Skoog (MS) medium with rotary shaking for 4 days under light (Geile and Wagner, 1980).

After the initial shaking, any large or unspoiled callus can be eliminated by filtration. The perfect initiation of cell suspension cultures depends on several factors including plant growth regulators, medium nutrients, biological factors and physical factors. The size of initial callus inoculum is determined by the critical initial cell density which is the effective density that maintains culture growth. In other words, it was the lowest inoculum density per volume of medium at which a cell culture will grow. Dixon and Gonzales (1994) assumed that 10% of initial cell density to the total volume was necessary to initiate suspension culture. They further noted that decreasing the inoculum size will affect the growth curve pattern, wherein a small inoculum size leads to a longer lag phase (Dixon, 1985). While increasing the inoculum size make cells enter the stationary phase earlier

TABLE 6.2 Examples of Secondary Metabolites Production from Callus Cultures.

Plant species	Medium + PGRs (mg/L)	Explants used	Light	Culture period (d)	Products	Yield	References
Ambrosia tenuifolia	MS + 10 µM kin, 1 µM 2–4, D	Leaf	Continuous/ dark	35	Altamisine, Psilostachynolides B-C, Psilostachynolides	0.9 mg/L, 2.9 mg/L, 3.0 mg/L, DW	Goleniowski and Trippi (1999)
Arachis hypogea	MS + 4 NAA+ 1 BAP	Stem	Dark	30	Piceatannol, Resveratrol	5.31 µg/g, 11.97 µg/g	Ku et al. (2005)
Aronia melanocarpa	MS + 2 NAA + 2 BA	Bud	Continuous	28	Phenolic acids	83.84 mg/100 DW	Szopa and Ekiert (2014)
A. annua	MS + 0.5 NAA + 0.5 Kin	Seedling	16 h	nd	Artemisinin	96.8 mg/L	Baldi and Dixit (2008)
Aspidosperma ramiflorum	MS + 1 2,4-D + 1.5 BAP	Leaf/ Hypocotyl	16 h	140	Ramiflorin	0.014% DW	Olivira et al. (2001)
A. indica	MS+ 4 Indole-3-butyric acid (IBA)+ 1 BA	Leaf	Dark	42	Azadirachtin	0.0007% DW	Allan et al. (1994)
B. racemosa	WPM+ 2.0 2,4-D	Leaf	16 h	35	Lycopene	1.12 mg/g DW	Behbahani et al. (2011)
Capsicum annuum	MS + 2,4-D 2.0+0.5 Kin	Placenta	nd	21	Capsiacin	1.6 mg/g FW	Umamaheswari and Lalitha (2007)
Cassia senna	MS + 16 µM BA	Cotyledon	16 h	nd	Sennosides	0.13%	Shrivastava et al. (2006)
C. asiatica	MS + 2,4-D 2.0+1.0 Kin	Leaf	16 h	21	Asiaticoside	0.88 mg/g DW	Kiong et al., (2005)
Coscinium fenestratum	MS + 2.0 2,4-D + 2.0 BAP	Petiole	12 h	35	Berberine	1.788% DW	Khan et al. (2008)

TABLE 6.2 *(Continued)*

Plant species	Medium + PGRs (mg/L)	Explants used	Light	Culture period (d)	Products	Yield	References
C. sativus	B5+ IAA 2 + BA	Corm	Dark	21	Crocin	0.43 g/L	Chen et al. (2003)
Cynara cardunculus	MS+ 4.4 mm BA+ 16.1 mM NAA	Leaf	Dark	30	Cynarin, Chlorogenic acid	0.46 mg/g, 0.26 mg/g DW	Trajtemberg et al. (2006)
Hypericum perforatum	MS/B5 + BA 4.0	Apical segment	16 h	30	Hypericin, Pseudohypericin	20 μg/g, 180 μg/g DM	Gadzovska et al. (2005)
M. citrifolia	MS+ NAA 2.5 μM	Root	16 h	45	Anthraquinone	20.26 mg/g DW	Sreeranjini and Siril (2013)
Passiflora quadrangu-laris	MS + 2.0 kin + 3.0 2,4-D	Leaf	16 h	30	Orientin	1163 μg/g DW	Antognoni et al. (2007)
Pluchea lanceolata	MS + 1.0 NAA + 0.5 BAP	Leaf	16 h	42	Quercetin	0.23 mg/g DW	Arya et al. (2008)
P. lanceolata	MS + 1.0 NAA + 0.5 BAP	Leaf	16 h	42	Quercetin	1.86 mg/g	Arya and Patni (2013)
P. corylifolia	MS + IAA 5.71 μM + BAP 4.40 μM	Root	continuous	280	Daidzein, Genistein	2.28%, 0.21% DW	Shinde et al. (2009)
Pueraria lobata	MS + 25 μmol/L 2,4-D + 0.5 μmol/L BA	Root	16 h	168	Daidzin, Genistein, 3′-Methoxy-puerarin, Puerarin	8.67, 3.42, 25.61, 18.35 mg/100 g FW	Matkowski (2004)
Rheum ribes	MS + 1.0 IBA + 1.0 BA	Hypocotyl	16 h	42	Catechin	18.26 mg/100 g FW	Farzami and Ghorbanli (2005)

TABLE 6.2 *(Continued)*

Plant species	Medium + PGRs (mg/L)	Explants used	Light	Culture period (d)	Products	Yield	References
S. officinalis	MS + 0.1 NAA + 0.2 BA + 0.5 2, 4-D	Hypocotyl	Continuous	357	Carnosol, Rosmarinic acid	0.06 mg/g, 15.77 mg/g DW	Grzegorczyk et al. (2005)
Securinega suffruticosa	SH+ 0.5 IAA+ 5.0 KIN	nd	16 h	28	Securinine, Allosecurinine	1.73 mg/g, 3.11 mg/g DW	Raj et al. (2015)
S. striata	MS+ 0.5 NAA + 2.0 BA	Stem	Dark	60	Acteoside	0.0016 mg/g FW	Khanpour-Ardestani et al. (2015)
Solanum melongena	MS+ NAA 1 + Kin 0.25	Stem, Node, Leaf	16 h	56	Anthocyanin	70 µg/g FW	Chaudhary and Mukhopadhyay (2012)
Zataria multiflora	B5 + BAP 0.75	Node	16 h	42	Rosmarininc acid	158.26 mg/g DW	Francoise et al. (2007)
Zingiber officinale	MS + 0.5 2,4-D+ 0.1 BA	Shoot tip	Dark	56	Gingerol	30 µg/100 mg FW	El-Nabarawy et al. (2015)

PGRs: plant growth regulators, MS: Murashige and Skoog (1962), B5: Gamborg et al. (1968), WPM: Lloyd and McCown (1980), SH (Schenk and Hildebrandt, 1972), Nd: not determined.

(Mustafa et al., 2011). Higher uptake rates of ammonium, nitrate, and sugars were observed in the low inoculum-density (50 g FW/L) compared to the high inoculum-density (100 g FW/L) of *Catharanthus roseus* cells cultures. Moreover, the high-inoculum-density cultures produced higher ajmalicine concentrations compared to low inoculum-density, while catharanthine production was not affected by inoculum density (Lee and Shuler, 2000). The physical factors include light, temperature, agitation speed, and culture flask volume. Agitation conditions provide medium and cell mixing, aeration and oxygenation to minimize hypoxia, and hence, maintain proliferation. The high agitation speed (150 revolutions per minute (rpm)) induces nicotine accumulation in tobacco culture, but when normal speed was applied (110 rpm), it resulted in a decrease of nicotine synthesis (Alamgir, 2017). The size of the culture flask or bottle is determined by the volume of the medium. The proportion of liquid-volume relative to the flask size is essential for sufficient aeration which is considered to be about 20% of the total volume of the flask (Dixon, 1985). Various types of vessels have been used for shaking including conical flat-bottom round flasks, and bottle. For aeration without shaking, various devices can be used which include roller bottles, magnetic stirrers, and nipple flasks and tumble tubes. The envelope-shaped culture vessels named "culture bag" and box-shaped named "culture pack," made of fluorocarbon polymer film were used for the production of shikonin by *L. erythrorhizon* cell cultures (Fukui et al., 1999).

6.3.1.2.2 Maintenance of Cell Suspension Culture

Culturing of cell suspension in shaken flasks is usually named *batch culture*; limited by the amount of medium or exhaust carbon source during the culture period. Final biomass obtained is dependent on the quantity of the nutrient. However, when the culture medium is replenished during the culture, the culture system is named *continuous culture*. The continuous culture is usually carried out in bioreactors, where a continuous collection of cell biomass and replacement with the fresh medium are practicable.

The use of cell suspension cultures for secondary metabolite production is based on the concept of biosynthetic totipotency, where each cell could retain the complete genetic information for the production of a range of compounds found in the parent plant (Rao and Ravishankar, 2002).

There are several factors affecting the maintenance of cell cultures such as PGRs, nutrients, inoculum size, and media volume. Therefore, extensive optimization studies in cultured plant cells are necessary to increase the cell biomass and production of bioactive compounds. It was found that an increase in the sucrose concentration in a culture medium could result in an increase of secondary metabolite production (Collin, 2001). Among the different sucrose concentrations studied, the high concentration (5%) resulted in maximum anthraquinone production in *M. citrifolia* cell cultures (Sreeranjini and Siril, 2013). At an aggregate size of 250–500 μm, *Centella asiatica* cells gave the highest luteolin content compared to <250 μM and 500–750 μM. Production of flavonoid was high with the inoculum density of 0.3 g/25 mL compared to 0.1 g/25 mL and 0.5–1.5 g/25 mL (Tan et al., 2013).

A fine cell suspension culture can be obtained by filtering of cultures through pipetting or sieving, DeLong flasks, and the addition of a low concentration of pectinase (macerozyme) or cellulase. Mazarei et al. (2011) obtained three types of aggregate on suspension culture of *Panicum virgatum*. Filtering the initial suspension through a 210 μM mesh at 2-week intervals resulted in an *ultrafine type culture*. Then the culture was allowed to settle for a while prior to removing 6–8 mL of supernatant and replaced with 12–14 mL of fresh medium at 10–14 days intervals. The feeding with the fresh medium is sustained for about 2 months which resulted in a *sandy type culture*. Over time, the sandy type cultures become aggregated and release fine cells giving the supernatant a milky appearance, *milky type culture*. Pectinase can dissolve the intercellular pectins by breaking up the aggregates (Dixon, 1985).

The cell suspension cultures have diverse advantages compared to stationary cultures. 1) By growing in a liquid medium, each cell or aggregate consistently share the contents of nutrients, aeration, and growth regulators. In a callus culture, only cells in contact with the medium surface would directly acquire nutrient. 2) Cell cultivation of a plant offers immense opportunity for multi-investigation of that plant at physiological, biochemical and molecular levels. 3) Using continuous culture proffers the possibility of sustaining the high producer cells to be vigorous and steady in production for the desired period of time. 4) Cells are a source for selection of higher producer lines, mutant induction, and protoplasts isolation in large numbers. 5) Cells are relatively fast in growth, dividing every 22–70 h depending on the nutrient medium and may double within 15 h. 6) in solid media, the phenolic compounds released by oxidase enzyme from the explant when excised, will accumulate under the explants and cause browning on the medium surface. These phytotoxic products prevent explants to grow further, then turn necrotic and ultimately die. In liquid media, the phenolics would wash away from the explant and be diluted.

There are many reports of successful production of secondary metabolites in cell suspension culture. The first patent for the production of metabolites by cell cultures was reported in 1956 by Pfizer Inc. (Smetanska, 2008). The first industrial production of a compound by undifferentiated cell cultures of *L. erythrorhizon* was shikonin in 1983 by Mitsui Petrochemical Industries Ltd. (Fujita and Tabata, 1987). Cell suspension culture of *Maclura pomifera* showed a high level of metabolite accumulation (0.91%) than stems (0.26%), leaves (0.32%), and fruits (0.08%) of the parent plant (Monache et al., 1995). The tormentic acid content of the cell suspension culture of *Eriobotrya japonica* was determined to be 18.4 times greater than that of the leaves (Li et al., 2017).

The analysis of cell growth that was maintained in a batch culture type (finite medium) tends to develop a sigmoidal pattern of growth (S-shaped curve) during a given period of time (Jha and Ghosh, 2005; George, 2008; Santos et al., 2010). This kinetics growth contains five phases namely: (1) A lag phase, in which cells prepare to divide beginning with the metabolite mobilization, synthesis of proteins, and specific metabolites; (2) A period of exponential growth in which the cell division rate increases; (3) Linear growth in which the cell division is slow but the rate of the cell expansion increases; (4) Deceleration phase, a period when the rate of cell division decreases and cell expansion occurs; and (5) A stationary phase when growth ends and culture becomes inviable, that is, no cell division or increase in weight occurs.

Each phase of growth is separated from another according to the values of different measurable growth parameters, such as cell number, total DNA content and fresh/dry weights. Therefore, the total linked phases, when plotted, develop the S-shaped growth curve. Similar patterns of growth might occur in the organ cultures. During the period of stationary growth, some differentiation of cells may occur in cell cultures but generally, it is less complete than that which occurs in callus cultures (George, 2008). The consequences of relatively slow growth are that cell suspensions require long periods of culture before substantial amounts of biomass and products have accumulated (Constabel and Tyler, 1994). Cultures cannot be maintained in the stationary phase for long periods. Cells begin to die as the components of the medium become exhausted. Subculturing often becomes urgent when the density of cells, tissue or organs becomes excessive. However, high plant density may be acceptable as a biotic stress factor that could improve yield due to the high competition among plants for water and minerals (Yildis, 2012). Nevertheless, subculture is required to increase the volume of a culture or to increase the weight/number of cells. Likewise, the firm closed vessels used to maintain aseptic conditions for culturing plant material leads to the accumulation of toxic metabolites and the exhaustion of the medium, so subculturing is impressive (Varshney and Anis, 2014). Callus or suspension cultures are subdivided into new explants for re-culturing on fresh medium and are performed periodically. Consequently, the importance of establishing calli and cell growth curve when working with medicinal and aromatic plants not only helps to determine the correct time for media exchange and subculturing but also the time of secondary metabolites production (Santos et al., 2010).

The management of suspension cultures requires a high expenditure for labor, space, and equipment. Alternatively, the growth of callus on the solid medium has been appraised, principally when the depiction of large numbers of individual cultures is required.

6.3.2 SECONDARY METABOLITES PRODUCTION BY ORGAN CULTURES

Any in vitro or ex vitro plant organ can be used as explant to initiate an in vitro organ culture. In vitro explants, for organ culture, can be obtained from other culture types through embryogenic and organogenic redifferentiation, or direct induction from the node. Roots and, to a lesser extent, shoot is the most cultured organ for secondary metabolites production. Other organs such as flowers have also been reported (Matkowski, 2008). Like undifferentiated cells, when organs are cultured for the production of secondary metabolites, the aim is to achieve maximum growth rate and biomass gain. Although most of the valuable secondary metabolites are produced from cell and callus cultures, important medicinal plants such as *Atropa belladonna* and *Digitalis lanata* fail to accumulate considerable amounts of by-product when cultured as undifferentiated cells (Gaosheng and Jingming, 2012). Shoot culture of *Aronia melanocarpa* produced more phenolic acids than both its callus culture and intact fruit (Szopa and Ekiert, 2014). Similarly, saponin is specifically produced in the roots of *P. ginseng*, and hypericin and hyperforin are accumulated only in the foliar glands of *Hypericum perforatum* (Alamgir, 2017). In vitro differentiated cell cultures are more convenient for the large-scale production of valuable phytochemicals compared to undifferentiated cells cultures for several reasons. (1) Organ cultures generally display a lower sensitivity to shear stress in a bioreactor (Bourgaud et al., 2001). (2) Differentiated cultures are relatively more stable in the production of secondary metabolites (Rao and Ravishankar, 2002).

(3) Shoots and roots are more predictable in their behavior (Parr, 1989). (4) Organ cultures accumulate secondary products with concentrations that are often analogous to those of the intact plants (Oksman-Caldentey and Hiltunen, 1996). However, organ cultures in the bioreactor revealed nonuniform growth of biomass (Bourgaud et al., 2001). Also, organ cultures tend to grow slowly, and alteration of the yield and profile of a product is not easy (Oksman-Caldentey and Hiltunen, 1996). Therefore, up to date, the only commercial example of the use of plant organ cultures for secondary metabolite production is the cultivation of ginseng roots (Filová, 2014).

6.3.2.1 ROOT CULTURE

Different compounds are reported to be only induced by root systems of trees. Therefore, production of such compounds required cutting of the tree. Roots are the medicinal parts used for the extraction of many important medicinal plants such as *P. ginseng*, *Panax notoginseng*, *Coptis chinensis*, and *Salvia miltiorrhiza* (Gaosheng and Jingming, 2012). Moreover, in some manners, undifferentiated cells are unable to produce a target compound as it is specific to only root cells. To establish the protocol for root culture and production of secondary metabolites, there are three steps. Step 1 is the induction of the adventitious roots. Adventitious roots can be obtained from the leaf explant, cultivation of root explants, shoots or induced from callus. Auxin supplement is required, mostly Indole-3-butyric acid (IBA) or 1-Naphthaleneacetic acid (NAA) and to a less extent IAA. MS and B5 media are the most used medium cultures for induction and growth of roots. Step 2 is the culturing of adventitious roots in a liquid medium. After induction, adventitious roots can be directly harvested, or for more biomass growth and accumulation of phytochemicals, inoculated into liquid media and cultured in shaking flask or bioreactors. When roots are cultured, the aim is to increase production of secondary metabolites and this can be achieved by either raising the concentration of the compounds or increasing the total biomass. Both compounds and root biomass were affected by the medium contents, that is, sucrose concentration, PGRs types and concentration, and nutrients, as well as inoculum size and culture period (Table 6.3). For a bioreactor system, to uphold a continuous culture, growth kinetics was required for medium replacement or root harvest. While in the batch culture system, the medium is finite, therefore, establishing a growth curve is imperative in identifying the suitable day for subculture. Several studies reported that altering a medium during roots cultures will enhance metabolite accumulation. For example,

TABLE 6.3 Examples of Secondary Metabolites Production from Root Culture.

Plant species	Medium + PGRs (mg/L)	Explants used	Light regime	Culture period (d)	Products	Yield	References
Aloe vera	MS+0.3 IBA	Leaf	Continuous	35	Aloe emodin, Chrysophanol	4.42 µg/g, 63.65 µg/g	Lee et al. (2013)
Andrographis paniculata	MS+ 2.7 µM NAA	Leaf	Dark	28	Andrographolide	72.86 mg/g DW	Praveen et al. (2009)
Bupleurum Falcatum	B5+8 IBA	Root	Dark	56	Saikosaponin-a, Saikosaponin-b	420 mg/L, 350 mg/L	Kusakari et al. (2000)
Cephaelis ipecacuanha	MS+ 1 IAA, 3 IAA	Leaf	Dark	70	Emetine, cephaeline	0.514%, 1.319% DW	Teshima et al. (1988)
Datura metel	B5+12 µM IAA	Leaf	16 h	35	Hyoscyamine, Scopolamine	4.35 mg/g, 0.28 mg/g DW	Ajungla et al. (2009)
Echinacea angustifolia	½ MS + 2.0 IBA	Root	Dark	28	Total phenol and flavonoids	65.5 mg/g, 39.2 mg/g DW	Wu et al. (2009)
H. perforatum	1/2 MS + 0.1 kin + IBA	Root	Dark	35	Chlorogenic acid, Hypericin	0.97 mg/g, 1.389 mg/g	Cui et al. (2010)
M.citrifolia	MS+ 5 IBA	Leaf	Dark	28	Anthraquinone	251.89 g/L DW	Baque et al. (2011)
Panax ginseng	SH + 5 IBA	Root	Dark	28	Ginsenosides	3.5 mg/g DW	Marsik et al. (2014)
Peritassa campestris	WPM + 4.0 IBA	Cotyledons	Dark	7	Maytenin	972.11 µg/g DW	Paz et al. (2013)
Plumbago indica	B5+0.1 NAA	Leaf	Dark	24	Plumbagin	1.64 mg/g DW	Jaisi et al. (2013)
P. indica	B5+0.1 NAA	Leaf	Dark	20	Plumbagin	12.5 mg/g DW	Jaisi and Panichayupakaranant (2016)

TABLE 6.3 *(Continued)*

Plant species	Medium + PGRs (mg/L)	Explants used	Light regime	Culture period (d)	Products	Yield	References
Plumbago rosea	B5 + 1.0 NAA + 0.1 kin	Leaf	16 h	48	Plumbagin	0.129% DW	Panichayupakaranant and Tewtrakul (2002)
Polygonum multiflorum	MS+ IBA 9.84 μM	Leaf	Dark	28	Phenolics, Flavonoids	53.87 mg/g, 27.96 mg/g DW	Ho et al. (2018)
Prunella vulgaris	MS+ 0.5 NAA	Callus	nd	49	Phenolics, Flavonoids	0.995 mg/g, 6.615 mg/g-DW	Fazal et al. (2014)
P. corylifolia	MS+ NAA 0.5 + IAA 1.0 + IBA 1.5	Leaf	16 h	28	Psoralen	3.73 mg/ml	Siva et al. (2015)
Raphanus sativus	1/2 MS + 0.5 IBA	Root tip	14 h	28	Anthocyanin	250 mg/100 ml	Betsui et al. (2004)
Rhus javanica	LS+ $10^{-6\,M}$ IAA	Leaf	Dark	21	Galloylglucoses, Riccionidin A	30 mg/g, 0.32 mg/g FW	Taniguchi et al. (2000)
Talinum paniculatum	MS + 2.0 IBA	Leaf	Dark	28	Saponin	12.56 mm^2/0.01 g DW (spot area)	Manuhara et al. (2014)
Withania somnifera	1/2 MS + 0.5 IBA	Leaf	16 h	35	Withanolide-A	8.8 mg/g	Praveen and Murthy (2010)

PGRs: plant growth regulators, MS: Murashige and Skoog (1962), B5: Gamborg et al. (1968), WPM: Lloyd and McCown (1980), SH (Schenk and Hildebrandt, 1972), nd: not determined.

root biomass and formation of tanshinone and protocatechuic aldehyde in *S. miltiorrhiza* adventitious roots increased with the rise in sucrose to 60 g/L in MS medium (Guo et al., 2005). In contrast, maximum production of anthraquinone, phenolics, and flavonoids was achieved in the root culture of *M. citrifolia* when sucrose was decreased to 10 g/L (Baque et al., 2011). The source of nitrogen, that is, nitrate and ammonium nitrogen, in the medium was reported to affect secondary metabolites accumulation. The maximum secondary metabolite production was achieved with nitrate as the sole nitrogen source (Guo et al., 2005). However, increasing NH_4^+:NO_3^- ratios to 10:20 in the medium lead to decrease in the pH, and interrupted the mineral absorption which all resulted in low biomass in *Eleutherococcus koreanum* culture (Lee and Paek, 2012). Culture period can affect the root growth as with time, depletion of auxin and sucrose forms the medium and in the same time, produce compound accumulated in the medium, which might hamper root growth. Ishimaru and Shimomura (1995) reported that the concentration of sangulin H-6 reached a maximum level at week 4 of root cultures of *Sanguisorba officinalis*, and then decreased, while the amount of sanguiin H-11 increased, presuming there is a biosynthetic conversion from sangulin H-6 into sanguiin H-11. On the other hand, the root inoculum size must be manipulated. Ho et al. (2018) studied the effect of inoculum density (3–15 g/L) and found that the 5 g/L density resulted in the highest root dry weight and the highest concentration of bioactive compounds in the root culture of *Polygonum multiflorum*. Table 6.3 shows some of these protocols. Step 3 is to enhance accumulation of metabolites with the addition of elicitors, precursor feeding, or biotransformation.

6.3.2.2 SHOOT CULTURE

Shoot cultures (aerial parts) are usually used for the micropropagation of medicinal plants. However, many metabolites can be produced directly in shoot cultures of plant materials. For example, *Artemisia annua* did not produce artemisinin in callus or hairy root cultures but produced only in shoot cultures (Kim et al., 2002). Moreover, in vitro shoot multiplication of *Frangula alnus* produced the highest anthraquinone content (Namdeo, 2007). Shoots once established, reveal genetic stability and high capability for accumulation and production of secondary metabolite (Table 6.4). However, the problem with shoot cultures is the requirement for exogenous supply of plant growth regulators.

TABLE 6.4 Examples of Secondary Metabolites Production from Shoot Culture.

Plant species	Medium+PGRs (mg/L)	Explant used	Light regime	Culture period (d)	Products	Yield	References
A. melanocarpa	MS+0.5 NAA+1 BA	Bud	Continuous	28	Hydroxybenzoic acid, Salicylic acid, Coumaric acid	50.66 mg/100 g, 91.86 mg/100, 54.44 mg/100 DW	Szopa and Ekiert (2014)
A. indica	1/2MS+IBA 0.5	Embryo	nd	28	Azadirachtin, Nimbin	0.008 mg/g, 0.003 mg/g DW	Srividya et al. (1998)
H. perforatum	MS/B5+BA 1.0	Apical segment	16 h	30	Hypericin, Pseudohypericin	50 µg/g, 350 µg/g DM	Gadzovska et al. (2005)
H. perforatum	LS+0.1 NAA+0.1 BA	Seed	Continuous	21	Neochlorogenic acid, 3,4-Dihydroxyphenyl-acetic acid,	118.81 mg/100 g, 129.29 mg/100 g DW	Kwiecien et al. (2015)
Myristica fragrans	MS+26.85 NAA+4.44 BA	Callus (leaf)	Continuous	35	Myristin, methyl eugenol	4.33%, 84.62%	Indira Iyer et al. (2009)
Ophiorrhiza rugosa	MS+5 BA+0.5 NAA	Leaf	12 h	60	Camptothecin	0.065%	Vineesh et al. (2007)
P. corylifolia	MS+8 µM TDZ	Cotyledonary nodes	16 h	28	Daidzein, Genistein	1.23%, 0.38% DW	Shinde et al. (2009)
Rehmannia glutinosa	MS+1.0 BAP+0.1 IAA	Callus (hypocotyl)	16 h	35	Catalpol	45 mg/g DW	Piątczak et al. (2015)
S. officinalis	MS+IAA 0.1+BA 0.45	Shoot tip	Continuous	420	Carnosic acid, Carnosol, Rosmarinic acid	4.77 mg/g, 0.63 mg/g, 16.3 mg/g DW	Grzegorczyk et al. (2005)
S. suffruticosa	HM+0.3 mg/L NAA+3. 0 mg/L 2iP+1.0 mg/L BA	Callus (cotyledon)	16 h	28	Securinine, Allosecurinine	6.02 mg/g, 3.7 mg/g DW	Raj et al. (2015)
Thymus vulgaris	MS+BA4	Seed	16 h	30	Flavonoids	0.64 mg/g FW	Karalija and Parić (2011)

PGRs: plant growth regulators, MS: Murashige and Skoog (1962), B5: Gamborg et al. (1968), LS: Linsmaier and Skoog (1965), HM: Huang and Murashige (1976), Nd: not determined.

6.3.3 SECONDARY METABOLITE PRODUCTION BY TRANSGENIC ORGANS

Plant cell cultures are the most popular types of in vitro techniques that have been investigated because they are easier to manipulate especially in a bioreactor. But the plant cell cultures are subject to somaclonal variations which may result in the loss of productivity with culture age. Also, many cultured undifferentiated cells did not produce secondary metabolites. The ordinary root of many medicinal plants is basically the source of bioactive ingredients, but generally, roots exhibit slower growth than cultures of plant cells and are difficult to harvest. Although organ cultures are reported to produce valuable compounds, they are still hormone-dependent. To overcome this problem, several alternatives were explored which resulted in the use of organized or semiorganized tissue of hairy roots, shooty teratomas or crown galls cultures. These transformed organs have been obtained by genetic transformation with *Agrobacterium rhizogenes* or a mutated *Agrobacterium tumefaciens*. Production of secondary metabolites from transformed tissue was reported to be high yielding, stable, and promising.

6.3.3.1 HAIRY ROOT CULTURE

Hairy root cultures can be obtained from various host plants but mainly from dicotyledonous. The part that can be infected includes leaf, other organs or even protoplasts. Typically, culturing root explants involves the exogenous supply of phytohormone with a very slow growth, resulting in the poor synthesis of secondary metabolite (Rao and Ravishankar, 2002). The increase of biomass of hairy roots is resultant of the rate of elongation, lateral branching, and diameter thickening of roots (Oksman-Caldentey and Hiltunen, 1996).

There are several advantages of using hairy root culture for production of secondary metabolites. The hairy root phenotype is characterized by (1) hormone-independence, (2) fast growth (0.1–2.0 g dry weight/L/day) as unorganized cell suspension, (3) absence of geotropism, (4) extensive root branching, (5) genetically and biochemically stable, (6) expression of specific metabolic pathways as normal roots with similar or higher yields, (7) capability of transforming inert xenobiotics into bioactive metabolites, (8) maintaining the stability of yields, (9) the possibility of clone selection for high-yielding stable hairy root lines, and (10) like adventitious roots, hairy roots secrete metabolites into the liquid medium, making it easy for collection (Flores et al., 1993; Oksman-Caldentey and Hiltunen, 1996; Anand, 2010; Alamgir, 2017). Some hairy roots, when exposed to light, turn green and can be grown photoautotrophically, and these photoautotrophic roots show much higher levels of total alkaloids than the dark-grown roots (Flores et al., 1993).

Culturing of hairy roots in bioreactors showed some disadvantages associated with medium agitation such as sensitivity to shear stress or related to space as hairy roots grow actively hence occupy full space in the vessel. Bourgaud et al. (2001) described different techniques to overcome these problems such as to protect the roots from agitation by using screens or wire meshes, and immobilization of hairy roots into a polymer matrix. Moreover, secondary metabolites produced by hairy roots are limited to those synthesized in roots of the intact plants (Oksman-Caldentey and Hiltunen, 1996). Table 6.5 is an example of some secondary metabolites produced from the hairy root and crown gall cultures.

6.3.3.2 CROWN GALL AND SHOOTY TERATOMA CULTURES

The insertion of a tumor-inducing (Ti) plasmid by *A. tumefaciens* into a plant causes crown gall disease to appear as unorganized tumor at the part of the infection. Transfer DNA (T-DNA) encodes the enzyme that regulates the plant growth hormones (i.e., auxins and cytokinins) and has been detected in the transformed tissues. Endogenous phytohormones produced can affect the secondary pathway, therefore, crown gall tissue has been used for the production of various phytochemicals.

Different types of *A. tumefaciens* strains (e.g. wild-type or mutant strains Ti plasmids) used outcomes in different hormonal imbalance after infection. Consequently, the resultant morphology of crown gall tumors is formed either by amorphous callus or teratomas containing organized stem and leaf-like structures, the so-called shooty teratomas (Floryanowicz-Czekalska and Wysokinska, 2000). The shooty teratomas are formed due to overexpression of the cytokinin biosynthetic gene, that is, decrease in the auxin/cytokinin ratio in the transformed crown gall tissue leading to leaf and shoot formation. Shooty teratoma induction is highly desired as it provides a possibility to culture shoots independent of hormones for production of phytochemicals that are synthesized only in the aerial parts of plants. The number of plant species forming stable fully developed shooty teratomas is limited. The proper establishment of shooty teratomas requires several demands such as shoots that must be fully differentiated, rootless and callus

TABLE 6.5 Some Secondary Metabolites Produced from Hairy Root and Crown Galls Cultures.

Plant species	Medium	Explant	Culture type	Light regime	Culture period (d)	Products	Yield	References
A. indica	MS	Leaf, Stem	Hairy root	Dark	30	Azadirachtin	3.6 μg/g, 2.7 μg/g DW	Sundaram and Curry (1996)
Calendula officinalis	½ MS	Cotyledon, Hypocotyls	Hairy root	Dark	30	Oleanolic acid	8.42 mg/g DW	Długosz et al. (2013)
Cannabis sativa	B5	Callus	Hairy root	Dark	35	Cannabinoid	2.0 μg/g DW	Farag and Kayser (2015)
Coleus forskohlii	B5	Leaf	Hairy root	Dark	84	Forskolin	2.36 mg/g DW	Pandey et al. (2014)
Datura stramonium	½ B5	nd	Hairy root	Dark	33	Hyoscyamine	211.2 mg/L	Hilton and Rhodes (1993)
Portulaca Oleracea	½ MS	Cotyledon	Hairy root	16 h	28	Dopamine	1.21 mg/g	Moghadam et al. (2014)
T. paniculatum	MS	Leaf	Hairy root	Dark	14	Saponin	71 365 mg/L/g DW	Manuhara et al. (2015)
Valeriana officinalis	MS	Leaf	Hairy root	Dark	48	Valerenic acid	3.02 mg/g DW	Torkamani et al. (2014)
Salvia miltiorrhiza	6,7-V	Node	(Teratoma) cell suspension	Dark	16	Tanshinone	2.22 mg/250 mL	Chen et al. (1997)
S. miltiorrhiza	6,7-V	Node	(Teratoma) cell suspension	Dark	12	Cryptotanshinone, Tanshinone I, Tanshinone IIA, Rosmarinic acid, Lithospermic acid B	150 mg/L, 20 mg/L, 50 mg/L, 530 mg/L, 216 mg/L	Chen and Chen (1999)

PGRs: plant growth regulators, MS: Murashige and Skoog (1962), B5: Gamborg et al. (1968), 6,7-V: Veliky and Martin (1970), Nd: not determined.

free, and capable of growing in a liquid medium without browning, callusing or hyperhydricity (Subroto et al., 1996). Shooty teratomas can produce typical shoot-derived metabolites such as mint oil from *Mentha citrata* (Spencer et al., 2009) as well as biotransformation of root-derived metabolites such as nicotine and hyoscyamine (Saito, 1993). The shooty teratomas of *C. roseus* epicotyls and stem nodal explants displayed a 10-fold yield of vincristine over the untransformed cultures (Begum et al., 2009). The main advantage of shooty teratoma cultures over untransformed shoots cultures is that exogenous growth regulators are not required (Subroto et al., 1996). The co-culture of shooty teratomas and hairy roots of *A. belladonna* in a hormone-free medium produced scopolamine with an amount 3–11 times higher than that produced by the leaves of the intact plant (Floryanowicz-Czekalska and Wysokinska, 2000).

6.3.4 BIOREACTOR FOR PRODUCTION OF SECONDARY METABOLITES

The bioreactor is a physical/thermal system for the maintenance of cells in the best culture conditions for a fast growth (Ruffoni et al., 2010). It helps: (1) provide a pilot or large-scale production of biochemicals compared to shake flasks. Bioreactors vary considerably in the volume size which ranged between 1 and 5 L lab scales to 75,000 L industrial scale. The production of secondary metabolites in large bioreactors is preferred over the ordinary in vitro cultures for several reasons. (2) Bioreactor culture offers the benefits of using a liquid medium compared to static cultures. (3) Automatic controlling of the whole production process including optimizing the medium conditions, such as temperature, pH, dissolved oxygen, carbon dioxide, carbohydrates, and mineral nutrients. 4) Online measurements of the growth of the culture.

6.3.4.1 BIOREACTOR TYPES

A wide type of bioreactors has been designed so that they can fit the different types of cultures and can be grouped into three types depending on the agitation way; *mechanically-agitated* bioreactors, *pneumatically*-driven bioreactors, and *non-agitated* bioreactors. Mechanical bioreactors or stirred tank has a mechanical device for stirring medium, including a turbine impeller, helical ribbon impeller, and vibrating perforated plates. Wave reactors are mechanically agitated bioreactors, although they have no direct impeller agitation, they provide a wave motion within the liquid medium that is caused by swinging of the vessel (Georgiev et al., 2009; Ruffoni et al., 2010). Pneumatic bioreactors are vessels lacking a stirring device and agitation of the medium is put to function by air flow. These types of bioreactors can be alienated, depending on the means of providing the airflow, into two kinds, airlift and bubble column reactors. In airlift bioreactor, the medium is agitated and aerated by the introduction of air through the top of the column. While in the bubbling reactor the medium is agitated and aerated by introducing air from the bottom of the column. Airlift and bubble column reactors have been utilized for the cultivation of photoautotrophic or photomixotrophic cell suspension cultures (Georgiev et al., 2009).

Non-agitated bioreactors were considered the third group of bioreactors although they lack a means of agitation. However, the air is also mixed with media prior delivering to the cultures. These include temporary immersion and nutrient mist bioreactors. In temporary immersion bioreactors, the media is pumped to the culture section and kept for a short time, and then returned to the storage tank. In nutrient mist bioreactors, the sterilized mix of air and media is sprayed above the surface of cultures.

The numerous advantages that have been shown by the different bioreactor designs can be used as a guide to choose the type that fits the desired kind and purpose of the in vitro cultures. Helical ribbon impeller was found to be efficient for mass transfer of medium and gasses, and less damaging to cells than other used impellers (Smith, 1995). Rotary drum reactors are characterized by sustained suspension homogeneity, low shear stress, and higher oxygen transfer ability (Chattopadhyay et al., 2002). Stirred tank bioreactors are commonly used due to large-scale production, use with highly viscous cultures, high oxygen allocation and good culture mixing (Yue et al., 2014). Bubble column bioreactors are typified by low capital and operational costs, low shear stress and uncomplicated system (Ruffoni et al., 2010) due to the absence of stirring part.

Collectively, the main considerations for choosing a bioreactor should be adequate oxygen availability, low shear stress to cells, adequate nutrient supply, and product removal from cells (Yue et al., 2014).

Several modifications and enhancements have been applied to the bioreactors for better performance such as minimum shear stress, good aeration and adapted impeller blades to ensure no damage to cultures. A new agitated bioreactor named the centrifugal impeller has been developed for shear-sensitive in vitro cultures in which a conventional vessel is agitated by a centrifugal-pump-like impeller (Georgiev et al., 2009). To improve the homogenization of culture medium, an airlift mesh-draught reactor with wire helixes was designed for large-scale hairy root culture of *Solanum chrysotrichum* (Ruffoni et al., 2010). Increasing blade size has been found to reduce shear stirred-tank bioreactor. The accomplishment of the optimization of a bioreactor system for a type of culture indicates that the production of secondary metabolites is ready for scaling up to a commercial level (Smith, 1995). Cells of *Podophyllum hexandrum,* when cultured in a 3 L stirred tank bioreactor, showed an increase of 27% in productivity compared to shake flask culture (Chattopadhyay et al., 2002). *Digitalis purpurea* cell line cultured in airlift bioreactors improved the yield of digitoxin up to 430 mg/L (Gaosheng and Jingming, 2012).

6.4 ANALYSIS OF CULTURE GROWTH

For the production of secondary metabolites using in vitro cultures, the measurement of growth parameters is required. Such measurements are imperative to verify what is needed for the optimization of media contents, cultural conditions or other components, to maintain a high growth rate and/or yields. In addition, bioassays of plant growth hormones and comparisons of genotype performance can be performed by evaluating the growth characteristics. The detailed analysis of the biochemistry of plant in vitro cultures will certainly allow for improved manipulation of natural product biosynthesis.

These measurements involve a growth curve for the cultures by plotting the measured values. When the inoculum material is cultured in the medium, there is a lag period preceding growth then followed by exponential and linear growth continuing until a gradual deceleration is reached and finally, the culture enters a stationary phase. This pattern of growth is the so-called S-shaped curve.

Measuring growth parameters of batch cultures is imperative to ensure the reproducibility of production for experiments both in the laboratory and on industrial scales. Based on different parameters, the culture growth can be measured by several methods. These methods can be grouped into categories depending on the way of sampling or measuring a culture, *destructive methods,* and *nondestructive methods.*

6.4.1 DESTRUCTIVE METHODS

These methods involve harvesting of whole or samples of the biomass so sacrificing the cells. This includes various procedures such as measuring the fresh and dry weights (DWs), cell number, cell viability, and protein estimation (Dixon, 1985; Schripsema et al., 1990; Dixon and Gonzales, 1994; Doležel et al., 2007; Mustafa et al., 2011).

6.4.1.1 FRESH WEIGHT (FW) AND DRY WEIGHT (DW)

Fresh weight (FW) and DW are the most common parameters that are usually measured to monitor the growth of cells per volume cultured. The measurement of FW is less accurate because of variations in the adhering water (Schripsema et al., 1990). Measurement of DW is most frequently used because it is considered to be more precise. DW is usually used for the preparation of a growth curve, target compound yield, enzyme activity curve, and gene expression curve (Gaosheng and Jingming, 2012).

6.4.1.1.1 Organ and Callus Cultures

For FW, the biomass harvested from the culture ensuring no medium is attached, is placed on a pre-weighed piece of aluminum foil. When the culture is harvested, the weight must be acquired immediately to reduce variations caused by water evaporation. To obtain DW, there are different methods to dry the biomass harvested. (1) The biomass can be air-dried under lab conditions (25–30°C) by exposing the samples to fresh air until complete evaporation of the water content. This method is suitable for small biomass and it takes a long time. (2) Heating in a hot air oven at 40–60°C for 12–24 h is also reported for thermostable compounds. This is followed by placing the sample in a desiccator until cooling (15–20 min) and then recording the DW. The process needs to be repeated until constant weight is reached. 3) Drying in a freeze dryer is preferred because it is quick, and to guarantee that no compound will be affected by heating as in the oven method, or due to microorganism contamination of the cells during the air-drying method. Freeze-drying retains higher levels of phenolics content in plant samples than in air-drying (Liu et al., 2008).

Monitoring root growth (normal adventitious or hairy roots) can be invasive if precise measurements are required. After harvesting, root numbers (primary and laterals), root length (primary and laterals), total length (primary + laterals), and root growth unit (cm per root tips) are obtainable.

6.4.1.1.2 Cell Culture

For acquiring the FW of cell suspension, an appropriate sample volume of cells is collected on a pre-weighed Whatman filter paper or a nylon fabric placed in a funnel. The cell is then washed with sterile distilled water to remove the medium. After draining under vacuum, the cells with the filter are reweighed immediately before the cell loses fluid. For DW measurement, the cells and the nylon together with the cells are dried at 45–80°C for 12–24 h, which are then cooled in a desiccator and weighed to a constant weight (e.g. 10% moisture). The FW and DW can be expressed as per milliliter culture.

The obtained FW and DW values can be used to calculate the growth efficiency indices such as growth index, relative DW, FW increment, growth rate, root-growth ratio, growth ratio, and biomass doubling time. These growth indices can be used to measure the growth of all types of cultures but mainly they are used for callus and root cultures because they require tedious work in weighing and calculations. Some of the most used equations for calculation of growth indices are provided.

1. Growth index % $(Gi) = (G_1 - G_0)/(G_0) \times 100$
   where G_1 is the FW after specified cultivation period, and G_0 is the FW of the inoculum.
2. The relative DW% $(RDW) = DW/FW \times 100$
3. FW increment $(FWi) = FW_1 - FW_0$
   where fw_1 is the final FWafter every cycle per time and fw_0 is the initial FWat the beginning of each cycle.
4. Growth rate $(\mathrm{Gr}) = (W_1/W_0)$ -1 per unit time
   where W_1 is the final weight, W_0 is the inoculum weight.
5. Average growth rate $(\mathrm{AGR}) = ln\ Wf - ln\ Wi/t$
   where *ln* is Naperian (natural) logarithm, Wf = final weight of the fresh matter, Wi is inoculum weight, t is specific cultivation period.
6. Specific growth rate $(\mu) = In\ X_t - In\ X_0/t$
   where X_0 is the initial cell density, Xt is the cell density at time t.
7. Growth ratio $(\mathrm{GR}) = DWh - DWi/DWi$
   where DWh is the harvested DW, DWi is the inoculated DW.
8. Doubling time growth $(\mathrm{Dt}) = ln2/m$
   where $ln2$ is a natural logarithm, m is slope of the line.
9. Callus induction frequency $(\mathrm{Cif}) = PN/TN \times 100$
   where PN is the number of explants producing callus, TN is the total number of cultured explants.

10. Callus index (CI) $= 100n \times G/N$
    where n = number of explants initiating callus, G is visual callus rating of initiated explants, N = total number of explants planted. Visual callus rating: 1=25%, 2=50%, 3=75%, 4=100%
11. Secondary metabolites yield (SMY) = *DW* (g/L) × *content* (mg/g DW).

After the biosynthesis of target compounds, it might be accumulated in the cells (*intracellular*) or secreted into liquid media (*extracellular*) and in some cases, in both. To determine the yield of a compound, both contents should be summed to represent the producing ability.

In addition to the abovementioned weight-dependent parameters, cell suspensions have special measurements of growth reported in various research works (Hahlbrock, 1975; Sung, 1976; Dixon, 1985; David et al., 1989; Dixon and Gonzales, 1994; Mustafa et al., 2011). These methods include packed cell volume, cell counting, or cellular protein content. These techniques involve tedious preparation of the cells.

6.4.1.1.3 Packed Cell Volume

Cell division leads to a rise in the number of cells which cause an increase in the proportion of cells per milliliter of suspension and hence can be used to estimate growth of the cell in cultures. For estimating PCV, a sample (e.g. 10 mL) of uniformly dispersed suspension culture needs to be transferred into graduated centrifuge tubes (e.g. 15 mL) and centrifuged at 2000 rpm for 5–10 min. The measurement is conducted after cells are allowed to completely sediment in the tube. PCV was normally expressed as a percentage of the compacted volume of the cell pellet to the total culture volume. PCV can be considered as a partly-distractive method because it involves sacrificing only a sample of the culture.

6.4.1.1.4 Cell Viability

Throughout the period of culture, cell death may occur in suspension cultures because of, for example, the exhaust of medium and accumulation of toxic substances. Determining the viability of cells before cell counting is very important to ensure that data on the number of cells is correct. Cell viability can be carried out by the examination of protoplasmic streaming and the presence of an intact nucleus under a microscope. Cell viability can be determined by stains such as Evans methylene blue (10%). Nonviable cells become blue in color, while viable cells turn colorless. Cell viability may also be analyzed by other methods such as fluorescein diacetate, Tetrazolium test (2,3,5-triphenyl tetrazolium chloride), 3-[4,5-dimethylthiazol-2yl]-2,5-diphenyl tetrazolium bromide, and the mitotic index depending on the activity of reductase enzyme. The percentage of viability is usually recorded by taking 10 mL of sample. The measurement of cell concentration by cell counting has also shown a reasonably good correlation with DW parameter.

6.4.1.1.5 Number of Cells

The increase in the number of cells due to cell division is a measurable indicator of growth through the culture period. However, this can be performed only with fine cell suspension cultures. Cell suspension cultures containing large cell aggregates, therefore, must be broken down into individual cell components before cell counting. Several treatments are used for the dissociation of aggregates into individual cells. The most reported is digesting the suspension with chromic acid (Cr_2O_3 $0.5H_2O$) or chromium trioxide (CrO_3). A sample of the cell suspension (e.g. 1 mL) is added to a solution (e.g. 2 mL) of 2.5% chromic acid or 8% chromium trioxide heated to 60–70°C for 5–15 min. The mixture is cooled and vigorously shaken for 15 min for effective cell separation.

Hydrolytic enzymes such as cellulase and pectinase are also reported. The enzyme method can be applied by mixing 1 mL of the cell suspension with 0.5 mL of 10% cellulase and 0.5 mL of 5% pectinase. The mixture is then incubated for 30 min at 25°C with rotatory agitation at 100 rpm.

Then the suspension sample is dispersed with hypodermic needles on a hemocytometer slide. The cell count is measured under a microscope using a cell counter. Cell counting chamber such as the Sedgewick Rafter cell or the Neubauer chamber can be used. A sample with fixed volume (e.g. 10 μL) of the suspension is spread over a defined area (e.g. 10 squares). The number of cells counted within the 10 squares represents the number of cells in 10 μL. By calculation, cell density is easy to determine per whole volume of suspension, that is, multiply by 100 for density per milliliter. The cell number is usually comparable to the DW, while the PCV is usually comparable to theFW.

Cell viability, by the exclusion of vital stains, can be performed in the same sample after using enzymes because cells stay viable. Although chromium trioxide method is quicker and less complicated than the use of enzymes, cell viability cannot be estimated in the same sample due to cell death.

6.4.1.1.6 Nutrients and metabolite concentrations

Some nutrients/metabolites in the cell suspension culture medium show correlation with growth in a single culture flask. For example, the total nitrate and sugar levels in the medium can be used to measure growth.

6.4.1.1.7 Protein content

Protein content can be obtained by extraction of the whole harvested cells or in a sample of the culture. Cells collected on a Whatman glass fiber filter are washed twice with boiling 70% ethanol. Acetone is used to dry the material prior to the transfer to a solution of 1M NaOH followed by heating at 85°C for 1 h. Then hydrolyzed protein is determined in the filtrate. The total protein content is expressed per gram of cells. In general, the protein content per culture increases with the increase in growth, therefore showing the least values at the stationary phase.

6.4.2 NONDESTRUCTIVE METHODS

These methods include different procedures used to evaluate culture growth which allows quick estimations while maintaining sterile conditions. These measurements include several methods such as the culture optical density, residual electrical conductivity, and pH of the medium (Dixon, 1985; Schripsema et al., 1990; Dixon and Gonzales, 1994; Doležel et al., 2007; Mustafa et al., 2011).

6.4.2.1 CELL GROWTH MEASUREMENTS

6.4.2.1.1 Cell Volume after Sedimentation

Cell volume after sedimentation (CVS) involves the culture of cell suspension in 250 mL Erlenmeyer flasks. For performing the measurement, a CVS device was designed by Blom et al. (1992) to hold the 250 mL Erlenmeyer flask kept at an angle of 60°. Then the suspension is allowed to settle for at least 5 min. The height of the cell suspension from the bottom of the flask in the 60° position is measured to represent the volume of cells. Difficult to settle cells of fine and thick consistency of cell. According to Mustafa et al. (2011), the measurement of suspension cultures with volumes lower than 50 ml is less accurate because of the shape of the Erlenmeyer flask.

6.4.2.1.2 Settled Cell Volume

The total size of cells per milliliter of suspension is a result of the increase in the number of cells by cell division. Therefore, it can be used to estimate the growth of the cell in suspension cultures. For determination of SCV, the cells are transferred to 50 mL Falcon tubes and allowed to settle for 30 min. Then the volume of the tube which was occupied by the whole suspension was measured as SCV. To ensure that the measured value is accurate, a second reading after another 30 min can be done. If the variation between the two readings is higher than 5%, a third measurement is favored. SCV is usually comparable to the FW.

6.4.2.1.3 Dissimilation Curve

The dissimilation of sugars by cell culture causes a loss of weight of the contents of the culture flask. The value obtained can be used to follow the growth in a single culture flask. The important precaution is that culture flasks are closed firmly to ensure no evaporation occurs. To obtain the dissimilation curves, the cumulative loss of weight for every flask will be calculated. By weighing one culture flask regularly (during and after the experiment), information can be obtained about the different growth phases, for example, the length of the lag time, the doubling time, the moment the stationary phase is reached, the biomass yield and the amount of intracellularly stored carbohydrates. The dissimilation curves can be correlated to the concentration of sugars in the medium, the DW, and the FW.

6.4.2.1.4 Sidearm-Turbidity Method

Monitoring growth by measurement of turbidity of liquid cultures has been reported. The method involves measuring the turbidity of cultures grown in sidearm flasks. Sidewise tilting of the flask fills the sidearm so that turbidity can be read thoroughly in a photoelectric colorimeter with a blue filter at 400–465 nm. The turbidimetric measurement of cultures grown in sidearm flasks is a quick, easy and routine way of recording plant cell growth in batch cultures. The less accuracy in the measurement of cell concentration by turbidity (optical density) is because of the large variations in the cell size and cell aggregation. However, it has shown a reasonably good correlation with DW.

6.4.2.1.5 Electric Conductivity

The electric conductivity of the medium decreases with increase in the culture growth due to ion uptake by cells; that is, nitrate concentration. The measurement of this decrease is useful for the assessment of cell growth. This method offers several advantages over other methods, such as (1) continuous and online monitoring of cell growth, (2) no sampling is required, (3) it is economical and efficient, (4) it provides an accurate, reliable, and reproducible measurement of plant cell growth rate, and (5) it is independent of cell aggregation, growth morphology, and apparent viscosity.

The medium conductivity can give an impression of growth in a certain culture but is unsuitable for comparison of different cultures.

6.4.2.2 CALLUS FW

All the mentioned equations and methods provided above for callus growth measurements are *destructive sampling methods*, and in addition, require frequent handling of the calli. Therefore, to overcome these disadvantages, other methods were widely used including qualitative/quantitative index (McLean et al., 1992), concentric circles (Fowler and Janick, 1974), and surface area or volume of the callus as a basis for growth assessment (Mottley and Keen, 1987). Other methods for callus growth estimation were also reported using calculated quantities of the average callus diameter, the elliptical surface and the circular surface, determined from the measured linear callus dimensions (Berardi et al., 1993).

6.4.2.2.1 Qualitative and Quantitative Index

The callus growth and appearance were rated using numerical values 0, 1, 2, 3, and 4, which represent dead, poor, fair, good, and excellent, respectively

(Pua et al., 1985). A wide range of numerical values can also be used with a rating scale from 0 up to 9. For example, 0=no tissue growth, 1=initial callus growth from stem ends, 2=callus arising from one stem end, up to 9=callus growth 4 times the originally estimated mass.

Also, the score for callus induction as illustrated by Matkowski (2004) can be used such as: – no callus and poor growth, + good induction but poor growth, ++ good initiation and moderate growth, +++ best induction and vigorous growth.

6.4.2.2.2 The Concentric Circles

This method involves using a sequence of concentric circles of various sizes with a shared center. The concentric circles are drawn on transparent sheets, therefore, can be put, for example, on a Petri dish containing the callus to estimate its diameter. Then the correlation coefficient can be obtained between FW and the diameter. The disadvantage of this method is that calli always vary in shape which is irregular.

6.4.2.2.3 Callus Area Method

Different nondestructive methods based on the measurements of the callus area were also reported. These are point-counting method, electronic planimeter, callus standard width and callus greatest width.

The point-counting method can be done by placing callus pieces on the surface of 36 plates of NH4-S-RMOP agar medium and pressed slightly into the medium to obtain a satisfactory contact. This is important to prevent the calli from becoming disconnected from the medium surface when taking size measurements. Point counts were obtained by placing a transparent overlay at random on the base of the Petri dish. The overlay had points traced on its surface, arranged in a square pattern at intervals of 5.0, 2.5 or 1.0 mm. A minimum of six points per callus area were used in each case. Only those points with their centers exactly on or inside the edge of each callus area were counted as "in" and the areas of individual calli were calculated using the following formula:

$$A = N \times D^2$$

where A = calculated area, N = no. of "in" points, D = distance between the points.

6.4.2.2.4 Greatest and Standard Widths

Greatest width is obtained using a ruler to measure the distance between the two farthest points on each callus surface at a given time. Standard width was obtained using a ruler to measure the length of a line drawn at random through each callus surface on the base of each Petri dish at the beginning of the experiment.

6.4.2.2.5 Electronic Planimeter

For electronic planimeter readings, the callus borders are first carefully traced onto a plastic transparency. Planimeter area readings are obtained by tracing along the borders of each callus. Areas were automatically calculated and displayed.

6.4.2.2.6 Linear Callus Dimensions

From above the Petri dish cover surface, two linear callus dimensions of, the maximum diameter (MD) and the greatest length at the right angle (PD). MD and PD are used to calculate the average callus diameter, callus surface as an ellipse and as a circle.

6.4.2.3 ORGAN CULTURES GROWTH MEASUREMENTS

The growth of shoot and root in cultures can be monitored by special parameters. Such measurements can be conducted from out of the culture flask without losing sterilization. Growth in shoot culture is usually measured mainly using parameters such as the number of shoots, shoot length, and so forth. Similarly, root growth (normal adventitious or hairy roots) can be monitored by estimation of root numbers (primary and laterals), root length (primary and laterals), total length (primary + laterals) and the morphological features such as thickness and secondary root formation.

6.5 EXTRACTION AND ANALYSIS OF SECONDARY METABOLITES

The extraction of bioactive compounds from plant materials is the first step in the utilization of phytochemicals (Dai and Mumper, 2010). Preparation of plant sample in some cases is important. For example, the flavonoid quercetin can be obtained from the extraction of the quercetin glycosides followed by hydrolysis to release the aglycone and subsequent purification (Harwood et al., 2007). Secondary metabolites can be extracted from fresh, frozen or dried plant samples. Usually, before extraction, plant samples are preferred to be firstly air-dried or freeze-dried. The dried materials are then treated by milling, grinding, and homogenization. Usually, the traditional techniques such as Soxhlet, maceration, reflux, and hydro-distillation, which have been used for decades, form the first choice for extraction of phytochemicals. There are a number of factors that influence extraction of compounds from the plant matrix such as the chemical nature of the solvent, the sample to solvent ratio, sample particle size, disruption techniques, temperature as well as the time of exposure. For example, maceration with alcoholic solvents and plant solvent ratio of 1.5:10 can yield a greater level of quercetin (Nobre et al., 2005). Solvent extractions with methanol (particularly), ethanol, acetone, ethyl acetate, often with different proportions of water, are the most commonly used procedures of plant extracts. Weak organic acids, such as formic acid, acetic acid, citric acid, tartaric acid and phosphoric acid, and low concentrations of strong acids, such as trifluoroacetic acid and hydrochloric acid are recommended to minimize peak tailing (Dai and Mumper, 2010). After homogenization and selection of solvent, the extraction should be performed at temperatures that do not permit degradation of compounds of interest. This is done simply by allowing mixtures to macerate for a time (24–48 h) so that the solvent can penetrate all parts of the ruptured cells and solubilize compounds with similar polarity.

For accurate measurements and reliable quantitative determination of the phytochemical contents in raw plant materials, chromatographic methods with appropriate detection are commonly used. High-performance liquid chromatography (HPLC) currently represents the most popular and reliable technique for analysis of compounds. Liquid chromatography (LC) of flavonoids is usually carried out in the reversed-phase mode, on C8- or C18-bonded silica columns (Dai and Mumper, 2010) ranging from 100–250 mm in length and usually with an internal diameter of 3.9–4.6 mm (Liu et al., 2008). Ultra performance liquid chromatography instruments are based on the use of small particle size chromatographic columns (less than 2 μm) and offer substantial resolution enhancement resulting in more efficient separation of the compounds. This is applicable for monitoring of secondary metabolites production in vitro which is characterized by a small amount. In addition, it greatly reduces the analytical time and can withstand high pressure (Liu et al., 2008). Moreover, it has been known to consume less solvent than HPLC.

Gradient elution is generally performed with a binary solvent system (Liu et al., 2008). LC is usually performed at room temperature, but temperatures up to 40°C are sometimes required to reduce the time of analysis and because thermostated columns give more repeatable elution times. However, the constant column temperature is recommended for reproducibility (Dai and Mumper, 2010). If the main aim of the study is to determine the major flavonoids in a sample, the run time of 0.5–1 h is usually sufficient to separate the 5–10 compounds of interest (Rijke et al., 2006).

All flavonoid aglycones contain at least one aromatic ring and, consequently, efficiently absorb UV light. The first maximum, which is found in the 240–285 nm range, is due to the A-ring and the second maximum, which is in the 300–550 nm range, is due to the substitution pattern and conjugation of the C-ring (Rijke et al., 2006). UV detection is the recommended tool in all LC-based analysis types, and LC with multiple wavelength or diode–array detection is a reasonable tool for various studies such as quantification of the main aglycones or for interim subgroup classification. Flavonoids detection is usually carried out at 250, 265, 290, 350, 370 or 400 nm, and 500–525 nm for anthocyanidins (Rijke et al., 2006; Dai and Mumper, 2010). The other colored compounds such as carotenoid and quinoid pigments or UV-absorbing phenolics are commonly estimated by this technique (Matkowski, 2008). In flavonoid analysis, fluorescence detection is used only infrequently because few classes of flavonoids have innate fluorescence, including the isoflavones and flavonoids with OH group in the 3-position, such as 3-hydroxyflavone and catechin. However, the techniques involve spectrophotometry that is suitable for some groups of compounds and is inappropriate for other types.

Under the usual reversed-phase conditions, the more polar compounds are generally eluted first. Thus, diglycosides precede monoglycosides, which precede aglycones. The elution pattern for flavonoids containing equivalent substitution patterns is flavanone followed by flavonol and flavones. This elution pattern holds for both aglycones and glycosides for isomeric compounds, which differ in the structure of the saccharine attached at the 7-position, the rutinoside being eluted ahead of the neohesperidoside (Robards and Antolovich, 1997).

The use of hyphenated techniques such as LC–mass spectrometry and LC-nuclear magnetic resonance (NMR) or Two-dimensional-NMRis the best means for structure determination of novel compounds detected only in in vitro cultures and not in intact plants. (Matkowski, 2008).

6.6 STRATEGIES TO IMPROVE PRODUCTION

The tissue culture cells typically accumulate large amounts of secondary compounds only under specific conditions. This means that the maximization of the production and accumulation of secondary metabolites by plant tissue culture requires a strategy to enhance biosynthesis and production of secondary compounds. A number of reported methods (Kim et al., 2002; Rao and Ravishankar, 2002; James et al., 2008 Kuo et al., 2011; Cai et al., 2012) based on different environmental and nutritional factors are known to influence the biosynthetic pathways of secondary metabolites such as: (1) obtaining efficient cell lines for high growth, (2) selecting high yielding cell clones, (3) immobilization of cells to enhance yields of extracellular metabolites, (4) infusion of metabolites to facilitate downstream processing, (5) relationship with growth phase and subculturing, (6) manipulating the environment and medium, (7) adsorption of the metabolites to separate the products from the medium and to overcome feedback inhibition (8) biotransformation, (9) precursor feeding, and (10) elicitation.

6.6.1 SCREENING OF HIGH-GROWTH CELL LINE

Undifferentiated plant cells are genetically heterogeneous that makes it promising to select cell strains with superior metabolites production. Selection of a stable cell line and finding the optimum conditions for cell growth and maintenance, therefore, is fundamental. There are many reports on the selection of cultured cell strains that give high yields of useful compounds (Rao and Ravishankar, 2002). Selected cell strains have been obtained by various selection methods such as cell cloning, cell tolerance to stress agents, visual selection, fluorescence assay, HPLC technique, radioimmunoassay, and other bioassays selection. The selected cell lines can be cultivated in the lab to supply a continuous and reliable source of natural products.

The selected cell lines must be stable in growth and production of targeted compounds even after subculture or maintenance for a long period as variability in metabolite accumulation leads to a reduction in productivity. Variability in culture characteristics has been attributed to genetic changes by mutation or epigenetic changes due to physiological conditions (Yue et al., 2014).

Cell tolerance to stress and bioassays selection strategies involve exposure of a number of cells to a toxic or environmental stress, and only cells that are able to resist the selection procedures will survive (Rao and Ravishankar, 2002).

6.6.2 CELL IMMOBILIZATION

Immobilization is defined as the confinement of cells in or on a suitable matrix to enable the flux of the product in an extracellular medium (Anand, 2010). Generally, the cells are added to different types of gels such as agar, agarose, gelatin, polyacrylamide or calcium alginate (Rodríguez-Sahagún et al., 2012).

6.6.3 OPTIMIZATIONOFMEDIUMANDCULTURECONDITIONS

Several strategies have been adopted for the enhancement of bioactive metabolite production in in vitro cultures. The media constituents (source and concentration) namely, nutrients, carbohydrates, phytohormones, vitamins have to be optimized for both a maximum biomass gain and the accumulation of the targeted metabolite. The cultural conditions including temperature, pH, light, and oxygen also gradually affect the final yields. There are several types of in vitro culture media used widely for the growth of cultures and production of phytochemicals, such as MS (Murashige and Skoog, 1962), B5 (Gamborg et al., 1968), LS (Linsmaier and Skoog, 1965), SH (Schenk and Hildebrandt, 1972), and other improved liquid media according to the growth behavior of plant cells (Yue et al., 2014). The constituents of those media, i.e., carbon, nitrogen, phosphate, inorganic mineral and even pH, are well known in its level and type. A comparative analysis of the growth of *Artemisia annua* hairy roots in two medium formulations showed that the B5 medium was significantly optimum over MS for seven of eight factors studied (Kim et al., 2002). The higher total triterpene production achieved by culturing *E. japonica* cells in MS medium was likened to that of B5 or N6 medium (Ho et al., 2018). It is commonly known that the levels of inorganic nutrients in the MS medium are higher than in B5 medium. The in vitro culture is grown heterotrophically and depends only on sugar as a carbon source (Rao and Ravishanker, 2002). The sugar types that is, sucrose, glucose, and fructose and their concentrations have main effects in phytochemicals production. Rosmarinic acid production was found to increase by five times with increase of sucrose concentration from 3 to 5% (Alamgir, 2017). However, the critical factor, which directly affects both biomass production and phytochemicals accumulation, is the type and concentration of auxin or cytokinin or the auxin/cytokinin ratio (Lee et al., 2011). For example, NAA was superior to IAA and 2,4-Dichlorophenoxyacetic acid for the biosynthesis of anthocyanin in *Glehnia littoralis* cultures cell (Miura et al., 1998). The phytohormones are essential for the good stimulation of phytochemicals, except with a hormone-independent hairy root culture.

Light irradiation condition includes several factors namely, wavelength, intensity, and photoperiod which are reported to affect both the growth and production of secondary metabolites by the most grown in vitro cultures. For example, flavonoids production has been shown to affect positively with the good irradiation. Increasing light intensity doubles the growth yield of *A. annua* hairy roots (Kim et al., 2002). Hairy roots of *Acmella oppositifolia*, *Datura stramonium*, and *Lippia dulcis* turn green when exposed to light consequence to developing mature chloroplasts fully capable of photosynthesis (Flores et al., 1993). In addition to light, temperature, CO_2, and O_2 play an important role in controlling greening, growth and secondary product formation in hairy root cultures (Chandra and Chandra, 2011). However, Miura et al. (1998) established a light-independent system for anthocyanin production on the culture of *G. littoralis*, by optimizing CO_2 supply. The light regime for in vitro culture ranges between the ideal 16/8 h photoperiod to total darkness and continuous light. The pH of the medium is also important in regulation of secondary metabolites yield.

6.6.4 BIOTRANSFORMATION, PRECURSOR FEEDING, AND ELICITATION

Biotransformation is the enzymatic catalysis of new active components, which is stimulated by substrate feedings. The main enzymes are those that can undergo reactions such as reduction, oxidation, methylation, isomerization, acetylation, esterification, and glycosylations (Chandra and Chandra, 2011). There are two core reasons to choose plant cells for biotransformation: (1) cells catalyze the reactions stereospecifically, resulting in pure products, and (2) they can perform regiospecific modifications that are not easily synthesized by chemical or microorganisms (Smetanska, 2008). An alternative to biological transformation is a combined chemical and biological approach. This can be performed by using cell cultures to complete the difficult stages in a synthesis or using enzymes isolated from the cultured cells and the conversion is achieved in a cell-free environment (Collin, 2001). Plant in vitro cultures has been reported to transform exogenously supplied compounds into naturally existent and novel products. *S. rebaudiana* cell cultures are used to transform steviol into steviobioside, a glycoside 300 times sweeter than sucrose (Sasson, 1991). *Coffea Arabica* cell culture supplemented with vanillin and capsaicin has resulted in the production of vanillin glucosides and capsaicin glucoside, respectively (Smetanska, 2008).

Precursor feeding is based on the theory that any intermediary compound involved in the biosynthetic pathway of a product, represents an upright chance to heighten the final yield (Yue et al., 2014). A number of factors are to be considered when applying the precursor to the cell culture medium, such as the concentration and the time of addition of the precursor (Chattopadhyay et al., 2002). Problems related to feeding include a certain level of precursors being toxic to plant cells and inhibiting cell growth, in some cases, they inhibit secondary metabolism accumulation (Yue et al., 2014). Therefore, for one specific plant species, precursor concentration should be carefully adjusted, compared and optimized through the feeding experiment (Gaosheng and Jingming, 2012).

Elicitors are compounds which stimulate any type of physiological abnormality of the plant when introduced in a suitable concentration (Patel and Krishnamurthy, 2013). Therefore, the plant accumulates the secondary compounds as a defense mechanism against the stress induced by the elicitor. According to their origin and function, the elicitors are divided into abiotic and biotic. Abiotic elicitors are physical and chemical factors capable of inducing stress in the plant thus affecting the secondary metabolites accumulation. These include heavy metals, mineral salts and osmotic stress agents (chemicals elicitors), temperature, light, and UV, (environmental conditions), and wounding (physical elicitors). The biotic elicitors are those which have a biological origin, either from pathogenic microorganism or plant. The biotic elicitor may be extracted material (spores and cell wall) or toxins and compounds produced by an organism (polysaccharides, lipids, and glycoproteins). The sources are bacteria, yeast, fungal arthropods, and plants. Biosynthesis of flavonoids is induced either by light via phytochrome or/and UV-photoreceptors (abiotic elicitor), or by infection with a phytopathogenic organism (biotic elicitor) or compounds (abiotic/biotic elicitor) which induce the synthesis of antimicrobial compounds in plants (Sasson, 1991). Methyl jasmonate (MJ) is the most used elicitor in enhancing secondary metabolites accumulation and production. MJ was reported to maximize the production of paclitaxel, taxanes, and diterpenes from in vitro cultures of *Taxus* sp. (Patel and Krishnamurthy, 2013).

Before applying elicitors to the culture, several precautions and stages are required to get the intended results. These include elicitor specificity, the concentration of elicitor, stage and age of culture, elicitor fitting with the medium compositions, and the duration of elicitor contact. Elicitor treatment at late log phase results in higher biomass yield as well as secondary metabolite production, whereas during the early phase, it leads to the immediate increase in secondary metabolite production while lowering the biomass yield (Chandra and Chandra, 2011). High dosage of elicitor has been reported to induce a hypersensitive response leading to cell death, whereas an optimum level was required for secondary metabolite induction (Patel and Krishnamurthy, 2013).

6.6.5 RELATIONSHIP WITH GROWTH PHASE AND SUBCULTURING

To enhance the production of secondary metabolites, it is important to understand when in the growth phase a specific product is formed. For example, if a product is mainly formed during exponential growth, the batch culture can be used to keep the culture actively growing, for long-term maintainance and for maximization of the yields (Kim et al., 2002).

6.7 CONCLUSION

Plant in vitro culture is a complex and multiphase process which requires good management to maximize the production of desired compounds. This process includes three parts which are explant, medium, culture conditions, which must be managed through a time course for the highest degree of accumulation and maximum level of production. Each part can be subdivided into different components that require specific manipulation methods to achieve the goals of the process. The interaction between the components of one part and those of other parts during manipulation require careful management. All these characteristics are those that make in vitro culture systems attractive for production of secondary metabolites. A very wide variety of secondary products have now been demonstrated in the literature. However, for a process to be economically feasible, it has to outperform the conventional procedures. This can be achieved with the development and optimization of the process in all in vitro culture types for high daily productivity (see Chapter 7). As declared above, it requires several strategies varying in the means and time course of application. The modification of the medium compositions is the primary concern in those strategies. The selection of cell lines with stability and enhanced levels of product, either in continuous systems or in batch systems, is similarly important. Organized cultures have sizeable advantages over undifferentiated cultures which often tend to show circumscribed commercial production of secondary metabolites. The introduction of the transformation techniques so as to produce fast growth and phytohormone-dependent cultures, to regulate the biosynthetic pathways, is also likely to be a significant step towards making cell cultures more generally applicable to the commercial production of secondary metabolites.

KEYWORDS

- **plant cell culture**
- **in vitro production of phytochemicals**
- **secondary metabolites**
- **phytochemicals**
- **suspension culture**

REFERENCES

Abyari, M.; Nasr, N.; Soorni, J.; Sadhu, D. Enhanced Accumulation of Scopoletin in Cell Suspension Culture of *Spilanthes acmella* Murr. Using Precursor Feeding. *Braz. Arch. Biol. Technol.* **2016,** *59*. doi.org/10.1590/1678-4324-2016150533.

Ahmed, S. A.; Baig, M. M. Biotic Elicitor Enhanced Production of Psoralen in Suspension Cultures of *Psoralea corylifolia* L. *Saudi J. Biol. Sci.* **2014,** *21*(5), 499–504. DOI: 10.1016/j.sjbs.2013.12.008.

Alamgir, A. N. M. Cultivation of Herbal Drugs, Biotechnology, and in Vitro Production of Secondary Metabolites, High-Value Medicinal Plants, Herbal Wealth, and Herbal Trade. In *Therapeutic use of Medicinal Plants and Their Extracts;* Alamgir, A. N. M., Ed.; Progress in Drug Research, Vol. 73; Springer: Cham, 2017; Vol. 1, pp 379–452.

Alfermann, A. W.; Petersen, M.; Fuss, E. Production of Natural Products by Plant Cell Biotechnology: Results, Problems and Perspectives. In *Plant Tissue Culture 100 Years Since Gottlieb Haberlandt;* Laimer, M., Rücker, W., Eds.; Springer: Wien New York, 2003; pp 153–166.

Allan, E. J.; Eeswara, J. P.; Johnson, S.; Luntz, J. M.; Morgan, E. D.; Stuchbury, T. Tissue Cultures of Azadirachtin by in-Vitro of Neem, Azadirachta Indica. *Pestic. Sci.* **1994,** *42*, 147–152.

Anand, S. Various Approaches for Secondary Metabolite Production Through Plant Tissue Culture. *Pharmacia* **2010,** *1*(1), 1–7.

Antognoni, F.; Zheng, S.; Pagnucco, C.; Baraldi, R.; Poli, F.; Biondi, S. Induction of Flavonoid Production by UV-B Radiation in *Passiflora quadrangularis* Callus Cultures. *Fitoterapia* **2007,** *78,* 345–352.

Arya, D.; Patn, V.; Kant, U. In Vitro Propagation and Quercetin Quantification in Callus Cultures of Rasna (*Pluchea lanceolata* Oliver and Hiern.). *Ind. J. Biotechnol.* **2008,** *7*, 383–387.

Arya, D.; Patni, V. Micropropagation of *Pluchea lanceolata* (Oliver and Hiern.) – A Potent Anti-Arthritic Medicinal Herb. *Int. J. Med. Arom. Plants* **2013,** *3*, 55–60.

Baldi, A.; Dixit, V. K. Yield Enhancement Strategies for Artemisinin Production by Suspension Cultures of *Artemisia annua. Bioresour. Technol.* **2008,** *99*(11), 4609–4614.

Baque, M. A.; Elirban, A.; Lee, E. J.; Paek, K. Y. Sucrose Regulated Enhanced Induction of Antharquinone, Phenolics, Flavonoids Biosynthesis and Activities of Antioxidant Enzymes in Adventitious Root Suspension Cultures of *Morinda citrifolia* (L.). *Acta Physiol. Plant.* **2011,** *34*(2), 405–415 DOI: 10.1007/s11738-011-0837-2.

Begum, F.; Nageswara, R. S. S.; Rao, K.; Prameela, D. Y.; Giri, A.; Giri, C. C. Increased Vincristine Production from *Agrobacterium tumefaciens* C58 Induced Shooty Teratomas of *Catharanthus roseus* G. Don. *Nat. Prod. Res.* **2009,** *23*(11), 973–981.

Behbahani, M.; Shanehsazzadeh, M.; Hessami, M. J. Optimization of Callus and Cell Suspension Cultures of *Barringtonia racemosa* (*Lecythidaceae family*) for Lycopene Production. *Sci. Agric. (Piracicaba, Braz.)* **2011,** *68*(1), 69–76.

Berardi, G.; Ancherani, M.; Rosati, P. Estimation of Callus Growth from Petals of GF677 Peach × Almond Rootstock. *G. Bot. Ital.: Off. J. Soc. Bot. Ital.* **1993,** *127*(6), 1170–1172. DOI: 10.1080/11263509309429500.

Betsui, F.; Tanaka-Nishikawa, N.; Shimomura, K. Anthocyanin Production in Adventitious Root Cultures of *Raphanus sativus* L. cv. Peking Koushin. *Plant Biotechnol.* **2004,** *21*(5), 387–391.

Blom, T. J. M.; Kreis, W.; van Iren, F.; Libbenga, K. R.; A Non-Invasive Method for the Routine-Estimation of Fresh Weight of Cells Grown in Batch Suspension Cultures. *Plant Cell Rep.* **1992,** *11*, 146–149.

Bourgaud, F.; Gravot, A.; Milesi, S.; Gontier, E. Production of Plant Secondary Metabolities: A Historical Perspective. *Plant Sci.* **2001,** *161*, 839–851.

Chandra, S.; Chandra, R. Engineering Secondary Metabolite Production in Hairy Roots. *Phytochem. Rev.* **2011,** *10*(3), 371.

Chattopadhyay, S.; Srivastava, A. K.; Bhojwani, S. S.; Bisaria, V. S. Production of Podophyllotoxin by Plant Cell Cultures of *Podophyllum hexandrum* in Bioreactor. *J. Biosci. Bioeng.* **2002,** *93*(2), 215–220.

Chen, H.; Chen, F. Kinetics of Cell Growth and Secondary Metabolism of a High-Tanshinone-Producing Line of the Ti Transformed *Salvia miltiorrhiza* Cells in Suspension Culture. *Biotechnol. Lett.* **1999,** *21*(8), 701–705.

Chen, H.; Yuan, J. P.; Chen, F.; Zhang, Y. L.; Song, J. Y. Tanshinone Production in Ti-Transformed *Salvia miltiorrhiza* Cell Suspension Cultures. *J. Biotechnol.* **1997,** *58*, 147–156.

Chen, S. A.; Wang, X.; Zhao, B.; Yuan, X.; Wang, Y. Production of Crocin Using *Crocus sativus* Callus by Two-Stage Culture System. *Biotechnol. Lett.* **2003,** *25*, 1235–1238.

Collin, H. A. Secondary Product Formation in Plant Tissue Cultures. *Plant Growth Regul.* **2001,** *34,* 119–134.

Crozier, A.; Jaganath, I. B.; Clifford, M. N. Dietary Phenolics: Chemistry, Bioavailability and Effects on Health. *Nat. Prod. Res.* **2009,** *26*, 1001–1043.

Constabel, F.; Tyler, R. T. Chapter 11: Cell Culture for Production of Secondary Metabolites. In *Plant Cell and Tissue Culture;* Vasil, 1. K., Thorpe, T. A., Eds.; Kluwer Academic Publishers: Dordrecht, 1994; pp 271–289.

Dai, J.; Mumper, R. J. Plant Phenolics: Extraction, Analysis and Their Antioxidant and Anticancer Properties. *Molecules* **2010,** *15*, 7313–7352.

David, H.; Laigneau, C.; David, A. Growth and Soluble Proteins of Cell Cultures Derived from Explants and Protoplasts of *Pinus pinaster* Cotyledons. *Tree Physiol.* **1989,** *5*, 497–506.

Dixon, R. A. Isolation and Maintenance of Callus and Cell Suspension Cultures. In *Plant Cell Culture: A Practical Approach;* Dixon, R. A., Ed.; IRL Press: Oxford, 1985; pp 1–20.

Dixon, R. A.; Gonzales, R. A. *Plant Cell Culture: A Practical Approach,* 2nd ed.; Oxford University Press: New York, 1994; pp 87–97.

Długosz, M.; Wiktorowska, E.; Wiśniewska, A.; Pączkowski, C. Production of Oleanolic Acid Glycosides by Hairy Root Established Cultures of *Calendula officinalis* L. *Acta Biochim. Pol.* **2013,** *60*(3), 467–473.

Doležel, J.; Greilhuber, J.; Suda, J. Estimation of Nuclear DNA Content in Plants Using Flow Cytometry. *Nat. Protoc.* **2007,** *2*, 2233–2244.

Farag, S.; Kayser, O. Cannabinoids Production by Hairy Root Cultures of *Cannabis sativa* L. *Am. J. Plant Sci.* **2015,** *6*(11). 10.4236/ajps.2015.611188.

Farjaminezhad, R.; Zare, N.; Asghari-Zakaria, R.; Farjaminezhad, M. Establishment and Optimization of Cell Growth in Suspension Culture of *Papaver bracteatum*: A Biotechnology Approach for Thebaine Production. *Turk. J. Biol.* **2013,** *37*(6), 689–697.

Farzami, M. S.; Ghorbanli, M. Formation of Catechin in Callus Cultures and Micropropagation of *Rheum ribes* L. *Pak. J. Biol. Sci.* **2005,** *8*, 1346–1350.

Fazal, H.; Abbasi, B. H.; Ahmad, N. Optimization of Adventitious Root Culture for Production of Biomass and Secondary Metabolites in *Prunella vulgaris* L. Appl. Biochem. Biotechnol. **2014,** *174*(6), 2086–2095. DOI: 10.1007/s12010-014-1190-x.

Fedoreyev, S. A.; Kulesh, N. I.; Glebko, L. I.; Pokushalova, T. V.; Veselova, M. V.; Saratikov, A. S.; Vengerovskii, A. I.; Chuchalin, V. S. Maksar: A Preparation Based on *Amur maackia. Pharm. Chem. J.* **2004,** *38*, 605–610.

Filová, A. Production of Secondary Metabolities in Plant Tissue Cultures. *Res. J. Agric. Sci.* **2014,** *46*(1), 236–245.

Flores, H. E.; Dai, Y.; Cuello, J.; Maldonado-Mendoza, E.; Loyola-Vargas, V. M. Green Roots: Photosynthesis and Photoautotrophy in an Underground Plant Organ. *Plant Physiol.* **1993,** *101*, 363–371.

Floryanowicz-Czekalska, K.; Wysokińska, H. Transgenic Shoots and Plants as a Source of Natural Phytochemical Products. *Acta Soc. Bot. Pol.* **2000,** *69*(2), 131–136.

Fowler, C. W.; Janick, J. Non-Destructive Estimation of Callus Growth. *Hortscience* **1974,** *9*(6), 552.

Françoise, B.; Hossein, S.; Halimeh, H.; Zahra, N. F. Growth Optimization of *Zataria multiflora* Boiss. Tissue Cultures and Rosmarinic Acid Production Improvement. *Pak J. Biol. Sci.* **2007,** *10*(19), 3395–3399.

Fujita, Y.; Hara, Y.; Suga, C.; Morimoto, T. Production of shikonin derivatives by cell suspension cultures of *Lithospermum erythrorhizon*: II. A new medium for the production of shikonin derivatives. *Plant Cell Rep.*, **1981,** 1, 61-63.

Fujita, Y.; Tabata, M. Secondary Metabolites from Plant Cells: Pharmaceutical Applications and Progress in Commercial Production. In *Plant Tissue and Cell Culture;* Green, C. E., Somers, D. A., Hackett, W. P., Biesboer, D. D., Eds.; Alan R. Liss: New York, 1987; pp 169–185.

Fukui, H.; Feroj Hansan, A. F. M.; Ishii, Y.; Tanaka, M. An Envelope-Shaped Film Culture Vessel for Shikonin Production by Lithospermum Erythrorhizon Hairy Root Cultures. *Plant Biotechnol.* **1999,** *16*, 171–174.

Gadzovska, S.; Maury, S.; Ounnar, S.; Righezza, M.; Kascakova, S.; Refregiers, M.; Spasenoski, M.; Joseph, C.; Hagège, D. Identification and Quantification of Hypericin and Pseudohypericin in Different *Hypericum perforatum* L. in Vitro Cultures. *Plant Physiol. Biochem.* **2005,** *43*(6), 591–601.

Gamborg, O. L.; Miller, R. A.; Ojima, K. Nutrient Requirements of Suspension Cultures of Soybean Root Cells. *Exp. Cell Res.* **1968,** *50,* 151–158.

Gaosheng, H.; Jingming, J. Production of Useful Secondary Metabolites through Regulation of Biosynthetic Pathway in Cell and Tissue Suspension Culture of Medicinal Plants. In *Recent Advances in Plant in Vitro Culture;* Leva, A., Ed.; InTech, 2012; DOI: 10.5772/53038.

Geile, W.; Wagner, E. Rapid Development of Cell Suspension Cultures from Leaf Sections of *Chenopodium rubrum* L. *Plant, Cell Environ.* **1980,** *3,* 141–148. DOI: 10.1111/1365-3040.ep11580923.

George, E. F. Plant Tissue Culture Procedure – Background. In *Plant Propagation by Tissue Culture, The Background,* 3rd ed.; George, E. F.; Hall, M. A.; De Klerk, G.-J.; Ed; Springer: Dordrecht, the Netherlands, 2008; Vol. 1, pp 1–28.

Georgiev, V. Mass Propagation of Plant Cells – An Emerging Technology Platform for Sustainable Production of Biopharmaceuticals. *Biochem. Pharmacol. (Los Angel)*, **2015,** *4*, e180. DOI: 10.4172/2167-0501.1000e180.

Georgiev, M. I.; Kuzeva, S. L.; Pavlov, A. I.; Kovacheva, E. G.; Ilieva, M. P. Elicitation of Rosmarinic Acid by *Lavandula vera* MM Cell Suspension Culture with Abiotic Elicitors. *World J. Microbiol. Biotechnol.* **2007,** *23*(2), 301–304.

Georgiev, M. I.; Weber, J.; Maciuk, A. Bioprocessing of Plant Cell Cultures for Mass Production of Targeted Compounds. *Appl. Microbiol. Biotechnol.* **2009,** *83*, 809–823.

Goleniowski, M.; Trippi, V. S. Effect of Growth Medium Composition on Psilostachyinolides and Altamisine Production. *Plant Cell, Tissue Organ Cult.* **1999,** *56*(3), 215–218.

Grzegorczyk, I.; Bilichowski, I.; Mikiciuk-Olasik, E. B; Wysokińska, H. In Vitro Cultures of *Salvia officinalis* L. as a Source of Antioxidant Compounds. *Acta Soc. Bot. Pol.* **2005,** *74*(1), 17–21.

Guo, X. H.; Gao, W. Y.; Chen, H. X.; Huang, L. Q. Effects of Mineral Cations on the Accumulation of Tanshinone II a and Protocatechuic Aldehyde in the Adventitious Root Culture of *Salvia niltiorrhiza. Zhongguo Zhong Yao Za Zhi.* **2005,** *30*(12), 885–888.

Hahlbrock, K. Further Studies on the Relationship Between the Rates of Nitrate Uptake, Growth and Conductivity Changes in the Medium of Plant Cell Suspension Cultures. *Planta (Berl.)* **1975,** *124*, 311–318.

Harwood, M.; Danielewska-Nikiel, B.; Borzelleca, J. F.; Flamm, G. W.; Williams, G. M.; Lines, T. C. A Critical Review of the Data Related to the Safety of Quercetin and Lack of Evidence of in Vivo Toxicity, Including Lack of Genotoxic/Carcinogenic Properties. *Food Chem. Toxicol.* **2007,** *45*, 2179–2205.

Hilton, M. G.; Rhodes, M. J. C. Factors Affecting the Growth and Hyocyamine Production During Batch Culture of Transformed Roots of *Datura stramonium. Planta Med.* **1993,** *59,* 340–344.

Ho, T. T.; Lee, J. D.; Jeong, C. S.; Paek, K. Y.; Park, S. Y. Improvement of Biosynthesis and Accumulation of Bioactive Compounds by Elicitation in Adventitious Root Cultures of *Polygonum multiflorum. Appl. Microbiol. Biotechnol.* **2018,** *102*(1), 199–209. https://doi.org/10.1007/s00253-017-8629-2.

Ionkova, I. Optimization of Flavonoid Production in Cell Cultures of *Astragalus missouriensis* Nutt. (Fabaceae). *Phcog. Mag.* **2009,** *5*, 92–97.

Ishimaru, K.; Shimomura, K. Phenolics in Root Cultures of Medicinal Plants. In *Studies in Natural Products Chemistry;* Atta-ur-Rahman, Ed.; Elsevier Science B.V.: Amsterdam, the Netherlands, 1995; Vol. 17, pp 421–449.

Jaisi, A.; Panichayupakaranant, P. Increased Production of Plumbagin in *Plumbago indica* Root Cultures by Biotic and Abiotic Elicitors. *Biotechnol. Lett.* **2016,** *38*(2), 351–355. https://doi.org/10.1007/s10529-015-1969-z.

Jaisi, A.; Sakunphueak, A.; Panichayupakaranant, P. Increased Production of Plumbagin in *Plumbago indica* Root Cultures by Gamma Ray Irradiation. *Pharm. Biol.* **2013,** *51*(8), 1047–1051. DOI: 10.3109/13880209.2013.775163.

James, J. T.; Meyer, R.; Dubery, I. A. Characterization of Two Phenotypes of *Centella asiatica* in Southern Africa Through the Composition of Four Triterpenoids in Callus, Cell Suspensions and Leaves. *Plant Cell, Tissue Organ Cult.* **2008,** *94*, 91–99.

Jha, T. B.; Ghosh, B. *Plant Tissue Culture: Basic and Applied;* Universities Press: Hyderabad, India, 2005; p 206.

Karalija, E.; Parić, A. The Effect of BA and IBA on the Secondary Metabolite Production by Shoot Culture of *Thymus vulgaris* L. *Biologica Nyssana* **2011,** *2*(1), 29–35.

Khan, T.; Krupadanam, D.; Anwar, Y. The Role of Phytohormone on the Production of Berberine in the Calli Culture of an Endangered Medicinal Plant, Turmeric (*Coscinium fenustratum* L.). *Afr. J. Biotechnol.* **2008,** *7*, 3244–3246.

Khanpour-Ardestani, N.; Sharifi, M.; Behmanesh, M. Establishment of Callus and Cell Suspension Culture of *Scrophularia striata* Boiss.: An in Vitro Approach for Acteoside Production. *Cytotechnology* **2015,** *67*(3), 475–85. DOI: 10.1007/s10616-014-9705-4.

Khosh, M.; Singh, K. Callus Induction and Culture of Roses. *Sci. Hort.* **1982,** *17*(4), 361–370.

Kim, Y.; Wyslouzil, B. E.; Weathers, P. J. Secondary Metabolism of Hairy Root Cultures in Bioreactors. *In Vitro Cell. Develop. Biol. – Plant* **2002,** *38*, 1–10.

Ku, K. L.; Chang, P. S.; Cheng, Y. C.; Lien, C. Y. Production of Stilbenoids from the Callus of *Arachis hypogaea*: A Novel Source of the Anticancer Compound Piceatannol. *J. Agric. Food Chem.* **2005,** *53*, 3877–3881.

Kumar, R.; Sharma, N.; Malik, S.; Bhushan, S.; Sharma, U. K.; Kumari, D.; Sinha, A. K.; Sharma, M.; Ahuja, P. S. Cell Suspension Culture of *Arnebia euchroma* (Royle) Johnston – A Potential Source of Naphthoquinone Pigments. *J. Med. Plants Res.* **2011,** *5*(25), 6048–6054.

Kuo, C.; Chang J.; Chang, H.; Gupta, S. K.; Chan, H.; Chen, E. C.; Tsay, H. In Vitro Production of Benzylisoquinoline from *Stephania tetrandra* Through Callus Culture Under the Influence of Different Additives. *Bot. Stud.* **2011,** *52*, 285–294.

Kusakari, K.; Yokoyama, M.; Inomata, S. Enhanced Production of Saikosaponins by Root Culture of *Bupleurum falcatum* L. Using Two Step Control of Sugar Concentration. *Plant Cell Rep.* **2000,** *19*, 1115–1120.

Lee, C. W. T.; Shuler, M. L. The Effect of Inoculum Density and Conditioned Medium on the Production of Ajmalicine and Catharanthine from Immobilized *Catharanthus roseus*cells. *Biotechnol. Bioengr.* **2000,** *67*, 61–71.

Lee, E. J.; Paek K. Y. Effect of Nitrogen Source on Biomass and Bioactive Compound Production in Submerged Cultures of *Eleutherococcus koreanum* Nakai Adventitious Roots. *Biotechnol. Prog.* **2012,** *28*(2), 508–514. DOI: 10.1002/btpr.1506.

Lee, Y.; Dong-Eun, L.; Hak-Soo, L.; Kim, S.; Woo, S. L.; Soo-Hwan, K.; Myoung-Won, K. Influence of Auxins, Cytokinins, and Nitrogen on Production of Rutin from Callus and Adventitious Roots of the White Mulberry Tree (*Morus alba* L.). *Plant Cell, Tissue Organ Cult.* **2011,** *105*, 9–19.

Lee, Y. S.; Ju, H. K.; Kim, Y. J.; Lim, T.-G.; Uddin, M. R.; Kim, Y. B.; et al. Enhancement of Anti-Inflammatory Activity of *Aloe vera* Adventitious Root Extracts Through the Alteration of Primary and Secondary Metabolites Via Salicylic Acid Elicitation. *PLoS ONE* **2013,** *8*(12), e82479. https://doi.org/10.1371/journal.pone.0082479.

Li, H.-H.; Su, M.-H.; Yao, D.-H.; Zeng, B.-Y.; Chang, Q.; Wang, W.; Xu, J. Anti-Hepatocellular Carcinoma Activity of Tormentic Acid Derived from Suspension Cells of *Eriobotrya japonica* (Thunb.) Lindl. *Plant Cell Tiss Organ Cult.* **2017,** *130*, 427–433. DOI: 10.1007/s11240-017-1221-8.

Linsmaier, E. M.; Skoog, F. Organic Growth Factor Requirement of Tobacco Tissue Cultures. *Physiologica Plantarum* **1965,** *18*, 100–127.

Liu, H.; Qi, L.; Cao, J.; Li, P.; Li, C.; Peng, Y. Advances of Modern Chromatographic and Electrophoretic Methods in Separation and Analysis of Flavonoids. *Molecules* **2008,** *13*, 2521–2544.

Lo, K. Y.; Nadali, B. J.; Chan, L.-K. Investigation on the Effect of Subculture Frequency and Inoculum Size on the Artemisinin Content in a Cell Suspension Culture of *Artemisia annua* L. *Aust. J. Crop Sci.* **2012,** *6*(5), 801–807.

Manuhara, Y.; Sri, W.; Sri Saputri, N. O.; Kristanti, A. N. Production of Adventitious Root and Saponin of *Talinum paniculatum* (Jacq.) Gaertn. in Temporary Immersion Bioreactor. *Scholars Acad. J. Biosci.* **2014,** *2*(4), 246–250.

Manuhara, Y. S. W.; Saputri, N. O. S.; Kristanti, A. N.; Utami, E. S. W.; Yachya, A. Effect of Sucrose and Potassium Nitrate on Biomass and Saponin Content of *Talinum paniculatum* Gaertn. Hairy Root in Balloon-Type Bubble Bioreactor. *Asian Pac. J. Trop. Biomed.* **2015,** *5*(12), 1027–1032.

Marsik, P.; Langhansova, L.; Dvorakova, M.; Cigler, P.; Hruby, M. et al. Increased Ginsenosides Production by Elicitation of in Vitro *Cultivated Panax Ginseng* Adventitious Roots. *Med. Aromat. Plants* **2014,** *3*, 147. DOI: 10.4172/2167-0412.1000147.

Matkowski, A. In Vitro Isoflavonoid Production in Callus from Different Organs of *Pueraria lobata* (Wild.) Ohwi. *J. Plant Physiol.* **2004,** *161*(3), 343–346.

Matkowski, A. Plant in Vitro Culture for the Production of Antioxidants—A Review. *Biotechnol. Adv.* **2008,** *26*, 548–560.

Meena, M. C.; Patni, V. Isolation and Identification of Flavonoid "Quercetin" from *Citrullus colocynthis* (Linn.) Schrad. *Asian J. Exp. Sci.* **2008,** *22*(1), 137–142.

McLean, K. S.; Lawrence, G. W.; Reichert, N. A. Callus Induction and Adventitious Organogenesis of Kenaf *(Hibiscus cannabinus* L.). *Plant Cell Rep.* **1992,** *11*, 532–534.

Miura, H.; Kitamura, Y.; Ikenaga, T.; Mizobe, K.; Shimizu, T.; Nakamura, M.; et al. Anthocyanin Production of Glehnia Littoralis Callus Cultures. *Phytochemistry* **1998,** *48*, 279–283.

Moghadam, Y. A.; Piri, K.; Bahramnejad, B.; Ghiasvand, T. Dopamine Production in Hairy Root Cultures of *Portulaca oleracea* (Purslane) Using *Agrobacterium rhizogenes*. *J. Agric. Sci. Technol.* **2014,** *16*(2), 409–420.

Monache, G. D.; De Rosa, M. C.; Scurria, R.; Vitali, A.; Cuteri, A.; Monacelli, B.; Pasqua, G.; Botta, B. Comparison Between Metabolite Productions in Cell Culture and in Whole Plant of *Maclura pomifera*. *Phytochemistry* **1995,** *39*, 575–580.

Mottley, J.; Keen, B. Indirect Assessment of Callus Fresh Weight by Non-Destructive Methods. *Plant Cell Rep.* **1987,** *6*, 389–392.

Murashige, T.; Skoog, F. A Revised Medium for Rapid Growth and Bioassays with Tobacco Tissue Cultures. *Physiol. Plant.*, **1962,** 15, 473– 497.

Mustafa, N. R.; de Winter, W.; van Iren, F.; Verpoorte, R. Initiation, Growth and Cryopreservation of Plant Cell Suspension Cultures. *Nat. Protoc.* **2011,** *6*(6), 715–742.

Namdeo, A. G. Plant Cell Elicitation for Production of Secondary Metabolites: A Review. *Pharmacog. Rev.* **2007,** *1*, 69–79.

Nandani, D. V.; Narayan, R.; Batra, A. Isolation and Identification of Quercetin and Emodin from *Cassia tora* L. *Ann. Phytomed.* **2013,** *2*(2), 96–104.

Nobre, C. P., Raffin, F. N.; Moura, T. F. Standardization of Extracts from *Momordica charantia* L. (Cucurbitaceae) by Total Flavonoids Content Determination. *Acta Farm. Bonaerense* **2005,** *24*(4), 562–566.

Oksman-Caldentey, K.-M.; Hiltunen, R. Transgenic Crops for Improved Pharmaceutical Products. *Field Crops Res.* **1996,** *45*, 57–69.

Olivira, A. J. B.; Koika, L.; Reis, F. A. M.; Shepherd, S. L. Callus Culture of *Aspidosperma ramiflorum* Muell.-Arg. Growth and Alkaloid Production. *Acta Sci.* **2001,** *23*, 609–612.

Ong, S. L.; Ling, A. P. K.; Poospooragi, R.; Moosa, S. Production of Flavonoid Compounds in Cell Cultures of *Ficus deltoidea* as Influenced by Medium Composition. *Int. J. Med. Arom. Plants* **2011,** *1*(2), 62–74.

Pandey, R.; Krishnasamy, V.; Kumaravadivel, N.; Rajamani, K. Establishment of Hairy Root Culture and Production of Secondary Metabolites in Coleus (*Coleus forskohlii*). *J. Med. Plants Res.* **2014,** *8*(1), 58–62.

Panichayupakaranant, P.; Tewtrakul, S. Plumbagin Production by Root Culture of *Plumbago rosea. Electron. J. Biotechnol.* **2002,** *5*, 11–12.

Praveen, N.; Murthy, H. N. Production of Withanolide a from Adventitious Root Cultures of *Withania somnifera. Acta Physiol. Plant.* **2010,** *32*, 1017–1022.

Praveen, N.; Manohar, S. H.; Naik, P. M. Production of Andrographolide from Adventitious Root Cultures of *Andrographis paniculata. Curr. Sci.* **2009,** *96*, 694–697.

Parr, A. J. The Production of Secondary Metabolites by Plant Cell Cultures. *J. Biotechnol.* **1989,** *10*, 1–26.

Patel, H.; Krishnamurthy, R. Elicitors in Plant Tissue Culture. *J. Pharmacogn. Phytochem.* **2013,** *2*(2), 60–65.

Prakash, G.; Srivastava, A. K. Statistical Media Optimization Forcell Growth and Azadirachtin Production in *Azadirachta indica* A. Juss. Suspension Cultures. *Process Biochem.* **2005,** *40*, 3795–3800.

Pua, E.-C.; Ragosky, E.; Thorpe, T. A. Retention of Shoot Regeneration Capacity of Tobacco Callus by Na_2SO_4. *Plant Cell Rep.* **1985,** *4*, 225–228.

Raj, D.; Kokotkiewicz, A.; Drys, A.; Luczkiewicz, M. Effect of Plant Growth Regulators on the Accumulation of Indolizidine Alkaloids in *Securinega suffruticosa* Callus Cultures. *Plant Cell, Tissue Organ Cult.* **2015,** *123*(1), 39–45.

Rao, S. R.; Ravishankar, G. A. Plant Cell Cultures: Chemical Factories of Secondary Metabolites. *Biotechnol. Adv.* **2002,** *20*(2), 101–153.

Ratnadewi, D.; Satriawan, D.; Sumaryono. Enhanced Production Level of Quinine in Cell Suspension Culture of *Cinchona ledgeriana* Moens by Paclobutrazol. *J. Biotropia* **2013,** *20*(1), 10–18.

Rijke, E.; Out, P.; Niessen, W. M.A.; Ariese, F.; Gooijer, C.; Udo, A. T.; Brinkman, P. Analytical Separation and Detection Methods for Flavonoids. *J. Chromatogr. A* **2006,** *1112*, 31–63.

Robards, K.; Antolovich, M. Analytical Chemistry of Fruit Bioflavonoids – A Review. *Analyst* **1997,** *122*, 11R–34R.

Rodríguez-Sahagún, A.; Del Toro-Sánchez, C. L.; Gutierrez-Lomelí, M.; Castellanos-Hernández, O. A. Plant Cell and Tissue Culture as a Source of Secondary Metabolites. In *Biotechnological Production of Plant Secondary Metabolites,* Chapter 1; Orhan, I. E., Ed.; Bentham Science Publishers: Sharjah, UAE, 2012; pp 3–20.

Ruffoni, B.; Pistelli, L.; Bertoli, A.; Pistelli, L. Plant Cell Cultures: Bioreactors for Industrial Production. In *Bio-Farms for Nutraceuticals, Advances in Experimental Medicine and Biology;* Giardi, M. T., Rea, G., Berra, B., Eds.; Springer: Boston, MA, 2010; pp 203–221.

Sae-Lee, N.; Kerdchoechuen, O.; Laohakunjit, N. Enhancement of Phenolics, Resveratrol and Antioxidant Activity by Nitrogen Enrichment in Cell Suspension Culture of *Vitis vinifera. Molecules* **2014,** *19*(6), 7901–7912. DOI: 10.3390/molecules19067901.

Saito, K. Genetic Engineering in Tissue Culture of Medicinal Plants. *Plant Tissue Cult. Lett.* **1993,** *10*(1), 1–8.

Santos, M. R. A.; Ferreira, M. D. R.; Sarubo, V. N. Determination of Callus Growth Curve in Conilon Coffee. *Revista Caatinga, Mossoróo,* **2010,** *23*(1), 133–136.

Sasson, A. Production of Useful Biochemicals by Higher-Plant Cell Cultures: Biotechnological and Economic Aspects. *CIHEAM-IAMZ, Options Méditerranéennes – Série Séminaires,* **1991,** *14*, 59–74.

Schripsema, J.; Meijer, A. H.; van Iren, F.; Hoopen, H. J. G.; Verpoorte, R. Dissimilation Curves as a Simple Method for the Characterization of Growth of Plant Cell Suspension Cultures. *Plant Cell, Tissue Organ Cult.* **1990,** *22,* 55–64.

Sharma, N.; Patni, V. Comparative Analysis of Total Flavonoids, Quercetin Content and Antioxidant Activity of in Vivo and in Vitro Plant Parts of *Grewia asiatica* Mast. *Int. J. Pharm. Pharm. Sci.* **2013,** *5*(2), 464–469.

Shinde, A. N.; Malpathak, N.; Fulzele, D. P. Induced High Frequency Shoot Regeneration and Enhanced Isoflavones Production in *Psoralea corylifolia. Rec. Nat. Prod.* **2009,** *3*, 38–45.

Shrivastava, N.; Patel, T.; Srivastava, A. Biosynthetic Potential of in Vitro Grown Callus Cells of *Cassia senna* L. Var. Senna. *Curr. Sci.* **2006,** *90*(11), 1472–1473.

Siva, G.; Sivakumar, S.; Premkumar, G.; Kumar, T. S.; Jayabalan, N. Enhanced Production of Psoralen Through Elicitors Treatment in Adventitious Root Culture of *Psoralea corylifolia* L. *Int. J. Pharm. Pharm. Sci.* **2015,** *7*(1) 146–149.

Smetanska, I. Production of Secondary Metabolites Using Plant Cell Cultures. *Adv. Biochem. Eng./Biotechnol.* **2008,** *111*, 187–228.

Smith, M. A. L. Large Scale Production of Secondary Metabolites. In *Current Issues in Plant Molecular and Cellular Biology;* Terzi, M., et al.; Eds.; Kluwer Academic Publishers: Dordrecht, the Netherlands, 1995; pp 669–674.

Spencer, J. P. E.; Vanzour, D.; Rendeiro, C. Flavonoids and Cognition: The Molecular Mechanisms Underlying Their Behavioural Effects. *Arch. Biochem. Biophys.* **2009,** *492*, 1–9.

Sreeranjini, S.; Siril, E. A. Production of Anthraquinones from Adventitious Root Derived Callus and Suspension Cultures of *Morinda citrifolia* L. in Response to Auxins, Cytokinins and Sucrose Levels. *Asian J. Plant Sci. Res.* **2013,** *3*(3), 131–138.

Srividya, N.; Sridevi, B. P.; Satyanarayana, P. Azadirachtin and Nimbin Content in in Vitro Cultured Shoots and Roots of *Azadiracta indica* A. Juss. *Ind. J. Plant Physiol.* **1998,** *3*, 129–134.

Stalman, M.; Koskamp, A. M.; Luderer, R.; Vernooy, J. H.; Wind, J. C.; Wullems, G. J.; Croes, A. F. Regulation of Anthraquinone Biosynthesis in Cell Cultures of *Morinda citrifolia. J. Plant Physiol.* **2003,** *160*(6), 607–614.

Subroto, M. A.; Hamill, J. D.; Doran, P. M. Development of Shooty Teratomas from Several Solanaceous Plants: Growth Kinetics, Stoichiometry and Alkaloid Production. *J. Biotechnol.* **1996,** *45*(1), 45–57.

Sundaram, K. M. S.; Curry, J. Effect of Some UV Light Absorber on the Photostabilization of Azadirachtin, a Neem Based Pesticide. *Chemosphere* **1996,** *32*, 649–659.

Sung, Z. R. Turbidimetric Measurement of Plant Cell Culture Growth. *Plant Physiol.* **1976,** *57*, 460–462.

Szopa, A.; Ekiert, H. Production of Biologically Active Phenolic Acids in *Aronia melanocarpa* (Michx.) Elliott in Vitro Cultures Cultivated on Different Variants of the Murashige and Skoog Medium. *Plant Growth Regul.* **2014,** *72*, 51–58

Tan, S. H.; Musa, R.; Ariff, A.; Maziah, M. Effect of Plant Growth Regulators on Callus, Cell Suspension and Cell Line Selection for Flavonoid Production from Pegaga (*Centella asiatica* L. Urban). *Am. J. Biochem. Biotechnol.* **2010,** *6*, 284–299.

Tan, S. H.; Ariff, A.; Mahmood, M. Synergism Effect Between Inoculum Size and Aggregate Size on Flavonoid Production in *Centella asiatica* (L.) Urban (Pegaga) Cell Suspension Cultures. *Int. J. Res. Eng. Technol.* **2013,** *2*(10), 243–253.

Teshima, D.; Ikeda, K.; Satake, M.; Aoyama, T.; Shimomura, K. Production of Emetic Alkaloids by in Vitro Culture of *Cephaelis ipecacuanha* A. Richard. *Plant Cell Rep.* **1988,** *7*, 278–280.

Torkamani, M. R. D.; Jafari, M.; Abbaspour, N.; Heidary, R.; Safaie, N. Enhanced Production of Valerenic Acid in Hairy Root Culture of *Valeriana officinalis* by Elicitation. *Cent. Eur. J. Biol.* **2014,** *9*(9), 853–863.

Trajtemberg, S. P.; Apostolo, N. M.; Fernadez, G. Calluses of *Cynara cardunculus* Var. *Cardunculus* Cardoon (Asteraceae): Determination of Cynarine and Chlorogenic Acid by Automated High-Performance Capillary Electrophoresis. *In Vitro Cell. Dev. Biol. Plant* **2006,** *42*, 534–537.

Umamaheswari, A.; Lalitha, V. In Vitro Effect of Various Growth Hormones in *Capsicum annuum* L. on the Callus Induction and Production of Capsaicin. *J. Plant Sci.* **2007,** *2*(5), 545–551. DOI: 10.3923/jps.2007.545.551.

Vanisree, M.; Tsay, H. Plant Cell Cultures – An Alternative and Efficient Source for the Production of Biologically Important Secondary Metabolites. *Int. J. Appl. Sci. Eng.* **2004,** *2*(1), 29–48.

Varshney, A.; Anis, M. Trees: Propagation and Conservation: Biotechnology Approaches for Propagation of a Multipurpose Tree *Balanites aegyptica* Del. Springer: New Delhi, 2014; p 116.

Winkel-Shirley, B. Biosynthesis of Flavonoids and Effects of Stress. *Curr. Opin. Plant Biol.* **2002,** *5*(3), 218–223.

Yildiz, M. The Prerequisite of the Success in Plant Tissue Culture: High Frequency Shoot Regeneration. In *Recent Advances in Plant in Vitro Culture;* Leva, A.; Ed.; In Tech: Croatia, 2012; pp 63–90.

Zhong, J. J. Biochemical Engineering of the Production of Plant Specific Secondary Metabolites by Cell Suspension Cultures. *Adv. Biochem. Eng./Biotechnol.* **2001,** *72*, 1–26.

CHAPTER 7

PRACTICAL PROCESSES INVOLVED IN THE PRODUCTION OF PHYTOCHEMICALS BY PLANT TISSUE CULTURES

HANAN M. AL-YOUSEF

Department of Pharmacognosy, College of Pharmacy, King Saud University, Riyadh, Saudi Arabia, Tel.: +966555287629, E-mail: halyousef@ksu.edu.sa

*ORCID: *https://orcid.org/0000-0002-2607-0918*

ABSTRACT

Plant tissue culture (PTC) has wide applications in many areas. These applications are categorized into three; basic research, environmental aspects, and commercial items. Current research in PTC is highly magnified on commercial applications like crop development, secondary metabolite induction, and many strategies for involving genetic interference. Plant biotechnology has a key role to play in solving problems related to development of farms and fruit trees. *In vitro* techniques are being potentially applied to supplement the traditional methods of vegetative propagation and production of plants. Micropropagation *in vitro* techniques have advantages over traditional methods of vegetative propagation; small spaces needed, high multiplication rate, seasonal-free dependence under controlled culture condition, and plant-free microbes.

7.1 INTRODUCTION

Plant tissue culture (PTC) refers to the *in vitro* cultivation of all parts of a plant under aseptic circumstances. Any PTC techniques must contain many basic facilities. These include rooms/area for washing and preparation of media, sterilization, storage, collection of data, controlled incubators, and so forth. PTCs should be incubated under specific temperature, humidity, air ventilation, light/dark quality, and for a fixed duration. The PTC technique requires many organic and inorganic substances for culture media preparation. Growth room is a critical area where PTCs are maintained under controlled circumstances to achieve most favorable growth. Plants regenerated from *in vitro* PTCs are transplanted to vermiculite container (pots containing a yellow or brown mineral which shown as an alteration product of mica and other minerals and used for insulation or as a moisture-retentive medium for growing plants). The potted plants are transferred to growth cabinets or greenhouses and kept for further observations under controlled circumstances (Bhatia and Dahiya, 2015).

PTC system is used to study basic issues related to differentiation and growth under ultimate reproducible circumstances. It has also been applied in various practical applications in many areas such as horticulture, agriculture, and in research centers. It is interesting to know that PTCs are more economical and safe than classical method. There is upswing evidence that it might be possible to store precious germplasm of plant in culture media under low temperature. Recent techniques used such as gene transfer mediated by *Agrobacterium* and transgenic plants regeneration were established (Herrera-Estrella et al., 1983; De Block et al., 1984), which have been proven to be helpful after inducing desirable agronomic traits to transgenic plants (Shah et al., 1986). The concept "tissue culture" is utilized to include numerous variations, for example, meristem tissue culture for propagation of strawberry, orchids, potato, and grape (virus-free plants), cell suspension culture (CSC), protoplast tissue culture, organs (Gamborg, 2002), also pollen or anther tissue culture for inducing haploid plants (Guha and Maheshwari, 1968). One of the most common practical application of PTC techniques include the micropropagation (MP) of medicinal plants, agriculture, horticultural crops, and ornamental by regeneration of plant (Bhatia, 2015). Therefore, the goal of this chapter is to critically estimate the practical applications involved with the use of plant cell culture (PCC), organ culture, and others *in vitro* as a valuable tool for many researches and also for crop amelioration by biotechnology.

7.1.1 MAIN LABORATORY SETUP

Laboratories that can handle PTC experiments need glassware and disposable plasticware, reagents/chemicals (which serve as mineral nutrients for media culture preparation), distilled or deionized water, pH meter, autoclave, magnetic stirrer, filter sterilization units, weighing balance, oven, refrigerator, and so forth. Instrument such as laminar flow, a sterile air ventilation are required to keep aseptic media, explants and surrounding environment. Incubation of the cultures can be carried out on shelves fitted with lighting. Cultures might also be incubated in rotary shakers or growth chambers (for cell suspensions). For collecting and recording of the data as well as image capture, cameras and microscopes with photography hyphenates will be required (Sharma et al., 2015).

7.1.2 PREPARATION OF CELLS/TISSUES FOR CULTURING

Any part of the plant which is enucleated and placed in culture is claimed as the explant. This might be root, leaf disks, cotyledons, shoot tips, hypocotyls, axillary buds, and zygotic embryos. The chosen explants must be aseptic, which always include surface sterilization by using many dilutions (10–30% v/v) of Clorox or any bleach which have sodium hypochlorite (5.25% w/v) as the main ingredient. Chemicals such as silver nitrate or alcohol can also be used for surface sterilization. Prior to inoculating the explants onto the culture medium, it must be rinsed with autoclaved distilled/deionized water to get rid of chemical traces and then trimmed to remove the dead cells at the edges due to harsh chemicals used for sterilizing. There are many surface sterilization methods which are simplified and modified where the explant donor tissues, such as floral buds and seed pods, might be directly dipped into 70% alcohol with light flamed. The anthers or seeds are then enucleated aseptically for culture. Through this procedure, the explants free from chemical agents leads to a high survival rate of the explants. This procedure is useful for orchids (intact seed pods or anthers) in closed floral buds of many species.

Presurface sterilization is very important treatment especially for field-grown plants such as guava; scions were acquired from chosen field-grown plants and grafted to seedling rootstocks (Loh and Rao, 1989). Grafted plants were served in the laboratory for gathering nodal explants. To eliminate apical predominance and enhance propagation of the axillary buds, sanitary scion branches were decapitated 5–8 days before excision of the nodular explants. Surface sterilized of nodular segments were done by using 80% alcohol followed by Clorox solutions (5 and 3%) prior to successful setup of cultures. Physiological state and age of the explant donor plant might have an important influence on the success of plants regeneration. Many studies have reported that cotyledons (3–6 days old) seedlings of *Brassica spp.* are known as the important sources of regenerative explants for adventitious (transverse) shoot and genetic transformation mediated by *Agrobacterium* (Sharma, 1990). In petunia, the leaves are the main sources of explant, the first entire expanded leaf is chosen. A woody tree species such as *mangosteen*, solely young red leaves induced shoot buds in tissue culture. Moreover, *mangosteen* leaf segments (3-mm transverse sections) observed a significant polarity of regeneration with shoot buds driving from the midrib beside the apical cut end of leaf segments (Goh et al., 1994). Hypocotyls and seedling roots are also used in many species as the explant. In few of the cereals (rice and corn) and numerous grasses (Frame et al., 2002), also, in many of the coniferous trees (Lu et al., 1991), the zygotic embryo is preferred explant for tissue culture initiation. When an appropriate explant is chosen and prepared for tissue culture, it should be incubated on a suitable nutrient medium for growth and differentiation.

7.1.3 NUTRIENT MEDIA

Numerous mineral preparations are available to PTC. The major media include Murashige and Skoog medium (MSO or MS0 (MS-zero) medium) (Murashige and Skoog, 1962) and Gamborg's B5 medium (Gamborg et al., 1968). PTC media are made up of macro and micronutrients, phytohormones, vitamins, adjuvants like coconut water, and sucrose (2–3% w/v). The nutrient media is prepared by mixing stock solutions of many chemical substances or from manufactories mixed powder. Adjuvants like vitamin C, polyvinyl pyrrolidone, and activated charcoal which might be needed for few species that show ultimate cases of browning tissue on excision and release of polyphenolic compounds form the damaged cells. The pH of the medium culture is adjusted to 5.8 and an appropriate gelling material is added if a semisolid matrix is preferred. Agar (8–10 g/L) and the Gellangum such as Phytagel or Gelrite (2–3 g/L) are most common gelling agents used for PTC media.

The culture medium is sterilized by using autoclave around 20 min. Cell culture may be in the form of a liquid suspension (small clusters of cells), or in semisolid nutrient medium (apart from callus culture). If a liquid nutrient medium is needed it might be similarly prepared but without adding gelling agent and sterilized by using an autoclave or by filter sterilization (0.22-μm pore size). Furthermore, heat labile substances of the media like some phytohormones such as indoleacetic and gibberellic acid as well as antibiotics, when used, should be filter sterilized and put into an autoclaved medium that is cooled to about 60°C prior to aliquot the medium to aseptic culture vessels.

The choice of a suitable nutrient medium for a selected tissue/species is generally provided by empirical trials. Therefore, the medium ingredients should be classified into four categories and use three different concentrations for each (low, medium, high) category and prepare many combinations of the substances. However, one can begin from the standard MS medium culture and vary the ingredicnts of the many macro and micronutrients, and phytohormones and vitamin. Moreover, one of the major substances that have a potent effect on regeneration is the concentration and type of phytohormones in the culture medium (Skoog and Miller, 1957). In addition, a high ratio of cytokinin to auxin in the explant preferable shoot regeneration, a comparatively high auxin to cytokinin ratio preferable root regeneration, and the intermediate ratio causes callus propagation. Usually, phytohormones concentration in the medium is higher (normally 10±7–10±5 M), this is due to the endogenous concentration depending on the efficiency of uptake of the substance by the explant from the external medium. Thereby, optimization of the suitable phytohormone concentrations in the medium may also be empirically defined in the earlier set of investigational experiments. Once an optimum medium combination is determined, it may be used as an identified medium for the species/closely related species of plants.

7.2 PRODUCTION OF NATIVE PLANT CONSTITUENTS

In PTC, the rate of cell growth and biosynthesis in cultures initiated from a very small amount of plant material is quite high and the final product may be produced in brief period. PCCs are maintained under controlled conditions both environmental and nutritional which ensure the continuous yields of metabolites. CSC offers a more effective mechanism of incorporative precursors into cells that are found in the whole plant. It is possible to cite some more examples of cell cultures which synthesize comparatively high amount of natural plant products, but in many other cases PCCs either do not produce the natural compounds or do so only in very small amounts. This could be attributed to the following facts:

1. PCC is different from the intact plants in many ways, morphologically, cytologically, and physiologically and thus lack modifying the interaction of the intact organism.

2. Inadequate knowledge of the nutrients and other culture nutrition to support the synthesis of the product in question is another probable reason for the deficient performance of the PCCs in terms of secondary metabolite production, for example, the yield of alkaloids in cell, cultures are known to be affected by the growth phase of the cultures, composition of the medium, incubation conditions such as light and the genotype of the cell.
3. The genetic and epigenetic instability of the cells are considered the most serious problems in the production of the natural compounds by the PCCs.

This requires constant selection of the cells capable of synthesisizing the compounds to sustain production. If the above problems are solved or minimized, PCCs could become a practical method for the industrial production of some important natural compounds.

A few but well-established examples of secondary compounds synthesizing in a high amount by PCCs are known.

1. CSCs of *Coleus blumei* have been reported to accumulate rosmoric acid up to 15% of the dry weight of the cell which is five times higher than the alkaloid content in the intact plant (Zenk et al., 1977).
2. Cell and callus cultures of *Catharanthusroseus* have been reported to synthesize the relatively high amount of serpentine and ajmalicine (as high as 1%). Cell cultures derived from high-yielding strains also produce copious quantities of the alkaloids. Cell cultures from some low-yielding strain of *C. roseus* also accumulated elevated level of the alkaloids. Other reports showed that stem calli of *C. roseus* continued to synthesize serpentine even after 12 years of their initiation (Verpoorte et al., 1993).
3. *Morinda citrifolia* is a commercial source of anthraquinones. PCCs of the *C. citrifolia* contained 20 times more anthraquinones content than the roots (Zafar et al., 1992).

7.2.1 LOW PRODUCTION OF SECONDARY METABOLITES WAS COUNTERED BY SEVERAL TRYERS

1. Addition of precursors, for example, mevalonic acid increase steroidal synthesis.

2. Use of Zenk et al. media in cultured cells have been investigated to increase both biomass and secondary metabolites as for ajmalicine production in *C. roseus*.
3. Addition of precursor L-tryptophan to the culture media of *Cinchona ledegriana* increases its quinoline alkaloid content.
4. Addition of thiosemicarbazide to CSC of *Panax ginseng* promote biosynthesis of saponin and inhibit phytosterol.
5. Addition of colchicine to CSC of *Valeriana* spp. increases the valepotriates (60 folds).
6. Addition of copper sulfate to the CSC of various Solanaceae induced formation of sesquiterpene.

7.3 SOMATIC EMBRYOGENESIS (SEG)

In somatic embryogenesis (SEg), cells are developed into plants during embryogenetic stages without gametes fusion. After the first report of SEg in PTC of carrot, the importance of SEg in joining effective cloning of favorable genotypes has been recognized. It is interesting to say that plants regenerated via direct SEg are usually more uniform than plants regenerated from callus tissues. SEg could also generate secondary SEg from their surfaces. Secondary SEg occurs when primary SEg gives rise to successive cycles of embryos. Secondary embryogenesis supplied a way to induce considerable populations of vegetative propagules in a brief period (Lee et al., 1997). Therefore, secondary embryos might be helpful for recovering many plants from the genetic transformation, clonal propagation (CP), and produced mutation. Promoting embryogenic cells might be faced with microprojectile bombardment (genetic transformation), then the transformed cells might be chosen and regenerated inside plants. So, cassava (secondary embryos) were used for the production of mutation in vitro via γ-irradiation and the mutant plants have altered starch constituent were obtained (Joseph et al., 2004).

7.4 MICROPROPAGATION (MP)

MP may be known as a technique in which any meristematic (vegetative) part of plant-like shoot bud and tip, and so forth is occurred aseptically (cultured on sterile media) under controlled circumstances to produce plantlet which is same copy of its parent plant. MP can be determined as CP in vitro. The "clone" term was first used by Webber for cultivated plants that were propagated vegetatively. The term derived from Greek (clone = twig, broken off like propagules for multiplication). It signifies that plants developed from meristematic parts are simply transplanted parts of the identical individual and these plants are typical. This technique of culturing plants has a wide applied including morphology, biochemistry physiology, genetic engineering, and molecular biology through SEg, axillary bud, and adventitious budding (Bonga et al., 1987; Bonga and Aderkas, 1992).

7.4.1 GENERAL TECHNIQUE OF MP

MP is one of the major techniques of PTC. It is the practice of rapidly multiplying stock plant material to produce many progeny plants by using advance PTC methods. MP is used to multiply new plants like those that have been genetically manipulated or breed via classical plant breeding methods. Moreover, it is used to provide enough plantlets for planting from a stock plant which has no seeds, or does not well respond to vegetative reproduction. Interestingly, the use of this method for CP of plants is due to the success in this field with orchids. During progress in this area, it has been reported that multiplication of various fruit and ornamental cultivars is practiced on a commercially practical method of CP. So, CP is the multiplication of genetically similar individuals via asexual reproduction. Plant regeneration may be accomplished by culturing different tissue sections either via lacking adventitious origin (preformed meristem) such as axillary bud proliferation approach or through de novo origin (callus and PCCs). The stimulation of axillary buds, (which are often found in the axil of each leaf) lead to provide a shoot. This technique exploits the normal ontogenic path for branch development by lateral meristem. In nature, these buds stay recumbent for many periods based upon the growth pattern of the plant.

In many species, abstraction of terminal bud is substantial to break the apical predominance and motivate the axillary bud to grow into a shoot. Due to perpetually applied of cytokine in a cultured medium, the shoot grown by the bud, which is found on explants (shoot tip cutting/nodal segment) develops axillary buds. Then, the shoot is separated and rooted to induce plants or shoots and are handled as propagules for propagation. The importance of using axillary bud proliferation from meristem, bud culture, or shoot tip regeneration in an incipient shoot has been already differentiated in vivo. So, only root differentiation and elongation are needed to establish an entire plant. Also, this technique preserves the precise arrangement of whole layers necessary if a chimeral plant's genetic part is to be protected.

In an identical chimera, the surface layers of grown meristem are of differing genetic foundation and it is their contribution arrangement to the plant organ that produces the desisted properties. If the integrity of the meristem keeps intact and improvement is normal in vitro, therefore the chimeral pattern will be protected. However, callus tissue was permitted to form shoot proliferation thereafter and was from the adventitious origin; subsequently, there might be a risk that the chimeral layers of original explants might not all be represented in the specially need from in the adventitious shoots (Das and Mitra, 1990).

PTC is a useful technique for removing viruses from infected plantlets and for inducing virus-free plant seedlings. Although shoot-tip culture has been utilized for this purpose, the propagation rate of virus-free plantlets is low, and it is time-consuming. Many PTC techniques have been established to improve the efficiency of propagation, however, all have inherent defects as practical methods, it also needs period for cultivation, low propagation rates, and the need of mastering highly versatile skillful techniques. Ayabe and Sumi have established a new PTC method for garlic that utilizes the stem disc as an explant. These findings show that the stem disc culture method is of practical use for the MP of garlic plants, especially as virus-free seed plants induced by shoot-tip culture. Moreover, this method has improved a new system, epoch making garlic cultivation, in which seedlings instead of cloves are used for propagation. Due to seedlings much more easily cultivated by machinery than cloves, this culture system is functional for the practical cultivation of garlic, especially in large-scale cultivation (1998).

7.4.2 MP STAGES

Plant MP method aims to induce clones (true identical copies of a plant in copious quantities). This process is often divided into the following stages (Durzan, 1988):

7.4.2.1 STAGE 0 PRE-PROPAGATION STAGE

The pre-propagation stage needs suitable maintenance of the parent plants in the clean enclosed areas free from insect and disease conditions and with little dust. Glass greenhouse, plastic tunnels, and net covered tunnels, supplied high-quality explant source plants with low infection level.

Collection of explants for CP should be made after suitable pretreatment of the parent plants with pesticides and fungicides to decrease contamination in the in vitro cultures. This develops growth and multiplication rates of in vitro cultures. The control of contamination starts with the pretreatment of the parent plants. The selection of explant depends on the methods of shoot multiplication. All organs of plant namely nodal segment, internodal segments, shoot and root tip. For axillary bud production, callus culture, SEg explants nodal segments, internodes, and leaves are collected.

7.4.2.2 STAGE 1 INITIATION OF ASEPTIC CULTURE

Sterilization and establishment of explants (plant organ used to initiate a culture) were done. Select explant based on the procedure of shoot multiplication to be followed. For MP and callus culture work, the explants of choice are nodes and internodes/leaves, respectively. For SEg work, the explant of choice is internodes and leaves.

7.4.2.3 STAGE 2 MULTIPLICATION OF CULTURE

It is an important stage; the rate of multiplication was detected by the significant success of MP system this can be provided by enhanced axillary branching via adventitious bud and callusing formation. For enhancement of axillary branching, the axillary bud found in the axil of each leaf either grow into a single or cluster of shoots in the presence of cytokinins (BAP 1.0 mg/L) in the culture medium. For adventitious bud formation, the buds derived from the part other than leaf axils or shoot apex are called adventitious buds. Through callusing, plant cells are totipotent. In PTC, the mass of differentiated cells are known as callus. This either produced shoot bud or bipolar structure like SEg. This technique is used when the goal is to produce change especially in self-pollinating species with a narrow genetic dependent.

7.4.2.4 STAGE 3 IN VITRO ROOTING OF SHOOTS

Grown shoots lack root system in vitro. For the production of roots, they were transferred to rooting medium. For rooting half strength MS culture medium supplemented with 1.0 mg/Ls auxin hormone was used.

7.4.2.5 STAGE 4 HARDENING AND ACCLIMATIZATION OF TISSUE CULTURE PLANTLETS

This is the final stage and needs appropriate handling of plants. The transplantation from completely controlled circumstances should be gradual. This process of gradually preparing the plants to grow in the area conditions is known acclimatization. The plants induced in tissue culture, despite green in color, cannot prepare enough food for their own survival. Furthermore, inside the culture vessels humidity is high and therefore the natural protective covering of cuticle is not fully grown. Thus, immediately after transfer plants were kept under high humidity. The optimum environment was supplied to plants in greenhouse.

7.4.3 ADVANTAGES OF MP

MP has many advantages over conventional plant propagation techniques; the main advantage of MP is the induction of several plants which are clones of each other. MP can be utilized to produce infection/disease-free plants. MP also induces rooted plantlets suitable for growth, time-saving for the grower if cuttings and/or seeds are slow to grow. It has a substantially high-frequency rate, producing numerous of propagules while traditional techniques may only produce a few a number. Furthermore, it is the only viable technique of regenerating genetically manipulated cells or cells after fusion of protoplast. Also, it is helpful in multiplying plants which induce seeds in uneconomical quantities, or if plants are sterile and do not produce good seeds or if cannot be stored. MP usually produces robust plants, owing to accelerated growth when compared to typical plants produced by traditional methods. Few plants with tiny seeds such as most orchids are effectively grown from seed in sterile culture. A considerable number of plants may be produced/m^2 and the propagules may be stored longer period and in a smaller area (Sharma et al., 2015).

7.4.4 DRAWBACKS OF MP

MP is not always the excellent methods of multiplying plants, circumstances that limit its use are as follows (Verpoorte et al., 1993):

1. It is very expensive and may have an excessive cost more than 70%.

2. A monoculture is produced after MP, owing to a lack of overall infection/disease resilience (might be vulnerable to the same infections).
3. An infected plant may release infected progeny.
4. Not all plants could be successfully cultured as the proper culture medium is not known and/or the plants release secondary metabolites that may kill the explant.

7.5 BIOTRANSFORMATION

Biotransformation (BT) is a technique which uses the enzyme located in the plant callus to transform the externally supplied less active compounds (substrate) to a more active product by a certain chemical reaction such as hydroxylation or glycosylation. Two approaches are being followed in the BT studies using cell cultures. First: cells are supplied with substrate compounds normally not available to the plant such as synthetic compound analogs of intermediate or products from other species with the objective of obtaining compounds unknown in nature. Second: enhancement of production of a natural compound is being attempted by feeding nature intermediates of the plants (precursors of the compound in question) (Sommer and Brown, 1979).

Plant cells have been shown to glycolysate added substrates. Glycoside can be of higher commercial value than the aglycones. For example, aglycon steviol is not sweet, whereas the glycoside steviobioside can be used as a sweetening agent. Cell cultures of *Stevia rebaudiana* and *Digitalis purpura* have been reported to glycolysate steviol to steviobioside, in addition to stevioside. Other compounds glycolysated by cell cultures are diphenols, steroids, cardiac aglycons, and cardiac glycosides (Zafar et al., 1992).

Cell cultures of *Digitalis lanata* have been reported to increase the activity of a compound which is digitoxin by its conversation to digoxin. BT of digitoxin (less active and more toxic) to digoxin by the B-12-hydroxylation reaction is affected by an enzyme located in the cell of *D. lanata*. Commercial exploitation of this process would enable utilization of the large stocks of digitoxin which accumulate as a by-product in the manufacture of digoxin from *D. lanata* (Nmila, 2000).

The potentiality to produce anticancer agents are explicated by the BT of synthetic di-benzylbutanolides to lignans appropriate for conversion to etoposide including cultures of *Podophyllum peltatum* by using a semi-continuous method (Kutney et al., 1993). Interestingly, hydroxylation and oxidation reactions have also been determined for the BT of *podophyllum* lignans in CSCs of Forsythia intermedia (Broomhead and Dewick, 1991). Some BT are stereospecific and have the possibility for the isolation of optically active substances from the racemate mixture, so, *Nicotinia tabacum* PCCs can specifically hydrolyze the R-configuration forms of monoterpenes like bornyland isobornyl acetate (Zafar et al., 1992). Various biochemical transformations by PCCs have been determined, and contain hydroxylation, isomerization, epoxidations, ester formation and saponification, glycosylation, methylation, demethylation, and oxidation. For this technique to be commercially valuable the product must be sufficient in good amounts and the reaction should be not more than one which is more easily performed by microbes or by chemical reaction.

7.6 TRANSFORMED HAIRY ROOT CULTURE

Bhatia has been reported that the production of a transgene and its expression via PTC supported by many genetic materials which is the most crisis point argument nowadays. Incorporation of genes which induces stress tolerant plants will improve the production of secondary metabolite (2015). Some soil bacteria such as *Agrobacterium* can trigger a transformation of plant cells by incorporating into their genome t-DNA via the bacterial plasmid. Such transformed roots, formed by inoculating the host plant, when developed in a hormone-free medium to give copious roots claimed as "hairy roots or transformed root." Elimination of the *Agrobacterium* leads to enhance growth of the root profusely. Some plants which normally induce secondary metabolites, the hairy roots accumulate these metabolites in quantities like those presented in the intact plant.

Agrobacterium tumefaciens and *Agrobacterium rhizogenes* are most commonly used to effect on transformation. With normal roots and cells cultures, it is possible to use transformed roots to perform biological conversions not associated with the whole plant normally. The rapid hairy roots growth rate offers the probability of rapid conversions. Ginseng hairy root cultures have been found to convert digitoxigenin by esterification at C-3 with stearate, myristate, and palmitate into new compounds, and by the formation of sophorosides and gentiobioside. Parr et al., have studied on the tropane alkaloids biosynthesis fed on the S-analogue of tropinone (8-thiabicyclo (3.2.1.) octan-3-one) to transform root cultures of *Datura stramonium* and gave rise S-analogue of tropine, with 3-O-acetylester (1991).

7.7 IMMOBILIZATION OF PLANT CELLS

Immobilized plant cells (IPC) can be utilized in a comparable way as immobilized enzymes influence complicated chemical reactions. Petersen et al have reported on the IPC of *D. lanata* cells by suspending cells in a sodium alginate solution, the alginate precipitating and entrapped cells with calcium chloride ($CaCl_2$) solution become pellet allowing the product to get hard. These granules were catalyzed by the conversion of digitoxin to purpurea glycoside A and hydroxylated β-methyldigitoxin to give rise β-methyldigoxin. Despite the hydroxylating effect of the entrapped cells was around half that of suspended cells, the pellets have the advantage which the biocatalyst was reusable for periods extending to 2 months (1987).

A technique which has been established useful for the research on alkaloid formation in *Coffea arabica* is to utilize a polypropylene sheeting membrane of specified porosity, pore size, and thickness on which to cells immobilized in a 3-mm thick layer; the nutrient medium circulates under the membrane. *C. roseus* cells have also been studied and developed methods have been done for the release of alkaloids sequestrated in the cell vacuoles without damaging the culture (Zafar et al., 1992).

7.8 ORGAN CULTURE

Organs can be gained in the culture either by using growing points from intact plants, or sterilized roots or seedlings; or by differentiation obtained from callus tissue cultures by appropriate hormones. Usually, cultured organs will be synthesized secondary metabolites which might be either in poor yield or non-existent in the normal PCC. Therefore, quantities of cardenolide isolated from *D. purpurea* and *D. lanata* cultures increment as tissue differentiation yields.

Enhanced induction of alkaloids takes place when roots grow from the tropane alkaloid (Solanaceae) callus cultures. *C. roseus* leaf cultures and *Rauwolfia serpentina* synthesize a diversity of alkaloids. Dimeric alkaloids have been estimated in organ cultures of *C. roseus*, postulating the probability of an efficient induction system for these worthy alkaloids. The dimers occurred solely in those cultures contained catharanthine and vindoline. Whereas CSCs of *Papaver bracteatum* were obtained to synthesize sanguinarine and orientalidine, the shoot and root cultures induced thebaine. In *Hyoscyamus muticus,* the normal and hairy root cultures after treatment with jasmonic acid and its methyl ester induces enormous quantities of conjugated polyamines and methyl putrescin. Never the less, the increment of tropane alkaloid induction was not remarkable (Bionde et al., 2000).

7.9 FLOWERING IN VITRO

One of the recent applications of PTC is to accelcrate the breeding cycle of various ornamental species that have extended period such as orchids which require more than 3 years of vegetative development prior flowering. Under control conditions, flowering might be observed 5 months after germination of the seed instead of 3 years needed in field-development of plants, as well as separation of flower colors was found in in vitro flowers. This reduces labor costs and maximizes the space needed for orchid breeding. Moreover, flowers produced in culture might be pollinated with pollen grains collected from field-developed plants or self-pollinated in vitro trigger the formation of seed pod in culture (Sim et al., 2007; Hee et al., 2007).

7.10 CONCLUSION

The previous discussion has shown that the PTC promises to be a worthy tool for physiology, morphogenesis, molecular biology, and cell signaling research, furthermore, crop development via biotechnology. With the prediction of plant crop yield to be expanded by 2050 due to sustain consumption of the food and fuel needs with increasing population, it is secure to predict a firmly improved technology of PTC will be continued to encourage research as well as to agricultural biotechnology in the next decades.

KEYWORDS

- **plant tissue culture**
- **production of phytochemicals**
- **biotransformation**
- **organ culture**
- **micropropagatlon**

REFERENCES

Ayabe, M.; Sumi, S. Establishment of a Novel Tissue Culture Method, Stem-Disc Culture, and its Practical Application to Micropropagationof Garlic (Allium Sativum L.). *Plant Cell Rep*. **1998,** *17*, 773–779.

Bhatia, S. Application of Plant Biotechnology. In *Modern applications of plant biotechnology in pharmaceutical sciences*. Bhatia, S., Sharma, K.; Dahiya, R.; Bera, T. (Eds). Academic press: Boston. 2015, 157-207.

Bhatia, S.; Dahiya, R. Laboratory Organization. In *Modern Applications of Plant Biotechnology in Pharmaceutical Sciences*. Bhatia, S.; Sharma, K.; Dahiya, R., Bera, T., Eds; Academic Press: Boston, 2015, pp 109–120.

Biondi, S.; Fornalé, S.; Oksman-Caldentey, K. M.; Eeva, M.;Agostani, S.;Bagni, N. Jasmonates Induce Over-Accumulation of Methylputrescineand Conjugated Polyamines in *Hyoscyamus muticus* L. Root Cultures. *Planta Cell Rep*. **2000,** *19*(7), 691–697.

Bonga, J.M.; Durzan, D.J. (Eds). *Cell and Tissue Culture in Forestry*. 1,2,3, Martinus, Nijhoff Publishers, Dordrecht, 1987.

Bonga, J.M.; Aderkas, P.V. *In vitro culture of trees*; Khmer forestry publishers: Netherlands, 1992.

Broomhead, A. J.; Dewick, P. M.; Biotransformation of *Podophyllum*Lignansin Cell Suspension Cultures of Forsythia Intermedia. *Phytochemistry*. **1991,** *30*, 1511–1517.

Das. T.; Mitra, G.C. Micropropagation of Eucalyptus Tereticornis Smith, Plant Cell, Tissue Organ Cul. **1990,** *22,* 95–103.

De Block, M; Herrera-Estrella, L.; Van Montagu, M.; Schell, J.;Zambryski, P. Expression of Foreign Gene in Regenerated Plants and Their Progeny. *EMBO Journal*. **1984,** *3*, 1681–1689.

Durzan, D.J. Application of Cell and Tissue Culture in Tree Improvement. In*Application of Plant Tissue Culture*; Bock, G., Marsh, J., Eds.; John Wiley and Sons: New York, 1988.

Frame, B. R.; Shou, H.; Chikwamba, R. K.; Zhang, Z.; Xiang, C.;Fonger, T. M. *Agrobacterium tumefaciens* Mediated Transformation of Maize Embryos Using a Standard Binary Vector System. *Plant Physiology*. **2002,** *129*, 13–22.

Gamborg, O. L. Plant Tissue Culture. Biotechnology. Milestones. *In Vitro Cellular and Developmental Biology-Plant*. **2002,** *38,* 84–98.

Gamborg, O. L.; Miller, R. A.; Ojima, K. Nutrient Requirements of Suspension Cultures of Soybean Root Cells. *Exp. Cell Res*. **1968,** *50,* 151–158.

Goh, C. J.; Lakshmanan, P.; Loh, C. S. High Frequency Direct Shoot Bud Regeneration from Excised Leaves of Mangosteen (Garciniamangostana L.). *Plant Science*. **1994,** *101*, 173–180.

Guha, S.;Maheshwari, S. C. Cell Division and Differentiation of Embryos in the Pollen Grains of Daturain Vitro. *Nature*. **1966,** *212*, 97–98.

Hee, K. H.; Loh, C. S.; Yeoh, H. H. Early in Vitro Flowering and Seed Production in Culture in Dendrobium Chao Praya Smile (Orchidaceae). *Plant Cell Rep*. **2007,** *26*, 2055–2062.

Herrera-Estrella, L.; Depicker, A.; Van Montagu, M.; Schell, J. Expression of Chimaeric Genes Transferred in to Plant Cells Using a Ti Plasmid-Derived Vector. *Nature*. **1983,** *303*, 209–213.

Joseph, R.; Yeoh, H. H.; Loh, C. S. Induced Mutations in Cassava Using Somatic Embryos and the Identification of Mutant Plants with Altered Starch Yield and Composition. *Plant Cell Rep*. **2004,** *23,* 91–98.

Lee, K. S.; Van Duren, M.; Mopurgo, R. Somatic Embryogenesis in Cassava: A Tool for Mutation Breeding. In *Improvement of Basic Food Crops in Africa Through Plant Breeding, Including the use of use of Induced Mutations*; Ahloowalia, B. S. Ed., International Atomic Energy Agency: Vienna-TECDOC-951, Austria, 1997; pp 55–60.
Loh, C. S.;Rao, A. N. Clonal Propagation of Guava (PsidiumGuajava l.) from Seedlings and Grafted Plants and Adventitious Shoot Formation in Vitro. *Sci.Hortic.* **1989,***39*, 31–39.
Lu, C–Y.; Harry, I. S.; Thompson, M. R.; Thorpe, T. A. Plantlet Regeneration from Cultured Embryos and Seedling Parts of Red Spruce (Picea Rubens Sarg.). *Botanical Gazette*. **1991,** *152*, 42–50.
Murashige, T.; Skoog, F. A. Revised Medium for Rapid Growth and Bioassays with Tobacco Tissue Cultures. *PhysiologiaPlantarum*. **1962,** *15*, 473–497.
Nmila, R.; Gross, R.; Rchid, H.; Roye, M.; Manteghetti, M.; Petit, P.; Tijane, M.; Ribes, G.;Sauvaire, Y. Insulinotropic Effect of CitrullusColocynthis Fruit Extracts. *Planta Med.* **2000,** *66*(5),418-423.
Ochoa-Villarreal, M.; Howat, S.; Hong, S.; Jang, M. O.; Jin, Y-W.; Lee, E. K.; Loake, G. J. Plant Cell Culture Strategies for the Production of Natural Products. *BMB Rep.* **2016,** *49*(3), 149–158.
Petersen, M.; Alfermann, A. W.; Reinhard, E.; Seitz, H. U. Immobilization of Digitoxin 12β-Hydroxylase, A Cytochrome P-450-Dependent Enzyme from Cell Cultures of *Digitalis Lanata* EHRH. *Plant Cell Rep.* **1987,** *6*(3), 200–203.
Shah, D. M.; Horsch, R. B.; Klee, H. J.; Kishore, G. M.; Winter, J. A.; Tumer, N. E. Engineering Herbicide Tolerance in Transgenic Plants. *Science*. **1986,** *233*, 478–481.
Sharma, K. K.; Bhojwani, S. S.; Thorpe, T. A. Factors Affecting High Frequency Differentiation of Shoots and Roots from Cotyledon Explants of Brassica Juncea (L.) Czern. *Plant Science*. **1990,** *66*, 247–253.
Sharma, G. K.; Jagetiya, S.; Dashora, R. *General Techniques of Plant Tissue Culture*; Ed.; Lulu Press Inc. Raleigh: North Carolina, United States. 2015; pp 1–31.
Sim, G. E.; Loh, C. S.; Goh, C. J. High Frequency Early in Vitro Flowering of Dendrobium Madame Thong-In (Orchidaceae). *Plant Cell Rep.* **2007,** *26,* 383–393.
Skoog, F.; Miller, C. O. Chemical Regulation of Growth and Organ Formation in Plant Tissues Cultured in Vitro. *Symp. Soc. Exp. Biol.* **1957,** *11,* 118–130.
Sommer, H. E.; Brown, C. L. Application of Tissue Culture and. Forest Tree Improvement. In*Plant Cell and Tissue Culture, Principle and Applications;* Sharp, W.R., Larsen, P.O., Paddock, E.F., Raghavan, V. Eds.; Ohio State Univ. Press: Colitinbits, 1979; pp 461–491.
Verpoorte, R.; van der Heijden, R.; Schripsema, J. Plant Cell Biotechnology for the Production of Alkaloids: Present Status and Prospects. *J. Nat. Prod.* **1993,** *56,* 186–207.
Zafar, R.; Aeri, V.; Datta, A. Application of Plant Tissue and Cell Culture for Production of Secondary Metabolites. *Fitoterapia*. **1992,** *63,* 33–43.
Zenk, M. H; El-Shagi, H.; Ulbrich, B. Production of Rosmarinic Acid by Cell Suspension Culture of *Cocusblumei*. *Naturwissenschaften*. **1977,** *64,* 585–586.

CHAPTER 8

MEDICINAL AND INDUSTRIAL APPLICATIONS OF BROMELAIN

RAMESH KUMAR and ABHAY K. PANDEY*

Department of Biochemistry, University of Allahabad, Allahabad, Uttar Pradesh 211002, India, Mob.: +91 98395 21138

**Corresponding author. E-mail: akpandey23@rediffmail.com*

ABSTRACT

Proteases are a unique class of enzymes which occupy an important position with respect to their enormous physiological and commercial applications. Bromelain is a proteolytic enzyme present in pineapple along with closely related proteinases. Bromelain have found application in the food, animal feed, and textile industries. It has gained importance as a phytotherapeutic agent because of its safety and efficacy coupled with lack of unwanted side effects after oral administration. Numerous therapeutic advantages have been stated for bromelain including improved absorption of antibiotics and other drugs, platelet aggregation inhibition, surgical traumas, angina pectoris, bronchitis, sinusitis, pyelonephritis, and thrombophlebitis. Bromelain also modulates immune functions and has the potential to remove burn debris, accelerates wound healing, and acts as an anticancer agent. Bromelain will earn wide recognition as an antimetastatic drug, platelet aggregation inhibitor, skin debridement facilitator, along with other therapeutic applications after advanced clinical trials.

8.1 INTRODUCTION

Bromelain (EC 3.4.22.32) is a proteolytic enzyme derived from the fruit and stem of pineapple plant (*Ananas comosus*) in the aqueous extract containing many closely related proteinases and other compounds exhibiting various medicinal activities (Onken et al., 2008; Hale et al., 2010). Pineapple, a tropical fruit, is used as a food item and a medicinal supplement in many countries. It is native to Central and South America that is grown in many tropical and subtropical countries namely India, South Africa, Kenya, China, Hawaii, Malaysia, the Philippines, and Thailand. Several native cultures such as the Philippines, Hawaii, and so forth, use it as a folk remedy for the treatment of many diseases (Pavan et al., 2012). The beneficial effects of bromelain (Fig. 8.1) have been reported in varied health-related studies in lowering inflammation, swelling, pain, and bruising related to trauma and surgery. Bromelain has lesser undesirable effects in contrast to nonsteroidal anti-inflammatory drugs (Lapeyre-Mestre et al., 2013; de la Barrera-Núñez et al., 2014).

Bromelain primary component is a sulfhydryl proteolytic fraction. It also contains acid phosphatase, a peroxidase, many protease inhibitors, and organically bound calcium. It shows stability over a large pH range. Therefore, it is not necessary to protect protease from stomach acid. Nevertheless, it may be essential to defend the enzyme from digestion in the gut by acid proteases. It may be administered with a buffering agent such as bicarbonate or with water/solution containing nutrients to assist with absorption of fluid and nutrients (Tochi et al., 2008). Aqueous extract of pineapple contains a complex mixture of proteases and non-protease components. Bromelain is used in food processing for meat tenderization. It directly influences pain mediators such as bradykinin (Omojasola et al., 2008). However, its analgesic properties are associated with its anti-inflammatory properties (Brien et al., 2004). Edema reabsorption in the blood circulation has been shown to be promoted by the fibrinolytic action of bromelain (Maurer et al., 2001; Gaspani et al., 2002). It reduces swelling, bruising, pain, and healing time after trauma and surgical procedures (Taussig, 1980). Bromelain increases the prothrombin to thrombin conversion time indirectly and consequently activating plasmin formation from plasminogen which results in the prevention of fibrin formation (Tochi, 2008). All these cause a reduction in vascular permeability. Besides, the pro-inflammatory prostaglandin (especially PGE2) synthesis is inhibited by bromelain (Hale et al., 2005; Maurer, 2001). Bromelain is active over a pH range of 4.5–9.5. Fruit derived bromelain contains a lower amount of proteases in comparison with stem bromelain (White et al., 1988). It has been reported that the beneficial physiological effects of bromelain are due to multiple factors rather than due to a single proteolytic fraction (Walsh et al., 2002). Bromelain is also popular as a health-promoting nutritional supplement. The half-life of bromelain is about 6–9 h. It is absorbed in the human intestine without losing its biological activity. The highest concentration of bromelain in the blood was recorded 1 h after its administration (White et al., 1988). The focus of the current chapter is to present industrial and pharmacological activities of bromelain.

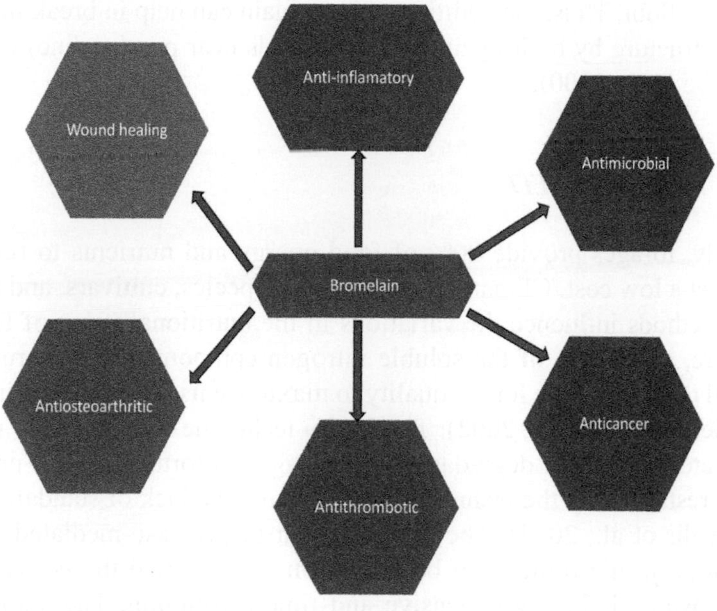

FIGURE 8.1 Pharmacological activities of bromelain.

8.2 INDUSTRIAL APPLICATIONS OF BROMELAIN

Bromelain is a pineapple protease having numerous industrial applications. It is used mainly in tenderization, foods, detergents, and textile industry. Bromelain is also an active ingredient of skin products and tooth-whitening dentifrices.

8.2.1 BAKING INDUSTRY

Gluten is an important functional component of wheat food products, such as flour. It consists of two major proteins, namely gliadin and glutenin. Upon hydration gluten forms lattice-like structures and becomes insoluble. Therefore, it is necessary to degrade gluten to evade resistance during dough stretching (Walsh, 2002). The utilization of bromelain, a proteolytic enzyme can improve dough formation, augment solubility, and stop dough shrinkage.

Hence, it permits the even rise of dough during the baking procedure (Kong et al., 2007). Bromelain has also been used in the production of hypoallergenic flour that is appropriate for utilization by wheat-allergic patients. The immunoglobulin E-binding epitope, Gln–Gln–Gln–Pro–Pro, is a major allergen in flour. Thus, the addition of bromelain can help in breaking down epitope structure by hydrolyzing peptide bonds near pro (proline) residues (Watanabe et al., 2000).

8.2.2 ANIMAL FEED

Generally, forages provide 90% of food energy and nutrients to ruminant animals at a low cost. Climatic factors, forage species, cultivars, and preservation methods influence the variations in the nutritional value of forages. Therefore, evaluation of the soluble nitrogen components in the rumen is essential to measure the forage quality to maximize its consumption in ruminants diet (Givens et al., 2002). The in situ technique is extensively used to investigate the protein degradability of forage. Unfortunately, its practicability is restricted by the technical problems and the lack of standardization (Abdelgadir et al., 2013). The measurement of protease-mediated protein degradation in the rumen can be an option to substitute the conventional method, which is highly expensive and time-consuming. The addition of protease to animal feed can enhance protein availability and decrease the price of animal feed. The use of bromelain in the evaluation of protein degradation in cereals, hays, forages, protein concentrates, and silages in ruminants have been successfully performed (Polaina and MacCabe, 2007).

8.2.3 TEXTILE INDUSTRY

Recently, the utilization of proteases in the silk industry has increased enormously, particularly the cocoon cooking method which uses strong alkaline agents and chemicals. However, this conventional technique has a harmful effect on the silk thread quality. Hence, by using enzyme treatment an effective cocoon cooking method can be developed which will decrease softening time coupled with rising production and energy economy. Use of pineapple extract with 9.8 mM of Na_2CO_3 has been shown to reduce the softening time from 20 h to 30 min at 60°C (Singh et al., 2003). Tactile behavior and wettability of silk has been improved by the pretreatment of wool and silk with bromelain (Koh et al., 2006). These properties increase the dye uptake by the silk fibers and wool and simultaneously maintain their tensile characteristics.

8.3 MEDICINAL USE OF BROMELAIN

Bromelain is an immunomodulator and acts as a detoxifier of the system. It eliminates gastritis induced by drug and other harmful effects. Hence, it is suggested for use in adjuvant therapy with antibiotics in chemotherapy. It has also been shown to help in the management of several ailments during clinical studies.

8.3.1 EFFECT OF BROMELAIN ON REGULATORS OF INFLAMMATION

Bromelain has been approved as a pharmaceutical product since 1956 as an anti-inflammatory agent after surgery and infection. The immunomodulatory action of bromelain is brought about by the induction of CD-2-mediated T-cell stimulation and increases T-lymphocyte multiplication in splenocyte. However, it has an insignificant effect on purified $CD4^+$ and $CD8^+$ T cells. On contrary, bromelain downregulates the discharge of pro-inflammatory cytokines and chemokines produced by the inflamed tissues, that is, IL-2/4/6, G-CSF, and IFNγ (Onken et al., 2008). Another study reported the release of inflammatory cytokines was induced in peripheral blood mononuclear cells sequestered from healthy donors as a result of IFNγ stimulation in addition to IFNγ release by activated NK cells (Engwerda et al., 2001). These observations suggested that bromelain exhibited the immunostimulatory effect only on the healthy immune system against foreign antigens. Upregulation of the Bax/B-cell lymphoma 2 (Bcl-2) ratio and induction of caspases 3 and 9 as well as inhibition NF-κB and COX-2 expression by bromelain have been shown to induce apoptosis in mouse skin papilloma in vivo suggesting the cytotoxic and antitumor effects of bromelain (Kalra et al., 2008). Müller et al. (2016) have reported that bromelain possesses comparatively better cytotoxic action against TFK-1 and SZ-1 (human cholangiocarcinoma cell lines) in vitro than papain. Expression of CD^{44} surface marker, a marker of tumor proliferation and migration, is diminished in presence of bromelain. In glioma cells, bromelain treatment reduces the invasion, migration, and adhesion abilities without showing any adverse effect on the normal surrounding cells (Mayer et al., 2008).

There is accumulating evidence showing the role of NF-κB signaling in many types of cancers. Among multiple target genes of NF-κB is Cox-2, involved in the synthesis of prostaglandin E2 (PGE2), a pro-inflammatory lipid that also acts as an immunosuppressant and facilitator of cancer proliferation by promoting conversion of arachidonate into PGE2. Inhibition of NF-κB, Cox-2, and PGE2 activity has been considered as a potential treatment of cancer and chronic inflammatory diseases. Bromelain down-regulates NF-κB and Cox-2 expression. Additionally, in human monocytic leukemia and murine microglial cell lines, bromelain was shown to inhibit bacterial endotoxin (LPS)-induced NF-κB activity and the expression of PGE2 as well as Cox-2 (Kalra et al., 2008). One of the interesting possibilities to investigate is whether bromelain generates cell-permeable peptide fragments similar to the synthetic NF-κB essential modulator binding domain peptides that possess NF-κB suppressing capacity. Bromelain can stimulate the innate immune system by activating neutrophils to produce ROS. Bromelain, as an ingredient of a polyenzyme preparation, stimulates the production of ROS and cancer cell killing potential in neutrophils in vitro. Similar activities are also exhibited in the neutrophils isolated from healthy volunteers taking same polyenzyme preparation (Brakebusch et al., 2001). ROS is also involved in intracellular regulation of functional activity in other cell types. Bromelain capacity to amend the levels of intracellular ROS would have a direct influence on the signaling pattern in immune and cancer cells. It is established that activated neutrophils and unwarranted ROS production bring about DNA damage and cancer pathogenesis. Thus excessive production of ROS is front-runner of oxidative stress conditions which are advantageous for cancer (Roessner et al., 2008). Recent reports have proposed that cancer cells induce the functional activity of neutrophils together with ROS production. However, in view of overall cytotoxic/anti-cancer activities of bromelain, it could be predicted that bromelain activity on ROS production in cells obtained from cancer patient may be focused towards inhibition of cancer. Further studies are essential to reveal these mechanisms (Klink et al., 2008).

8.3.2 BROMELAIN RELIEVES OSTEOARTHRITIS

Osteoarthritis is commonly occurring form of arthritis in Western world and in the United States and its prevalence ranges from 3.2 to 33% depending on the joint (Lawrence et al., 1998). Comparative study of diclofenac and a combination of bromelain, trypsin, and rutin in about

100 patients having osteoarthritis of the knee for 6 weeks treatments resulted in considerable and similar reduction in the pain and inflammation (Akhtar et al., 2004). As a food supplement, bromelain may act as a substitute for nonsteroidal anti-inflammatory drugs. It plays a vital role in the pathogenesis of arthritis (Brien et al., 2004). Bromelain has analgesic properties which result from its direct influence on pain mediators such as bradykinin (Kumakura et al., 1988).

8.3.3 COAGULATION REGULATORY ROLE

Oral administration of bromelain significantly lowers adenosine phosphate induced platelet aggregation ex vivo (Heinicke et al., 1972). In the study on the effect of bromelain on plasma fibrin (ogen) and blood coagulation, it displayed twin activity on blood coagulation, that is, at low concentration it showed a procoagulant effect while at higher concentration anticoagulant effect was observed (Errasti et al., 2016). Surgeons need to pay attention while prescribing bromelain to the patients with bleeding disorders. However, some researchers reported contrary to the above findings that in healthy volunteers, bromelain does not have a significant effect on the mechanism of blood clotting. Clinical study on breast cancer patients and healthy volunteers with oral bromelain treatment showed increment in the activated partial thromboplastin time while prothrombin time and plasminogen remained unaltered (Eckert et al., 1999). In another clinical trial, patients with edema and inflammation were treated with 40-mg oral bromelain four times daily for 1 week. No significant therapeutic effect was observed on prothrombin time, bleeding, and coagulation which suggested that used dose of bromelain did not affect blood clotting (Cirelli and Smyth, 1963). Bromelain increases the serum fibrinolytic ability and inhibits the synthesis of fibrin, and thereby affects blood coagulation. Dose-dependent effect of bromelain on serum fibrinogen level is observed in rats. At the higher dose of bromelain, prothrombin time, as well as activated partial thromboplastin time, is markedly prolonged. Studies have proved that bromelain is an effective fibrinolytic agent (Taussig and Batkin, 1988).

8.3.4 SKIN WOUND HEALING ACTIVITY

Bromelain topical application to burns and skin wounds has been demonstrated to be an effective and safe method for necrotic tissue debridement, an alternative to surgical debridement (Cordts et al., 2016; Krieger et al., 2012). It also finds support from the reports of other workers who have proved bromelain local applications to be noninvasive, safe and effective, and promotes natural wound healing (Koller et al., 2008). Debridement of necrotic tissue is due to a non-proteolytic component escharase having a molecular weight of 45,000 Da and is present in bromelain extract which also helps in healing. Method for isolation of escharase from pineapple stem is known. Escharase assists in digestion and separation of devitalized eschar tissue from burn injury (Houck et al., 1983). In a multicenter, open-label, controlled and randomized clinical study, patients having deep partial and complete thickness burns were treated with a bromelain-rich topical agent NexoBrid which was applied for 4 h or by standard of care. There was reduced time to complete debridement, need for surgery and need for autografting in bromelain treatment group (Rosenberg et al., 2014).

8.3.5 ANTIMICROBIAL ACTIVITY

Bromelain supplementation protects animals against *Escherichia coli* and *Vibrio cholerae* enterotoxin-mediated diarrhea. Bromelain acting as anti-adhesion molecule modifies the receptor attachment sites and hence affects the secretory signaling pathways in the intestine (Chandler and Mynott, 1998). Bromelain efficacy against specific infections has been attributed to its capability to resist certain effects of specific intestinal pathogens as well as its synergistic action with antibiotics. It also shows antihelminthic activity against the intestinal nematodes in vitro (Stepek et al., 2005; Stepek et al., 2006). On the other hand, in vitro antifungal activity of bromelain in presence of trypsin against *Candida albicans* is accounted for stimulation of phagocytosis and respiratory burst killing. An infectious skin disease condition, pityriasis lichenoides chronica, has been shown to be resolved completely by bromelain (Massimiliano et al., 2007). In humans it also elevates the levels of some antibiotics in blood and urine (Shahid et al., 2002). Antibiotic therapy combined with bromelain has shown better efficacy than treatment with antibiotics alone in bronchitis, pneumonia, sinusitis, cutaneous *Staphylococcus* infection, thrombophlebitis, cellulitis, pyelonephritis, urinary tract infections, and in rectal and perirectal abscesses (Mori et al., 1972). In children with sepsis, bromelain, trypsin, and rutin combination as an adjuvant therapy with antibiotics has produced good results (Shahid et al., 2002). An improvement in protein utilization has been observed in elderly nursing home patients administered with a blend of bromelain and *Aspergillus niger* derived enzymes (Glade et al., 2001). Further combination of bromelain with sodium bicarbonate, sodium alginate, and essential oils has been shown to improve dyspeptic symptoms considerably. Success of bromelain administration as a digestive enzyme for the treatment of exocrine pancreas insufficiency, pancreatectomy, and intestinal disorders has also been reported. A mixture of bromelain, ox bile, and pancreatin is effective in reducing stool fat elimination in pancreatic steatorrhea patients, resulting in symptomatic improvements in pain, flatulence, and stool frequency (Pellicano et al., 2009).

8.3.6 CELL GROWTH MODULATION BY BROMELAIN

Impaired the cell cycle in normal cells might proceed to uncontrolled cellular growth and result in transformation to cancer cells. Concerted interaction of various pathways inside the cells provides protection to their DNA from ensuing injury due to genomic instability and toxicity (Chobotova et al., 2010). Checkpoint proteins are critical for monitoring the normal cell cycle activity. Checkpoint controls are often lost in tumor cells and thus for cancer chemotherapy, control of cell cycle is used as one of the essential tactics (Beuth et al., 2005). Bromelain inhibits NF-κB translocation through G2/M arrest to apoptosis in human epidermoid carcinoma and melanoma cells. The process of apoptosis is fundamental in the developmental and homeostatic maintenance of complex biological systems (Báez et al., 2007). The apoptotic changes are brought about by shrinkage of the cell, chromatin condensation, and fragmentation of DNA and the activation of caspases, the cysteine proteases. Generally, apoptosis is achieved by either mitochondrial pathways (intrinsic) or death receptor pathways (extrinsic). The mitochondrial pathway is characterized by the upregulation of the expression of a pro-apoptotic protein, Bcl-2-like protein 4 (Bax) through p53 acting as a transcription factor. Bax antagonizes an anti-apoptotic protein Bcl-2 present in the mitochondrial membrane (Snowden et al., 2001). In case of an increase in Bax/Bcl-2 ratio, the protection provided by Bcl-2 on the mitochondrial membrane is interrupted. This facilitates the release of cytochrome c into the cytoplasm and attaches with apoptotic protease activating factor-1 to form an apoptosome complex. It activates caspase-9 that causes commencement of the caspase cascade resulting in the enzyme-mediated destruction of cytoplasmic proteins and DNA damage and ultimately leads to cell death (Guimarães-Ferreira et al., 2007).

Bromelain upregulates expression of p53 and increases Bax expression causing the release of cytochrome *c* in tumor cells which selectively induces the mitochondrial apoptotic pathway (Tysnes et al., 2001). Furthermore, bromelain diminishes the activity of Akt and extracellular signal-regulated kinases, the cell survival regulators and thereby encourages apoptosis mediated tumors cell death (Mantovani et al., 2008). Bromelain treatment has been shown to cause matrigel invasion capacities as well as cell growth inhibition in mouse tumor cell lines in vitro (Juhasz et al., 2008). In addition, bromelain treatment has been shown to considerably reduce the growth of gastric carcinoma Kato-III cell lines.

8.3.7 EFFECT ON ANGIOGENESIS AND METASTASIS

High mortality rates associated with cancer results because of the metastatic migration of cancer cells from the original site. Four interconnected biological events are essential for tumor metastasis namely cell invasion, cell proliferation, cell adhesion, and the angiogenesis (Kleef et al., 1996). Interestingly, the antitumor activity of bromelain is associated with its obstructive effect on tumor cell metastasis as it potentially hampers the metastatic progression of tumor at an array of critical points. Bromelain activity is mediated by inhibition of cell surface adhesion proteins, the key elements responsible for important pro-cancer events such as cell adhesion, migration, and inflammation. This inhibition is predominantly imposed by suppression of NF-κB activation. Furthermore, bromelain inhibits the invasiveness of human cancer cells by suppressing matrix metalloproteinase (MMP)-9 expression (Philchenkov, 2004; Li et al., 2005) through inhibiting activator protein 1 (AP-1) and NF-κB signaling pathways. A study conducted on bromelain reported that it primarily inhibits the phosphorylation of NF-κB leading to a reduction in the c-Jun N-terminal kinases' phosphorylation and consequently activation of AP-1. A relationship between platelets and tumor cells are commonly observed in malignancies. Platelet activation and the platelet-based production of numerous factors enabling angiogenesis is initiated by tumor cells. In addition, tumor cells have the capability to cover themselves with the platelets, making tumor-platelet aggregates which provide protection to tumor cells from immune recognition. Oral administration of bromelain has been shown to reduce platelet aggregation and activation in vitro (Garbin et al., 1994). Moreover, in vitro bromelain treatment is associated with a reduction in platelet count in healthy volunteers (Gläser and

Hilberg, 2006). Proteolytic activity of the bromelain has been accounted for inhibition of platelet activation. Thus, bromelain obstructs platelet-mediated tumor growth and development, and thwarts the production of tumor-platelet aggregates by uncovering cancer cells and revealing them to the immune system (Kalra et al., 2008). The induction of growth of new blood vessel is a necessary step for tumor development and metastasis so as to arrange for the metabolic requirements of briskly proliferating malignant cells. Angiogenesis is regulated by numerous pro-angiogenic genes and signaling molecules. Anti-angiogenic effect of bromelain has been displayed against many cancer cell lines (Karlsen et al., 2011). Bromelain regulates a range of pro-angiogenic growth factors, enzymes, and transcription factors (Wu et al., 2012). Bromelain also prevents the angiogenic response produced by FGF-2 arousal in endothelial cells of mouse and reduces the MMP-9 expression, an enzyme associated with tissue remodeling that is important for the growth and development of new blood vessels (Wallace, 2002). Furthermore, bromelain treatment has been shown to decrease the levels of COX-2 and VEGF, the angiogenic biomarkers in hepatocellular carcinoma cells, and caused a decline in tumor neo-capillary density when compared with untreated cells. Bromelain has also been proven to affect several cellular adhesion molecules linked with the processes of tumor development and metastasis (Juhasz et al., 2008).

8.4 CONCLUSION

Bromelain occupies the vital position with respect to its vast medicinal and industrial applications. It has received growing acceptance among patients and researchers as a phytotherapeutic drug. Bromelain provides numerous therapeutic benefits including anticancer, antimicrobial, anti-inflammatory, antithrombotic, coagulation regulator, and immunomodulatory activities.

ACKNOWLEDGMENT

Ramesh Kumar acknowledges financial support from CSIR as Junior Research Fellow. Authors acknowledge UGC-SAP and DST-FIST Facilities of the Department of Biochemistry, University of Allahabad, Allahabad for providing necessary infrastructure.

KEYWORDS

- **bromelain**
- **enzyme**
- ***Ananas comosus***
- **phytochemicals**
- **industrial applications**

REFERENCES

Abdelgadir, I. E.; Cochran, R. C.; Titgemeyer, E. C.; Vanzant, E. S. In Vitro Determination of Ruminal Protein Degradability of Alfafa and Prairie Hay Via a Commercial Protease in the Presence Or Absence of Cellulase Or Driselase. *J. Anim. Sci.* **2013,** *75*, 2215–2222.

Akhtar, N.M.; Naseer, R.; Farooqi, A.Z.; Aziz, W.; Nazir, M. Oral Enzyme Combination Versus Diclofenac in the Treatment of Osteoarthritis of the Knee—A Double-Blind Prospective Randomized Study. *Clin. Rheumatol.* **2004,** *23*, 410–415.

Báez, R.; Lopes, M. T.; Salas, C. E.; Hernández, M. In Vivo Antitumoral Activity of Stem Pineapple (*Ananas comosus*) Bromelain. *Planta Med.* **2007**, *73*, 1377–1383.

Beuth, J.; Braun, J. M. Modulation of Murine Tumor Growth and Colonization by Bromelaine, an Extract of the Pineapple Plant (*Ananas comosus*). *In Vivo* **2005,** *19,* 483–485.

Brakebusch, M.; Wintergerst, U.; Petropoulou, T.; Notheis, G.; Husfeld, L.; Belohradsky, B.H.; Adam, D. Bromelain is an Accelerator of Phagocytosis, Respiratory Burst and Killing of *Candida albicans* by Human Granulocytes and Monocytes *Eur. J. Med. Res.* **2001,** *6*, 193–200.

Brien, S.; Lewith, G.; Walker, A.; Hicks, S. M.; Middleton, D. Bromelain as a Treatment for Osteoarthritis: A Review of Clinical Studies. *Evid. Based Complement Alternat. Med.* **2004,** *1,* 251–257.

Chandler, D. S.; Mynott, T. L. Bromelain Protects Piglets from Diarrhoea Caused by Oral Challenge with K88 Positive Enterotoxigenic *Escherichia coli. Gut.* **1998,** *43*, 196–202.

Chobotova, K.; Vernallis, A. B.; Majid, F. A. Bromelain's Activity and Potential as an Anti-Cancer Agent: Current Evidence and Perspectives. *Cancer Lett.* **2010,** *290*, 148–156,

Cirelli, M. G.; Smyth, R. D. Effects of Bromelain Anti-Edema Therapy on Coagulation, Bleeding, and Prothrombin Times. *J. New Drugs* **1963,** *3*, 37–39.

Cordts, T.; Horter, J.; Vogelpohl, J.; Kremer, T.;Kneser, U.; Hernekamp, J. F. Enzymatic Debridement for the Treatment of Severely Burned Upper Extremities–Early Single Center Experiences. *BMC Dermatol.* **2016,** *16*(8), 1–7.

de la Barrera-Núñez, M. C.; Yáñez-Vico, R. M.; Batista-Cruzado, A.; Heurtebise-Saavedra, J. M.; Castillo-de Oyagüe, R.; Torres-Lagares, D. Prospective Double-Blind Clinical Trial Evaluating the Effectiveness of Bromelain in the Third Molar Extraction Postoperative Period. *Med. Oral. Patol. Oral Cir. Bucal.* **2014,** *19*, 157–162.

Eckert, K.; Grabowska, E.; Stange, R.; Schneider, U.; Eschmann, K.; Maurer, H. R. Effects of Oral Bromelain Administration on the Impaired Immunocytotoxicity of Mononuclear Cells from Mammary Tumor Patients. *Oncol. Rep.* **1999,** *6*, 1191–1199.

Engwerda, C. R.; Andrew, D.; Ladhams, A.; Mynott, T. L. Bromelain Modulates T cell and B cell Immune Responses In Vitro and In Vivo. *Cell Immunol.* **2001,** *210,* 66–67.

Errasti, M. E.; Prospitti, A.; Viana, C. A.; Gonzalez, M. M.; Ramos, M. V.; Rotelli, A. E.; Caffini, N. O. Effects on Fibrinogen, Fibrin, and Blood Coagulation of Proteolytic Extracts from Fruits of *Pseudananasmacrodontes, Bromelia balansae*, and *B. Hieronymi* (Bromeliaceae) in Comparison with Bromelain. *Blood Coagul. Fibrinolysis* **2016,** *27*, 441–449.

Garbin, F.; Harrach, T.; Eckert, K.; Maurer, H. R. Bromelain Proteinase-F9 Augments Human Lymphocyte-Mediated Growth-Inhibition of Various Tumor-Cells In-Vitro. *Int. J. Oncol.* **1994,** *5*, 197–203.

Gaspani, L.; Limiroli, E.; Ferrario, P.; Bianchi, M. In Vivo and In Vitro Effects of Bromolain on PGE2 and SP concentrations in the Inflammatory Exudate in Rats. *Pharmacol.* **2002,** *65*, 83–86.

Givens, D. I.; Owen, E.; Axford, R. F. E.; Omed, H. M. *Forage Evaluation Inruminant Nutrition;* CABI Publishing: Wallingford, UK, 2002.

Glade, M. J.; Kendra, D.; Kaminski, M. V. Jr. Improvement in Protein Utilization in Nursing-Home Patients on Tube Feeding Supplemented with an Enzyme Product Derived from *Aspergillus niger* and Bromelain. *Nutrition* **2001,** *17*, 348–350.

Gläser, D.; Hilberg, T. The Influence of Bromelain on Platelet Count and Platelet Activity In Vitro. *Platelets* **2006**, *17*, 37–41.

Guimarães-Ferreira, C.A.; Rodrigues, E.G.; Mortara, R.A.; Cabral, H.; Serrano, F.A.; Ribeiro-dos-Santos, R.; Travassos, L.R. Antitumor Effects In Vitro and In Vivo and Mechanisms of Protection Against Melanoma B16F10-Nex2 Cells by Fastuosain, a Cysteine Proteinase from *Bromelia fastuosa*. *Neoplasia* **2007,** *9*, 723–733.

Hale, L. P.; Greer, P. K.; Trinh, C. T.; James, C. L. Proteinase Activity and Stability of Natural Bromelain Preparations. *Int. Immunopharmacol.* **2005,** *5*, 783–793.

Hale, L. P.; Chichlowski, M.; Trinh, C. T.; Greer, P. K. Dietary Supplementation with Fresh Pineapple Juice Decreases Inflammation and Colonic Neoplasia in IL-10-Deficient Mice with Colitis. *Inflammatory Bowel Dis.* **2010,** *16*, 2012–2021

Heinicke, R. M.; van der Wal, L.; Yokoyama, M. Effect of Bromelain (Ananase) on Human Platelet Aggregation. *Experientia* **1972,** *28*, 844–5.

Houck, J. C.; Chang, C. M; Klein, G. Isolation of an Effective Debriding Agent from the Stems of Pineapple Plants. *Int. J. Tissue React.* **1983,** *5*, 125–34.

Juhasz, B.; Thirunavukkarasu, M.; Pant, R.; Zhan, L.; Penumathsa, S. V.; Secor, E. R. Jr.; Srivastava, S.; Raychaudhuri, U.; Menon, V. P.; Otani, H.; Thrall, R. S.; Maulik, N. Bromelain Induces Cardioprotection Against Ischemia-Reperfusion Injury Through Akt/FOXO Pathway in Rat Myocardium. *Am. J. Physiol. Heart Circ. Physiol.* **2008,** *294*, H1365–H1370.

Kalra, N.; Bhui, K.; Roy, P.; Srivastava, S.; George, J.; Prasad. S.; Shukla, Y. Regulation of P53, Nuclear Factor KappaB and Cyclooxygenase-2 Expression by Bromelain Through Targeting Mitogen-Activated Protein Kinase Pathway in Mouse Skin. *Toxicol. Appl. Pharmacol.* **2008**, *226*, 30-37.

Karlsen, M.; Hovden, A. O.; Vogelsang, P.; Tysnes, B. B.; Appel, S. Bromelain Treatment Leads to Maturation of Monocyte-Derived Dendritic Cells But Cannot Replace PGE2 in a Cocktail of IL-1β, IL-6, TNF-α and PGE2. *Scand. J. Immunol.* **2011,** *74*, 135–143.

Kleef, R.; Delohery, T. M.; Bovbjerg, D. H. Selective Modulation of Cell Adhesion Molecules on Lymphocytes by Bromelain Protease 5. *Pathobiology* **1996,** *64*, 339–346.

Klink, M.; Jastrzembska, K.; Nowak, M.; Bednarska, K.; Szpakowski, M.; Szyllo, K.; Sulowska, Z. Ovarian Cancer Cells Modulate Human Blood Neutrophils Response to Activation In Vitro. *Scand. J. Immunol.* **2008**, *68*, 328–336.

Koh, J.; Kang, S. M.; Kim, S. J.; Cha, M. K.; Kwon, Y. J. Effect of Pineapple Protease on the Characteristics of Protein Fibers. *Fibers Polym.* **2006,** *7,* 180–185.

Koller, J.; Bukovcan, P.; Orsag, M.; Kvalteni, R.; Graffinger, I. Enzymatic Necrolysis of Acute Deep Burns–Report of Preliminary Results with 22 Patients. *Acta. Chir. Plast.* **2008,** *50,* 109–14.

Kong, X.; Zhou. H.; Qian, H. Enzymatic Hydrolysis of Wheat Gluten by Proteases and Properties of the Resulting Hydrolysates. *Food Chem.* **2007,** *102,* 759–763.

Krieger, Y.; Bogdanov, B. A.; Gurfinkel, R.; Silberstein, E.; Sagi, A.; Rosenberg, L. Efficacy of Enzymatic Debridement of Deeply Burned Hands. *Burns* **2012,** *38,* 108–112.

Kumakura, S.; Yamashita, M.; Tsurufuji, S. Effect of Bromelain on Kaolin-Induced Inflammation in Rats. *Eur. J. Pharmacol.* **1988,** *150,* 295–301.

Lapeyre-Mestre, M.; Grolleau, S.; Montastruc, J. L.; Association Française Des Centresrégionaux De Pharmacovigilance (CRPV). Adverse Drug Reactions Associated with the Use of NSAIDs: A Case/Noncase Analysis of Spontaneous Reports from the French Pharmacovigilance Database 2002–2006. *Fundam. Clin. Pharmacol.* **2013,** *27,* 223–30.

Lawrence, R. C.; Helmich, C. G.; Arnett, F.; Deyo, R. A.; Felson, D. T.; Giannini, E. H.; Heyse, S. P.; Hirsch, R.; Hochberg, M. C.; Hunder, G. G.; Liang, M. H.; Pillemer, S. R.; Steen, V. D.; Wolfe, F. Estimates of Prevalence of Arthritis and Selected Musculoskeletal Disorders in the United States. *Arthritis Rheum.* **1998,** *41,* 778–799.

Li, Q.; Withoff, S.; Verma, I. M. Inflammation-Associated Cancer: NF-KappaB is the Lynchpin. *Trends Immunol.* **2005,** *26,* 318–325.

Mantovani, A.; Allavena, P.; Sica, A.; Balkwill, F. Cancer-Related Inflammation. *Nature* **2008,** *454,* 436–444.

Massimiliano, R.; Pietro, R.; Paolo, S.; Sara, P.; Michele, F. Role of Bromelain in the Treatment of Patients with Pityriasis lichenoides chronica. *J. Dermatolog. Treat.* **2007,** *18,* 219–222.

Maurer, H. R. Bromelain: Biochemistry, Pharmacology and Medical Use. *Cell Mol. Life Sci.* **2001,** *58,* 1234–1245.

Mayer, S.; ZurHausen, A.; Watermann, D. O.; Stamm, S.; Jäger, M.; Gitsch, G.; Stickeler, E. Increased Soluble CD44 Concentrations are Associated with Larger Tumor Size and Lymph Node Metastasis in Breast Cancer Patients. *J. Cancer Res. Clin. Oncol.* **2008,** *134,* 1229–1236.

Mori, S.; Ojima, Y.; Hirose, T.; Sasaki, T.; Hashimoto, Y. The Clinical Effect of Proteolytic Enzyme Containing Bromelain and Trypsin on Urinary Tract Infection Evaluated by Double Blind Method. *Acta Obstet.Gynaecol. Jpn.* **1972,** *19,* 147–153.

Müller, A.; Barat, S.; Chen, X.; Bui, K. C.; Bozko, P.; Malek, N. P.; Plentz, R. R. Comparative Study of Antitumor Effects of Bromelain and Papain in Human Cholangiocarcinoma Cell Lines, *Int. J. Oncol.* **2016,** *48,* 2025–2034.

Omojasola, P.; Folakemi, J.; Omowumi, P.; et al. Cellulase Production by Some Fungi Cultured on Pineapple Waste. *Nature Sci.* **2008,** *6,* 64–79.

Onken, J. E.; Greer, P. K.; Calingaert, B.; Hale, L. P. Bromelain Treatment Decreases secretion of Pro-Inflammatory Cytokines and Chemokines by Colon Biopsies In Vitro. *Clin. Immunol.* **2008,** *126,* 345–352.

Pavan, R.; Jain, S.; Shraddha, Kumar, A. Properties and Therapeutic Application of Bromelain: A Review. *Biotechnol. Res. Int.* 2012, Article ID 976203, pp 1–6. http://dx.doi.org/10.1155/2012/976203

Pellicano, R.; Strona, S.; Simondi, D.; Reggiani, S.; Pallavicino, F.; Sguazzini, C.; Bonagura, A. G.; Rizzetto, M.; Astegiano, M. Benefit of Dietary Integrators for Treating Functional Dyspepsia: a Prospective Pilot Study. *Minerva Gastroenterol Dietol.* **2009,** *55,* 227–235.

Philchenkov, A. Caspases: Potential Targets for Regulating Cell Death. *J. Cell Mol. Med.* **2004,** *8*, 432–444.

Polaina, J.; MacCabe, A. P. *Industrial Enzymes: Structure, Function and Applications*; Springer: Netherland, 2007.

Roessner, A.; Kuester, D.; Malfertheiner, P.; Schneider, S. R. Oxidative Stress in Ulcerative Colitis-Associated Carcinogenesis. *Pathol. Res. Pract.* **2008,** *204*, 511–524.

Rosenberg, L.; Krieger, Y.; Bogdanov, B. A.; Silberstein, E.; Shoham, Y.; Singer, A. J. A Novel Rapid and Selective Enzymatic Debridement Agent for Burn Wound Management: a Multi-Center RCT. *Burns* **2014,** *40*, 466–74.

Shahid, S. K.; Turakhia, N. H.; Kundra, M.; Shanbag, P.; Daftary, G. V.; Schiess, W. Efficacy and Safety of Phlogenzym—A Protease Formulation, in Sepsis in Children. *J. Assoc. Physicians India* **2002,** *50*, 527–531.

Singh, L. R.; Devi, Y. R.; Devi, S. K. Enzymological Characterization of Pineapple Extract for Potential Application in Oak Tasar (*Antheraea proylei* J.) Silk Cocoon Cooking and Reeling. Electron. *J. Biotechnol.* **2003,** *6,* 198–207.

Snowden, H. M.; Renfrew, M. J.; Woolridge, M. W. Treatments for Breast Engorgement During Lactation. *Cochrane Database Syst. Rev.* **2001,** *2,* CD000046.

Stepek, G.; Buttle, D. J.; Duce, I. R.; Lowe, A.; Behnke, J. M. Assessment of the Anthelmintic Effect of Natural Plant Cysteine Proteinases Against the Gastrointestinal Nematode, *Heligmosomoides polygyrus*, In Vitro. *Parasitology* **2005,** *130*, 203–211.

Stepek, G.; Lowe, A. E.; Buttle, D. J.; Duce, I. R.; Behnke, J. M. In vitro and In vivo Anthelmintic Efficacy of Plant Cysteine Proteinases Against the Rodent Gastrointestinal Nematode, *Trichurismuris*. *Parasitology* **2006,** *132,* 681–689.

Taussig, S. J. The Mechanism of the Physiological Action of Bromelain. *Med Hypotheses.* **1980,** *6*, 99–104.

Taussig, S. J.; Batkin, S. Bromelain, the Enzyme Complex of Pineapple (*Ananas comosus*) and its Clinical Application: An Update. *J. Ethnopharmacol.* **1988,** *22*, 191–203.

Tochi, B. N.; Wang, Z.; Xu, S-Y.; Zhang, W. Therapeutic Application of Pineapple Protease (Bromelain): A Review. *Pak. J. Nutr.* **2008,** *7*, 513–520.

Tysnes, B. B.; Maurer, H. R.; Porwol, T.; Probst, B.; Bjerkvig, R.; Hoover, F. Bromelain Reversibly Inhibits Invasive Properties of Glioma Cells. *Neoplasia.* **2001,** *3*, 469–479.

Wallace, J. M. Nutritional and Botanical Modulation of the Inflammatory Cascade-Eicosanoids, Cyclooxygenases, and Lipoxygenases as an Adjunct in Cancer Therapy. *Integr. Cancer Ther.* **2002,** *1,* 7–37.

Walsh, G. *Proteins: Biochemistry and Biotechnology*; John Wiley and Sons Ltd: England, 2003.

Watanabe, M.; Watanabe, J.; Sonoyama, K.; Tanabe, S. Novel Method for Producing Hypoallergenic Wheat Flour by Enzymatic Fragmentation of the Constituent Allergens and its Application to Food Processing. *Biosci., Biotechnol., Biochem.* **2000,** *64*, 2663–2667.

White, R. R.; Crawley, F. E.; Vellini, M.; Rovati, L. A. Bioavailability of 125I Bromelain After Oral Administration to Rats. *Biopharm. Drug Dispos.* **1998,** *9*, 397–403,

Wu, S.Y.; Hu, W.; Zhang, B.; Liu, S.; Wang, J. M.; Wang, A. M. Bromelain Ameliorates the Wound Microenvironment and Improves the Healing of Firearm Wounds. *J. Surg. Res.* **2012,** *176*, 503–509.

CHAPTER 9

CYSTEINE PROTEASES FROM PLANTS AND THEIR APPLICATIONS

JUAN ABREU PAYROL[1*], WALTER DAVID OBREGÓN[2], JULIANA COTABARREN[2], T. B. MUTSAURI[1], and INIDIA RUBIO VARGAS[1]

[1]*Departamento de Farmacia, Instituto de Farmacia y Alimentos, Universidad de La Habana, Calle 222, entre 23 y 29, # 2317, La Coronela, La Lisa, CP 13600, La Habana, Cuba, Tel: 5372020930/2716789/2679207*

[2]*Departamento de Ciencias Biológicas, Facultad de Ciencias Exactas, Centro de Investigación de Proteínas Vegetales (CIPROVE), Universidad Nacional de La Plata, 47 y 115s/N, B1900AVW, La Plata, Argentina, Tel: 542214226977/6979/6981, Telefax: 542214226947*

[*]*Corresponding author. E-mail: jabreu@ifal.uh.cu; japayrol@gmail.com*

ABSTRACT

Cysteine proteases are everywhere in nature. In the plants, they perform multiple functions associated with growth and development. This chapter addresses the essential aspects associated with the main botanical families studied by the presence of these enzymes, their classification in clans, families and subfamilies, and other subgroups; fundamental structural features associated with each group and their relationship with the mechanism of action; the main functions that they perform in plants and applications they have today in social life, as well as other potentialities that systematic study can provide. In general remarks, the principal applications and potentialities of these enzymes are shown, especially of those more studied: papain and bromelain. The chapter also identified the major sources of information about cysteine proteases in web databases; also a general bibliography about the theme supports these comments, useful for those academics interested in deeper knowledge about these interesting enzymes.

9.1 INTRODUCTION

Due to the various ways in which proteolytic enzymes affect the health and well-being of humanity, this century has seen a remarkable acceleration on the pace of research in peptidases, revealed in a number of annual publications on their study which already exceeded 1885 citations in the PubMed database of the US National Center of Biotechnology Information, only in the course of 2017.

The MEROPS database (https://www.ebi.ac.uk/merops/), major web database on proteolytic enzymes, their inhibitors, and substrates, which reached 20 years in 2016, increasing the number of peptidase sequences registered in its systematic updates: 413,834 (August 2013), 523,871 (July 2015), and 912,290 (September 2017). The analysis of complete sequences of several genomes has shown that approximately 2% of the information encoded by genes are peptidases, indicating that this is one of the larger functional groups of proteins (Barrett et al., 2012).

Cysteine proteases of plants are a well-characterized group of proteolytic enzymes, among which are those in clan CA, a superfamily of papain (family C1) has been studied. This family includes endopeptidases with different specificities, aminopeptidases, exopeptidases, and some members without catalytic activity, but the plant sources produce endopeptidases a widely applied in medicine and foods, among others fields.

The forecast for the 2022 market for enzymes of plant origin exceeds USD 41 billion, of which an important part is cysteine plant proteases. Due to its qualities and wide industrial application, this trend must be maintained. These arguments reveal the need to advance in the research of this group of natural products, of wide perspectives and potential impact in branches important for humanity as health and nutrition.

9.2 CLASSIFICATION/STRUCTURE

In cysteine-type peptidases, the sulfhydryl group of a cysteine residue attacks the peptide bond, as a nucleophile. Also, a proton donor and general base are required; in this case, a histidine residue (Azarkan et al., 1996). Among the plant peptidases, cysteines presently represent around 19.6% of the 912,

290 sequences annotated in the MEROPS database, the third in abundance after serine peptidases (36.6%) and metalloproteinases (32.7%) (Rawlings et al., 2016). Cysteine proteases are grouped into 92 families belonging to 16 different clans (Rawlings et al., 2016). In 2008, 76 families belonging to 13 different clans were recorded(Caffini, 2009), while in 2004 they had scored 40 families and 6 clans (Grudkowska and Zagdanska, 2004), which reveals a sustained increase in research in this field.

Forty-one families are belonging to the CA clan, which makes it the most important of all. Another 22 families are part of the CD, CE, CF, CL, CM, CN, CO, CP, CQ, and CR clans; all share the mechanism of catalysis that includes the nucleophilic cysteine. Another 18 families are belonging to clans PA, PB, PC, and PD, which include peptidases with other catalytic mechanisms (serine and threonine) and 11 remain without assignment to a clan. The majority, including the main and best-known cysteine proteases, are found in the CA clan particularly in the C1 family, the papain family, C01.001, EC 3.4.22.2, clan archetype. The C1 family is subdivided into two subfamilies such as C1A and C1B. The cysteine peptidases that are grouped in C1A have been evolutionarily very successful, represent the largest group of these enzymes in the eukaryotes and are much distributed in the vegetable kingdom, Including secreted and lysosomal (or vacuolar) enzymes, mainly endopeptidases. Along with them in this subfamily, there are endopeptidases of DNA viruses, protozoa, and animals. There are also some exopeptidases of bacteria, fungi, and animals.

The distinction between exopeptidases and endopeptidases in the subfamily is unclear. In some members, one or the other activity may predominate, although against some substrates they act in reverse. The sequences have been assembled in the same clan, considering that the structures whose crystallographic data are known are similar or because they contain motifs with similar sequences in the environment of the catalytic residues (Barrett et al., 2012). There are 40 peptidases of the C1 family that have data of the three-dimensional structure obtained by X-ray crystallography with different degrees of resolution, in some cases, forming complexes with inhibitors, including 12 of plant origin, it is worth mentioning papain, caricain, chymopapain, and stem bromelain. In total, 227 enzymes throughout the family have been completely sequenced(Rawlings et al., 2016). In Figure 9.1, it can be seen that the simple polypeptide chain of papain forms two structural and between them the active site cleft. The N-terminal domain widely is a set of α helices, while the C-terminal domain contains a β-barrel. A long helix is along the upper center of the molecule and the catalytic cysteine is at the start of this (Barrett et al., 2012).

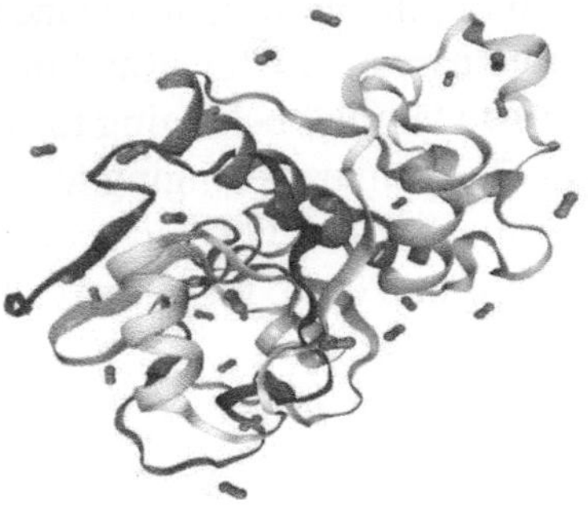

Color	Meaning
	N – terminal end
	N-terminal domain
	Long helix along the upper center of the molecule and active site cleft
	C-terminal domain
	C – terminal end
	Methanol molecule

FIGURE 9.1 **(See color insert.)** Structure of papain refined at 1.65 Å resolution.

Source: Adapted from Kamphuis et al. (1984). (The image was prepared from the protein data bank entry 9PAP.)

9.2.1 STRUCTURAL CHARACTERISTICS OF SUBFAMILY C1A TYPE PAPAÍNA

Some basic structural characteristic features of the peptidases of C1A subfamily, particularly those of plant origin, stand out as common elements in this group (Barrett et al., 2012):

- They are α/β proteins, with the nucleophilic Cys at the beginning of a helix and the catalytic His at the start of a β-sheet. A typical feature is the presence of 3 disulfide bonds, sometimes more.
- Many are inhibited by the compound E-64 (Fig. 9.2) irreversibly and by proteins of the cystatin family, although some cystatins can inhibit legumain, a CD clan peptidases, because they have a second reactive site and some inhibit also metallopeptidases (Alvarez-Fernandez et al., 1999; Valente et al., 2001).
- Those that enter in the secretory pathway usually exist as inactive precursors, with N-terminal propeptides (signal peptides); for mature (active) enzyme they also function as inhibitors. Propeptides homologous exist in most members of the C1A family, similar to that of papain, with 100 or more residues (those of cathepsin B are shorter and of different sequence) and must act the same, blocking the active site when joining it in an inverted position to which a substrate would make it. The papain-type propeptides can be identified by the presence of the ERFNIN motif, in which some of the following residues are conserved (numbered according to the propeptide of

papain): Glu64, Arg68, Phe72, Asn75, Asn83, Phe96, Asp98, and Glu103 (Novinec and Lenarcic, 2013). It is emphasized that the Pro2 residue is frequently conserved in mature peptidases, this can prevent the attack by aminopeptidases since the Xaa-Pro bond is resistant to many such enzymes.

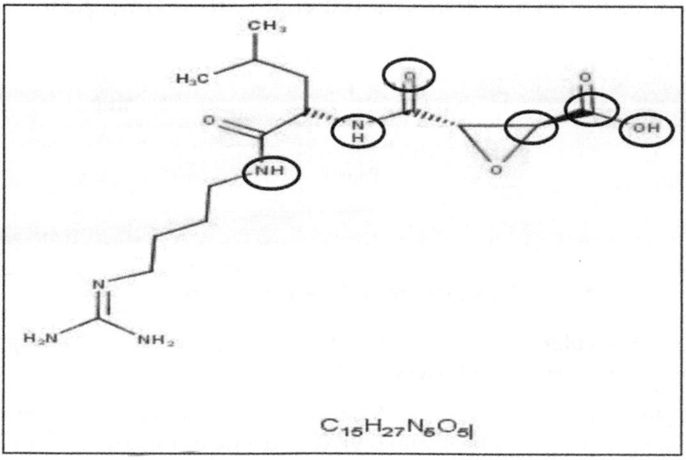

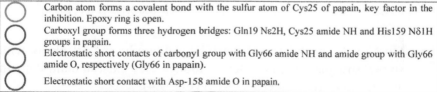

Carbon atom forms a covalent bond with the sulfur atom of Cys25 of papain, key factor in the inhibition. Epoxy ring is open.

Carboxyl group forms three hydrogen bridges: Gln19 Nε2H, Cys25 amide NH and His159 Nδ1H groups in papain.

Electrostatic short contacts of carbonyl group with Gly66 amide NH and amide group with Gly66 amide O, respectively (Gly66 in papain).

Electrostatic short contact with Asp-158 amide O in papain.

FIGURE 9.2 **(See color insert.)** Structure of E-4.

Source: The image was created with MarvinSketch 17.29.0 from Chemaxon (https://www.chemaxon.com).

- Most C1A cysteine peptidase propeptides consist of two parts and share a similar fold. The N-terminal portion is formed by two α-helices and an extended β-sheet and interacts with a "binding pro-union loop" located superficially on the mature protease. There is a long central α-helix of 25–30 residues that contain the ERFNIN motif. The C-terminal segment links the two domains of the enzyme, being anchored to the S′ sites by a short α-helix. This arrangement of the substrate binding site prevents contacts with the catalytic site of the enzyme. However, the modes of binding of the substrate and the propeptide occur in opposite directions: the side chains of the propeptide must use the same binding sites of the substrates, but the reverse orientation of the peptide chain results in such a position of the peptide bond that it makes it resistant to rupture (Harrison et al., 1997; Rzychon et al., 2004).

- Plant peptidases appear to have homologous C-terminal extensions to papain (*Lycopersicon esculentum*, *Arabidopsis thaliana*, and α and β oryzains of *Oryza sativa*) (Barrett et al., 2012) (Fig. 9.3).

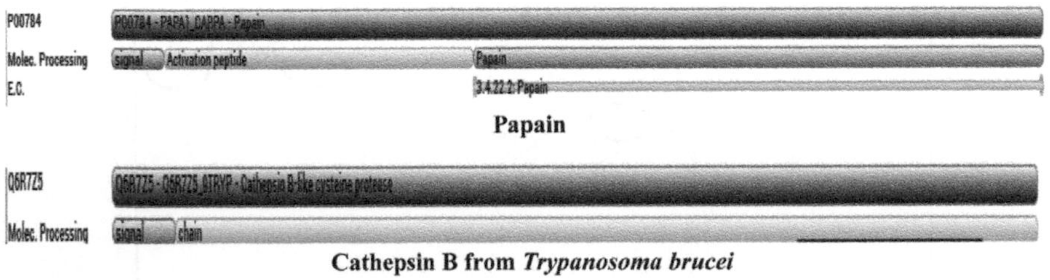

FIGURE 9.3 (See color insert.) Full protein feature view of papain and cathepsin B from Trypanosoma brucei showing propeptides length.

Source: Adapted from Kamphuis et al. (1984) and Koopmann et al. (2012). (The image was prepared from the Protein Data Bank entries 9PAP and 3MOR, using de entries P00784 and Q6R7Z5 from UniprotKB database. In grey all length sequence, in green signal peptide + activation peptide (propeptide domain) and peptidase chain (Ec 3.4.22.2 for papain).

- Most of the peptidases of the C1A subfamily and all plants with known structure are monomers, although they exist in multi-domain organizations (Barrett et al., 2012) (Fig. 9.4).

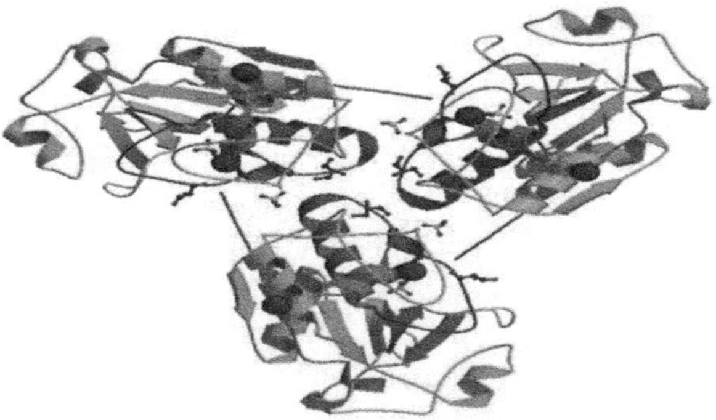

FIGURE 9.4 (See color insert.) Structure of multi-domain protease from Crocus sativum refined at 1.31 angstroms resolution. (The image was prepared from the Protein Data Bank entry 3U8E. There are three identical units join by weak electrostatic interactions.)

From an evolutionary point of view, several groups can be distinguished within the enzymes of the C1A subfamily, two main groups are the cathepsin L (papain type) and the cathepsin B type, presents in Eukaryotes. Enzymes from the cathepsin B group have a shorter propeptide than cathepsin L group and the ERFNIN motif is not conserved in these cathepsin B type peptidases propeptides (Novinec and Lenarcic, 2013).

In the C1A subfamily, cathepsin-L type peptidases are expanded between plants with modifications, while two other groups, cathepsin X and dipeptidyl peptidase I groups are absent (Richau et al., 2012).

9.2.1.1 OTHER PLANTS CYSTEINE PROTEASES IN CLAN CA

Other families in the CA clan contain plant peptidases. The enzymes from C12 family are structurally very similar to papain. The molecules have two lobes, one consisting mainly of helices, the other containing a β-barrel surrounded by helices. The catalytic Cys is at the beginning of one of the helices and the catalytic His is at the beginning of a β strand. One difference with papain is that the first strand of the β-barrel precedes the helix in the sequence carrying the catalytic Cys. The peptidases of this family have no propeptides and are intracellular. They are peptidases that hydrolyze the ubiquitin-conjugated glycine link wherever there is a α-peptide or isopeptide bond, with diverse specificities.

The C19 family is the second group of C-terminal ubiquitin hydrolases. Their structures are more complicated than those of C12, many are multidomain proteins, have a greater variety and are intracellular, but they are capable of releasing ubiquitin from much larger polyubiquitinated peptides.

9.2.1.2 OTHER PLANTS CYSTEINE PROTEASES

Other clans and families group cysteine proteases of plant origin, but in much less relevance than the clan CA and especially family C1, subfamily C1A.

Among the families of the CD clan is C13, which includes endopeptidases that break asparaginyl bonds. Among them, legumain, which has been found in a great variety of dicotyledonous plants, in legume seeds and is responsible for the posttranslational processing of seed proteins before storage. It is not inhibited by the E - 64.

In the remaining families, cysteine peptidases of plant origin are rare or have not been found.

9.3 CATALYTIC MECHANISM

A complete review of the catalytic mechanism of clan peptidases CA is cited in Polgár (2013), which explain the role of residues Cys25, His159, Gln19, and Asn175 in the catalysis. In mature papain, the catalytic dyad consists of residues Cys25 and His159, which are respect to the active site in opposite domains of the cleft. Also, they are functionally important residues Gln19 and Asn175 (Fig. 9.5).

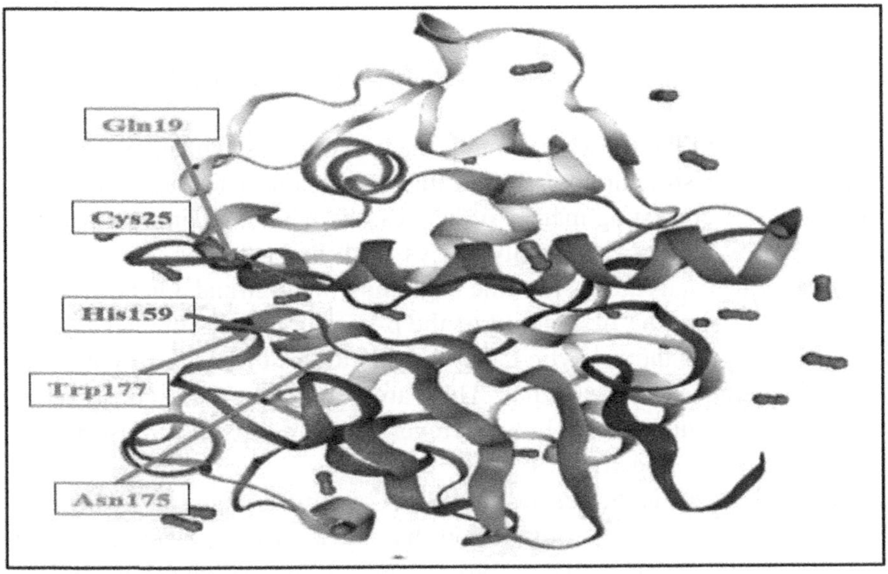

FIGURE 9.5 **(See color insert.)** Tridimensional structure of papain and position of the residues involved in catalysis Cys25, His159, Gln19 y Asn175, and Trp177.

Source: Adapted from Kamphuis et al. (1984). (The image was prepared from the Protein Data Bank entry 9PAP.)

The sulfur atom of Cys25 and the imidazole ring of His159 are in the same plane, atoms of sulfur and nitrogen are separated by 3.4 Å, the distance corresponding to a contact van der Waals. The imidazole ring is hydrogen bonded to the side chain of Asn175 and the hydrogen bridge is protected from the solvent by the indole ring of Trp177, aiding the convenient orientation of the imidazole ring in His159.

The thiol group in the active site is deprotonated by histidine, starting the catalysis of the CA peptidases, with a basic side chain, forming the thiolate-imidazolium ion pair. Then the thiolate anion of the deprotonated cysteine nucleophilically attacks the sessile peptide bond over the carbonyl carbon (Fig. 9.6A). The oxygen atom, negatively charged, allows to form the first tetrahedral state of transition. Oxyanion is stabilized by hydrogen bonding with the NH groups of the side chain of Gln19 and the skeleton of Cys25, which results in the formation of oxyanion hole (Fig. 9.6B), an electrophilic center that stabilizes the tetrahedral intermediary. Following rotation of the His159 residue allows proton transfer of the imidazolium cation to the peptidic nitrogen in the bond to be hydrolyzed and that is when the break occurs. The newly formed amine substrate is bounded by a hydrogen bond to His159, while the carboxylic part of the substrate is linked to Cys25 through a thioester bond, forming the acyl-enzyme intermediate (Fig. 9.6C).

The next reaction step involves the exit of a fragment of the substrate with an amino-terminal and the attack of a water molecule. The histidine residue is reconverted to its deprotonated form and imidazole nitrogen contributes to the polarization of the water molecule, which then attacks the acyl-enzyme over the carbonyl carbon (Fig. 9.6D), resulting in the second tetrahedral intermediate (Fig. 9.6E). In the final step, the deacylation of the thioester leads to the recovery of the carboxyl group in the hydrolyzed substrate, at the same time of the release of the active enzyme (Fig. 9.6F) (Harrison et al., 1997; Rzychon et al., 2004). An interesting feature is that when the active site has accommodated the substrate, the slot is extended by 1 Å.

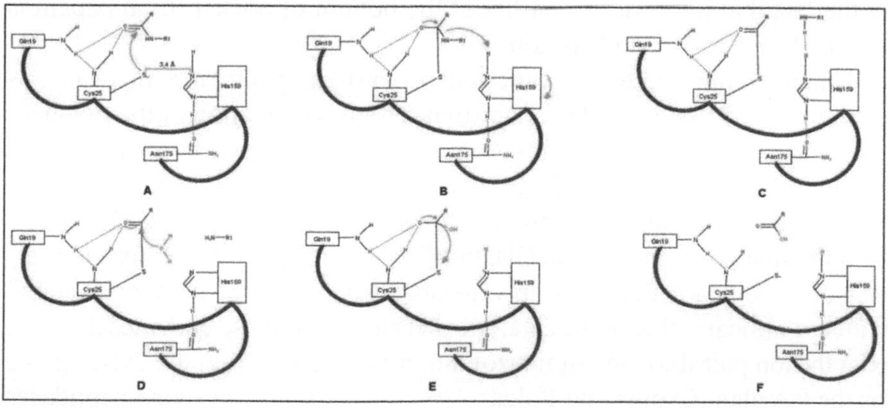

FIGURE 9.6 **(See color insert.)** Schematic representation of the catalytic mechanism of papain.

Source: The image was created with MarvinSketch 17.29.0 from Chemaxon (https://www.chemaxon.com).

Most papain-type peptidases have a broad specificity, and the main determinant is the residue at P2 position in the substrate (Berger and Schechter, 1970; Novinec and Lenarcic, 2013) (Fig. 9.7). They accept in P2 position residues with a voluminous and hydrophobic side chain not charged, although there are variations in this behavior.

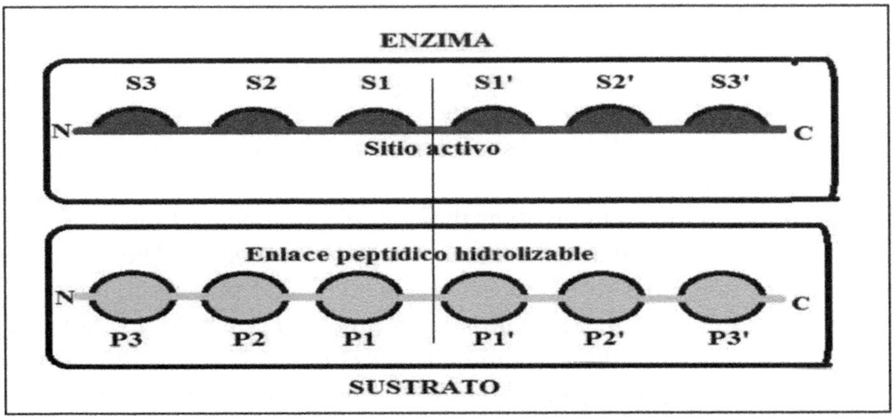

FIGURE 9.7 (See color insert.) Nomenclature of schechter y berger (1970) for the specificity of the substratum of a peptidase.

Source: Adapted from Berger and Schechter (1970).

The enzyme cathepsin B readily accepts Arg, which can be explained by the fact that the residue that lies at the bottom of pocket S2 in papain is Ser205, but in cathepsin B is Gln.

Among some interesting variations in cysteine peptidases mechanisms are the Asn 175 residue, which contributes to the orientation of the imidazolium ring of the catalytic His159, is occasionally replaced by Asp in the C12 family and others. Also, the catalytic Cys25 is usually followed by a hydrophobic aromatic amino acid, and in all the known ones of the C12, glycine occupies that position. In Clan CD, the C13 family is of interest for the presence of cysteine peptidases from vegetable origin, legumains. Experimental evidence indicates that in the catalytic mechanism of these enzymes does not exist the ion pair thiolate—imidazolium or is different from the existing one for the CA clan (Csoma and Polgár, 1984). Papain-type cysteine peptidases from plants are usually endopeptidases but may exhibit other activities as result of structural modifications to the folding of papain, which restrict the access of substrate to the active site in some side of its cleft, probably as an evolutionary strategy of the organisms in which they exist. This is the cause of that we find total or partial activity as exopeptidases, carboxypeptidases, and aminopeptidases (Novinec and Lenarcic, 2013).

Because the intensity of research in cysteine peptidases, the number of clans, families, and structures that continue to appear is growing. Although in plants predominate the features described, apparently for evolutionary reasons; particularly in bacteria and viruses appear not only different folds but different catalytic entities have been found. It would not be surprising that novel studies on peptidases of the vegetal kingdom have similar results.

9.4 ROLE IN NATURE

Plant proteases take part in almost all life processes in plants. They are implied in several physiological processes, including protein degradation, digestion, maintenance of cells, signaling, differentiation, growth, development, apoptosis, maturation, synthesis, degradation of reserve proteins during the germination of seeds, circadian rhythms, senescence, and programmed cell death (PCD). They play fundamental roles to regulate the biological processes, such as recognition of pests and pathogens (Konno et al., 2004) and in the effective induction of defensive responses and in resistance to unfavorable conditions that include the attack of herbivores, water, and environmental stress (García-Lorenzo, 2007; Caffini, 2009).

Many of plant enzymes of the C1 family are essentials in protein degradation in vacuoles. They appear in fruits, particularly immature; their activity prevents insects feeding and hydrolyzes endogenous proteins during the maturation of fruits (Turk et al., 2012).

In the natural selection process some families of plant cysteine proteases have been diversified in the competition between plants and their pathogens: plants produce proteases that suppress the growth of fungi, fungi generate inhibitors specific to these proteases and these are diversified to favor the immune response (Kaschani et al., 2010).

Perhaps, the most important function is their involvement in proteosomes, related to various metabolic processes such as hormonal signaling, cell cycle, embryogenesis, morphogenesis, floral development, and oxidative stress (Watanabe and Lam, 2005). It is usually considered that these proteases have cleaning functions ("housekeepers"), eliminating nonfunctional proteins and recycling the amino acids released in the hydrolysis. However, some appear to be part of a signal cascade (Sasabe et al., 2000), others seem to act in presence of predators by different mechanisms: (a) liberating elicitors of the invader who, when recognized, unleash the defense mechanism; (b) binding of the elicitor to the protease causing the activation thereof, triggering a cascade of reactions involving the breakdown of proteins involved in the defensive process; and (c) binding of the elicitor to the protease could inhibit its activity, acting on elicitor—protease complex as a signal to unleash the defensive mechanism (van der Hoorn and Jones, 2004).

Peptidases type cathepsin L represent the majority of the repertoire of peptidases of the C1 family in plants, the most recognized are the papain (papaya, *Carica papaya* L.), bromelains (pineapple, *Ananas comosus* L.), and ficain (figs, *Ficus* sp.), produced by plants in large quantities and very used for medicinal products, in food industry and for numerous other applications (González-Rábade et al., 2011).

Papain and bromelain protect plants from parasites, such as fungi or insects (Konno et al., 2004) (Lopez-Garcia et al., 2012). For other homologous peptidases also have been described roles in plants immunity (Shindo et al., 2012). Xylem-specific peptidases implicated in PCD related with xylogenesis have been found (Avci et al., 2008) and others with general senescence of plants (Otegui et al., 2005).

Peptidases of type cathepsin L (papain), B, H, and F are mainly responsible for the proteolytic activity during the senescence of the leaves. In this crucial process, nutrients from leaf are relocated to storage or growing tissues. Massive protein degradation involves extensive metabolic networks, different subcellular compartments, and various types of proteases and regulators (Diaz-Mendoza et al., 2014).

9.5 APPLICATIONS OF VEGETABLE CISTEIN PEPTIDASES

Historically, peptidases have had multiple applications, in many cases as mixtures and not as purified enzymes. In ancient times, fig juice was used to coagulate the milk (contains ficaina) and rennet from the stomach of cattle to make cheese (contains chymosin). Industrially they are used to remove hair from skins and other modifications in the leather industry, to tenderize meat, clarify beers, enhance the flavors of cheeses, and others foods, as biological detergents and cleaning liquids for contact lenses, among other applications. In the area of medicine, they are used to eliminate gastrointestinal parasites, removal of dead skin of burn patients, determination of blood groups, and so forth. They are of relevant value in current medical research, molecular biology, and biotechnology.

The beginning of its great commercial boom was marked in the 80 s of the last century, global enzyme trade in the middles of 80 was well above the 500 million annual dollars, at that time an annual growth of 5% was predicted, estimated that was the real growth that was reaching in subsequent years, for example, in 1997 the total value traded was close to 1500 million dollars (Caffini, 2009).

Towards the end of 1990s, it was reported that the increase in those years was of the order of 6.5% per year, initially was estimated that for 2009 would reach a figure close to 5100 million dollars; being the proteases among the enzymes more required, the fundamental reason due to the wide use of these enzymes in the processing of materials of natural origin, but also was foresaw the development of novel applications, in particular pharmaceuticals, such forecast result are accurate, given the multiple applications that have gradually reached such enzymes (Caffini, 2009).

On the other hand, these enzymes are capable of activating the target protease receptors and in this way, they will act as important pharmacological and toxicological agents (Domsalla and Melzig, 2008). Cysteine peptidases are usually obtained from fruits such as papaya (*C. papaya*), kiwi (*Actinidia chinensis*), and pineapple (*A. comosus*). However, the most come from microbial sources, although several plant peptidases remain irreplaceable for some applications, in particular, papain, bromelain, and ficain. Nowadays, the interest in them grows due to the wide variety of their medical and industrial applications and research reports. However, the number of plant proteases isolated and characterized continues relatively very low (Caffini, 2009).

9.5.1 PAPAIN TYPE ENZYMES IN GENERAL

The fruit of green papaya (*C. papaya*), the leaves and the latex of the bark are rich in enzymes known as papain, the better well-known and the most applied.

In the area of foods, the papain-like cysteine peptidases have been used in the manufacture of chewing gum, toothpaste, meat tenderizers, beer's clarification (for its value for foam production and malting of beer as result of the fermentation of barley or basic cereal), cheese production, preservation of species, food supplements (its positive effect on casein and cow whey protein degradation in the stomach of children is used), and so forth. In addition, it is also believed that these enzymes have antifungal, antiviral, and also antibacterial properties (Berger and Asenjo, 1940; Buttle et al., 2011; Esti et al., 2013; He et al., 2014).

In December 2017, a review of World Intellectual Property Organization (WIPO) patents database registers 5143 hits related to papain, 108 of them in 2017, an excellent number in this group of compounds.

In medicine, they are applied to treat digestive problems, wound, and burns healing (improve epithelialization and reduce wound size) (Gurung and Škalko-Basnet, 2009; Singh and Singh, 2012). There are studies in other directions, such as the removal of kidney stones, hypertension, urinary tract problems, menstrual pains, analgesia, dysentery, diarrhea, and fever (Hasimun and Ernasari, 2014) (Berger and Asenjo, 1940; He et al., 2014).

They seem to have an essential role in the degenerative and invasive diseases of the immune system (e.g., cathepsin K catalyzes bone degradation in osteoclasts, its selective inhibition could be valuable in osteoporosis, some forms of arthritis) (Lecaille et al., 2002). Papaya leaf extracts significantly inhibit proliferative responses of solid tumor cell lines taken from cervical carcinoma, in addition, for example, remove adenocarcinomas, hepatocellular carcinomas, lung adenocarcinoma, pancreatic epitheloid carcinoma, and mesotheliomas (Ikram et al., 2015).

They are applied in many other areas, such as cosmetics, textiles, detergents, food industry, baking, obtaining of modified proteins (protein hydrolysates) destined to food industry, manufacture of leather, recovery of silver, and the treatment of industrial waste with high protein concentration (such as "tails"of fishmeal industry) (Berger and Asenjo, 1940; Caffini, 2009; Amri and Mamboya, 2012).

Papains (a mixture of papaya peptidases) helps to protect immature fruits, for its action in the control of diseases of plants produced by parasites such nematodes and arthropods (Miller and Sands, 1977; Konno et al., 2004; Stepek et al., 2007).

Cysteine peptidases from papaya are much more likely to succeed in terms of safety and tolerability than other medications that are used as anthelmintics because they are part of the current human food (Stepek et al., 2006).

They are also used in the production of peptides, synthesis of molecules, and pharmaceutical products industry (Berger and Asenjo, 1940; He et al., 2014). The relatively recent and novel application in the synthesis of peptides in nonaqueous media (obtaining of aspartame sweetener) opens a road to growth (Bordusa, 2002).

9.5.2 OTHER PLANTS CYSTEINE PEPTIDASES

Bromelain is the second phytoprotease in importance, after papain and the most studied in *Bromeliaceae*, is found in leaves, stem, and fruits of pineapple (*A. comosus*). In 2005, more than 320 patents on their industrial applications and pharmaceutical companies were published, of them about 130 were American, 95 were Japanese, and almost all the others from European countries, concentrated in the two decades prior to that date. In December of 2017, a revision in WIPO patent database records 529 entries, 12 of them in 2017, a notable rythm in last 12 years.

They are much applied in various areas, such as food industry and cosmetics. Highlight their potential in medicine (Maurer, 2001), mainly, because of its anti-inflammatory and anticancer properties, in addition to its ability to induce cellular apoptosis (Arshad et al., 2014).

It has been applied to treat the rheumatoid arthritis, circulatory disorders (bruising, thrombophlebitis, and coagulation), oral, rectal and perirectal inflammation, ulcers, diabetes, angina, bronchitis, sinusitis, wound healing, surgical traumas, pyelonephritis, relieves pain, and swelling and to strengthen the absorption of drugs such as antibiotics. It is considered nontoxic and without side effects, it is possible to use it in doses between 200 and 2000 mg/kg for long periods (Taussig and Batkin, 1988; Maurer, 2001; Salas et al., 2008; Pavan et al., 2012).

Other therapeutic areas are now actively exploring, some with results known from traditional medicine (anthelmintic) and its presence in the market grows continuously (Arshad et al., 2014).

Ficain, from fig (*Ficus* sp.) is another cysteine protease used in the food processing (brewery, meat, and so forth.) (Homaei et al., 2014). Unfortunately, it has not been well characterized, partly because of it self-hydrolyzes (Baeyens-Volant et al., 2015).

Pinguinain has been slightly studied. It is obtained from the fruits of *Bromelia pinguin*. It has been successfully tested to clean the devitalized tissue in bedsores, it can be useful as fibrinolytic, clot breaker, and anti-inflammatory (Toro-Goyco et al., 1968), although do not appear in scientific literature studies that endorse them directly. On the other hand, an effective procedure was developed to separate schistosoma eggs (*Schistosoma mansoni*) from tissues of infected animals, as part of a diagnostic procedure of the infection with this parasite (Toro-Goyco and Rodriguez-Costas, 1976; Toro-Goyco et al., 1980).

Its capacity as an anthelmintic was evaluated and in the synthesis of nonaqueous systems, with encouraging results. It is expected that pinguinain behavior would be similar to the proteases of *A. comosus*, in particular to fruit bromelain, with which keeps the greatest similarities in composition and properties (Payrol et al., 2005, Caffini, 2008).

KEYWORDS

- plant cysteine proteases
- clan CA
- family C1
- papain
- bromelain

REFERENCES

Alvarez-Fernandez, M.; Barrett, A. J.; Gerhartz, B.; Dando, P. M.; Ni, J.; Abrahamson, M. Inhibition of Mammalian Legumain by Some Cystatins is Due to a Novel Second Reactive Site. *J. Biol. Chem.* **1999,** *274*(27), 19195–19203.

Amri, E.; Mamboya, F. Papain, a Plant Enzyme of Biological Importance: A Review. *Am. J. Biochem. Biotechnol.* **2012,** *8*(2), 99–104.

Arshad, Z. I.; Amid, A.; Yusof, F.; Jaswir, I.; Ahmad, K.; Loke, S. P. Bromelain: An Overview of Industrial Application and Purification Strategies. *Appl. Microbiol. Biotechnol.* **2014,** *98*(17), 7283–7297.

Avci, U.; Petzold, H. E.; Ismail, I. O.; Beers, E. P.; Haigler, C. H. Cysteine Proteases XCP1 and XCP2 Aid Micro-Autolysis Within the Intact Central Vacuole During Xylogenesis in Arabidopsis Roots. *Plant J.* **2008,** *56*(2), 303–315.

Azarkan, M.; Maes, D.; Bouckaert, J.; Thi, M. H. D.; Wyns, L.; Looze, Y. Thiol Pegylation Facilitates Purification of Chymopapain Leading to Diffraction Studies At 1.4 Å Resolution. *J. Chromatogr. A.* **1996,** *749*(1–2), 69–72.

Baeyens-Volant, D.; Matagne, A.; El Mahyaoui, R.; Wattiez, R.; Azarkan, M. A Novel Form of Ficin from Ficus Carica Latex: Purification and Characterization. *Phytochemistry* **2015,** *117,* 154–167.

Barrett, A. J.; Woessner, J. F.; Rawlings, N. D. *Handbook of Proteolytic Enzymes;* Elsevier: USA, 2012.

Berger, A.; Schechter, I. Mapping the Active Site of Papain with the Aid of Peptide Substrates and Inhibitors. *Philos. Trans. R. Soc. Lond. B Biol. Sci.* **1970,** *257*(813), 249–264.

Berger, J.; Asenjo, C. F. Anthelmintic Activity of Crystalline Papain. *Science* **1940,** *91*(2364), 387–388.

Bordusa, F. Proteases in Organic Synthesis. *Chem. Rev.* **2002,** *102*(12), 4817–4868.

Buttle, D.J.; Behnke, J. M.; Bartley, Y.; Elsheikha, H. M.; Bartley, D. J.; Garnett, M. C.; et al. Oral Dosing with Papaya Latex is an Effective Anthelmintic Treatment for Sheep Infected with Haemonchus Contortus. *Parasites Vectors* **2011,** *4*(1), 36.

Caffini, N. *Enzimas Proteolíticas De Vegetales Superiores: Aplicaciones Industriales;* 2009, 9879641361.

Caffini, J. Purification and Characterization of Four New Cysteine Endopeptidases from Fruits of *Bromelia pinguin* L. Grown in Cuba. *Protein J.* **2008,** *27*(2), 9.

Csoma, C.; Polgár, L. Proteinase from Germinating Bean Cotyledons. Evidence for Involvement of a Thiol Group in Catalysis. *Biochem. J.* **1984,** *222*(3), 769–776.

Diaz-Mendoza, M.; Velasco-Arroyo, B.; Gonzalez-Melendi, P.; Martinez, M.; Diaz, I. C1a Cysteine Protease-Cystatin Interactions in Leaf Senescence. *J. Exp. Bot.* **2014,** *65*(14), 3825–3833.

Domsalla, A.; Melzig, M. F. Occurrence and Properties of Proteases in Plant Latices. *Planta Med.* **2008,** *74*(07), 699–711.

Esti, M.; Benucci, I.; Lombardelli, C., Liburdi, K.; Garzillo, A. M. V. Papain from Papaya (*Carica papaya* L.) Fruit and Latex: Preliminary Characterization in Alcoholic–Acidic Buffer for Wine Application. *Food Bioprod. Process* **2013,** *91*(4):595–598.

García-Lorenzo, M. The Role of Proteases in Plant Development. Ph.D. Thesis; Umea University, Sweden, 2007.

González-Rábade, N.; Badillo-Corona, J. A.; Aranda-Barradas, J. S.; Oliver-Salvador Mdel, C. Production of Plant Proteases in Vivo and in Vitro—A Review. *Biotechnol. Adv.* **2011,** *29*(6), 983–996.

Grudkowska, M.; Zagdanska, B. Multifunctional Role of Plant Cysteine Proteinases. *Acta Biochim. Pol.* **2004,** *51*(3), 609–624.

Gurung, S.; Škalko-Basnet, N. Wound Healing Properties of *Carica Papaya* Latex: In Vivo Evaluation in Mice Burn Model. *J. Ethnopharmacol.* **2009**, *121*(2), 338–341.

Harrison, M. J.; Burton, N. A.; Hillier, I. H. Catalytic Mechanism of the Enzyme Papain: Predictions with a Hybrid Quantum Mechanical/Molecular Mechanical Potential. *J. Am. Chem. Soc.* **1997,** *119*(50), 12285–12291.

Hasimun, P.; Ernasari, G. Analgetic Activity of Papaya (*Carica papaya L.*) Leaves Extract. *Procedia Chem.* **2014,** *13,* 147–149.

He, Y., bin Tuan Chik, S.M.S.; Chong, F.C. Purification of Papain from Unclarified Papaya Juice Using Reversed Phase Expanded Bed Adsorption Chromatography (RP-EBAC). *J. Ind. Eng. Chem.* **2014,** *20*(6), 4293–4297.

Homaei, A.; Barkheh, H.; Sariri, R.; Stevanato, R. Immobilized Papain on Gold Nanorods as Heterogeneous Biocatalysts. *Amino Acids* **2014,** *46*(7), 1649–1657.

Ikram, E. H. K.; Stanley, R.; Netzel, M.; Fanning, K. Phytochemicals of Papaya and Its Traditional Health and Culinary Uses–A Review. *J. Food Compos. Anal.* **2015,** *41,* 201–211.

Kamphuis, I. G.; Kalk, K.; Swarte, M.; Drenth J. Structure of Papain Refined At 1.65 Å Resolution. *J. Mol. Biol.* **1984,** *179*(2), 233–256.

Kaschani, F.; Shabab, M.; Bozkurt, T., Shindo, T., Schornack, S., Gu, C. et al. An Effector-Targeted Protease Contributes to Defense Against Phytophthora Infestans and is Under Diversifying Selection in Natural Hosts. *Plant Physiol.* **2010,** *154*(4), 1794–1804.

Konno, K.; Hirayama, C.; Nakamura, M.; Tateishi, K.; Tamura, Y.; Hattori, M. et al. Papain Protects Papaya Trees from Herbivorous Insects: Role of Cysteine Proteases in latex. *Plant J. cell Mol. Biol.* **2004,** *37*(3), 370–378.

Koopmann, R.; Cupelli, K.; Redecke, L.; Nass, K.; DePonte, D. P.; White, T. A.;et al. In Vivo Protein Crystallization Opens New Routes in Structural Biology. *Nat. Methods* **2012,** *9*(3), 259–262.

Lecaille, F.; Kaleta, J.; Brömme, D. Human and Parasitic Papain-Like Cysteine Proteases: Their Role in Physiology and Pathology and Recent Developments in Inhibitor Design. *Chem. Rev.* **2002,** *102*(12), 4459–4488.

Lopez-Garcia, B.; Hernandez, M.; Segundo, B. S. Bromelain, a cysteine protease from pineapple A Cysteine Protease from Pineapple (Ananas comosus) Stem, is an Inhibitor of Fungal Plant Pathogens. *Lett. Appl. Microbiol.* **2012,** *55*(1), 62–67.

Maurer, H. Bromelain: Biochemistry, Pharmacology and Medical Use. *CMLS Cell Mol Life Sci.* **2001,** *58*(9), 1234–1245.

Miller, P.; Sands, D. Effects of Hydroclytic Enzymes on Plant-Parasitic Nematodes. *J. Nematol.* **1977,** *9*(3), 192.

Novinec, M.; Lenarcic, B. Papain-Like Peptidases: Structure, Function, and Evolution. *Biomol. Concepts* **2013,** *4*(3), 287–308.

Otegui, M. S.; Noh, Y. S.; Martinez, D. E.; Vila Petroff, M. G.; Staehelin, L. A.; Amasino, R. M. et al. Senescence-Associated Vacuoles with Intense Proteolytic Activity Develop in Leaves of Arabidopsis and Soybean. *Plant J. Cell Mol. Boil.* **2005,** *41*(6), 831–844.

Pavan, R.; Jain, S.; Shraddha.; Kumar, A. Properties and Therapeutic Application of Bromelain: A Review. *Biotechnol. Res. Int.* **2012.** Article ID 976203, 1–6. http://dx.doi.org/10.1155/2012/976203

Payrol, J. A.; Obregon, W. D.; Natalucci, C. L.; Caffini, N. O. Reinvestigation of the Proteolytically Active Components of *Bromelia Pinguin* Fruit. *Fitoterapia.* **2005,** *76*(6), 540–548.

Polgár, L. *Catalytic mechanisms of cysteine peptidases. Handbook of Proteolytic Enzymes;* 3rd Ed.; Elsevier: USA, 2013; pp 1773–1784.

Rawlings, N. D.; Barrett, A. J.; Finn, R. Twenty Years of the MEROPS Database of Proteolytic Enzymes, their Substrates and Inhibitors. *Nucleic Acids Res.* **2016,** *44*(D1), D343–D350.

Richau, K. H.; Kaschani, F; Verdoes, M.; Pansuriya, T. C.; Niessen, S.; Stuber, K.; et al. Subclassification and Biochemical Analysis of Plant Papain-Like Cysteine Proteases Displays Subfamily-Specific Characteristics. *Plant Physiol.* **2012,** *158*(4), 1583–1599.

Rzychon, M.; Chmiel, D.; Stec-Niemczyk, J. Modes of Inhibition of Cysteine Proteases. *Acta Biochim. Pol.* **2004,** *51*(4), 861–873.

Salas, C. E.; Gomes, M. T.; Hernandez, M.; Lopes, M. T. Plant Cysteine Proteinases: Evaluation of the Pharmacological Activity. *Phytochemistry.* **2008,** *69*(12), 2263–2269.

Sasabe, M.; Takeuchi, K.; Kamoun, S.; Ichinose, Y.; Govers, F.; Toyoda, K. et al. Independent Pathways Leading to Apoptotic Cell Death, Oxidative Burst and Defense Gene Expression in Response to Elicitin in Tobacco Cell Suspension Culture. *Eur J Biochem.* **2000,** *267*(16), 5005–5013.

Shindo, T.; Misas-Villamil, J. C.; Horger, A. C.; Song, J.; van der Hoorn, R. A Role in Immunity for Arabidopsis Cysteine Protease RD21, the Ortholog of the Tomato Immune Protease C14. *PloS one* **2012**, *7*(1), e29317.

Singh, D.; Singh, R. Papain Incorporated Chitin Dressings for Wound Debridement Sterilized by Gamma Radiation. *Radiat. Phys Chem.* **2012,** *81*(11), 1781–1785.

Stepek, G.; Curtis, R.; Kerry, B.; Shewry, P.; Clark, S.; Lowe, A.; et al. Nematicidal Effects of Cysteine Proteinases Against Sedentary Plant Parasitic Nematodes. *Parasitology* **2007,** *134*(12), 1831–1838.

Stepek, G.; Lowe, A. E.; Buttle, D. J.; Duce, I. R.; Behnke, J. M. In Vitro and in Vivo Anthelmintic Efficacy of Plant Cysteine Proteinases Against the Rodent Gastrointestinal Nematode, Trichuris Muris. *Parasitology* **2006**, *132*(Pt 5), 681–689.

Taussig, S. J.; Batkin, S. Bromelain, the Enzyme Complex of Pineapple (*Ananas comosus*) and its Clinical Application. An Update. *J. Ethnopharmacol.* **1988,** *22*(2), 191-203.

Toro-Goyco, E.; Maretzki, A.; Matos, M. L. Isolation, Purification, and Partial Characterization of Pinguinain, the Proteolytic Enyzme from *Bromelia pinguin* L. *Arch. Biochem. Biophys.* **1968,** *126*(1), 91–104.

Toro-goyco, E.; Rodríguez-Costas, I.; Ehrig H. Structural Studies on Pinguinain. Changes Induced by Carboxamidomethylation. *Biochim. Biophys. Acta.* **1980,** *622*(1), 151–159.

Toro-Goyco, E.; Rodriguez-Costas, I. Immunochemical Studies on Pinguinain, a Sulfhydryl Plant Protease. *Arch. Biochem. Biophys.* **1976,** *175*(2), 359–366.

Turk, V.; Stoka, V.; Vasiljeva, O.; Renko, M.; Sun, T.; Turk, B. et al. Cysteine Cathepsins: from Structure, Function and Regulation to New Frontiers. *Biochim. Biophys. Acta.* **2012,** *1824*(1), 68–88.

Valente, R. H.; Dragulev, B.; Perales, J.; Fox, J. W.; Domont, G. B. BJ46a, a Snake Venom Metalloproteinase Inhibitor. *Eur. J. Biochem.* **2001,** *268*(10), 3042-3052.

van der Hoorn, R. A.; Jones, J. D. The Plant Proteolytic Machinery and Its Role in Defence. *Curr. Opin. Plant Biol.* **2004,** *7*(4), 400–407.

Watanabe, N.; Lam, E. Two Arabidopsis Metacaspases AtMCP1b and AtMCP2b are Arginine/Lysine-Specific Cysteine Proteases and Activate Apoptosis-Like Cell Death in Yeast. *J. Biol. Chem.* **2005,** *280*(15), 14691–14699.

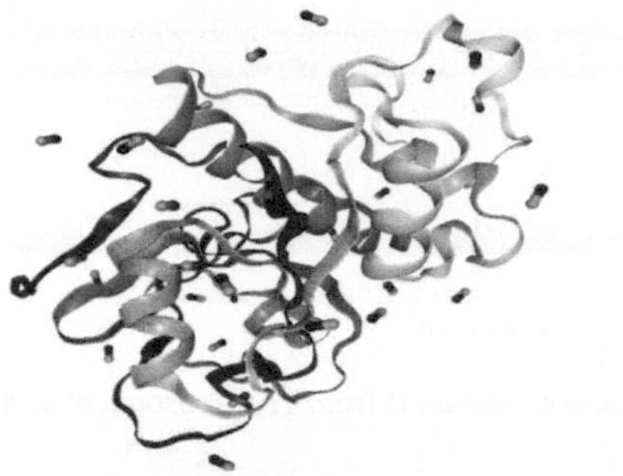

Color	Meaning
	N – terminal end
	N-terminal domain
	Long helix along the upper center of the molecule and active site cleft
	C-terminal domain
	C – terminal end
	Methanol molecule

FIGURE 9.1 Structure of papain refined at 1.65 Å resolution.

Source: Adapted from Kamphuis et al. (1984). (The image was prepared from the protein data bank entry 9PAP.)

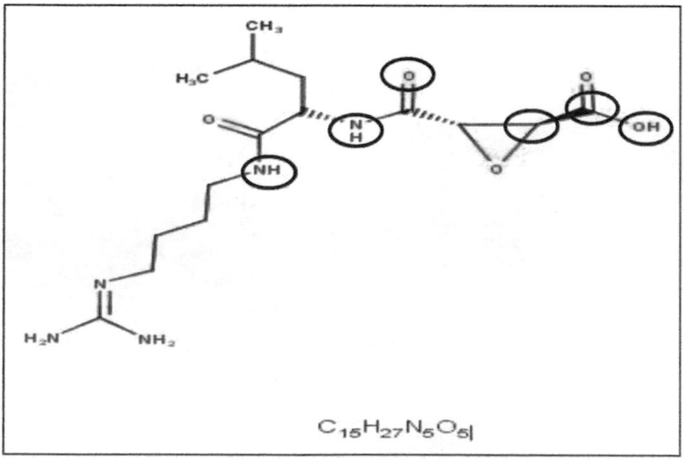

◯	Carbon atom forms a covalent bond with the sulfur atom of Cys25 of papain, key factor in the inhibition. Epoxy ring is open.
◯	Carboxyl group forms three hydrogen bridges: Gln19 Nε2H, Cys25 amide NH and His159 Nδ1H groups in papain.
◯	Electrostatic short contacts of carbonyl group with Gly66 amide NH and amide group with Gly66 amide O, respectively (Gly66 in papain).
◯	Electrostatic short contact with Asp-158 amide O in papain.

FIGURE 9.2 Structure of E-4.

Source: The image was created with MarvinSketch 17.29.0 from Chemaxon (https://www.chemaxon.com).

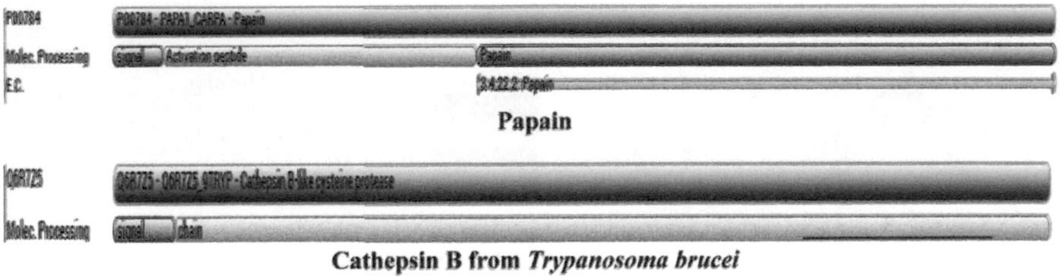

FIGURE 9.3 Full protein feature view of papain and cathepsin B from Trypanosoma brucei showing propeptides length.

Source: Adapted from Kamphuis et al. (1984) and Koopmann et al. (2012). (The image was prepared from the Protein Data Bank entries 9PAP and 3MOR, using de entries P00784 and Q6R7Z5 from UniprotKB database. In grey all length sequence, in green signal peptide + activation peptide (propeptide domain) and peptidase chain (Ec 3.4.22.2 for papain).

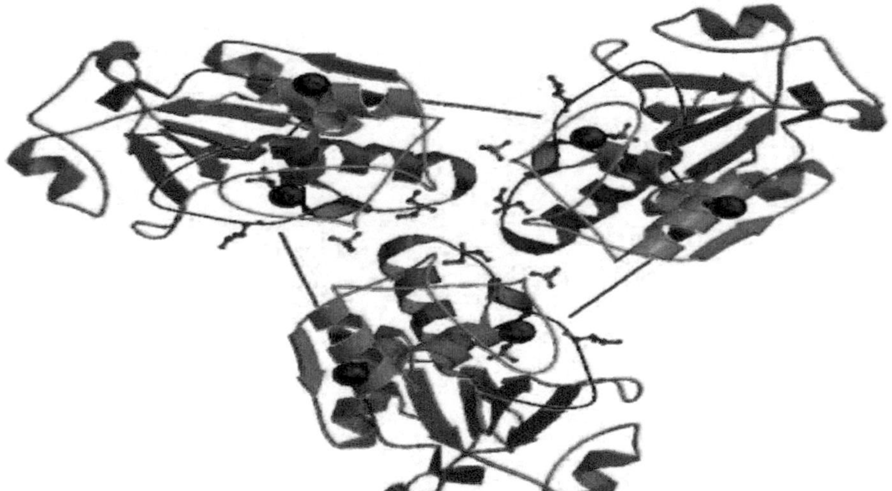

FIGURE 9.4 Structure of multi-domain protease from Crocus sativum refined at 1.31 angstroms resolution. (The image was prepared from the Protein Data Bank entry 3U8E. There are three identical units join by weak electrostatic interactions.)

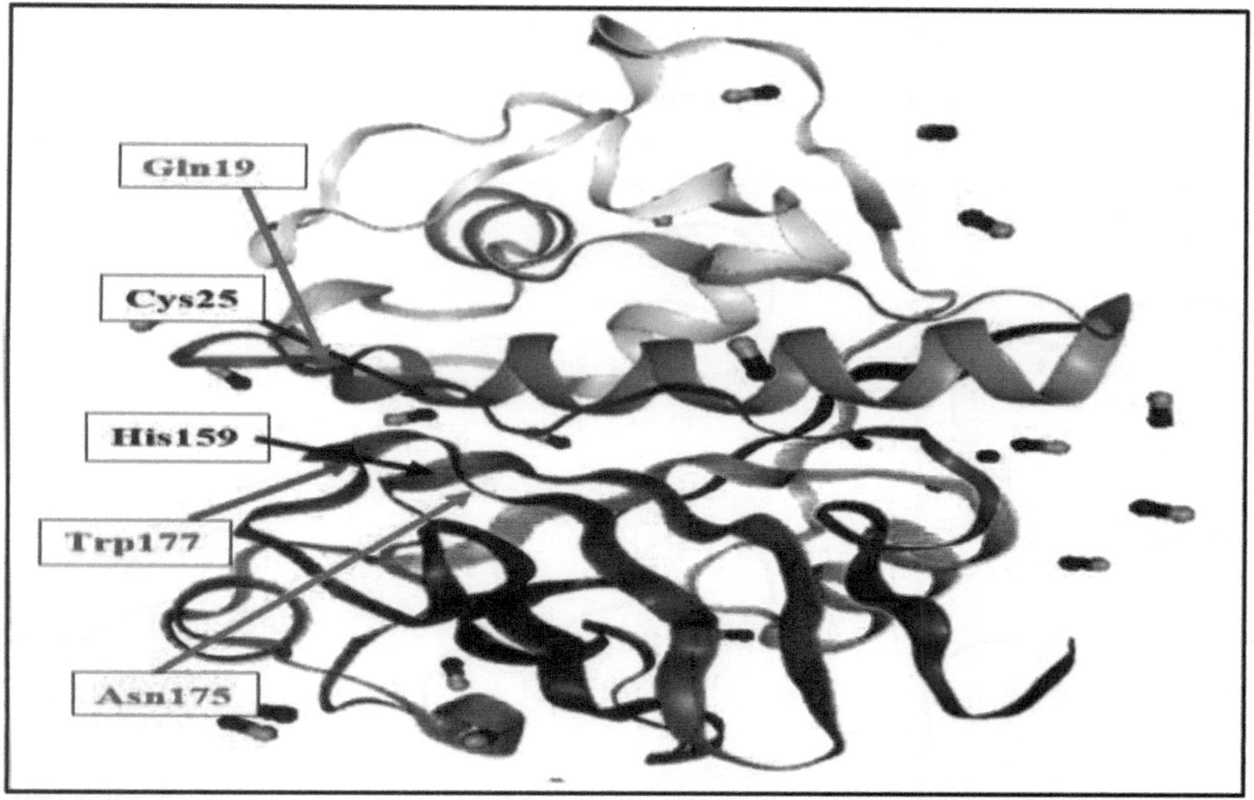

FIGURE 9.5 Tridimensional structure of papain and position of the residues involved in catalysis Cys25, His159, Gln19 y Asn175, and Trp177.

Source: Adapted from Kamphuis et al. (1984). (The image was prepared from the Protein Data Bank entry 9PAP.)

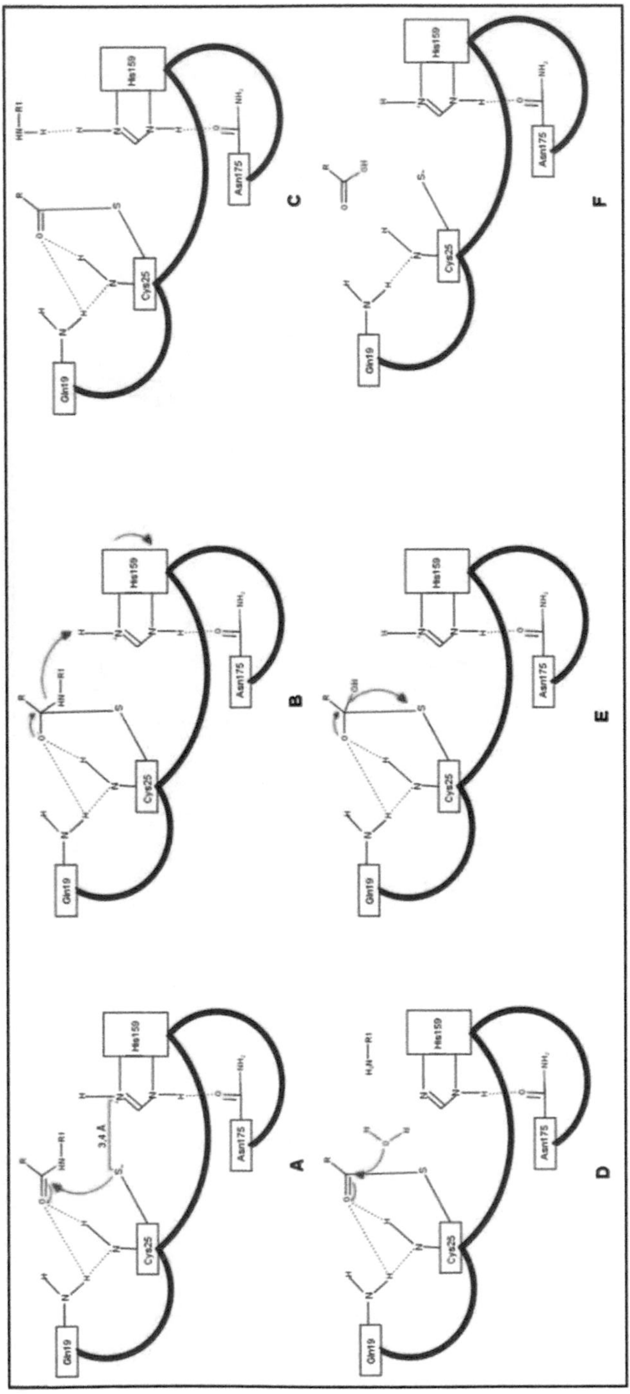

FIGURE 9.6 Schematic representation of the catalytic mechanism of papain.

Source: The image was created with MarvinSketch 17.29.0 from Chemaxon (https://www.chemaxon.com).

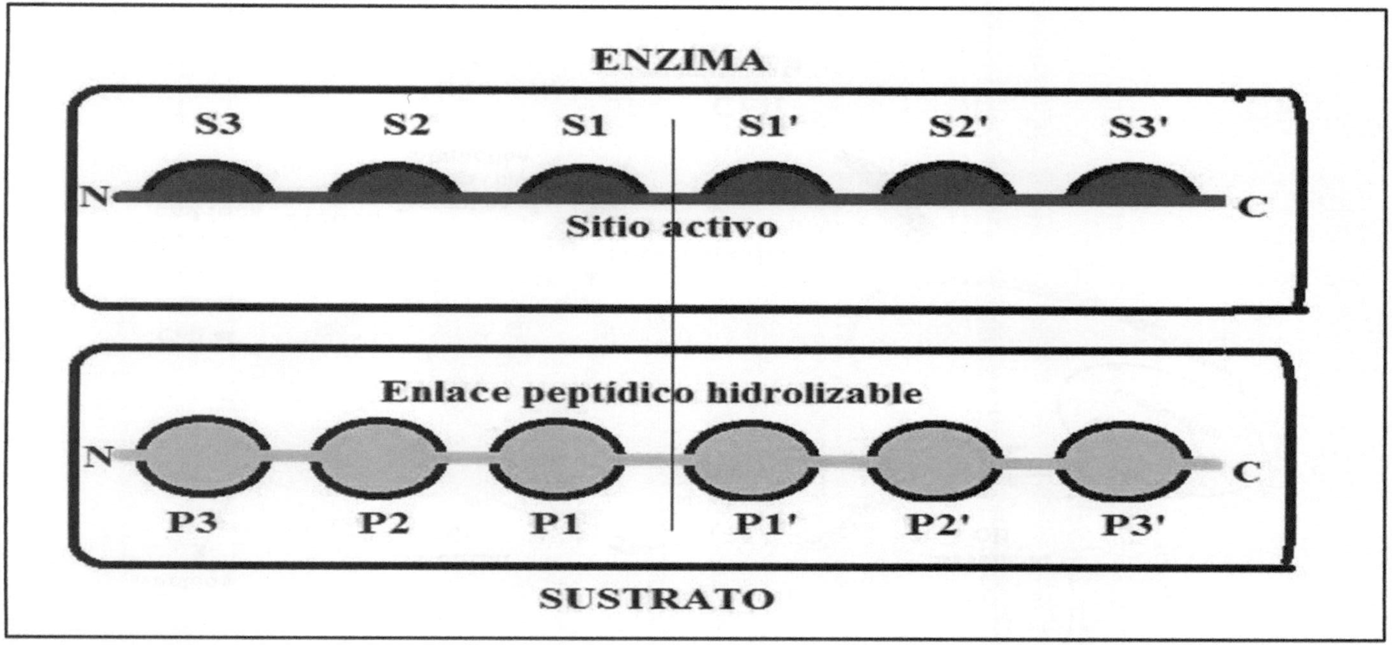

FIGURE 9.7 Nomenclature of schechter y berger (1970) for the specificity of the substratum of a peptidase.

Source: Adapted from Berger and Schechter (1970).

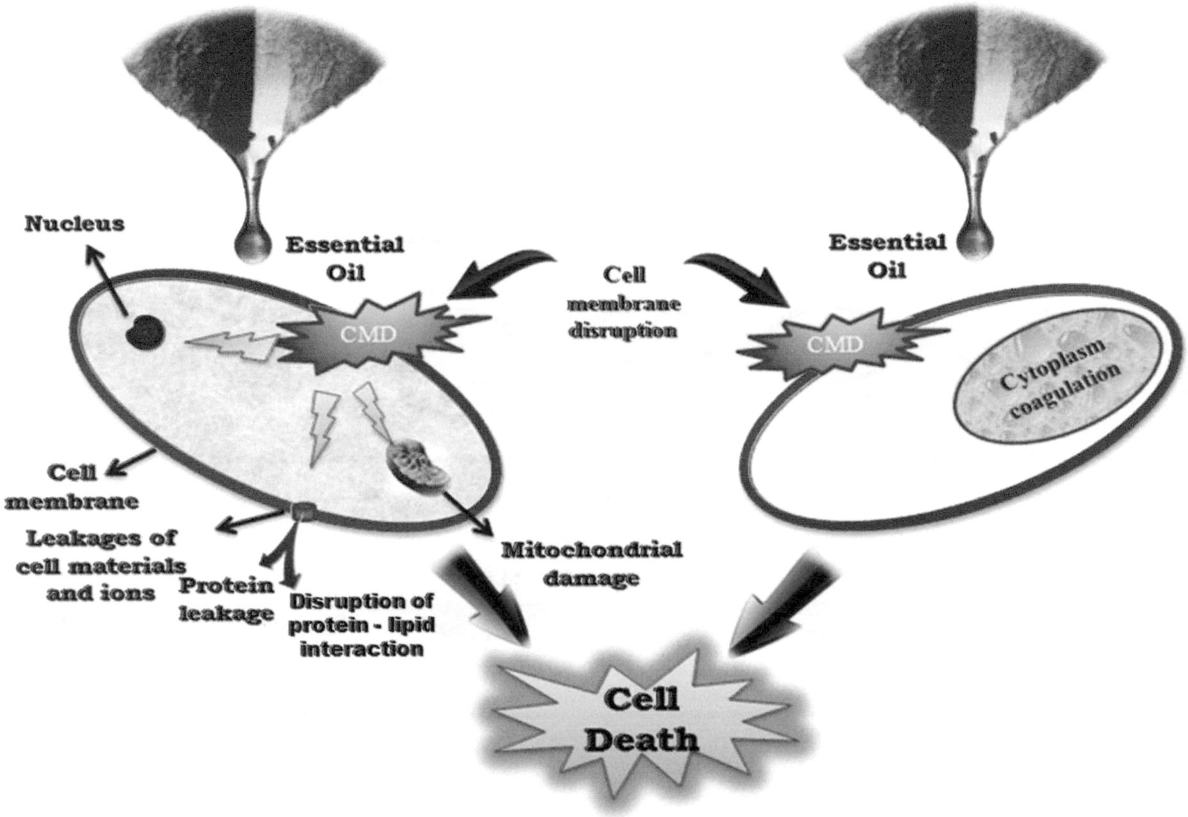

FIGURE 17.4 Diagrammatic representation of the antifungal mode of action of essential oil (EO).

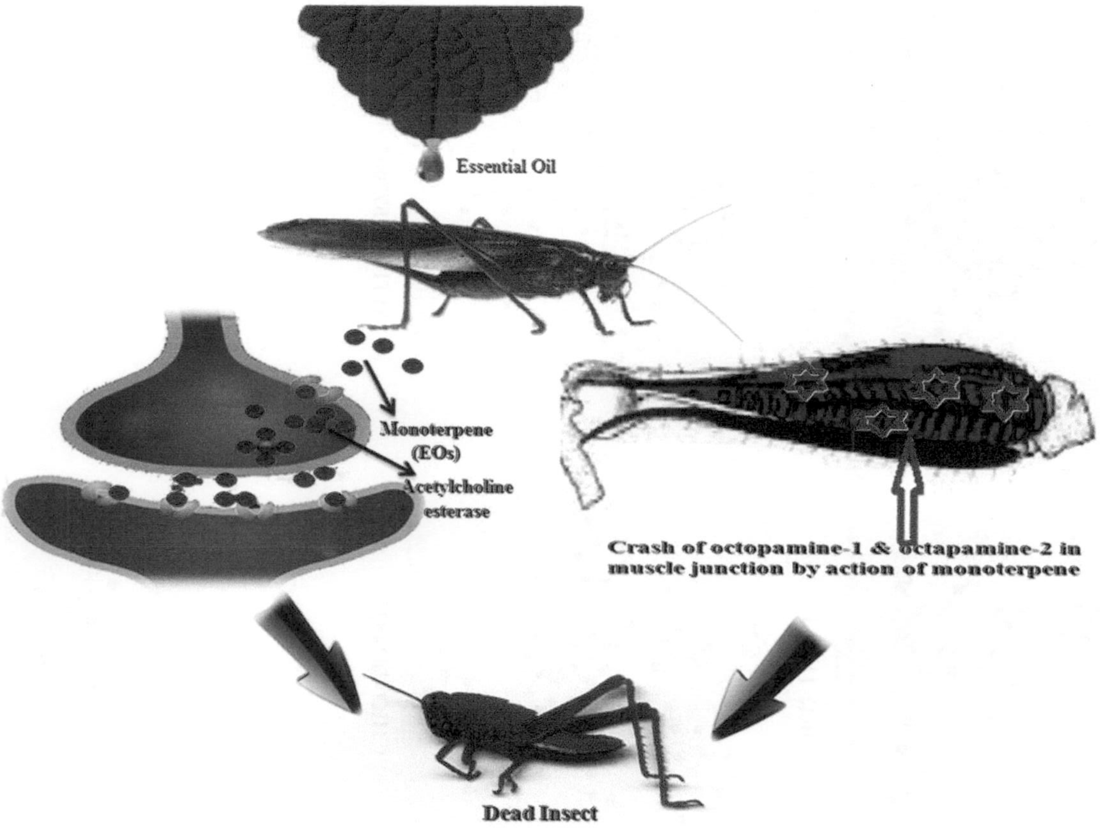

FIGURE 17.5 Target sites in insects as a possible neurotransmitter-mediated toxic action of essential oils.

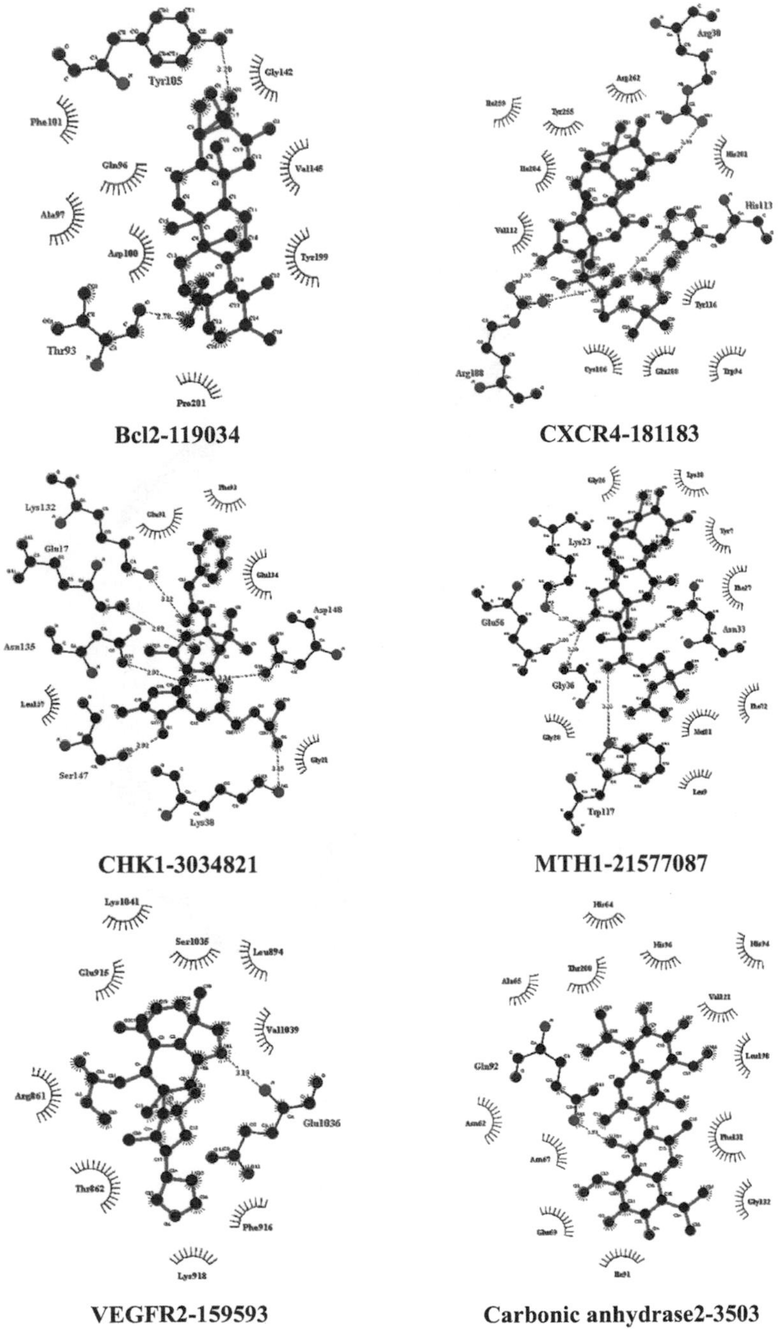

FIGURE 19.12 LigPlot of lead terpenoids with Bcl2, VEGFR2, CXCR4, MTH1, CHK1 and Carbonic anhydrase 2 proteins.

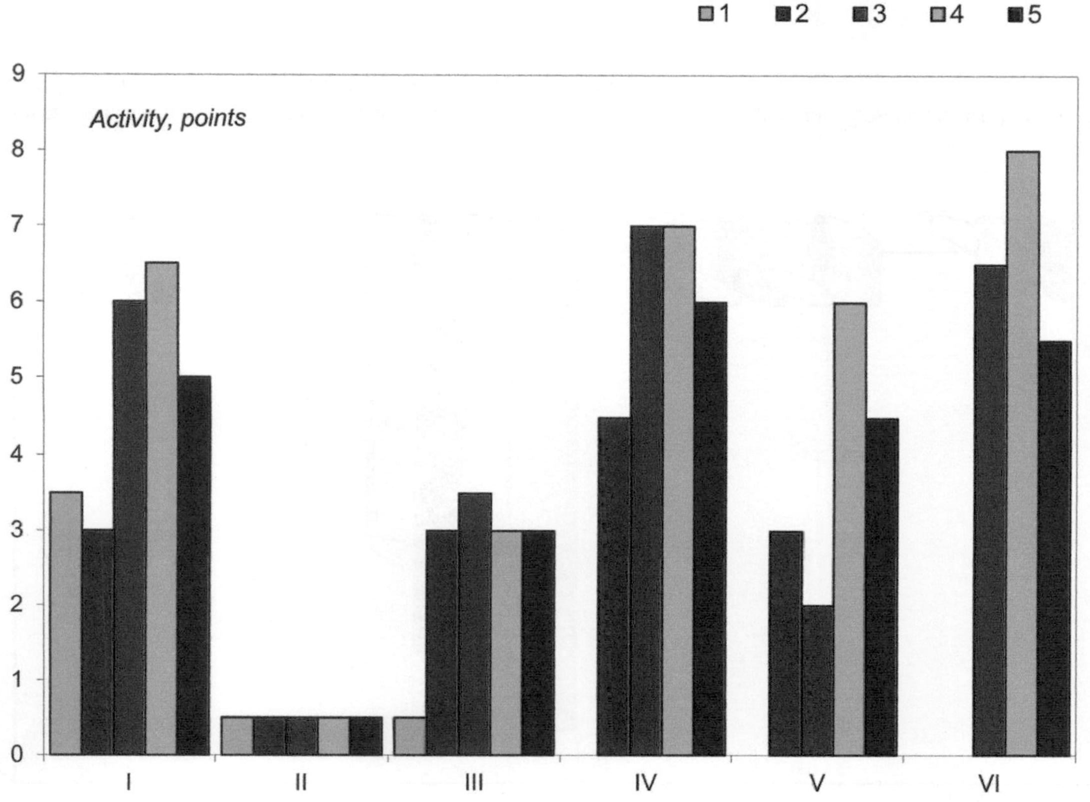

FIGURE 20.5 Dynamics of activity of lectins of *E. purpurea* of the first year of vegetation. I—root system; II—leaf blade; III—leafstalk; IV—stems; V—not blossoming inflorescences; VI—blossoming inflorescences. Sampling time: 1 June; 2 July; 3 August; 4 September; 5 October.

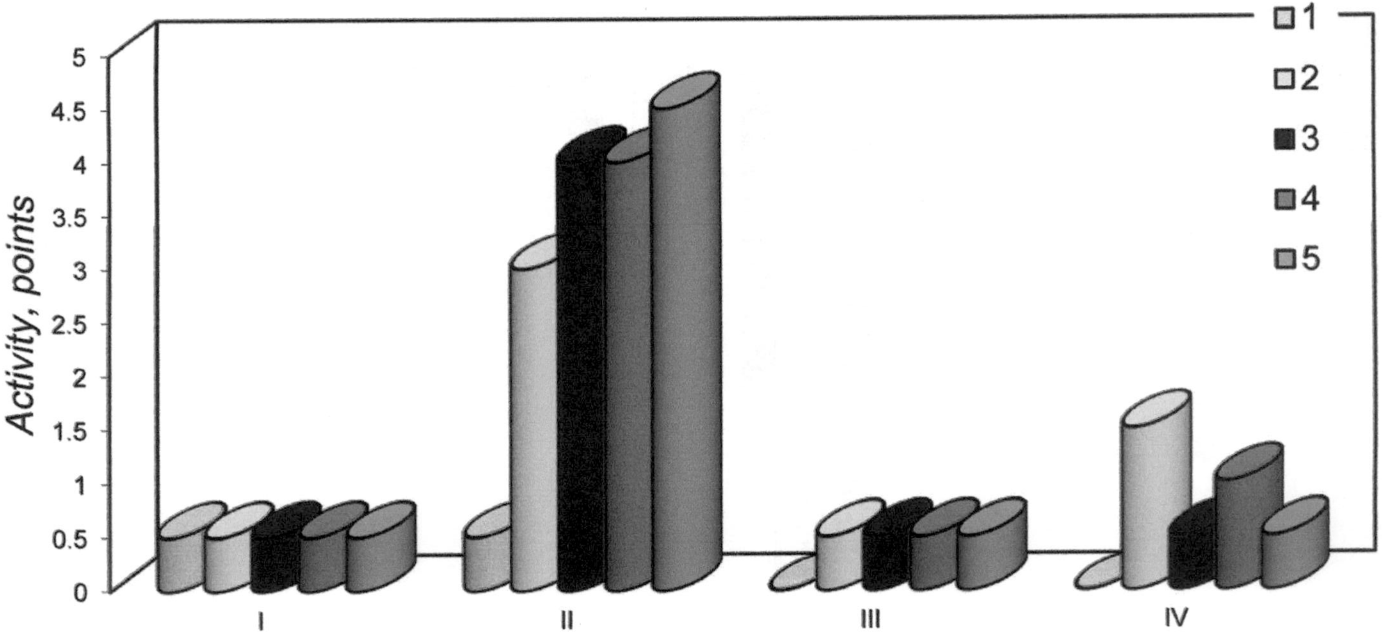

FIGURE 20.6 Dynamics of activity of lectins in leaves of *E. purpurea* of the first year of vegetation. Rosette leaves: I-blade; II-leafstalk; Stem leaves: III- blade; IV-leafstalk. Sampling time: 1-June; 2-July; 3-August; 4-September; 5-October.

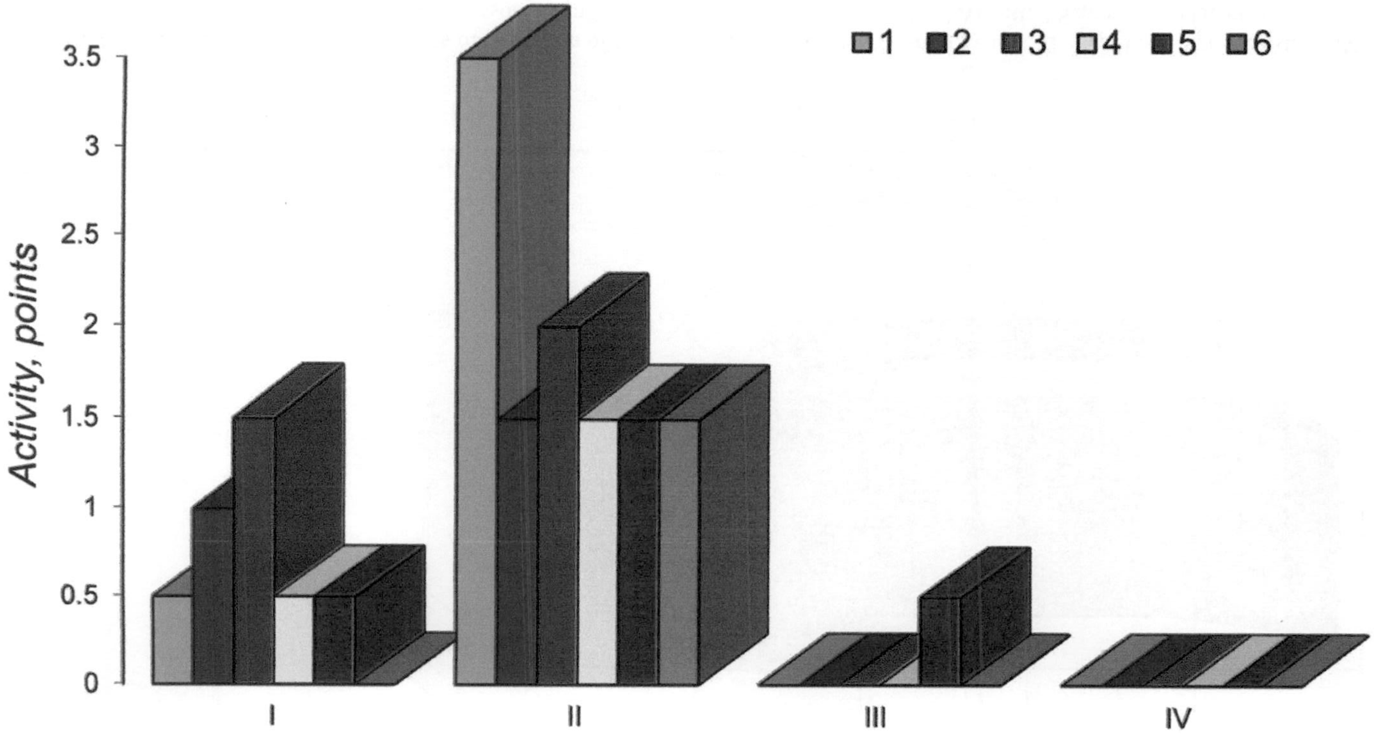

FIGURE 20.8 Dynamics of activity of lectins in leaves of *E. purpurea* of generative period of ontogenesis. Rosette leaves: I—blades; II—stems; Stem leaves: III—blade; IV—leafstalk; Sampling time: 1—renewal of vegetation; 2—regrowth; 3—formation of inflorescences; 4—flowering; 5—fruit formation; 6—ripening of fruits.

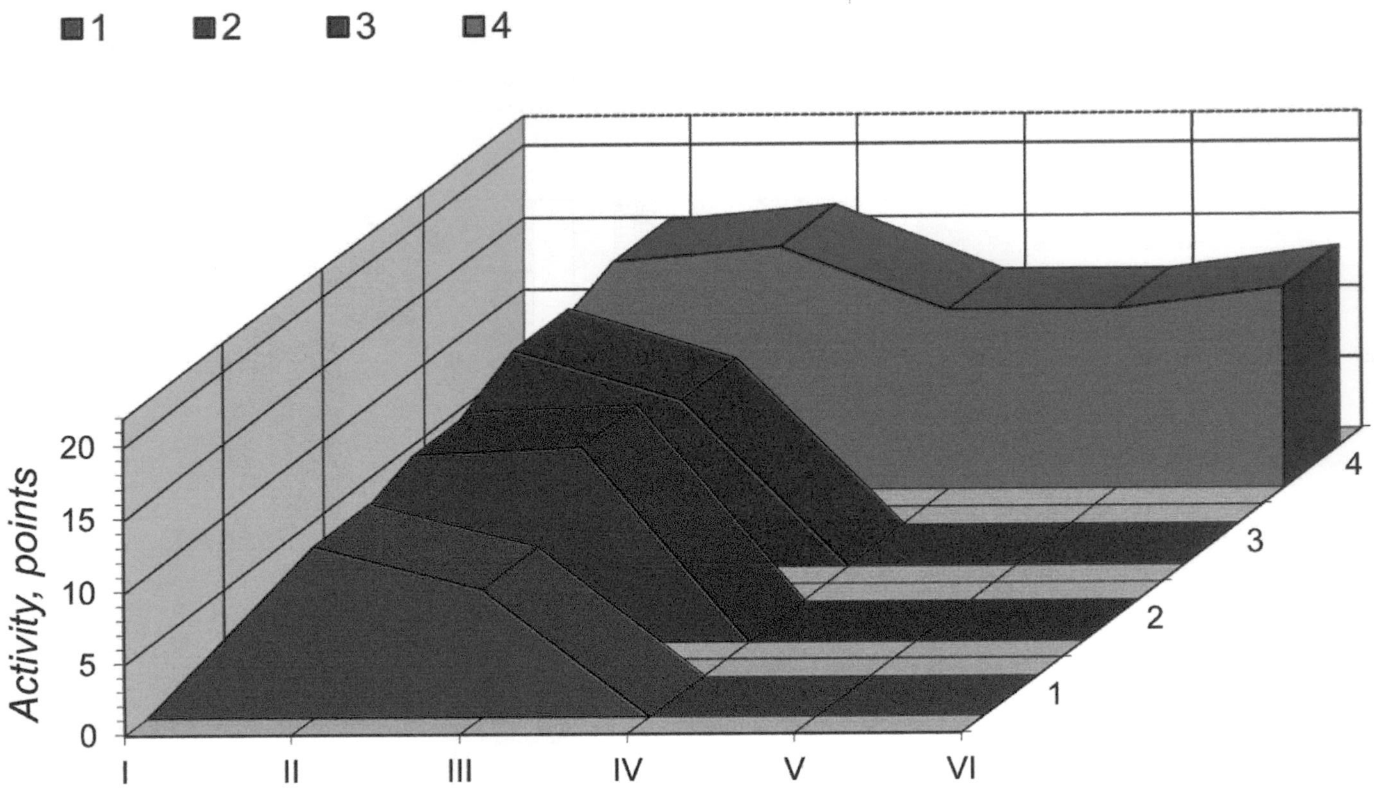

FIGURE 20.9 Dynamics of activity of lectins of *E. pallida* of the first year of vegetation. I—root system; II—leaf blade; III—leafstalk; IV—stems; V—not blossoming inflorescences; VI—blossoming inflorescences. Sampling time: 1 July; 2 August; 3 September; 4 October.

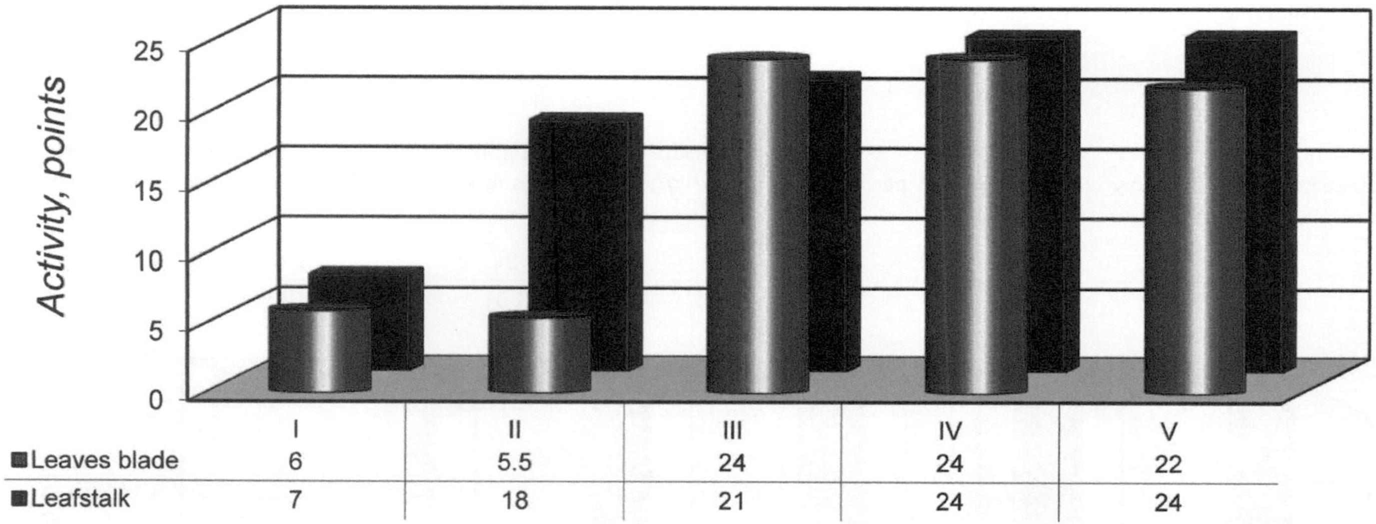

FIGURE 20.10 Dynamics of activity of lectins in rosette leaves of *E. pallida* of the second year of vegetation. Sampling time: I—regrowth; II—formation of inflorescences; III—flowering; IV—fruit formation; V—ripening of fruits.

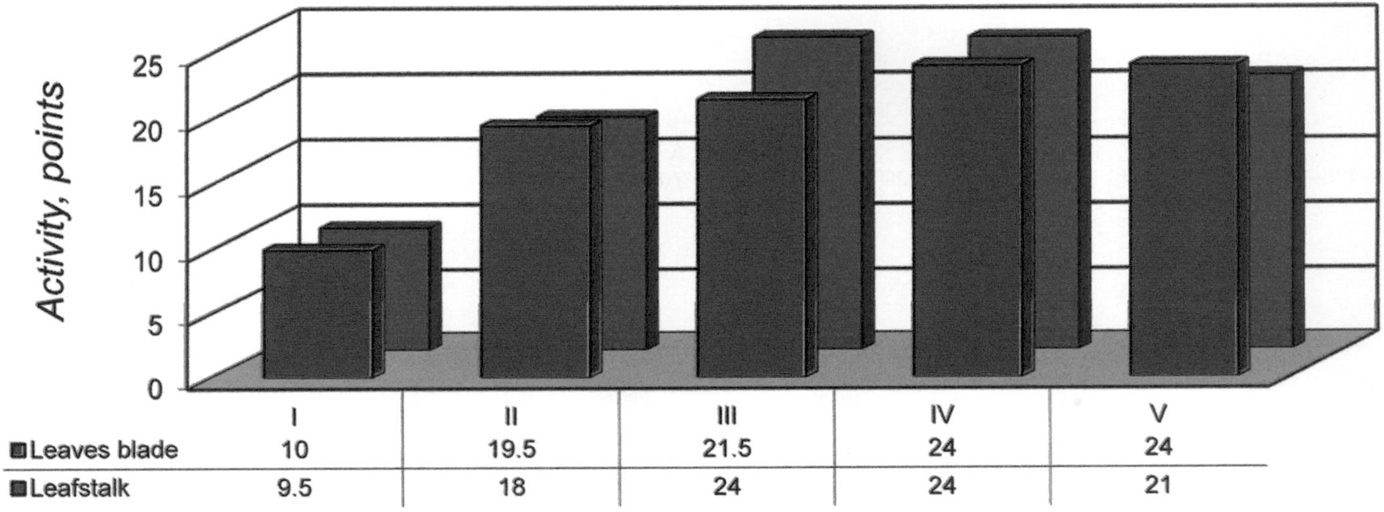

FIGURE 20.11 Dynamics of activity of lectins in stem leaves of *E. pallida* of the second year of vegetation. Sampling time: I–regrowth; II–formation of inflorescences; III–flowering; IV–fruit formation; V–ripening of fruits.

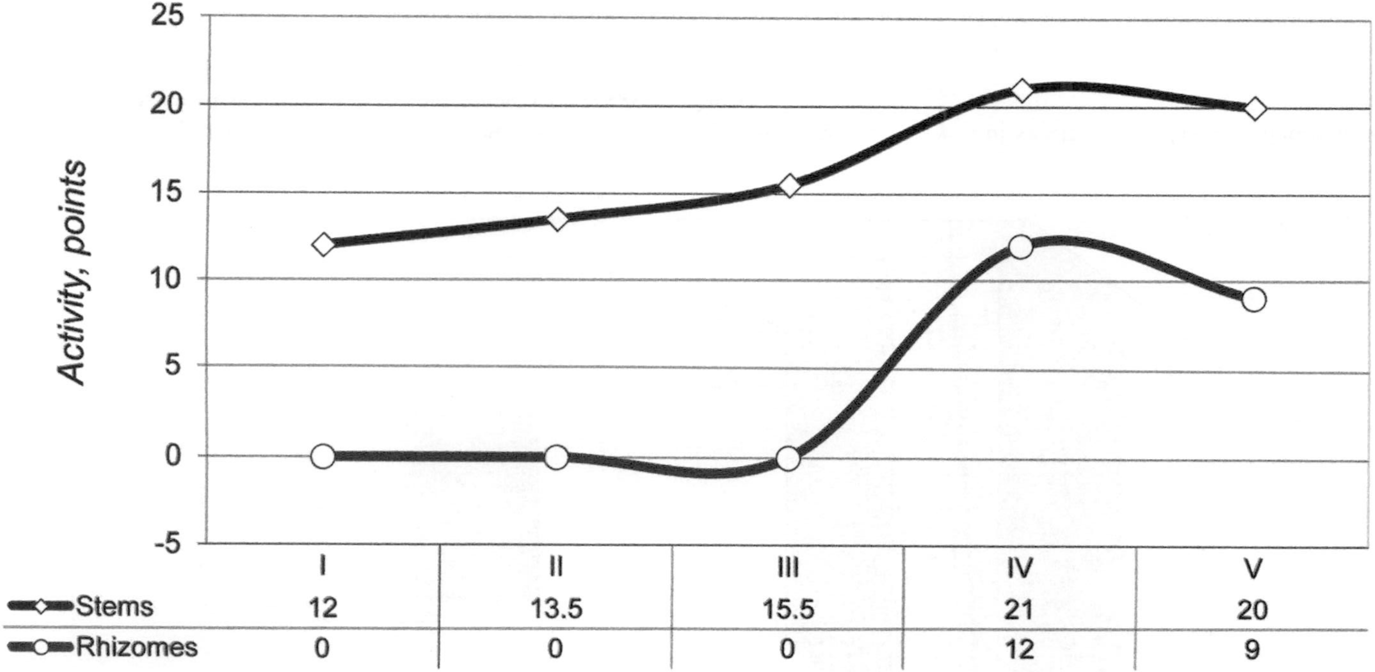

FIGURE 20.12 Dynamics of activity of lectins in stems and rhizomes of *E. pallida* of the second year of vegetation. Sampling time: I—regrowth; II—formation of inflorescences; III—flowering; IV—fruit formation; V—ripening of fruits.

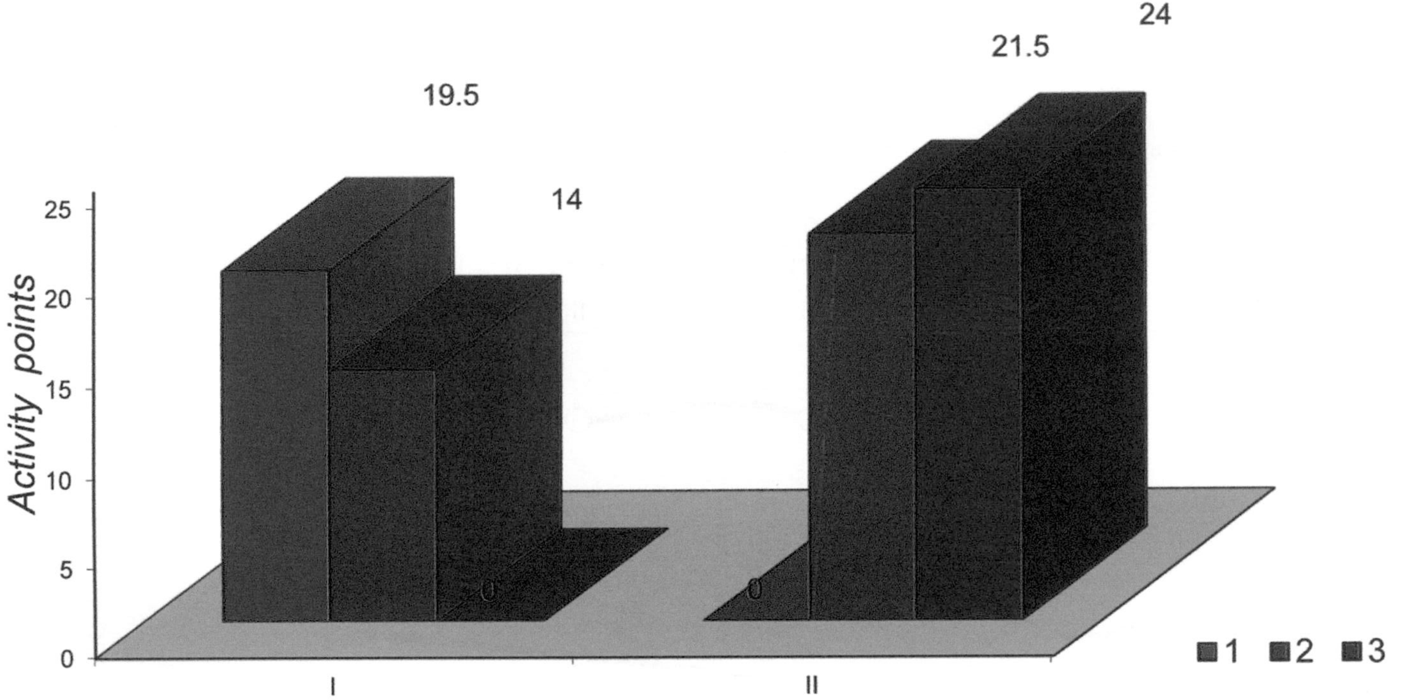

FIGURE 20.13 Dynamics of activity of lectins in inflorescences of *E. pallida* of the second year of vegetation. I—date of inflorescences forming; II—blossoming inflorescences Sampling time: 1 June; 2 July: 3 August.

CHAPTER 10

PHYTOTHERAPY AND ENCAPSULATION

ŞABAN KESKIN[1], MERVE KESKIN[2,*], and SEVGI KOLAYLI[2]

[1]*Department of Chemistry, Faculty of Science and Literature, Bilecik Şeyh Edebali University, Bilecik, Turkey*

[2]*Department of Chemistry, Faculty of Science, Karadeniz Technical University, Trabzon, Turkey, Tel.: +902282141641*

[*]*Corresponding author. E-mail: merveozdemirkeskin@gmail.com*
[*]*ORCID: https://orcid.org/0000-0001-9365-334X*

ABSTRACT

Phytotherapy can be defined as a treatment for preventing from exact complaint or for assistive application to a modern remedy. Encapsulation could be defined as coating a phytochemical with a suitable polymeric material. This technology is widely used in the pharmaceutical industry since the solubility and stability of a phytochemical could be increased by this technology. Controlled release properties of phytochemicals could be improved by this technique as well. Targeting the phytochemicals to the right place in a body is the main scope of encapsulation. Encapsulation also contributes for the phytotherapy practitioners to administer a phytochemical in dose-controlled manner because encapsulation provides a determined composition for a product. Deciding on the method to achieve better encapsulation is principally conditioned by the chemical constituents of the extract and the solvent used for extraction.

The current chapter discusses encapsulation methods used in phytotherapy. The comparison of encapsulation methods by telling its advantageous and disadvantageous sides was also discussed. In the present chapter, one can find the necessity of encapsulation of phytochemical(s) as well.

10.1 INTRODUCTION

Phytotherapy is a treatment either for preventing from exact complaint or for assistive application to a modern remedy (Choubey et al., 2013). Phytotherapeutic applications go back to ancient times. From the beginning of prehistoric age to date, plants or herbs are used as medicines. It was estimated that one million plant species were grown all around the world and only 20,000 of them could be used for phytotherapeutic purposes (Parıldar et al., 2011). In future, the number of plants will be increased with the increase of researches being conducted on plants and herbs.

The usage of whole plant or plant part was the main phytotherapeutic application till the beginning of 19th century. Phytotherapeutic applications have shifted to purify the active compound(s) from the plant with the exploration of extraction techniques and put them into a formulation alone or in combination. Phytotherapeutic compounds such as saponins, polyphenols, flavonoids, volatile oils, and so forth, are not enduring after extraction (Arriola et al., 2016). They may undergo some modification as they are highly susceptible to pH, humidity, oxygen concentration, and light or they may give side reactions with active ingredients put in the formulation together. Encapsulation of these active components could prevent them from these side effects.

As mentioned above, phytochemicals are highly susceptible to environmental condition after extraction, the stability of them could be ensured by encapsulation processes. When encapsulated a phytochemical could maintain its activity for a long time. This increased shelf life makes the capsules potential drug or drug additive. In addition to shelf life increasing, encapsulation also provides a phytotherapist to arrange the concentration of phytochemicals. This is because one can calculate the amount of phytochemical(s) in the capsules after encapsulation process. This makes it easy for the phytotherapy practitioner to estimate and prescribe the amount of daily intake for the patient. Moreover, encapsulation also provides us to target a phytochemical to the right place of the body by the ability of controlled release of the encapsulated compound(s) (Desai and Park, 2005; Nedovic et al., 2011). Encapsulation can also be used to mask any off-flavors of a phytochemical (Stojanovic et al., 2012; McClements, 2015).

10.2 ENCAPSULATION AS BIOTECHNOLOGICAL TOOL

Encapsulation, an immobilization technique, is the packaging of solid, liquid, or gaseous components such as phytochemicals, enzymes, cells, and other substances with a protein, lipid, or carbohydrate-based coating material. Macro, micro, or nanoscale capsules could be obtained, depending on the technique used and process conditions. The material in the capsule is expressed as core, internal phase, or filler. However, the wall can sometimes be a shell, a coating, or a membrane. The core could be a crystal, rough absorbent particle, emulsion, suspension, or suspension of smaller capsules (Gökmen et al., 2012)

Encapsulation has many underground practices in the fields of pharmacy, veterinary, biotechnology, food industry, chemical, agriculture, feed, and medicine. The selection of encapsulation method, an encapsulant or wall material mainly relies on the properties of phytochemicals. By the help of current knowledge and technology, varied size of particles can be obtained based on the various properties of the core, wall material, and encapsulation technique (Gharsallaoui et al., 2007). The morphology of capsules can be described as mononuclear, poly/multinuclear, matrix, multiwall, and irregular. Figure 10.1 represents the morphology of capsules (Peanparkdee et al., 2016).

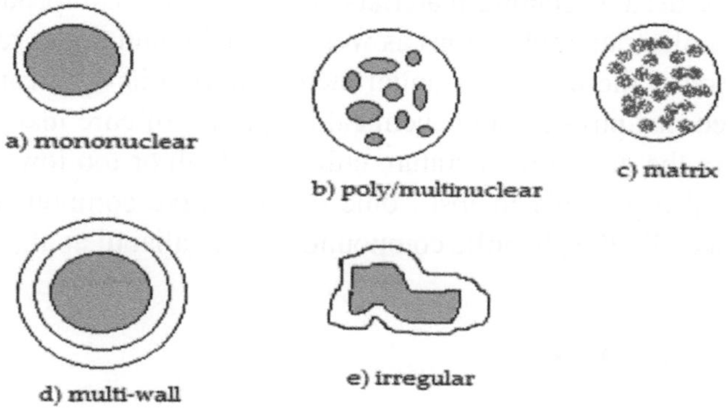

FIGURE 10.1 Representation of the morphology of capsules.

Source: Adapted from Peanparkdee et al. (2016). Open Access. http://www.agrsci.jp/ras/article/view/23/48

10.3 ENCAPSULATION TECHNIQUES

Choosing of encapsulation technique mainly depends on the physical and chemical properties of the core material. There are three classes of encapsulation techniques, namely as chemical, physical, and physicochemical methods (Jyothi et al., 2010). Chemical methods cover in situ polymerization and liposomes; physical methods range from spray-drying to fluidized bed coating and physicochemical methods include coacervation and solgel encapsulation (Gibbs, 1999; Gouin, 2004). The capsules produced by using these methods separately have different properties and application field (Fang and Bhandari, 2010).

10.3.1 SPRAY-DRYING METHOD

Spray-drying is an encapsulation method which requires the homogenization of core material (phytochemical) into an aqueous solution of encapsulating agent. The homogenate is then converted to a powder form by heating and spraying. Out of the spray nozzle, the solvent (water) is quickly evaporated and powder capsules are formed. Obtained capsules are highly enduring to chemical or microbial deterioration as a result of a reduced amount of water. This is one of the advantageous properties of spray-drying method. Reduction of water amount in the capsules also contributes to lower storage and transportation costs. Hydrocolloids such as gelatin, modified starch, or dextrin are used as coating materials. The technique is reproducible and suitable for industrial applications as well. The inlet and outlet temperature in this method is the most substantial factor limiting its application. It has been reported that physical and chemical properties of core material can be effected from the drying temperature either too high or too low (Tan et al., 2015). It is also possible to lose some of the active components of core material especially the phenolic compounds (Gharsallaoui et al., 2007).

10.3.2 LIPOSOMES

Liposomes are formed by using nontoxic phospholipids and cholesterol. The spherically shaped capsules can carry hydrophobic and hydrophilic molecules. Physicochemical properties like surface charge and size of a liposome are mainly derived from lipid composition used for the production. Liposomes are generally used in the pharmaceutical and food industries for entrapment of an aqueous solution within a phospholipid bilayer. Liposomes are microscopic pockets formed by phospholipid bilayers surrounding aqueous compartments. Liposomal entrapment can protect phytochemicals from environmental and chemical stresses, including the presence of enzymes or reactive chemicals and exposure to extreme pH, temperature, and high ion concentrations (Gouin, 2004).

10.3.3 COACERVATION/PHASE SEPARATION METHOD

Simple coacervation is the process that occurs when a hydrophilic polymer is put into two phases. In this method, a polymer rich phase and dilute liquid phase are formed. Coacervation can be induced by various means like a change in temperature, pH, and electrolyte balance of the system or addition of non-solvent. Complex coacervation is the complexation reaction. Two different polymers oppositely ionized or crosslinking agents like glutaraldehyde should be used for complex coacervation. Once the coacervation process is completed, phase separation could be carried out by using one of the separation techniques such as filtration or centrifugation. Then the separated particles are washed and dried (Schmitt et al., 1998).

10.3.4 SOLGEL ENCAPSULATION

Solgel chemistry started with the hydrolysis and condensation of metal alkoxides. The solgel encapsulation technique can occur in two steps. First is the generation of a sol by the hydrolysis of alkoxides. The second step is the synthesis of a gel through polycondensation to create metal-oxo-metal or metal-hydroxy-metal bonds. Phytochemicals can be encapsulated by using the solgel technique. Relatively mild process conditions like temperature and pH make this method advantageous. The temperature required for the process is often close to room temperature. So this method minimizes the thermal degradation of phytochemicals. The controllable particle formation in concern with particle and pore size also makes this method valuable (Flora and Brennan, 2001; Gupta and Chaudhury, 2007).

10.3.5 FREEZE-DRYING METHOD

Freeze drying takes place in three stages; freezing, basic drying phase, and second drying step. The first step is to freeze the mixture of phytochemical and shell material. The second step is the sublimation of ice known as lyophilization, under vacuum. Finally, bound water is removed by evaporation under reduced pressure. In some situation preheating could be required to obtain a uniform mixture of shell and core material depending on the solubility of shell matrix. Although this processing has some benefits like decreased heat deterioration, controllable water content of end product but high operation cost, longer process time, and requiring a freeze dryer makes the method inapplicable for industrial scale.

10.3.6 EXTRUSION-EMULSION METHOD

Extrusion technique is the oldest and most universal method used in making capsules with hydrocolloids. In this method, alginate is the most used hydrocolloid. Encapsulation is performed in two steps by using extrusion process. The first step is the preparation of hydrocolloid solution in concentration range 0.6–2%. In this step phytochemical(s) should be homogenized into hydrocolloid solution. The second step is the addition of the homogenate to a divalent cation solution mostly Ca^{2+} solution in concentration range 0.005–1.5 M. Addition of the homogenate into hardening solution can be performed by passing it through the syringe needle. The shape and the size of obtained capsules mainly depend on the alginate solution viscosity and divalent cation concentration as well as the margin between the droplet and hardening solutions. Being a simple and cheap method, it is also advantageous as there is no damage to phytochemicals, and it does not require deleterious solvent. The difficulty of large-scale application, large size distribution, and limited choice of wall material are the disadvantages of this method (Koç et al., 2010).

In the emulsion technique, a small volume of phytochemical(s)/polymer slurry (dispersed phase) is added into a large volume of vegetable oil (continuous phase) like soy, sunflower, corn, and light paraffin oil. Emulsions could be obtained by two strategies, namely water in oil (W/O) or oil in water (O/W). After obtaining an emulsion, cross-linking should be carried out to form gels. Gelling can be obtained by different mechanisms such as ionic, enzymatic, and interfacial polymerization. This process can easily be scaled up and obtained beads are considerably smaller ranging from 25 μm to 2 mm. The cost of this method is a bit high due to the usage of vegetable oils, surfactant, and emulsifier (tween 80) (Krasaekoopt et al., 2003).

10.3.7 CO-CRYSTALLIZATION

Co-crystallization is an application of sucrose as a matrix surrounding the phytochemicals. Nanosucrose between 3 and 30 μm during dragging of materials between or within sucrose crystals is a spontaneous crystallization of varying microcrystalline clusters. The amount of saturated sucrose syrup is mixed with the preset core material. The encapsulated material is then transferred from the container, emptied and dried to the proper moisture content. The core material is primarily comprised of crystals formed among the cracks (Barbosa-Canovas et al., 2005).

10.4 COATING MATERIALS

The composition of the coating material specifies the final product functional properties. So an ideal coating material has the following properties (Bansode et al., 2010);

- Good rheological properties at high concentration and easy to encapsulate.
- It should be an emulsion and dispersing property and the emulsion stability must also be high.
- During the coating process with the core material and during storage, it should not react in such a way as to disrupt the core material.
- It should be able to coat the core material in a stable manner both during the processing and storage.
- Must be soluble in the desired solvent.
- It must be cheap.

10.5 APPLICATION FIELDS OF ENCAPSULATION

Encapsulation technology is a widely used in several industries, especially food and pharmaceutical industries since it can increase solubility, enhance stability, and improve the controlled release properties of compounds such as essential oils, antioxidants, enzymes, drugs, and so forth. Therefore, this section focuses on the applications of encapsulation in these industries. Table 10.1 represents the industrial applications of encapsulation.

As mentioned before, phytotherapy could be used either for preventing of exact illness or for assistive application to a modern remedy. In modern therapy, doctors have the consensus on the usage of phytochemicals in a dose-controlled manner. That is why scientists are searching for both the active compound(s) of medicinal plants and better extraction methods for them. After the extraction, the concentration of phytochemical(s) can be determined sensitively by using advanced analytical techniques like HPLC, LC-MS, and GC-MS, and so forth. Although it is possible to determine the concentration of phytochemical in extracts, still there are some limitation factors like solvent of the extract for prescribing them to a patient. Encapsulation of phytochemical(s) from the extract is a biotechnological way to solve this problem. At the end of this chapter, some examples of phytochemical encapsulation are given.

TABLE 10.1 Some Industrial Applications of Encapsulation.

Pharmaceutical industry	Food industry	Other industries
Specific drug delivery	Functional foods	Textile industries
Oral drug delivery	Probiotics	Fragrance finishing
Transdermal drug delivery	Antioxidants	Color change materials
Stomach-specific drug delivery	Vitamins	Fire retardants
Colon-specific drug delivery	Dietary fiber	
Small intestine-specific drug delivery	Food preservatives	Cosmetic industries
Bitter taste masking	Food colorants	Essential oils
	Food flavor	Polyphenolic compounds

Source: Adapted from Peanparkdee, et al. (2016). Open Acess. http://www.agrsci.jp/ras/article/view/23/48

Bidens pilosa L. is a South American medicinal plant with proved antimalaric, hepatoprotective, and antioxidant activities, generally linked to their secondary metabolites, flavonoids, and polyacetylenes. Increasing the stability of its phytochemicals, extract of *B. pilosa* was encapsulated by using spray-drying method. Obtained capsules were evaluated as stable for three different stress storage conditions both in open containers and in sealed sachets (Cortés-Rojas et al., 2016). Although it is not common sense to introduce phytochemicals to the body by injection since the complex nature of phytochemicals but an injectable nanoparticulate system was achieved. mPEG–PLGA–mPEG (PELGE) platform was reported to be used for the preparation of nanoparticles. Sustained release of co-encapsulated four active components of Ginkgo biloba extract was managed by Han et al. (2012). It was stated that the bitter melon (*Momordica charantia* L.) is a medicinal fruit mostly used for the handling of diabetes, due to its content of saponins, phenolics, and flavonoids and its antioxidant capacity. As mentioned before, extracted phytochemicals are highly susceptible to the environmental conditions. That is why encapsulation is a highly practical tool in order to improve the shelf life of phytochemicals extracted from the bitter melon. Tan et al. reported that water extract of bitter melon was encapsulated by a spray-drying method by using maltodextrin and gum arabic as an encapsulating agent. Improved shelf life and better handling were reported as well (Tan et al., 2015).

It was known that herbal essential oils such as *Cuminum cyminum*, are natural antifungal agents consisting of many different volatile compounds. In a study, ıt was reported that encapsulation by chitosan (CS)–caffeic acid (CA) system was used to improve antimicrobial activity and stability of the *C. cyminum* essential oils against *Aspergillus flavus*. An encapsulation efficiency of 85% was reported to be achieved. As revealed through the release kinetics studies, 78% of the encapsulated oils were released in 1 week. Reported results imply that because the oils are volatile and unstable due to the environmental factors, capsulated oils significantly showed better performance. A decreased minimum inhibitory concentration of encapsulated oils against *A. flavus* is the evidence of better performance of encapsulated oils (Zhaveh et al., 2015).

10.5.1 ENHANCING BIOAVAILABILITY OF PHYTOCHEMICALS

Bioavailability could be described as the amount of interested compound(s) that achieve the bloodstream after oral administration in its native form. Recently, the numbers of studies on phytochemicals have been growing around the world since their therapeutic effects and relatively smaller side effects as compared to the synthetic drugs. However, many phytochemicals in herbal extracts in spite of their efficacious in vitro activity exhibit poor or negligible in vivo activity since their poor bioavailability. This could be due to the low concentration of phytochemical(s) in the extract, the most often in microgram quantities in a liter of solution resulting in poor absorption. Weak lipid solubility of most phytochemicals could also contribute to their poor bioavailability. It is known that a small portion of phytochemical(s) administered orally can pass the membrane barrier in gastrointestinal (GI) as unaltered because of insufficient residence time, low permeability, and/or low solubility. The presence of a deforming agent in the GI tract (pH, enzymes, the presence of other nutrients, and so forth.), limits the activity and the potential health benefits of phytochemicals.

As stated before, encapsulation could protect the core material (phytochemicals) through GI track from the deforming agents. Encapsulation also provides an increased concentration for the core material. The concentration of phytochemicals in capsules could be hundred or thousand times more than its counter extract solution. By choosing the suitable encapsulant and encapsulation techniques it is possible to encapsulate a phytochemical to increase its bioavailability. It could be achieved by the ability of controlled release property of a capsule. For instance, alginate capsules pass through the stomach without any deformation, they release the core material in intestine since they are completely destroyed (Kang et al., 2009; Gupta and Kesarwani, 2013; Muttepawar et al., 2014).

KEYWORDS

- **encapsulation**
- **phytotherapy**
- **phytochemicals**
- **extrusion**
- **liposomes**

REFERENCES

Arriola, A. N.; Mattos de Medeiros, P.; Prudencio, E. S.; Müller, C. M. O.; Amboni, R. D. C. Encapsulation of Aqueous Leaf Extract of Stevia Rebaudiana Bertoni with Sodium Alginate and its Impact on Phenolic Content. *Food Bioscience*, **2016,** *13,* 32–40.

Bansode, S. S.; Banarjee, S. K.; Gaikwad, D. D.; Jadhav, S. L.; Thorat, R. M. Microencapsulation: A Review. *Int. J. Pharm. Sci. Rev. Res.* **2010,** *1*(2), 38–43.

Barbosa-Canovas, G. V.; Ortega-Rivas, E.; Juliano, P.; Yan, H. *Food Powders: Physical Properties, Processing and Functionality;* Kluwer Academic: New York, 2005; 199–219.

Choubey, J.; Patel, A.; Verma, M. K. Phytotherapy in the Treatment of Arthritis: A Review. *Int. J. Pharm. Sci. Res.* **2013,** *4*(8), 2853–2865.

Cortés-Rojas, D. F.; Souza, C. R. F.; Oliveira, W. P. Assessment of Stability of a Spray Dried Extract from the Medicinal Plant *Bidens pilosa* L. *J. King Saud Univ. Eng. Sci.* **2016,** *28,* 141–146.

Desai, K. G. H.; Park, H. J. Recent Developments in Microencapsulation of Food Ingredients. *Drying Technol.* **2005,** *23*(7), 1361–1394.

Fang, Z.; Bhandari, B. Encapsulation of Polyphenols—A Review. *Trends Food Sci. Technol.* **2010,** *21,* 510–523.

Flora, K. K.; Brennan, J. D. Effect of Matrix Aging on the Behavior of Human Serum Albumin Entrapped in a Tetraethyl Orthosilicate-Derived Glass. *Chem. Mater.* **2001,** *13,* 4170–4179.

Gharsallaoui, A.; Roudaut, G.; Chambin, O.; Voilley, A.; Saurel, R. Applications of Spray-Drying in Micro-Encapsulation of Food Ingredients: An Overview. *Food Res Int.*, **2007,** *40,* 1107–1121.

Gibbs, B. F.; Kermasha, S.; Alli, I.; Mulligan, C. N. Encapsulation in the Food Industry: A Review. *Int. J. Food Sci. Nutr.* **1999,** *50,* 213–224.

Gökmen, S.; Palamutoğlu, R.; Sarıçoban, C. Gıda Endüstrisinde Enkapsülasyon Uygulamaları. *Gıda Teknolojileri Elektron. Derg.* **2012,** *7*(1), 36–50.

Gouin, S. Microencapsulation: Industrial Appraisal of Existing Technologies and Trends. *Trends Food Sci. Technol.* **2004,** *15,* 330–347.

Gupta, R.; Chaudhury, N. K. Entrapment of Biomolecules in Solgel Matrix for Applications in Biosensors: Problems and Future Prospects. *Biosens. Bioelectron.* **2007,** *22,* 2387–2399.

Gupta, R.; Kesarwani, K. Bioavailability Enhancers of Herbal Origin: An Overview. *Asian Pac. J. Trop. Biomed.* **2013,** *3*(4), 253–266.

Han, L.; Fu, Y.; Cole, A. J.; Liu, J.; Wang, J. Co-encapsulation and Sustained-Release of Four Components in Ginkgo Terpenes from Injectable PELGE Nanoparticles. *Fitoterapia* **2012,** *83,* 721–731.

Jyothi, N. V. N.; Prasanna, P. M.; Sakarkar, S. N.; Prabha, K. S.; Ramaiah, P. S.; Srawan, G. Microencapsulation Techniques, Factors Influencing Encapsulation Efficiency. *J. Microencapsulation* **2010,** *27,* 187–197.

Kang, M. J.; Cho, Y. J.; Shim, B. H.; Kim, D. K.; Lee, J. Bioavailability Enhancing Activities of Natural Compounds from Medicinal Plants. *J. Med. Plants Res.* **2009,** *3*(13), 1204–1211.

Koç, M.; Sakin, M.; Kaymak-Ertekin, F. Microencapsulation and its Applications in Food Technology. *Pamukkale Üniv. Mühendislik Bilimleri Derg.* **2010,** *16*(1), 77–86.

Krasaekoopt, W.; Bhandari, B.; Deeth, H. Evaluation of Encapsulation Techniques of Probiotics for Yoghurt: A Review. *Int. Dairy J.* **2003,** *13*(1), 3–23.McClements, D. J. Encapsulation, Protection, and Release of Hydrophilic Active Components: Potential and Limitations of Colloidal Delivery Systems. *Adv. Colloid Interface Sci.* **2015,** *219,* 27–53.

Muttepawar, S. S.; Jadhav S. B.; Kankudate, A. D.; Sanghai, S. D.; Usturge, D. R.; Chavare, S. S. A Review on Bioavailability Enhancers of Herbal Origin. *World J. Pharm. Pharm. Sci.* **2014,** *3*(3), 667–677.

Nedovic,V.; Kalusevic, A.; Manojlovic, V.; Levic, S.; Bugarski, B. An Overview of Encapsulation Technologies for Food Applications. *Procedia Food Sci.* **2011,** *1,* 1806–1815.

Parıldar, H.; Ciğerli, Ö.; Kut, A.; Yeşilada, E. Medicinal Herbs in Clinical Practice: How to Prevent Adverse Effects. *Turk. J. Family Med. Primary Care* **2011,** *5,* 9–14.

Peanparkdee, M.; Iwamotoa, S.; Yamauchia, R. Microencapsulation: A Review of Applications in the Food and Pharmaceutical Industries. *Rev. Agric. Sci.* **2016,** *4,* 56–65.

Schmitt, C.; Sanchez, C.; Desobry-Banon, S.; Hardy, J. Structure and Technofunctional Properties of Protein-Polysaccharide Complexes: A Review. *Crit. Rev. Food Sci. Nutr.* **1998,** *38,* 689–753.

Stojanovic, R.; Belscak-Cvitanovic, A.; Manojlovic, V.; Komes, D.; Nedovic, V.; Bugarski, B. Encapsulation of Thyme (Thymus serpyllum L.) Aqueous Extract in Calcium Alginate Beads. *J. Sci. Food Agric.* **2012,** *92,* 685–696.

Tan, S. P.; Kha, T. C.; Parks, S. E.; Stathopoulos, C. E.; Roach, P. D. Effects of the Spray-Drying Temperatures on the Physiochemical Properties of an Encapsulated Bitter Melon Aqueous Extract Powder. *Powder Technol.* **2015,** *281,* 65–75.

Zhaveh, S.; Mohsenifar, A.; Beiki, M.; Khalili, S. T.; Abdollahi, A.; Rahmani-Cherati, T.; Tabatabaei, M. Encapsulation of *Cuminum cyminum* Essential Oils in Chitosan-Caffeic Acid Nanogel with Enhanced Antimicrobial Activity Against *Aspergillus flavus*. *Ind. Crops Prod.* **2015,** *69,* 251–256.

CHAPTER 11

EFFECTIVE PROCESSING METHODS FOR FRUITS AND VEGETABLES

MARIA ASLAM*, SIDRA KHALID*, and HAFSA KAMRAN

University Institute of Diet and Nutritional Sciences, Faculty of Allied Health Sciences, University of Lahore, Pakistan

**Corresponding author. E-mail: mnarz.aslam@gmail.com; sidrakhalid.uaf@gmail.com*
ORCID: https://orcid.org/0000-0002-5681-4260

ABSTRACT

Fruits and vegetables are rich sources of antioxidants namely vitamin C, carotenoids, and phenolic compounds; which have health-protective effects. Diet rich in fruits and vegetables pose low risk of degenerative diseases such as atherosclerosis, diabetes, cancers and neural disorders through the minimization of the risk of oxidative stress. Food processing has effects on fruits and vegetables from harvest, transport, and to storage in ways that can lead to adversarial variations in the physiological status. Moreover, the health-endorsing content of fruit and vegetables depends on their processing history. Vitamin C and polyphenols are more vulnerable to lose during processing and these health-promoting phytochemicals including antioxidants in fruits and vegetables should be well-preserved during storage and handling.

11.1 INTRODUCTION

Some food, especially fruits and vegetables, deteriorate as a result of physiological aging, metabolic alterations, increased respiration rate, and high production of ethylene gas. These aspects contribute to depigmentation, loss of firmness, development of off flavors, acidification, and microbial spoilage significantly. Simultaneously, food processors are using emerging approaches to process perishable commodities, along with enhanced nutritional and sensorial quality (Pasha et al., 2014). Phytochemicals are bioactive non-nutrient plant compounds present in numerous fruits, vegetables, grains, and other plant foods (Dembinska-Kiec et al., 2008). Most common fruits and vegetables including berry crops, many tree fruit crops, and onions are plentiful in phenolic antioxidants. In Western European diet, apples, onions, and tea make available the greatest of antioxidants flavonoids by giving benefits to their content and their rate of consumption. A number of studies have shown that in fully ripe fruits, pH and colored antioxidants (e.g., carotenoids and anthocyanins) often reach their highest level. Some methods such as freezing, cutting, drying, tempering, bleaching, sterilization, and extraction have been used in the food industries. The benefits of using ultrasound for food processing, includes more actual mixing and micromixing, high energy and mass transfer, lessened thermal and concentration gradients, decreased temperature, selective extraction, minimized apparatus size, quicker reaction to extraction control process, quick start up, improved production, and exclusion of process steps (Chemat and Khan, 2011). Fruits and vegetables are collected, shifted, and stored in ways that can carry out physiological stresses that lead to adverse changes in their optical quality and other chemical outlines. By using an effective method of processing, fruits and vegetable shelf life can be increased. Steps included in processing are raw material planning, cleaning, trimming, and peeling, and later cooking, canning, or freezing.

It is known that lower risks of several degenerative diseases are linked to a diet rich in fruit and vegetables. These outcomes have formed a new viewpoint relating to the potential of diet in preventing serious ailments in the future. Moreover, the health-endorsing content of fruit and vegetables severely depends on their processing history. Processing is predictable to affect activity and bioavailability of bioactive compounds (Nicoli et al., 1999). Antioxidants functions in human nutrition have increased interest, especially due to their link with health-positive effects for a number of chronic diseases, which include cardiovascular diseases and certain types of cancer. Fruits and vegetables are perishable and hard to preserve as fresh products. Dried fruits and vegetables can be simply stored, shifted at comparatively lowest cost, have cheap packing costs, and their low water content delays microbial spoilage. Drying methods using air, freezer, microwave, and solar energy are the most systematically studied among drying methods (Kamiloglu et al., 2016). Besides increasing the usefulness and accessibility of processed groceries, handling is also aimed at optimizing nutrient accessibility and to maintain product quality along with the decline of losses and wastes of products. It should be concluded that the value of the final products is directly linked to the processing operations and conditions and remarkably differ from natural non-processed commodities. Among possible effects of processing on the whole quality of fruit and vegetable products, the most important are naturally occurring components, development of original constituents with an increased antioxidative potential or prooxidant activity and connections between different compounds (Figiel and Michalska, 2016).

11.2 PROCESSING METHODS FOR FRUITS AND VEGETABLES

11.2.1 HIGH-PRESSURE PROCESSING

To increase shelf life of the product, high-pressure processing technique is used, that ranges from 100 to 900 MPa to inactivate microorganisms. The pressure is applied by two mechanisms (1) direct pressure (2) indirect pressure. In both cases pressure is maintained, which are extracted from product size and geometry, hence, decreases the adverse effect on texture, tissue rupture, and other quality parameters of the products (Table 11.1). The technique is skillful of preserving flavor, color pigments nutrient, and antioxidant content (Tewari et al., 2017); however, availability of carotenoids in different types of vegetables were found slightly altered (McInerney et al., 2007).

11.2.2 POWER ULTRASOUND TECHNIQUE

The use of power ultrasound to aid the freezing of fruits and vegetables is a comparatively new concept. Cavitation and a sponge effect produced by sound waves, affect the freezing rate and qualities of the frozen products. The practice of using ultrasound in the freezing process aids to eliminate enzymes and microbes and improves the ice crystal nucleation process (Table 11.1). High freezing rate, quicker crystallization, uniform distribution of ice crystals, better microstructure, and good product quality are the benefits of ultrasound-assisted freezing over conventional freezing. However, quite little is recognized about the fundamental thermodynamics, moisture diffusion, and heat transfer in the ultrasound-assisted freezing process. The design of proper transducer systems and freezers to suit the requirements of fruits and vegetables has not been taken into account yet. It seems that

TABLE 11.1 Processing Methods used for Fruits and Vegetables.

S/ No.	Processing method	Technique	Benefits	Limitations	References
1.	High-pressure processing	High pressure	Preserve color, flavor, nutrients, antioxidant	Altered availability of carotenoids	Tewariet al. (2017), McInerney et al. (2007)
2.	Power ultrasound technique	Ultrasound rays	Eliminates enzymes and microbes, improves the ice crystal nucleation	Altered physicochemical properties of food	Islam et al. (2017)
3.	Ozone	—	Mycotoxin and pesticide control	Losses in physical quality	Karaca and Velioglu (2007)
4.	Drying	Heat	Increase shelf life	Decrease heat sensitive nutrients quality, altered nutritional and physical properties	Rodríguez et al. (2017), Karam et al. (2016)
5.	Spray drying	Spray	Cost effective, maintain phytochemicals	Change biologically active compounds	Figiel and Michalska (2016)
6.	Thermosonication	Conventional thermal processing	Improve the microbial and enzymatic inactivation rates, shelf life, decrease effect on the nutritional content	—	Anaya-Esparza et al. (2017)
7.	Radiation processing	Irradiation process	Influences the antioxidant position	Change bioactive compounds	Xue et al. (2016)
8.	Ohmic heating	Electrical resistance heating	Less thermal damage	Depends on electrical conductivity of food product	Kaur et al. (2016)
9.	Minimally processed, fresh-cut fruits and vegetables	Physical change	Increase shelf life	Physical damage	Varoquaux and Wiley (2017)
10.	Minimally processed refrigerated fruits and vegetables	Freezing	Nutrition security	—	Yildiz (2017)

there is a vital need to observe the effect of the ultrasound-assisted freezing process on the physicochemical properties of frozen fruits and vegetables (Islam et al., 2017).

11.2.3 OZONE

Ozone is one of the powerful oxidants; it is effective against several kinds of microorganisms on fruits and vegetables. Expected results have been found in solving the food industry problems like mycotoxin and pesticide remains by ozone operation. Impulsive decay expects forming dangerous remains in the treatment medium makes ozone safe in food applications. If not used properly, ozone can cause some harmful effects on products, for example, losses in physical quality (Table 11.1). Treatment conditions should be in detail observed for all kinds of products for actual and safe use of ozone (Karaca and Velioglu, 2007).

11.2.4 DRYING

Drying allows the procurement of products with a long shelf life by dropping the water activity to a low level for the growth of microorganisms, enzymatic reactions, and other inactivation reactions to be inhibited. Despite the benefits of this operation, heat-sensitive products quality is decreased when high temperatures are in use (Table 11.1). The usage of low drying temperatures decreases the heat damage but being the drying time longer, oxidation reactions occur and a lessening of the quality is also observed. For this reason, alternative techniques are being studied. Power ultrasound measured a developing and favorable technology in the food industry. The latent of this machinery depends on its ability to speed up the mass transfer processes in solid–liquid and solid–gas systems. The strengthening of the drying practice by the use of power ultrasound can be accomplished by changing the product behavior during drying, using pretreatments like soaking in a liquid medium or by applying power ultrasound in the gaseous medium during the drying process (Rodríguez et al., 2017).

Drying is a food preservation process in which water removal minimizes many of the moisture-driven worsening reactions impacting the bioproduct quality. Dried fruits and vegetables and their use in powder form have enlarged attention in the food industry. During powder processing, drying and grinding conditions significantly influence the quality features of biological materials. It not only modifies the nutritional value but also results in changes in textures, sensory, functional, and physical properties. These changes are of abundant position and need to be controlled through retro-engineering methodologies (Karam et al., 2016).

11.2.5 SPRAY DRYING

Spray drying (SD) is a genuine technique in which liquid products are directly turned into powders. SD is used typically in industry, especially for pharmaceuticals making and in the processing of dairy and fruit products (Jain et al., 2012). This technique was set up to be 4–5 times low cost as likened to freeze drying (FD). Likewise, it is confirmed that application of SD process for dehydration of chokeberry juice into powders resulted in better maintenance of total phenolic compounds, total flavonoids, total monomeric anthocyanin's (Table 11.1) when likened to FD however, in the literature there are some point of data connected with connotation of both drying techniques in positions of the changes of the biologically active compounds (Figiel and Michalska, 2016).

Spray FD (SFD) is another FD technique that produces distinctively powdered products even as still including the incomes of conventionally freeze-dried products. In relations of product structure, quality, and the retention of volatiles and bioactive compounds, SFD has dormant applications in high-value products due to its edge over other drying techniques. In cases where other drying techniques cannot provide these product qualities, SFD stands out despite the costs and difficulties involved (Ishwarya et al., 2015). Between the techniques used, FD is considered as the best method because low-temperatures functional in this process allow the highest retention of bioactive compounds comparable with the raw material (Figiel and Michalska, 2016).

11.2.6 THERMOSONICATION

Thermosonication is a unique and workable technique that is working to replace the conventional thermal processing (Table 11.1). It can improve the microbial and enzymatic inactivation rates, lengthen product shelf lifespan and diminish the impact on the nutritional content and general quality of fruit and vegetable juices (Anaya-Esparza et al., 2017).

11.2.7 RADIATION PROCESSING

Irradiation treatment is a usable storage method in which ionizing or nonionizing radiation is exposed to food. G-rays, X-rays, or high-energy electrons are the basis of ionizing radiation, which carries higher energy to ionize molecules or atoms (Table 11.1). Nonionizing radiation is characterized primarily by microwaves, infrared, visible light, and ultraviolet rays (UV-A, UA-B, and UA-C). Radiation influences the antioxidant position by changing the gathering of antioxidant bioactive compounds (polyphenols, vitamin C, flavonoids, and so forth) or the activity of antioxidant-related enzymes. These effects change due to factors like energy carried by radiation, the exposure time, the type of product treated, and many other. Ultraviolet is the most normally used radiation form preservation of fruits and vegetables (Xue et al., 2016).

11.2.8 OHMIC HEATING

Ohmic heating, as well called electrical resistance heating, joule heating, or electroconductive heating, is an advanced thermal food processing technique when electric current is passed due to electrical resistance its heat is internally generated in a sample. It is a different technique which delivers quick and smooth heating, resulting in less thermal damage to the food product (Table 11.1). The recent literature stated that, plant products are most suitable and often used for ohmic heat processing. More than heating of fruits and vegetables, the practical electric field under ohmic heating causes various changes in quality and nutritional factors which consist of inactivation of enzymes and microorganisms, degradation of heat-sensitive compounds, changes in cell membranes, viscosity, pH, color, and rheology (Kaur et al., 2016).

11.2.9 MINIMALLY PROCESSED, FRESH-CUT FRUITS AND VEGETABLES

Physiological (due to the enzymatic and metabolic activity of the living plant tissue) and microbial activities (due to the proliferation of microorganisms) are connected to the nutritional value, phytochemical quality, sensory quality, safety quality, and spoilage of minimally processed, fresh-cut fruits and vegetables (Table 11.1). Processing of fresh fruits and vegetables destroys the inner compartmentalization that separates enzymes from substrates and removes the natural protection of the epidermis. Therefore, plant tissues undergo physical damages that make them much more perishable than when the original product is in one piece. Furthermore, processing outcomes in a stress reply by the produce characterized by an bigger respiration rate (wound respiration) and ethylene production, leading to faster metabolic rates; changes in metabolic rates and damage of the plant tissue lead to exposure to air, desiccation (transpiration), and gathering of enzymes with substrates, all leading to quality degradation. Proper processing and packaging reduce the changes and quality loss with increased shelf life (Varoquaux and Wiley, 2017).

11.2.10 MINIMALLY PROCESSED REFRIGERATED FRUITS AND VEGETABLES

Slightly fresh processed plants foods have fresh-like, living cells and active enzyme-containing qualities. They are packaged and a little processed and refrigerated (Table 11.1). All crops are grown, harvested, and transported, under progressive hygienic and sanitary practices. The raw materials are washed, cut and spin dried, processed, and packaged in cool factories with tremendously sanitized conditions. Minimally processed refrigerated fruits and vegetables food system covers the several activities and performers in food value chains involved in transforming inputs into outcomes, which for a sustainable food system should include food and nutrition security, convenience to the consumer, environmental quality, and human well being (Yildiz, 2017).

Epidemiological studies have established a positive link between the intake of fruits and vegetables and prevention of diseases like athero-sclerosis, cancer, diabetes, arthritis, and also aging. Fruits and vegetables help enhance good health by preventing diseases. Most studied antioxidants are phenolic flavonoids, lycopene, carotenoids, and glucosinolates. Antioxidants have also been recommended to have a distinct role as preservatives. These preservatives are defined by the US Food and Drug Administration as a substance used to preserve food by delaying decline, rancidity, or discoloration caused by oxidation. During processing and storage lipid peroxidation is a deteriorative reaction of foods (Kaur and Kapoor, 2001).

11.3 EFFECT OF PROCESSING METHODS ON PHYTOCHEMICAL CONTENT

The role of phytochemicals having antioxidant properties in reducing the effects of oxidative stress in the development of disease and aging process is well established and accordingly contribute to the health-protective role of fruits and vegetables (Alvarez-Suarez et al., 2014). Varying processing procedures such as dehydration or drying, canning, extrusion, high-hydrostatic pressure, ohmic heating, and pulsed electric field limit the availability of phytochemicals (Nayak et al., 2015).

Thermal degradation, air exposure due to disturbance of plant tissues and cells, and enzymatic activity within plants may affect phytochemical content during food processing. For instance, vitamin C being heat sensitive can be easily degraded during processing (Francisco et al., 2010). In contrast, fat-soluble compounds such as β-carotene exhibit normally a comparatively greater retention during thermal procedures (Svelander et al., 2011). In addition, the bioavailability of these health-related compounds can be subjective to processing circumstances due to the formation of certain microstructures (Parada and Aguilera, 2007). For example, as compared to unprocessed fruit, in vitro bioavailability of lycopene from tomato can be improved by mechanical and heat processing (Tibäck et al., 2009). Similarly, increased bioavailability of carotenes from both tomato and carrot has been observed by certain treatments to disturb plant tissues and cells, such as high-pressure homogenization (Svelander et al., 2011). β-cryptoxanthin present in certain fruits and vegetables including papaya and pumpkin has health-protective role in the prevention and treatment of certain diseases, especially cancer (Ma et al., 2011). Studies exploring the effect of drying on β-cryptoxanthin content discovered that drying usually reduces the β-cryptoxanthin content present in fruits and vegetables (Table 11.2). FD has been found to be an effective method in terms of retaining antioxidant compounds in contrast to the other drying techniques. Due to use of low temperatures, FD is better able to preserve heat-sensitive antioxidants. In addition, FD results in greater extraction capacities of antioxidants with the establishment of ice crystals within the plant matrix in freezing, which may lead to a larger interruption of cell structure, permitting more solvent infiltration into the matrix. Conversely, less cell damage is caused by other drying methods, as well as harmful effects of high-temperature processing, both of which support the loss of antioxidants (Kamiloglu et al., 2016). Thus, food processing methods can be used to improve the phytonutrients content and bioavailability of final food products based on fruits and vegetables (Sánchez-Campillo et al., 2012).

TABLE 11.2 Effect of Thermal processing on Phytochemicals.

S/ No.	Phytochemical	Food	Processing method	Effect	Reference
1.	Lycopene	Tomato	Heat processing	Improved bioavailability	Svelander et al. (2011)
2.	Carotenes	Tomato, carrot	High-pressure homogenization	Improved bioavailability	Parada and Aguilera (2007)
3.	β-cryptoxanthin	Fruits, vegetables; papaya, pumpkin,	Drying	Decreases content	Kamiloglu et al. (2016)

11.4 CONCLUSION

Fruits and vegetables have disease-preventive effect and processing methods can damage its disease-protective properties. These naturally occurring compounds impart bright color to fruits and vegetables and act as antioxidants in the body by destroying harmful free radicals, which are associated with most degenerative diseases. Fruits and vegetables should be minimally processed to retain its phytochemical activity.

KEYWORDS

- **processing method**
- **heat processing**
- **high-pressure homogenization**
- **drying**
- **fruits and vegetables**

REFERENCES

Alvarez-Suarez, J. M.; Giampieri, F.; Tulipani, S.; Casoli, T.; Di Stefano, G.; González-Paramás, A. M.; Santos-Buelga, C.; Busco, F.; Quiles, J. L.; Cordero, M. D.; et al. One-Month Strawberry-Rich Anthocyanin Supplementation Ameliorates Cardiovascular Risk, Oxidative Stress Markers and Platelet Activation in Humans. *J. Nutr. Biochem.* **2014,** *25*(3), 289–294.

Anaya-Esparza, L. M.; Velázquez-Estrada, R. M.; Roig, A. X.; García, H. S.; Sayago-Ayerdi, S. G.; Montalvo-González, E. Thermosonication: An Alternative Processing for Fruit and Vegetable Juices. *Trends Food Sci. Technol.* **2017,** *61,* 26–37.

Chemat, F.; Khan, M. K. Applications of Ultrasound in Food Technology: Processing, Preservation and Extraction. *Ultrason. Sonochem.* **2011,** *18*(4), 813–835.

Dembinska-Kiec, A.; Mykkänen, O.; Kiec-Wilk, B.; Mykkänen, H. Antioxidant Phytochemicals Against Type 2 Diabetes. *Br. J. Nutr.* **2008,** *99*(E-S1), ES109–ES117.

Figiel, A.; Michalska, A. Overall Quality of Fruits and Vegetables Products Affected by the Drying Processes with the Assistance of Vacuum-Microwaves. *Int. J. Mol. Sci.* **2016,** *18*(1), 71.

Francisco, M.; Velasco, P.; Moreno, D. A.; García-Viguera, C.; Cartea, M. E. Cooking Methods of Brassica Rapa Affect the Preservation of Glucosinolates, Phenolics and Vitamin C. *Food Res. Int.* **2010,** *43*(5), 1455–1463.

Ishwarya, S. P.; Anandharamakrishnan, C.; Stapley, A. G. Spray-Freeze-Drying: A Novel Process for the Drying of Foods and Bioproducts. *Trends Food Sci. Technol.* **2015,** *41*(2), 161–181.

Islam, M. N.; Zhang, M.; Adhikari, B. Ultrasound-Assisted Freezing of Fruits and Vegetables: Design, Development, and Applications. In *Global Food Security and Wellness;* Barbosa-Cánovas, G.V., Pastore, G.M., Candoğan, K. et al. Springer: New York, 2017; pp 457–487.

Jain, M. S.; Lohare, G.B.; Chavan, R.B.; Barhate, S.D.; Shah, C. B. Spray Drying in Pharmaceutical Industry: A Review. *Res. J. Pharm. Dos. Forms Technol.* **2012,** *4,* 74–79.

Kamiloglu, S.; Toydemir, G.; Boyacioglu, D.; Beekwilder, J.; Hall, R. D.; Capanoglu, E. A Review on the Effect of Drying on Antioxidant Potential of Fruits and Vegetables. *Crit. Rev. Food Sci. Nutr.* **2016,** *56*(supl), S110–S129.

Karaca, H.; Velioglu, Y. S. Ozone Applications in Fruit and Vegetable Processing. *Food Rev. Int.* **2007,** *23*(1), 91–106.

Karam, M. C.; Petit, J.; Zimmer, D.; Djantou, E. B.; Scher, J. Effects of Drying and Grinding in Production of Fruit and Vegetable Powders: A Review. *J. Food Eng.* **2016,***188,* 32–49.

Kaur, C.; Kapoor, H. C. Antioxidants in Fruits and Vegetables–the Millennium's Health. *Int. J. Food Sci. Technol.* **2001,** *36*(7), 703–725.

Kaur, R.; Gul, K.; Singh, A. Nutritional Impact of Ohmic Heating on Fruits and Vegetables—A Review. *Cogent Food Agric.* **2016,** *2*(1), 1–15.

Ma, G.; Zhang, L.; Kato, M.; Yamawaki, K.; Kiriiwa, Y.; Yahata, M.; Ikoma, Y.; Matsumoto, H. Effect of Blue and Red Led Light Irradiation on B-Cryptoxanthin Accumulation in the Flavedo of Citrus Fruits. *J. Agric. Food Chem.* **2011,** *60*(1), 197–201.

McInerney, J. K.; Seccafien, C. A.; Stewart, C. M.; Bird, A. R. Effects of High Pressure Processing on Antioxidant Activity, and Total Carotenoid Content and Availability, in Vegetables. *Innovative Food Sci. Emerging Technol.* **2007,** *8*(4), 543–548.

Nayak, B.; Liu, R. H.; Tang, J. Effect of Processing on Phenolic Antioxidants of Fruits, Vegetables, and Grains—A Review. *Crit. Rev. Food Sci. Nutr.* **2015,** *55*(7), 887–918.

Nicoli, M.; Anese, M.; Parpinel, M. Influence of Processing on the Antioxidant Properties of Fruit and Vegetables. *Trends Food Sci. Technol.* **1999,** *10*(3), 94–100.

Parada, J.; Aguilera, J. M. Food Microstructure Affects the Bioavailability of Several Nutrients. *J. Food Sci.* **2007,** *72*(2), R21–R32.

Pasha, I.; Saeed, F.; Sultan, M. T.; Khan, M. R.; Rohi, M. Recent Developments in Minimal Processing: A Tool to Retain Nutritional Quality of Food. *Crit. Rev. Food Sci. Nutr.* **2014,** *54*(3), 340–351.

Rodríguez, Ó.; Eim, V.; Rosselló, C.; Femenia, A.; Cárcel, J. A.; Simal, S. Application of Power Ultrasound on the Convective Drying of Fruits and Vegetables: Effects on quality. *J. Sci. Food Agric.* **2017,** *98*(5), 1660–1673.

Sánchez-Campillo, M.; Larqué, E.; González-Silvera, D.; Martínez-Tomás, R.; García-Fernández, M.; Avilés, F.; Wellner, A.; Bialek, L.; Parra, S.; Alminger, M.; et al. Changes in the Carotenoid Concentration in Human Postprandial Chylomicron and Antioxidant Effect in HepG2 Caused by Differently Processed Fruit and Vegetable Soups. *Food Chem.* **2012,** *133*(1), 38–44.

Svelander, C. A.; Lopez-Sanchez, P.; Pudney, P. D.; Schumm, S.; Alminger, M. A. High Pressure Homogenization Increases the in Vitro Bioaccessibility of α-and β-Carotene in Carrot Emulsions but Not of Lycopene in Tomato Emulsions. *J. Food Sci.* **2011,** *76*(9), H215–H225.

Tewari, S.; Sehrawat, R.; Nema, P. K.; Kaur, B. P. Preservation Effect of High Pressure Processing on Ascorbic Acid of Fruits and Vegetables: A Review. *J. Food Biochem.* **2017,** *41*(1), e12319.

Tibäck, E. A.; Svelander, C. A.; Colle, I. J.; Altskär, A. I.; Alminger, M. A.; Hendrickx, M. E.; Ahrné, L. M.; Langton, M. I. Mechanical and Thermal Pretreatments of Crushed Tomatoes: Effects on Consistency and in Vitro Accessibility of Lycopene. *J. Food Sci.* **2009,** *74*(7), E386-E395.

Varoquaux, P.; Wiley, R. C. Biological and Biochemical Changes in Minimally Processed Refrigerated Fruits and Vegetables. In *Minimally Processed Refrigerated Fruits and Vegetables;* Yildiz, F., Wiley, R. C., Eds.; Springer: USA, 2017; pp 153–186.

Xue, Z.; Li, J.; Yu, W.; Lu, X.; Kou, X. Effects of Nonthermal Preservation Technologies on Antioxidant Activity of Fruits and Vegetables: A Review. Food Science and Technology International, **2016,** *22*(5), 440–458.

Yildiz, F. Initial Preparation, Handling, and Distribution of Minimally Processed Refrigerated Fruits and Vegetables. In *Minimally Processed Refrigerated Fruits and Vegetables;* Yildiz, F., Wiley, R. C., Eds.; Springer: USA, 2017; pp 53–92.

PART III

Environmental Concerns and Eco-Friendly Control Measures

CHAPTER 12

EFFECTS OF ENVIRONMENTAL FACTORS ON THE ACCUMULATION OF PHYTOCHEMICALS IN PLANTS

SECHENE STANLEY GOLOLO

Department of Biochemistry, School of Science and Technology, Sefako Makgatho Health Sciences University, Ga-Rankuwa, Pretoria, South Africa, Tel.: +27 12 521 4372

E-mail: Stanley.gololo@smu.ac.za

ABSTRACT

The effects of environmental factors on phytochemical compositions of medicinal plants highlight some disparities in the manner in which they respond to different environmental conditions. In this chapter, the effects of different environmental factors such as geographical locations of different altitudes, seasonal variation, and different exposure levels to pollution on the phytochemical composition of selected medicinal plants are discussed. The accumulation of phytochemicals in medicinal plants as a response to the influences of different environmental factors appear to differ among different plants. Thus, the accumulation of phytochemicals in medicinal plants as a response to environmental factors follows a non-general trend.

12.1 INTRODUCTION

The use of medicinal plants for healthcare purpose is a very old practice that is as old as humankind. The knowledge of medicinal plants with healing properties has been passed along generations, which, contributed, to their continuous usage up to this modern age (Petrovska, 2012). It is estimated that the use of medicinal plants has tremendously increased with about 80% of the population worldwide reported to be relying on herbal remedies for their health care needs over the past decades (Ekor, 2014). The increased reliance or usage of herbal remedies emanates from several factors that include their perceived and proven effectiveness, preference over manufactured products, cost-effectiveness, and perceived safety (Bandaranayake, 2006). Medicinal plants are to be regarded as plants that possess properties or compounds that can be used for healthcare purposes or that may be used as leads in the development of important drugs (WHO, 2008). The compounds that contribute to the medicinal properties of these plants are known or referred to as phytochemicals.

Phytochemicals, also known as phytoconstituents, are found in different plant species and are classified based on their chemical and biological properties. Phytochemicals include compounds such as alkaloids, flavonoids, phytosterols, saponins, polyphenols, terpenes, lectins, and many others (Webb, 2013). Phytochemicals are also referred to as secondary metabolites, in the sense that they are not necessarily required for the growth of the plant. They are synthesized mainly to contribute to the adaptation and survival of the plants in their interaction with the environment as defenses against pathogens as well as herbivorous and symbiotic insects (Kennedy and Wightman, 2011). Furthermore, phytochemicals are defined as chemical compounds of natural occurrence that induce biological activities, which are of health benefits to humans and animals. Phytochemicals possess many inherent biological activities such as anti-inflammation, anticancerous, antimicrobial, and antioxidation (Graça et al., 2016).

Generally, these chemical compounds protect plants from environmental hazards such as pollution, stress, drought, ultraviolet exposure and pathogenic attack. It is this inherent function of phytochemicals in plants, the function of protecting the plants from hostile environmental conditions that informs their accumulation depending on the extent of the risk. Phytochemicals accumulate in different plant parts, such as the roots, stems, leaves, flowers, fruits, and seeds as a response to the growing conditions (Saxena et al., 2013). It is therefore apparent that the accumulation of phytochemicals in plant parts is dependent on its interaction with the environment. Environmental conditions that may influence the accumulation of phytochemicals in plants include altitude, seasonal variation, ecological factors such as soil pH, soil organic matter, and mineral content, and the geographical conditions such as climate (Liu et al., 2015). The aim of this review was to establish whether the accumulation of phytochemicals in plants as influenced by their interaction with different environmental factors follow a general trend among medicinal plants and whether that trend is adhered to different phytochemicals based on the available literature.

12.2 ENVIRONMENTAL INFLUENCES ON PLANTS PHYTOCHEMICALS

Environmental conditions may influence the types, the contents, and proportions of phytochemical constituents in plant species. Some constituents are only synthesized or their accumulation is increased or decreased under certain environmental conditions (Liu et al., 2016). Therefore, the comparison of the phytochemical compositions in plants under the influence of different environmental factors may be either qualitative, quantitative, or both. In this regard, different studies have determined the presence or amounts of specific phytochemicals in several plant species under different growing conditions and locations. Many of such studies have demonstrated significant differences in the amounts of phytochemicals of one plant or many plants as influenced by different environmental conditions such as geographical locations, seasonal variations, pollution, and several ecological factors.

12.2.1 EFFECT OF GEOGRAPHICAL LOCATION ON THE PHYTOCHEMICALS OF MEDICINAL PLANTS

Geographical location may be described in terms of altitude and climatic conditions. Studies have been conducted on several medicinal plants that demonstrated that their phytochemical compositions were affected by geographical location parameters from which they were collected. In the study by Liu et al., the contents of phytochemicals in the leaves of *Potentilla fruticosa* from different growing locations in China were determined, whereby phytochemical contents were found to be qualitatively and quantitatively different (2016). The qualitative differences in the extracts of the leaves of *P. fruticosa* from different locations were determined by High-performance liquid chromatography analysis. According to the study, the differences in the chromatographic profiles of the leaf extracts of the plant species samples from different locations were displayed by the presence of some peaks in extracts of samples from some locations that are absent in the extracts of other samples from different locations. The observed significant differences were attributed to altitude and temperature patterns of the growing locations.

Quantitatively, altitude was positively correlated with flavonoids, rutin, and total phenolic contents, while also negatively correlated to total tannin content. The temperature was positively correlated with flavonoids and rutin content, while negatively correlated to total phenolic content. In the same study, highest tannin, flavonoid, and rutin contents were found in leaves sample from the Kangding, Sichuan province, whereas lowest tannin and rutin contents were recorded in the leaves from Shangri-la, Yunnan. The lowest flavonoid content was found in the leaves from Jingyuan. However, in contrasting observation, the highest total phenolic content was recorded in leaves samples from Shangri-la, Yunnan province. The provinces differ in terms of altitudes, thus the different phytochemicals in the same plant respond differently to the same variable.

The effect of climate change on the phytochemical composition of *Aloe vera* was determined in a study by Kumar et al. (2017). In this study, extracts of samples from highland and semiarid zones showed higher total phenolic contents than those from tropical zones. Wild bush tea (*Athrixia phylicoides*) growing at locations differing in altitude, climate, and edaphic factors were shown to have differences in the amounts of phytochemicals by a study conducted by Nchabeleng et al. (2012). The highest polyphenol content was recorded in bush tea samples from Haenertsburg area, while the lowest was in samples from the Levubu area. In contrast, the samples of the same plant species from Levubu showed the highest amounts of tannins and lower tannins were recorded in samples from Khalavha area. In the same study, a positive correlation was shown between total polyphenol content and altitude, whereas climatic conditions, soil macroelements, and soil pH did not affect total polyphenols and tannins. Thus, the findings of this study suggest that high amounts of total polyphenols are found in wild bush tea growing at high altitudes. However, the findings of the same study suggest that the accumulation of tannins is high at low altitudes in wild bush tea.

The results of the cited studies depict a picture whereby some medicinal plants have high amounts of different phytochemicals under the influence of contrasting location factors. For example, a medicinal plant possesses high amounts of tannins at high altitude location and the same medicinal plant possesses high amounts of other phytochemicals such as flavonoids at low altitude location. The findings of these studies also demonstrate the possession of high amounts of a specific phytochemical group by some medicinal plants at relatively higher altitudes while the accumulation of similar phytochemicals is not affected by altitude in other different medicinal plants. While several studies indicate that geographical location does have an effect on the phytochemical compositions of medicinal plants, it appears that the effect is not in a general form. Examples of relative altitudes under which selected medicinal plants possess high amounts of specific phytochemicals are presented in Table 12.1. The altitudes are referred to as relative to the highest altitude of locations in one study was not necessarily the highest in other studies and the same applies to lower altitudes.

TABLE 12.1 Examples of Relative Altitudes Under which Selected Medicinal Plants have a High Accumulation of Specific Phytochemicals.

Medicinal plants	Alkaloids	Essential oils	Phenols	Tannins	Flavonoids	Saponins	References
Potentilla fruticosa	–	–	HA	LA	HA	–	Liu et al. (2016)
Aloe vera	–	–	HA	LA	–	–	Kumar et al. (2017)
Athrixia phylicoides	–	–	HA	LA	–	–	Nchabeleng et al. (2012)
Zanthoxylum alatum	–	LA	–	–	–	–	Gupta et al. (2011)
Primula denticulata	HA	–	HA	HA	–	IA	Khaleefa et al. (2015)
Sphagnum junghuhnianum	–	–	HA	–	LA	–	Majuakim et al. (2014)
Arnica montana	–	–	LA	–	HA	–	Clauser et al. (2014)
Matricaria chamomilla	–	–	HA	–	HA	–	Ganzera et al. (2008)

HA: relative high altitude; LA: relative low altitude; IA: relative intermediate altitude; (–): not determined.

12.2.2 EFFECT OF SEASONAL VARIATION ON THE PHYTOCHEMICAL COMPOSITION OF MEDICINAL PLANTS

Seasonal variations are characterized by fluctuations in mean temperatures and rainfalls. Several studies were conducted to determine the season during which high accumulation of phytochemicals is obtained in selected medicinal plants. To cite a few, Ncube et al. reported on the observed effect of seasonal variation on the phytochemical compositions of *Tulbaghia violacea*, *Hypoxis hemerocallidea*, *Drimia robusta*, and *Merwilla plumbea* (2011). The study showed total phenolic contents to be generally higher in spring in all plants, whereas tannins and flavonoids were either higher in spring or winter except for *H. hemerocallidea* whose tannin levels were higher in autumn. In the same study, saponins were higher in winter in all plants.

Effect of seasonal changes on the phytochemical quantity was also observed for the leaves of three medicinal plants from the Limpopo province of South Africa, namely *Barleria dinteri*, *Grewia flava*, and *Jatropha lagarinthoides* (Gololo et al., 2016). The three medicinal plants were found to have high amounts of alkaloids and tannins during colder seasons in South Africa (autumn and winter), whereas flavonoids were in high amounts during warmer seasons (spring and summer). Saponins were in high amounts during a warmer season in *G. flava* and *J. lagarinthoides* and were not significantly different among seasons in *B. dinteri*. However, phenols showed a different trend with high amounts recorded in autumn for *G. flava*, summer for *J. lagarinthoides* and no significant seasonal difference in *B. dinteri*.

Examples of different seasons during which selected medicinal plants have a high accumulation of specific phytochemicals are presented in Table 12.2. As seen in the geographical location, the accumulation of phytochemicals in medicinal plants is affected by seasonal variation. However, the findings of the cited studies indicate that some medicinal plants possess higher amounts of different phytochemicals during particular seasons and that different medicinal plants possess high amounts of similar phytochemicals during different seasons. Thus, the effect of seasonal variation on the accumulation of phytochemicals also does not follow a general trend for medicinal plants.

12.2.3 POLLUTIONONTHEPHYTOCHEMICALCOMPOSITION OF MEDICINAL PLANTS

Pollution may be described as the direct or indirect introduction of substances, as a result of human activity, into the air, water, or land that

TABLE 12.2 Examples of Different Seasons During which Selected Medicinal Plants have High Accumulation of Specific Phytochemicals.

Medicinal plants	Alkaloids	Phenols	Tannins	Flavonoids	Saponins	References
Tulbaghia violacea	–	S1	S1/W	–	W	Ncube et al. (2011)
Hypoxis hemerocallidea	–	S1	A	–	W	
Drimia robusta	–	S1	S1/W	–	W	
Merwilla plumbia	–	S1	S1/W	–	W	
Barleria dinteri	A/W	NSD	A/W	S1/S2	NSD	
Grewia flava	A/W	A	A/W	S1/S2	S1/S2	Gololo et al. (2016)
Jatropha lagarinthoides	A/W	S2	A/W	S1/S2	S1/S2	
I. montana	–	S1	–	S2	–	Roux et al. (2017)

A: autumn; S1: spring; S2: summer, W: winter; NSD: no significant difference; (–): not determined.

may affect living organisms (Trivedy, 1995). The disparities in the phytochemical compositions of selected medicinal plants as a result of exposure to pollutants have been shown through some studies. In this regard, Ujuwundu et al. investigated the effect of gas flaring on the phytochemical composition of *Treculia Africana* and *Vigna subterranean* (2013). The findings of such particular study demonstrated that tannins and cyanogenic glycosides were in higher amounts in samples from polluted areas as compared to those from unpolluted areas. In a separate study by Olivares, phenols were found to be in higher amounts in the samples of *Tithonia diversifolia* collected at heavy traffic roadside than in light traffic roadsides (2003). The findings of the study by Rezanejad also reported significantly higher levels of flavonoids in the pollen grains of *Thuja orientalis* from the industrial and agricultural polluted area rather than in samples from an unpolluted area (2009).

While the findings of the earlier cited studies project a scenario of a positive correlation between pollution and the accumulation of phenolic compounds, there are exceptions among medicinal plants as demonstrated by the findings of the study by Gierlych and Karolewski (2000). In contrast to the findings of the earlier cited studies, no significant differences were found in the total phenolic contents of *Pinus sylvestris* between samples from polluted and the unpolluted areas (Gierlych and Karolewski, 2000). Differences in exposure to air pollutants were also found not to influence flavonoid composition in the saplings of *Psidium guajava* (Myrtaceae) both qualitatively and quantitatively (Furlan et al., 2010). Thus, the findings of these studies suggest no generality in the effect of pollution on the phenolic contents of medicinal plants. The suggestion is supported by the contrasting findings of the cited studies regarding the accumulation of phytochemicals in different medicinal plants upon exposure to different levels of pollution.

12.2.4 NON-GENERALITY IN THE ENVIRONMENTAL INFLUENCES ON PLANTS PHYTOCHEMICALS

First, the screening of plants used as health remedies for the presence of specific phytochemicals is important to ascertain their medicinal value. In addition to screening, quantitative analysis of phytochemicals found in medicinal plants affords the determination of which plants are good sources of specific phytochemicals. Since different phytochemicals exert specific biological activities, the determination of plants from which specific phytochemicals are found in relative abundance is also of paramount importance. Such findings will enable the isolation of phytochemicals in high yields, a limitation that is often encountered in the study of medicinal plants. As demonstrated through a number of studies, the accumulation of most phytochemicals is influenced by environmental factors (Ncube et al., 2011; Nchabeleng et al., 2012; Saxena et al., 2013).

However, the findings of several studies paint a picture that the environmental conditions under which certain phytochemicals are found in abundance in one plant are not nccessarily a given scenario for the next plant. In other words, the response to environmental stimuli in terms of phytochemical accumulations does not follow a general trend for different plants. In addition, the environmental conditions under which a specific phytochemical is found in abundance in a particular plant species are not necessarily the same for other phytochemicals even in that same particular plant species. As such, the influence of environmental factors on the phytochemical composition of medicinal plants is mostly both plant species and phytochemical specific. The study of the phytochemical compositions of medicinal plants under the influence of different environmental conditions has immense potential to contribute to the quality assurance of the use of medicinal plants. It is important to determine the beneficial aspects or the potential toxicity of specific compounds that are present in medicinal plants under certain environmental conditions and absent in the same plants under different conditions.

12.3 CONCLUSIONS

The review of the effect of environmental factors on phytochemical compositions of selected medicinal plants highlights some disparities in the manner in which different medicinal plants response to different environmental factors. Disparities could be seen in the accumulation of phytochemicals in medicinal plants as a response to differences in geographical locations, seasonal variation, and different exposure levels to pollutants. The review, therefore, indicates non-generality in the accumulation of the phytochemicals of medicinal plants as a response to environmental factors. Based on these non-generality in the environmental factors-induced phytochemical composition of medicinal plants, the undertaking of more studies for the determination of environmental conditions under which important medicinal plants possess high amounts of phytochemicals is recommended.

KEYWORDS

- **medicinal plants**
- **phytochemical accumulation**
- **environmental factors**
- **seasonal variation**
- **pollution**

REFERENCES

Aslam, K.; Nawchoo, I. A.; Ganai, B. A. Altitudinal Variation in some Phytochemical Constituents and Stomatal Traits of *Primula denticulata*. *Int. J. Adv. Sci. Res.* **2015,** *1,* 93–101.

Bandaranayake, W. M. Quality Control, Screening, Toxicity, and Regulation of Herbal Drugs. In *Modern Phytomedicine. Turning Medicinal Plants into Drugs;* Ahmad, I., Aqil, F., Owais, M., Eds.; Weinheim: Wiley-VCH GmbH & Co. KgaA, 2006; p 25.

Clauser, M.; Aiello, N.; Scartezzini, F.; Innocenti, G.; DallAcqua, S. Differences in the Chemical Composition of *Arnica montana* Flowers from Wild Populations of North Italy. *Nat. Prod. Commun.* **2014,** *9*(1), 3–6.

Ekor, M. The Growing Use of Herbal Medicines: Issues Relating to Adverse Reactions and Challenges in Monitoring Safety. *Front. Pharmacol.* **2014,** *4,* 1–10.

Furlan, C. M.; Santos, D. Y. A. C.; Motta, L. B.; Domingos, M.; Salatino, A. Guava Flavonoids and the Effects of Industrial Air Pollutants. *Atmos. Pollut. Res.* **2010,** *1,* 30–35.

Ganzera, M.; Guggenberger, M.; Struppner, H.; Zidorn, C. Altitudinal Variation of Secondary Metabolite Profiles in Flowering Heads of *Matricaria chamomilla* cv. BONA. *Planta Med.* **2008,** *74,* 453–457.

Gierlych, M. J.; Karolewski, P. Phenolic Compounds Distribution Along the Length of Scots Spine Needles in a Polluted and Control Environment and its Connection with Necroses Formation. *Acta Soc. Bot. Pol.* **2000,** *69,* 127–130.

Gololo, S. S.; Shai, L. J.; Agyei, N. M.; Mogale, M. A. Effect of Seasonal Changes on the Quantity of Phytochemicals in the Leaves of Three Medicinal Plants from Limpopo Province, *South Africa. J. Pharmacogn. Phytother.* **2016,** *8,* 168–172.

Graça, V. C.; Ferreira, I. C. F. R.; Santos, P. F. Phytochemical Composition and Biological Activities of *Geranium robertianum* L. A Review. *Ind. Crops Prod.* **2016,** *87,* 363–378.

Gupta, S.; Bhaskar, G.; Andola, H. C. Altitudinal Variation in Essential Oil Content in Leaves of *Zanthoxylum alatum* Roxb. A High Value Aromatic Tree from Uttarakhand. *Res. J. Med. Plant* **2011,** *5,* 348–351.

Kennedy, D. O.; Wightman, E. L. Herbal Extracts and Phytochemicals: Plant Secondary Metabolites and the Enhancement of Human Brain Function. *Adv. Nutr.* **2011,** *2,* 32–50.

Kumar, S.; Yadav, A.; Yadav, M.; Yadav, J. P. Effect of Climate Change on Phytochemical Diversity, Total Phenolic Content and in Vitro Antioxidant Activity of *Aloe vera* (L) Burm.f. *BMC Res. Notes* **2017,** *10,* 1–12.

Liu, W.; Liu, J.; Yin, D.; Zhao, X. Influence of Ecological Factors on the Production of Active Substances in the Anti-Cancer Plant *Sinopodophyllum hexandrum* (Royle) T.S. Ying. *Plos One* **2015,** *10,* e0122981.

Liu, W.; Yin, D.; Li, N.; Hou, X.; Wang, D.; Li, D.; Liu, J. Influence of Environmental Factors on the Active Substance Production and Antioxidant Activity in *Potentilla fruticosa* L. and its Quality Assessment. *Sci. Rep.* **2016,** *6,* 28591.

Majuakim, L.; Ng, S. Y.; Abu Bakar, M. F.; Suleiman, M. Effect of Altitude on Total Phenolics and Flavonoids in *Sphagnum junghuhnianum* in Tropical Montane Forests of Borneo. *Sepilok Bull.* **2014,** *19–20,* 23–32.

Nchabeleng, L.; Mudau, F. N.; Mariga, I. K. Effects of Chemical Composition of Wild Bush Tea (*Athrixia phylicoides* DC.) Growing at Locations Differing in Altitude, Climate and Edaphic Factors. *J. Med. Plant Res.* **2012,** *6,* 1662–1666.

Ncube, B.; Finnie, J. F.; Van Staden, J. Seasonal Variation in Antimicrobial and Phytochemical Properties of Frequently Used Medicinal Bulbous Plants from South Africa. *S. Afr. J. Bot.* **2011,** *77,* 387–396.

Olivares, E. The Effect of Lead on the Phytochemistry of *Tithonia diversifolia* Exposed to Roadside Automotive Pollution or Grown in Pots of Pb-Supplemented Soil. *Braz. J. Plant Physiol.* **2003,** *15,* 149–158.

Petrovska, B. B. Historical Review of Medicinal Plants' Usage. *Pharmacogn. Rev.* **2012,** *6,* 1–5.

Rezanejad, F. Air Pollution Effects on Structure, Proteins and Flavonoids in Pollen Grains of *Thuja orientalis* L. (Cupressaceae). *Grana* **2009,** *48,* 205–213.

Roux, D.; Alnaser, O.; Garayev, E.; Baghdikian, B.; Elias, R.; Chiffolleau, P.; et al. Ecophysiological and Phytochemical Characterization of Wild Populations of *Inula montana* L. (Asteraceae) in Southeastern France. *Flora* **2017,** *236–237,* 67–75.

Saxena, M.; Saxena, J.; Nema, R.; Singh, D.; Gupta A. Phytochemistry of Medicinal Plants. *J. Pharmacogn. Phytochem.* **2013,** *1,* 168–182.

Trivedy, R. K. *Encyclopaedia of Environmental Pollution and Control;* Enviro-Media: Karad, 1995.

Ujuwundu, C. O.; Nwaogu, L. A.; Ujuwundu, F. N.; Belonwu, D. C. Effect of Gas Flaring on the Phytochemical and Nutritional Composition of *Treculia africana* and *Vigna subterranean.* *Br. Biotechnol. J.* **2013,** *3,* 293–304.

Webb, D. Phytochemicals' Role in Good Health. *Today's Dietitian* **2013,** *15,* 70.

WHO. *Traditional Medicine;* Fact Sheet No. 134; 2008. http://www.who.int/mediacentre/factsheets/2003/fs134/en/ (accessed Sept 12, 2017).

CHAPTER 13

EFFECTS OF ENVIRONMENT ON THE CHEMICAL CONSTITUENTS AND BIOLOGICAL CHARACTERISTICS OF SOME MEDICINAL PLANTS

VINESH KUMAR* and YOGITA SHARMA

Department of Sciences, Kids' Science Academy, Roorkee, Uttarakhand, India, Mob.: +91 9997228095

**Corresponding author. E-mail: vkresearch47@gmail.com*
ORCID: https://orcid.org/0000-0002-7560-7355

ABSTRACT

Environmental factors have significant effects on the growth and development of plants. Climate change is responsible for the variation in environmental conditions of different areas differently. The environmental circumstances like frequency and intensity of weather events, such as hurricanes, storms, floods, and droughts are life-threatening. These events might affect the flora and fauna of the place and also affects environmental factors such as atmosphere, water, temperature, light, fire, nutrients, grazers, and so forth. Change in environmental conditions has the effect on the habitat and growth of plants. The environmental factors have significant effects on the chemical constituents, generally on plant secondary metabolites. These plant constituents are responsible for biological and pharmaceutical activities. The results reveal that environment has the significant effects on the plant phenology, secondary metabolites, and biological properties of medicinal plants. This chapter describes the effects of environmental factors on the chemical constituents and biological characteristics of some medicinal plants.

13.1 INTRODUCTION

Environmental factors are of two types, that is, biotic and abiotic factors. These factors have significant effects on the growth and development of organisms. The abiotic components of environment include air, water, soil, minerals, light, rain, and climatic conditions while biotic components are all organisms including microorganisms. There is a continuous interaction between these biotic and abiotic components. Plants are the producer, which synthesize organic food from inorganic substances by several physiological processes including photosynthesis.

Medicinal plants are extremely valuable to human beings to cure diseases and maintain health. Medicinal plants are the backbone of traditional systems of medicine including herbal therapy, Ayurveda, and aromatherapy; and also have economic importance (Vinesh and Devendra, 2013). The lifecycle of the medicinal plant from the dormancy state to germination, vegetative propagation, growth, flowering, fruit and seed development and again when it goes into a new dormant state, affected by several environmental factors. The medicinal plants are very sensitive to their environment. The change in the environmental conditions of an area may affect the medicinal plant at any stage of their growth and development. The biogeochemical reactions occur in the plant affected by changes in the environmental conditions. These changes are also responsible for the nature of secondary metabolites synthesized by plants.

The wealth of herbs of any country has an influence on the medical sector as well as on the economics of any country (Vinesh and Devendra, 2013). The urbanization, transportation, industrialization, deforestation, and agricultural activities are the major contributors responsible for increasing the level of greenhouse gases in the atmosphere. The greenhouse gases are responsible for global warming and climate change. The climate change is responsible for the extreme weather events and environmental conditions of an area. The frequency and intensity of these extreme weather events increases which are life-threatening for all organisms including medicinal plants. The human population is increasing day by day and increasing the stress on medicinal plants.

Warming directly affects the rate of plant respiration, photosynthesis, and other biogeochemical processes. The predicted patterns of global climate change are the major concern in many areas of socioeconomic activities, such as agriculture, forestry,and so forth, and are a major threat to biodiversity and ecosystem function. Climate change has effects on the growth and production of *Saccharum officinarum* and *Mangifera indica* (Vinesh et al., 2011). Climate change is a result of the emission of greenhouse gases (e.g., CO_2, CH_4, and N_2O, etc.) in the past century that will cause atmospheric warming (IPCC, 2007a).

With environmental climatic factors, competition within the species is also responsible for plant species. The different plant species show different responses toward environmental factors.

13.2 CONSEQUENCES OF ENVIRONMENT CHANGE

The climate changes are responsible for the change in temperature, precipitation, and season duration of a particular area. These environmental changes could shorten the ripening period of the medicinal plants. The shortening in the ripening period may decrease the size, weight, and production of grains and fruits (Vinesh, 2011). The quick increasing concentration of greenhouse gases in the troposphere has significant changes in regional and seasonal climate pattern. These changes can strongly affect the distribution and diversity of plants (Huntley, 1999).

Different plant species will react differently to climate change. Some species of medicinal plants will stay in place but adapt to new climatic conditions through assortment. Other species will shift to higher latitudes or altitudes. Some species of medicinal plants may become extinct (Keutgen, 1997). The results of some studies showed that range shifts of individual species are likely to result in changes in community composition, as a result of local extinction and dispersal/migration (Benning, 2002). Salick states that due to rise in temperatures, some cold adopted plant species migrate upward until there are no higher areas to inhabit, at this tolerance point (altitude) these plant species may be faced with extinction (2009).

The plant autecology depends on temperature, water, atmosphere, light, and biotic factors (Daubenmire, 1974). Many authors have also reported different responses to environmental factor by plants with C_4 and C_3 photosynthetic pathways (Christie and Detling, 1982; Ehleringer, 1985; Cadwell, 1985). If the changes in environmental factors including temperature, precipitation, and drought are beyond the tolerance level, the pressure will increase on medicinal plants. These factors can also modify the secondary metabolites which can affect the medicinal properties of the species.

13.3 ENVIRONMENTAL FACTORS AND THEIR EFFECTS ON MEDICINAL PLANTS

The environmental factors which affect the growth, development, and productivity of medicinal plants are temperature, water, light, atmosphere, fire, nutrients, drought, and grazers.

13.3.1 TEMPERATURE

Researchers have recognized that temperature regulates the rate of physiological processes and effects the growth and development of medicinal plants. Each biological process occurs in a certain range of temperature and has an optimal (minimal and maximum) operating temperature (Larcher, 1980). The temperature response also depends on other environmental factors such as moisture and radiant energy (Laude, 1974).

According to Cooper and Tainton (1968), the suitable range of temperature lies between 20 and 25°C for almost all temperate C_3 grasses while for subtropical C_4 grasses, the range is in between 30 and 35°C. As noted by some authors, the increase in temperature with water stress is responsible for mineral deficiency in plants. The decrease in temperature below the tolerance level also affects the plant physiology.

This result in delaying starting of growth of leaves, the opening of stomata, restricts water movement to roots and decreasing the length of photosynthesis during spring. In grassland farming of some regions of the world, winter is a major cause of injury and death of forage plants (Smith, 1964).

The alternative change in above and below freezing temperature can cause damage to plant by frost heaving, acclimation, and freezing of plant cells. Freezing of plant parts due to low temperature is a major cause of plant death or loss and affect the distribution of plants.

According to Smith (1964), old plants are more sensitive to winter injury than a younger plant because of insects, diseases, and poor fertility of the land.

Winterkill (death of plants) due to low temperature has been reported in rangelands for several shrub species. These include *Caenothus velutinus* (Stickney, 1965), *Purshia tridentata* (Jensen and Urness, 1979), *Atriplex canescens* (Van Epps, 1975), and *Artemisia tridentata* (Hanson, 1982).

13.3.2 WATER

Water is an important liquid, which sustains life on earth planet. All living organisms including plants require water to sustain their life. The lack and excess of water create stress on plants. The availability of water affects the growth and development of water (Brown, 1977). He also describes that the water deficiency occurs in plant when the rate of transpiration is more than the rate of water absorption.

The prolonged stress of water on the shoot development effects leaf size and internode length. According to Slatyer (1974), the root growth reduces in proportion to shoot growth, delaye flowering time, reduces the size, number and capability, and ceased growth and development followed by death in severe water scarcity.

According to the study of Feldman (1984), in flooded areas oxygen supply decreases or get stopped and normal exchanges of gasses from roots may also get disturbed. The flooded environment also affects the metabolism and inhibits the plant growth. The tolerance level varies from one plant species to another species. The morphological and physiological adaptations also get affected by the flooded environment.

13.3.3 LIGHT

According to Smith (1982), light is an essential environmental factor, for the existence of higher photoautotrophic plants. The rate of photosynthesis depends on the intensity and duration of light. Decrease in the amount of light, effects the plant growth and physiology (Harper, 1977). The amount of light absorbed depends on several factors including the age, size and shape of leaves, the angle of incident light, and physiological conditions (Risser, 1985).

The leaf is the first place of the plant, which accepts and interacts with light. The growth rate of a plant depends on the leaf surface area. According to Brougham (1956), the maximum growth rate occurs when leaves absorb 95% of incoming solar light. The plants in limited light resources adjust their structure and growth rate in available light (Harper, 1977).

Therefore, light plays an essential role in the growth and development and is responsible for physiological changes in plants.

13.3.4 ATMOSPHERE

The blankets of gases include nitrogen 78%, oxygen 21%, and carbon dioxide 0.03%. The carbon dioxide is required for photosynthesis, oxygen is required for respiration, and nitrogen required for other physiochemical processes. The toxic pollutants from the atmosphere, hydrosphere, and lithosphere are also absorbed by the plant (Larcher, 1980). The cloud, wind, fog, and some other component of the troposphere can influence the plant growth and development.

13.3.5 FIRE

Medicinal plants are generally found in hilly and mountain areas. Fire can affect medicinal plants directly or indirectly through heat and gases. According to Scifres (1980), plant responses to fire are different with phenology and morphological stages of growth and development. The fire of forest severely destroys many plants species every year. The existence of these species is dependent upon the capacity to restore after losing of aerial stems.

13.3.6 GRAZERS

Grazers especially livestock, wildlife, and insects eat plant leaves and shoot tissues. This affects the growth and development of plants. The plants show responses with an increase in leaf replacement potential. This resistance depends upon the stage of growth as well as on the species of plant (Hyder, 1972). Grazers also affect the soil fertility and influence several other factors including soil erosion.

13.3.7 COMPETITION

Plants grow with different other plant species and have competition for resources (Miller, 1980). The growing conditions for different plant species differ from one species to another. The availability of resources affects the number and distribution of plant species.

13.4 EFFECTS OF ENVIRONMENT ON CHEMICAL CONSTITUENTS

Climatic factors include moisture, light, temperature, and so on (Yang, 2004). They regulate the processes of water, soil, and heat conditions. These are the primary factors for the growth and development of herbal medicine (Yang, 2001).

There are studies which noticed that climate change is causing visible effects on the distribution, growth, life cycles, and on secondary metabolites. The plants of high altitudes of the Himalayas, those remains under the snow cover for a significant period of time and unprotected to the severe environmental situations, clamps a vast potential to work as a medicine for some chronic illnesses (Kala, 2009).

The result of different studies showed that climate change has significant effects on natural resources and alter temperature ranges, weather events, seasonal patterns, and so forth (IPCC, 2007a, b; Root, 2003; Parmesan, 2003). The moments of climate change are now being felt in different areas across the world and its consequences on seasonal movement in terrestrial ecosystems are significant and well recognized (Root, 2003; Walther, 2002). Results suggest that range shifts of individual plant species are probable to outcome in deviations in community arrangement, as a consequence of native extinction and migration (Hansen, 2001; Benning, 2002).

In the Indian Himalayan region, predominantly in alpine areas, variations in temperatures and snow patterns are already affecting the phenology and distribution of some plant species (Nautiyal, 2004). The study of Khanduri (2008), has explored some phenological alterations in more than 650 temperate plant species.

Alpine ecosystems are more sensitive to climate warming since plant species have altitudinal limits of climatic limits and limitation of resources (Panigrahy, 2010). Thus, alpine plant species have various morphological and physiological modifications to adept against adverse climatic changes.

13.5 EFFECT OF ENVIRONMENT ON SECONDARY CHEMICAL PRODUCTION

Climate change influences weather patterns, temperature and result in loss of habitat, the shift of species distribution, altered species composition and has effects on growth and development of plant species. There has been little concern on medicinal plants and their secondary metabolite production. The changes in environmental conditions may directly change plant fitness

(Galen and Stanton, 1991; Wookey, 1993), as well as change the reproductive success of plants species and flowering phenology (Hughes, 2000).

The studies showed that change in environment could alter the chemical composition to change itself for the survival in high altitude region. Predominantly, the temperature stress can alter secondary plant metabolites and many other compounds that plants synthesis, which is basically responsible for medicinal activity (Salick, 2009; Zobayed, 2005). Normally when plants are under stress, secondary metabolite production may rise because growth is often self-conscious more than photosynthesis, and the carbon fixed not assigned to growth is in its place assigned to secondary metabolites (Mooney 1991).

Numerous studies have observed the effects of increased temperatures on plant's secondary metabolite production, but most of these studies have conflicting results (Jochum, 2007). Some reveal that secondary metabolites production increases with increase in temperatures (Litvak, 2002), while others report that these decrease with increase in the temperature (Snow, 2003).

According to Chaturvedi (2007), the increase in temperature and the CO_2 level will change growth cycles of alpine plants and active chemical constitutes of the plants as a result of physiological changes (Chaturvedi, 2007). The change in the secondary metabolites may affect the medicinal value and activities of the plant. For a long-term supply of quality raw material for curing illnesses, studies on the effects of environment on plant secondary metabolic production and composition become important.

Medicinal plants are the rich sources of many biologically active compounds including phenolic compounds, tannins, steroids, and flavonoids. Phenolic constituents and other secondary plant metabolites show a chemical interface between environment and plants. The synthesis and concentration of plant metabolites depend upon several environmental factors (Gobbo-Neto, 2007).

The tannin concentration has been found higher during spring and summer in species of lotus (Gobrehiwot, 2001). The same results were seen in *Alnus rubra* (Gonazlez, 2002). Bruno (2011) observed that the concentration of metabolites in the leaves of plant *Lafoensia pacari* influences by temperature, micronutrients, and other environmental factors. The concentration of phenolic compounds in plant tissues depend upon the surrounding temperature. It was founded that at low temperature, the concentration of phenolic compounds was maximum (Padda, 2008). He also suggested that high concentration of phenolic compounds at low temperature is due to the increased activity of phenylalanine ammonia lyase enzyme.

Júlio et al. (2006) found a close relationship between the rainfall level and tannins concentrations in plants *Myracrodruon urundeuva* and *Anadenanthera colubrina*.

According to Hatano et al. (1986), the ecological factors are responsible for qualitative and quantitative changes in the level of tannins. The environmental factors can change the biosynthetic pathways. In many species, the concentration of phenolic compounds increases at high temperature.

According to Gebrehiwot (2002), the change in the concentration of tannin occurs with changing in the seasons. Similar results were observed in the *A. rubra.* The study of Coley (2002) showed that the plants growing in fertile soil have a high concentration of total phenolic compounds and tannins in comparing the plants growth in poor soil. The concentration of phenol and tannin is high in *Ceratonia siliqua* in water stress.

The environmental conditions also affect the size of plant leaves, rhizome, and stem. Plants resist biological, physical, and chemical environmental stresses by regulating the accumulation of secondary metabolites in long periods of adaption to the environment. Ecological factors are the dominant factors affecting the secondary metabolites of the plants (Ncube, 2012).

Environmental conditions show a key part in describing the function and distribution of plants, in combination with other factors. There is already evidence that plant species are shifting their ranges in altitude and latitude as a response to changing regional climates. The timing of phenological events such as flowering is often related to environmental variables such as temperature. Changing environments are therefore expected to lead to changes in life cycle events, and these have been recorded for many species of plants (Parmesan and Yohe, 2003).

The weather or environmental conditions have a significant effect on phytochemical constituents, concentration, moisture contents, ash contents, and biological characteristics of the plants. India has tremendous causes to be worried about the impacts of climate change on plants especially medicinal herbs. In the future, research should be carried out on others plants worldwide.

Medicinal plants are the rich source of phytochemicals with interesting biological and medicinal properties (Gibson, 1998). These phytochemicals protect plants from disease and repair damaged cells. These plant metabolites protect plants cells and tissues from environmental hazards such as drought, ultraviolet exposure, pollution, and pathogenic attack (Gibson, 1998; Mathai, 2000).

About 4000 phytochemicals have been listed and are grouped by physical characteristics and chemical characteristics with their protective functions (Meagher, 1999). These phytochemicals are present in vegetables, stem, leaves, flowers, fruits, legumes, nuts, whole grains, spices, herbs, and seeds (Mathai, 2000; Costa, 1999). The environmental factors including soil nutrients, foliar nutrients, and climate affect the leaf of *Myrcia tomentosa* which has essential oil composition (Leonardo et al. 1980).

13.6 EFFECT OF ENVIRONMENT ON BIOLOGICAL ACTIVITIES

The primary chemical constituents include vitamins, proteins, sugars, amino acids, chlorophylls, and so forth. Secondary metabolites include flavonoids, alkaloids, lignans, terpenes, plant steroids, saponins, phenolics, curcumin, glucosides, and flavonoids (Hahn, 1998). The biological activities of these medicinal plants depend upon the nature and concentration of phytochemicals plant metabolites. These phytochemicals are also known as secondary plant metabolites and have biological properties including antimicrobial effect, antioxidant activity, decreasing of platelet aggregation, modulation of detoxification enzymes, stimulations of the immune system, anticancer property, and modulation of hormone metabolism. Plants synthesize these chemicals to protect themselves and can also be used by human to protect against diseases (Narasinga, 2003). The amounts of these phytochemicals depend upon the variety, processing, nutrients, and environmental conditions (King, 1999). Phytochemicals may also be used as food supplements (American Cancer Society, 2000). The change in the nature and concentration of secondary metabolites may alter the biological and medicinal properties of medicinal plants.

13.7 CONCLUSION

Environmental factors have significant effects on the growth and development of plants. Medicinal plants are extremely valuable to human beings to cure diseases and maintain health. Medicinal plants are the backbone of the traditional system of medicine and also have economic importance. The environmental factors which affect the growth, development, and productivity are temperature, water, light, atmosphere, fire, nutrients, drought, and grazers. The change in the environmental conditions of an area may affect the medicinal plant at any stage of their growth and development. The biogeochemical reactions occur in the plant affected by changes in the environmental conditions. These changes are also responsible for the nature of secondary metabolites synthesized by plants. Medicinal plants are the rich source of phytochemicals with interesting biological and medicinal properties. The change in the nature and concentration of secondary metabolites may alter the biological and medicinal properties of herbs.

KEYWORDS

- **environment**
- **climate change**
- **fauna and flora**
- **medicinal plants**
- **metabolites**

REFERENCES

Benning, T. L.; La Pointe, D.; Atkinson, C. T., Vitousek P. M. Interactions of climate change with biological invasions and land use in the Hawaiian Islands: modeling the fate of endemic birds using a geographic information system. *Pediatr. Acute onset Neuropsychiatr. Syndr. (PANS)*. **2002,** *99*(22), 14246–14249.

Brougham, R. W. Range Forage Production Changes on a Water Spreader in Southeastern Montana. *J. Range Manage* **1956,** *9*, 187–191.

Brown, R. W. Water Relations of Range Plants. In. *Rangeland plant physiology;* Issue 4 of Range science series. Sosebee, R. E. Ed.; Society for Range Management, Littleton, USA. 1977; pp 97–140.

Cadwell, M. M.; Cold Desert. In *Physiological Ecology of North American Plant Communities;* Chabot, B. F., Mooney, H. A., eds., Chapman and Hall: New York, 1985A, 199–212.

Chaturvedi, A. K.; Vashistha, R. K.; Prasad, P.; Nautiyal, M. C. Need of Innovative Approach for Climate Change Studies in Alpine Region of India. *Cur. Sci.* **2007,** *93*(12), 1648–1649.

Christie, E. K.; Detling, J. K. Analysis of Interference Between C3 and C4 Grasses in Relation to Temperature and Soil Nitrogen Supply. Ecology **1982,** *63*, 1277–1284.

Cooper, J. P.; Tainton, N. M. Light and Temperature Requirements for Growth of Tropical and Temperate Grasses. *Herb. Abstr.* **1968,** *38*, 167–176.

Costa, M. A.; Zia, Z. Q.; Davin, L. B.; Lewis, N. G. Chapter Four: Toward Engineering the Metabolic Pathways of Cancer-Preventing Lignans in Cereal Grains and Other Crops. In *Phytochemicals in Human Health Protection, Nutrition, and Plant Defense*; Recent Advances in Phytochemistry. Romeo, J. T., Ed.; Springer: New York, 1999; *33,* 67–87.

Daubenmire, R. F. *Plant and environment a text book of plant autecology*; John Willy and Sons: New York, 1974.

Ehleringer, J. Annuals and Perennials of Warm Deserts. In *Grasses and Grasslands;* Chabot, B. F., Mooney, A. Ed.; McMillan and Co Ltd.: New York, 1985; 162–180.

Feldman, L. J. Regulation of Root Development. *Ann. Rev. Plant Physiol.* **1984,** *35*, 223–242.
Galen, C.; Stanton, M. L. Consequences of Emergences Phenology for Reproductive Success in Ranunculus Adoneus (Ranunculaceae). *Am. J. Bot.* **1991,** *78*, 978–988.
Gebrehiwot, L.; Beuselink, P. R.; Roberts CA Seasonal Variations in Condensed Tannins Concentration of Three Lotus Species. *Agron. J.* **2002,** *94*, 1059–1065.
Gibson, E. L.; Wardel, J.; Watts, C. J. Fruit and Vegetable Consumption, Nutritional Knowledge and Beliefs in Mothers and Children. *Appetite* **1998,** *31*, 205–228.
Gobbo-Neto, L.; Lopes, N. P. Plantas Medicinais: Fatores De Influência No Conteúdo De Metabólitos Secundários. *Quim Nova* **2007,** *30*, 374–381.
González-Hernández, M. P.; Starkey, E. E.; Karchesy, J. Seasonal Variation in Concentrations of Fiber, Crude Protein and Phenolic Compounds in Leaves of Red Alder (Alnus Rubra): Nutritional Implications for Cervids. *J. Chem. Ecol.* **2000,** *26*, 293–301.
Hahn, N. I. Is Phytoestrogens Nature'S Cure for What Ails Us? A Look At the Rsearch. *J. Am. Diet. Assoc.* **1998,** *98*, 974–976.
Hansen, A. J.; Neilson, R. R.; Dale, V. H.; Flather, C. H.; Iverson, L. R.; Currie, D. J.; Global Change in Forests: Responses of Species, Communities, and Biomes. *Biosci.* **2001,** *51*, 765–779.
Hanson, C. L.; Morris, R. P.; Wight, J. R. Foliage Mortality of Mountain Big Sagebrush (Artemisia Tridentate Subsp. Vaseyana) in Southwestern Idaho During the Winter of 1976–77. *J. Range Manage* **1982,** *36*, 576–578.
Harper, J. L. *Polpulation Biology of Plants;* Academic Press: New York, 1977.
Hatano, T.; Kira, R.; Yoshizaki, M.; Okuda, T. Seasonal Changes in the Tannins of Liquidambar Formosana Refl Ectings Their Biogenesis. *Phytochemistry* **1986,** *25*, 2787–2789.
Hughes, L. Biological Consequences of Global Warming: is the Signal Already Apparent? *Trends Ecol. Evol.* **2000,** *15*, 56–61.
Huntley, B. The Responses of Vegetation to the Past and Future Climate Change. In *Global Change and Arctic Terrestrial Ecosystems;* Oechel, W. C. Ed.; Springer: New York, 1999.
Hyder, D. N. Defoliation in Relation to Vegetative Growth. In *Biology and Utilization of Grasses*; Younger, V. B., McKell, C. M. Eds.; Academic Press: New York, 1972; pp 304–317.
IPCC (Intergovernmental Panel on Climate Change). Working Group I Report *The Physical Science Basis*, Working Group II Report *Impacts, Adaptation and Vulnerability*, Working Group III Report *Mitigation of Climate Change.* 2007a. http://www.ipcc.ch
IPCC, Summary for Policymakers. In *Climate Change: Mitigation. Contribution of Working Group III to the Fourth Assessment Report of the Intergovernmental Panel on Climate Change;* Metz, B., Davidson, O. R., Bosch, P. R., Dave, R., Meyer, L. A. Eds., Cambridge University Press: Cambridge, United Kingdom and New York, NY, USA; 2007b.
Jensen, C. H.; Urness, P. J. Winter Cold Damage to Bitterbrush Related to Spring Sheep Grazing. *J. Range Manage* **1979,** *32*, 214–216.
Jochum, G. M.; Mudge, K. W.; Richard, B. T. Elevated Temperatures Increase Leaf Senescence and Root Secondary Metabolite Concentrations in the Understory Herb Panax Quinquefolius (Araliaceae). *Am. J. Bot.* **2007,** *94*(5), 819–826.
Júlio, M. M. et al. The Effects of Seasonal Climate Changes in the Caatinga on Tannin Levels in Myracrodruon Urundeuva (Engl.) Fr. All. and Anadenanthera Colubrina (Vell.) Brenan. *J. Pharmacognosy.* **2006,** *16*(3), 338–344.
Kala, C. P. Medicinal Plants Conservation and Enterprise Development. *Med. Plants* **2009,** *1*(2), 79–95.
Keutgen, N.; Chen, K.; Lenz, F. Responses of Strawberry Leaf Photosynthesis, Chlorophyll Fluorescence and Macronutrient Contents to Elevated Co2. *J. Plant Physiol.* **1997,** *150*, 395–400.

King, A.; Young, G. Characteristics and Occurrence of Phenolic Phytochemicals. *J. Am. Diet. Assoc.* **1999,** *24*, 213–218.

Larcher, W. *Physiology Plant Ecology*; Springer-Verlag: Berlin 1980.

Laude, H. M. In *Effect of Temperature on Morphogenesis as the Basis for Scientific Management of Range Resources*, Proceeding of the Workshop of the United States-Australia Rangelands Panel, March 29 April 5, 1971; Berkeley, C. A., Dep Agr Misc Publ No. *1271*: U.S., 1974.

Leonardo, L.; Borges; Suzana F; Alves; Maria TF; Bara; Edemilson C; Conceiçao; Levitt J.; Responses of Plants to Environmental Stress.; Vol 2, Water, Radiation, Salt and Other Stresses, Academic Press: New York, 1980.

Litvak, M. E.; Constable, J. V.; Monson, R. K. Supply and Demand Processes as Controls Over Needle Mononterpene Synthesis and Concentration in Douglas Fir [Pseudotsuga menziesii (Mirb.) Franco]. *Oecologia* **2002,** *132*, 382–391.

Mathai, K. Nutrition in the Adult Years. In *Krause's Food, Nutrition, and Diet Therapy;* 10th ed., Mahan, L.K. Escott-Stump, S. Eds.; Saunders: USA, 2000; 271, 274–275.

Meagher, E.; Thomson, C. Vitamin and Mineral Therapy. In *Medical Nutrition and Disease*, 2nd ed.; Morrison, G., Hark, L., Eds.' Blackwell Science Inc.: Malden, Massachusetts, 1999; 33–58.

Miller, R. F.; Findley, R. R.; Alderfer-Findley, J. Changes in Mountain Big Sagebrush Habitat Types Following Spray Release. *J. Range Manage* 1980, *33*, 278–181.

Mooney, H. A.; Winner, W. E.; Pell, E. J. *Response of Plants to Multiple Stresses;* Academic Press: San Diego, California, USA, 1991.

Narasinga, R. Bioactive Phytochemicals in Indian Foods and Their Potential in Health Promotion and Disease Prevention. *Asia Pac J. Clin. Nutr.* **2003,** *12*(1), 9–22.

Nautiyal, M. C.; Nautiyal, B. P.; Prakash, V. Effect of Grazing and Climatic Changes on Alpine Vegetation of Tungnath, Garhwal Himalaya, India. *Environ.* **2004,** *24*(2), 125–134.

Ncube, B.; Finnie, J. F.; van Staden, J. Quality From the Field: the Impact of Environmental Factors as Quality Determinants in Medicinal Plants. *South Afr. J. Bot.* **2012,** *82*, 11–20.

Padda, M. S.; Picha, D. H. Effect of Low Temperature Storage on Phenolic Composition and Antioxidant Activity of Sweet Potatoes. *Postharvest Biol. Technol.* **2008,** *47*, 176–180.

Panigrahy, S.; Anitha, D.; Kimothi, M. M.; Singh, S. P. Timberline Change Detection Using Topographic Map and Satellite Imagery. *Tropl. Ecol.* **2010,** *51*, 87–91.

Parmesan, C.; Yohe, G. A. Globally Coherent Fingerprint of Climate Change Impacts Across Natural Systems. *Nature* **2003,** *421*, 37–42.

Risser, P. G. In. *Physiological Ecology of North American Plant Communities*; Chabot, B. F., Mooney, H. A. Eds., Chapman and Hall: New York, 1985; 232–256.

Root, T. L.; Price, J. T.; Hall, K. R.; Schneider, S. H.; Rosenzweig, C.; Pounds, A. Fingerprints of Global Warming on Wild Animals and Plants. *Nature* **2003,** *421*, 57–60.

Salick, J.; Fangb, Z.; Byg, A. Eastern Himalayan Alpine Plant Ecology, Tibetan Ethnobotany, and Climate Change. *Global. Environ. Chang.* **2009,** *19*(2), 147–155.

Scifres, C. J. *Brush Management Principles and Practices for Texas and Southwest;* Texas A&M University Press: College Station, 1980.

Slatyer, R. O. In *Effects of Water Stress on Plant Morphogenesis, plant morphogenesis as the basis for scientific management of range resources,* Proceedings of the workshop of the United State- Australia rangelands panel, March 29-April 5, 1971; Krietlow, K. W., Hart, R. H., Berkey, C. A. Eds., Dep. Agr. Misc. Publ. No. 1271: U.S. 1974. P. 3–13.

Smith, D. Winter Injury and the Survival of Forage plants. *Herb. Abstr.* **1964,** *34*, 203–209.

Smith, D. Light Quality, Photoperception, and Plant Strategy. *Ann. Rev. Plant Physiol.* **1982,** *33*, 481–518.

Snow, M. D.; Bard, R. R.; Olszyk, D. M.; Minster, L. M.; Hager, A. N.; Tingey, D. T. Monoterpene Levels in Needles of Douglas Fir Exposed to Elevated CO2 and Temperature. *Physiol. Plantarum* **2003,** *117*, 352–358.

Stickney, P. F. Note on Winter Crown Kill of Ceanothus Velutinus. *Proc. Montana Academy Sci.* **1965,** *25*, 52–57.

Van Epps, G. W. Winter Injury to Fourwing Saltbush. *J. Range Manage* **1975,** *28*, 157–159.

Vinesh, K.; Devendra, T. Phytochemical Screening and Free-Radical Scavenging Activity of Bergenia Stracheyi. *J. Pharmacogn. Phytochem.* **2013,** *2*(2), 175–180.

Vinesh, K.; Yogita, S.; Sanyogita, C. Impact of Climate Change on the Growth and Production of Saccharum Officinarum and Magnifera Indica. I.J.S.T.M. **2011,** *2*(1), 42–47.

Yang, J. X.; Tian, Y. X. Medicinal Plant Cultivation. China Agriculture Press: Beijing, China, 2004.

Yang, M. H.; Lu, J.; Xiang, C. Z.; Yao, H. W. Soil Environmental Quality and Gap of Chinese Herbal Medicines. *China J. Chin. Mater. Med.* **2001,** *26*(8), 514–516.

CHAPTER 14

PHYTOCHELATINS AND HEAVY METAL TOLERANCE IN PLANTS

MARIA CATHERINE B. OTERO[1] and GENEVIEVE D. TUPAS[2,*]

[1] *College of Medicine Research Center, Davao Medical School Foundation, Inc., Davao City, Philippines.*

[2] *Department of Pharmacology, College of Medicine, Davao Medical School Foundation Inc., Davao City, Philippines, Tel.: +639175351638*

[*]Corresponding author. E-mail: gentupas@email.dmsf.edu.ph; ORCID: https://orcid.org/0000-0001-9322-2478

ABSTRACT

Heavy metal tolerance is an adaptation of plants to the terrestrial environment. Since most plants rely on the soil for nutrients and water, mechanisms to neutralize the effects of leached heavy metals on plant metabolism evolved. Chelation by heavy metal-binding ligands is the most common way plants respond to heavy metal toxicity. Phytochelatins (PCs) are cysteine-rich peptide ligands found in plants and yeast that bind and sequester toxic metal ions into vacuoles to detoxify the plant cells. Mounting evidence suggests that numerous plants are able to produce PCs. However, constitutively expressed PC synthase (PCs)-like genes were also reported in certain animals, but there is no evidence of animal gene products with PC functions, suggesting roles other than PC biosynthesis. PCs, glutathione, and O-acetyl-L-serine influence hyperaccumulation of heavy metals in certain plants. The ability of plants to clean up heavy metals from the soil and water contributes to phytoremediation in metal contaminated areas.

14.1 INTRODUCTION

There are several ways by which plants respond and adapt to heavy metal toxicity. These include exclusion, immobilization, activation of the general stress response in plants, and chelation and sequestration of metal ions (Cobbett, 2000). Among these responses, the most common is chelation of metal-binding ligands, and in certain cases, the localization of the resulting ligand–metal complex in the vacuole.

Metal-binding ligands include organic acids such as citrate and malate, and the peptides ligands (Cobbett, 2000). PCs are analogous to metallothioneins (MT), a class of metal-binding proteins, in terms of functions, but differ entirely in the structure and biosynthesis. MTs are expressed by the cell, while PCs are synthesized enzymatically and are not encoded in the plant genome. Bacteria and other prokaryotic cells produce MTs similar to mammalian MTs, but not PCs. PCs offer an advantage over MTs in metal binding since PCs also possess strong reactive oxygen species (ROS) scavenging activities (Tsuji et al., 2002).

There are two general characteristics of PCs. First, PCs are synthesized only when the plant cells are exposed to metal ions such as Cu^{2+}, Pb^{2+}, Zn^{2+}, and Ag^{+} and are thus heavy metal-inducible. Second, PCs are capable of binding to more than one type of metal or metalloid, hence, it is not very specific to a particular heavy metal.

14.1.1 PHYTOCHELATIN (PC) STRUCTURE

PCs are cysteine-rich peptides found in plants and yeast that bind and sequester toxic metal ions. The term was coined by Grill et al. (1985) when they found peptides with $(\gamma\text{-Glu-Cys})_n$-Gly general structure in plants exposed to Cd^{2+}, with variations only in the number of γ-Glu-Cys (γ-EC) repeats, denoted by *n* (Grill et al., 1985). PCs generally have the range 2–5, but studies have shown that the number of γ-EC repeats can go as high as 11 (Cobbett, 2000).

Table 14.1 list the general structure of PC and its variants. PC-like peptides have been reported in certain yeast species, where the glycine at the C-terminal was replaced by des-glycine. Other PC variants have been characterized as well, and differ from PC because the terminal glycine is replaced by either alanine, glutamate, serine, or glutamine. Homophytochelatins derived from homoglutathione were reported in several plants from the family Fabaceae and have the general formula of $(\gamma\text{-Glu-Cys})_n$-Ala. Iso-phytochelatins found in maize have glutamate instead of the terminal glycine, while those found in horseradish substituted the terminal glycine with glutamine. Hydroxymethyl-phytochelatins in plants from the Gramineae family have serine instead of the terminal glycine (Inouhe, 2005).

TABLE 14.1 General Structure of Phytochelatins and their Variants.

Type	General structure
Phytochelatin	$(\gamma\text{-Glu-Cys})_n$-Gly
Homophytochelatin	$(\gamma\text{-Glu-Cys})_n$-Ala
Iso-phytochelatin	$(\gamma\text{-Glu-Cys})_n$-Glu or
	$(\gamma\text{-Glu-Cys})_n$-Gln
Hydroxymethyl-phytochelatin	$(\gamma\text{-Glu-Cys})_n$-Ser

14.1.2 FUNCTIONS OF PCs

PCs relieve heavy metal stress and detoxify the plant cells in the presence of glutathione (GSH). Many other cellular processes are mediated by GSH, and elevated GSH levels alone do not always predict enhanced heavy metal tolerance (Xiang et al., 2001). In cyanobacteria, which are the ancestors of chloroplasts in plants, antioxidant activities are mainly carried out by GSH (Yadav, 2010).

PC and PC-related peptides have been reported in plants and yeast. Mounting evidence suggests that numerous plants are able to produce PCs. Based on expressed sequence tags, it is clear that phytochelatin synthase (PCS) genes can be found in all higher plants (angiosperms, gymnosperms, and bryophytes). PCS genes were also found to be expressed constitutively, suggesting roles other than PC biosynthesis (Yadav, 2010). PCS-like genes were also reported in the nematodes, roundworms, and schistosomes (Inouhe, 2005), but there is no evidence of animal gene products with PC functions (Cobbett, 2000).

14.1.3 PC BIOSYNTHESIS

GSH and PC biosynthesis overlap because GSH acts as a direct substrate in PC formation. PCs are non-translationally formed from the reduced form of GSH by transpeptidation, which is catalyzed by the PCS (Yadav, 2010).

The steps in PC biosynthesis are shown in Figure 14.1. First, the γ-glutamylcysteinesynthetase (γ-EC synthetase, γECS) mediates the formation of the γ-glutamylcysteine from cysteine and glutamate. The γ-ECS acts as the rate-limiting step and its activity is enhanced by Cd^{2+}. The next step is catalyzed by GSH synthetase, which adds a glycine to the γ-EC to form GSH. Lastly, the PCS (formerly called the γ-glutamylcysteine dipeptidyl transpeptidase) sequentially adds the γ-EC units of the GSH to form PCs (Cobbett, 2000; Inouhe, 2005). Cd^{2+} was found to be the best activator of PCS, followed by Ag^{+}, Bi^{3+}, Pb^{2+}, Zn^{2+}, Cu^{2+}, Hg^{+}, and Au^{+}. PC biosynthesis is regulated through a negative feedback mechanism, where the PC produced chelates the activating metal ions to terminate the reaction (Cobbett, 2000).

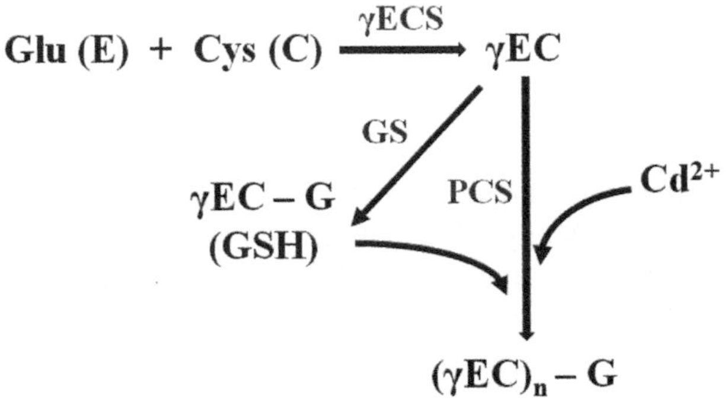

FIGURE 14.1 Glutathione-dependent synthesis of phytochelatins.

14.2 HEAVY METAL TOLERANCE IN PLANTS

The soil is the major sink of heavy metals that may come from various industrial and agricultural applications and the natural geochemical cycle (Wuana and Okieimen, 2011), and in order to survive, plants must respond to this environmental stress. The most common heavy metals in contaminated soils include arsenic (As), lead (Pb), zinc, (Zn), chromium (Cr), cadmium (Cd), mercury (Hg), nickel (Ni), and copper (Cu) (Evanko and David, 1997). Although normally found in low levels, anthropogenic activities catalyze the accumulation of heavy metals in soils. These activities include, but are not limited to, sewage sludge, use of fertilizers, emissions from machines and factories, metal mining, and metal smelting (Yadav, 2010). Because heavy metals are resistant to chemical or microbial degradation, they can persist in soils for a very long time, only changing their chemical forms and bioavailability (Kirpichtchikova et al., 2006; Adriano, 2003). Most plants rely on the soil for nutrients and water and so mechanisms to neutralize the effects of leached heavy metals on plant metabolism evolved. Thus, heavy metal tolerance is postulated to be an adaptation of plants to the terrestrial environment (Inouhe, 2005).

14.2.1 EFFECT OF HEAVY METALS ON PLANTS

Certain heavy metals and metalloids are essential for plants and animals. Copper, molybdenum, manganese, iron, zinc, and nickel are required for optimal growth and development of higher plants. Arsenic, lead, cadmium, and tin are also necessary, but in very low concentrations (Alloway, 2013). Once the concentrations of these heavy metals go above the threshold and accumulate in the cells, they can lead to toxicity in the plant cells since metals cannot be metabolized.

In general, once the plant is exposed to excess heavy metals, the cells experience oxidative stress and ROS are generated. Excess ROS in the cells can induce oxidation and consequent modification of membrane lipids, proteins and cellular amino acids, and DNA (Yadav, 2010). When not resolved, the ionic homeostasis will be disturbed and cellular damage can ensue (Singh et al., 2011; Demiral and Turkan, 2005). Indirect consequences of increased heavy metal concentration in the plant include the substitution of essential nutrients, effects on growth of beneficial microorganisms, and decreased soil fertility (Alloway, 2013). Taken together, both the direct and indirect consequences of high heavy metal concentration in plants will result in decreased plant growth and eventually, plant death (Fig. 14.2).

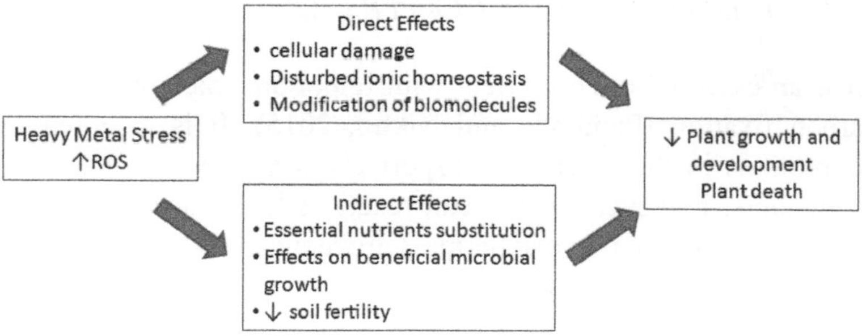

FIGURE 14.2 Consequences of heavy metal stress in plants.

Here we discuss the effects of elevated levels of specific heavy metals in the development of plants.

14.2.1.1 EFFECT OF EXCESS CADMIUM (CD)

Plants growing beyond the permissible limit of 100-mg cadmium level for every 1 kg of soil already show signs and symptoms of cellular injury such as browning of root tips, chlorosis, inhibition of growth, and death (Mohanpuria et al., 2007). Excess Cd interferes with transport, utilization, as well as uptake of water and Mg, K, Ca, and K by plants. It also alters the activity of the plant enzymes in the root and shoot, such as Fe(III) reductase, nitrate reductase, and even ATPases. Additionally, lipid peroxidation of the cell membrane is induced and chlorophyll biosynthesis is inhibited (Asati et al., 2016).

14.2.1.2 EFFECT OF EXCESS LEAD (PB)

One of the most abundant heavy metal in the soil is lead. Its effects on plants in excess concentrations may include morphology, plant growth, and photosynthesis disruption. Lead toxicity can result in interference with enzyme activity. This eventually causes inhibition of stem and root elongation, inhibition of leaf expansion, and induction of abnormal morphology, such as radial thickening and lignifications. In corn, lead was found to reduce the percentage of germination, suppress plant growth, reduce biomass, and decrease in protein content of plant cells (Asati et al., 2016).

14.2.1.3 EFFECTS OF EXCESS COPPER (CU)

Copper is an essential micronutrient with important roles in ATP synthesis and carbon fixation (Pichhode and Nikhil, 2015). It is also required in various proteins in the electron transport chain and the photosystems. In excess amounts, however, copper can result in leaf chlorosis and growth retardation. Seed production and biomass are reduced, as well as root growth (Yadav, 2010). Copper mostly accumulates in the roots. In tomato, the enzyme activities of guaiacol peroxidases, catalase, and polyphenol oxidase increased in response to increasing Cu. At higher concentrations of Cu, enzyme activities decreased, suggesting that other detoxification systems are already in place (Martins and Mourato, 2006).

14.2.1.4 EFFECTS OF EXCESS ARSENIC (AS)

Inorganic As in the form of arsenate or arsenite is easily taken up by plants. Arsenic competes directly with phosphate for the root plasmalemma uptake (Yadav, 2010). Besides transport, other phosphate-dependent pathways in metabolism can also be affected. Once As is translocated to the shoots, it can inhibit biomass accumulation and expansion and overall plant growth. Arsenic can also negatively affect plant reproduction by reducing fruit production and fertility (Garg and Singla, 2011). Certain plant species are able to tolerate increased As in the soil. In grasses, for example, As tolerance develops when the high-affinity phosphate/arsenic uptake system is suppressed. In this way, the influx of As is reduced so that the plant is detoxified through constitutive mechanisms (Meharg, 1994).

14.2.2 MECHANISMS OF HEAVY METAL TOLERANCE

Tolerance to various heavy metals can be achieved in several ways. One is to sequester the heavy metals into vacuoles, which was documented in plants and yeast. Sequestration of PCs to the vacuole was observed in tobacco plants in response to excess cadmium, where almost all of the Cd and low and high molecular weight PC–Cd complexes were localized in the vacuole. The transport of these complexes to the vacuolar membrane is through an ATP-dependent, protein gradient-independent transporter (Cobbett, 2000). Another mechanism is to pump the heavy metals out of the cell membrane, as in the proton gradient-dependent Cd/H^+ antiporter. Last is to chelate the toxic metals and bind them to thiol compounds that are found in the cytosol like GSH (Yadav, 2010).

Genetic manipulations in PC synthesis and GSH-related genes in plants have allowed investigations about tolerance in various heavy metals. Mishra et al. (2006) have shown that Pb tolerance is also mediated by PCs in coontail plants. However, overproduction of PCs may deplete GSH, and cause oxidative stress. Inorganic arsenic also induced PC synthesis in vitro and in intact land plants.

14.3 METAL HYPERACCUMULATION AND PHYTOREMEDIATION

14.3.1 HYPERACCUMULATOR PLANTS

There are over 400 species of plants that can hyperaccumulate trace metals, metalloids, and nonmetals in their shoots and more than 100 of these are heavy metal hyperaccumulators (Yadav, 2010). The plant family Brassicaceae accounts for the most number of metal hyperaccumulators, with 87 species across 11 genera showing activity against Ni, Zn, Cd, and Pb (Prasad and

Freitas, 2003). Five fern species from the family Pteridaceae have been found to be arsenic hyperaccumulators: *Pteris vittata, Pteris cretica, Pteris longifolia, Pteris umbrosa,* and *Pityrogramma calomelanos* (Meharg, 2002). The brake fern, *P. vittata*, can carry more than 20,000 mg/kg per dry weight of its fronds.

This ability of certain plants to store a large amount of metals coming from its environment highlights their potential in biogeochemical prospecting and phytoremediation. However, leached metals coming from exudates of hyperaccumulator plants can have a detrimental effect on the growth of neighboring plants (Prasad and Freitas, 2003). The safety of human consumption of these special plants is also an important issue that must not be overlooked and should be regulated.

14.3.2 PHYTOREMEDIATION

Hyperaccumulation of metals in certain plant species has been taken advantage in plant-based remediation of contaminated sites or phytoremediation. There are four mechanisms involved in phytoremediation in water, sediment, or soil: rhizofiltration, phytostabilization, phytovolatilization, and phytoextraction (Prasad and Freitas, 2003). These mechanisms depend largely on the bioavailability of the metals in the target site. But because of the slow speed at which contaminated sites can be cleaned by hyperaccumulators, whether genetically engineered or naturally occurring, phytoremediation is considered as a long-term solution.

14.4 BIOMARKERS FOR METAL HYPERACCUMULATION

In addition to PC and GSH, the levels of the cysteine intermediate O-acetyl-L-serine had been strongly correlated to metal hyperaccumulation in certain plants (Yadav, 2010). Hyperaccumulator plants possess long-distance transport systems for metals through the transpiration stream. This apoplastic route carries heavy metals from the roots to the shoots. This ability to suck out metals from the soil and water is said to contribute to phytoremediation in metal contaminated areas (Inouhe, 2005). Overexpression of the GSH1 gene was found to be a promising strategy in producing transgenic plants that have highly efficient Cd phytoremediation capacities (Yadav, 2010).

PCs and PC-related peptides can potentially be used as biochemical indicators of heavy metal contamination. Roots and shoots are sensitive to various metals, as influenced by the rapid changes in the levels of PCs, GSH, and cysteine. These changes can be harnessed to quantify heavy metal contamination in habitats. (Inouhe, 2005). But other less understood mechanisms for metal detoxification may affect such biochemical changes, interpretation must be made with caution.

KEYWORDS

- **phytochelatins**
- **heavy metal tolerance**
- **phytoremediation**
- **hyperaccumulation**
- **plants**

REFERENCES

Adriano, D. C. *Trace Elements in Terrestrial Environments: Biogeochemistry, Bioavailability, and Risks of Metals*, 2nd ed.; Springer: New York, USA, **2003**.

Alloway, B. J. Heavy Metals and Metalloids as Micronutrients for Plants and Animals. In *Heavy Metals in Soils;* Alloway, B., Ed.; Springer: Netherlands, 2013; 195–209.

Asati, A.; Pichhode, M.; Nikhil, K. Effect of Heavy Metals on Plants: An Overview. *Int. J. Appl. Innovation Eng. Manage* **2016,** *5*(3), 2319–2325.

Cobbett, C. S. Phytochelatins and their Roles in Heavy Metal Detoxification. *Plant Physiol.* **2000,** *123*(3), 825–832.

Demiral, T.; Türkan, I. Comparative Lipid Peroxidation, Antioxidant Defense Systems and Proline Content in Roots of Two Rice Cultivars Differing in Salt Tolerance. *Environ. Exp. Bot.* **2005,** *53*(3), 247–257.

Evanko, C. R.; Dzombak, D. A. Remediation of Metals-Contaminated Soils and Groundwater. Ground-Water Remediation Technologies Analysis Center: Pittsburg, USA, 1997.

Garg, N.; Singla, P. Arsenic Toxicity in Crop Plants: Physiological Effects and Tolerance Mechanisms. *Environ. Chem. Lett.* **2011,** *9*(3), 303–321.

Grill, E.; Winnacker, E. L.; Zenk, M. H. Phytochelatins: The Principal Heavy-Metal Complexing Peptides of Higher Plants. *Science* **1985,** *230,* 674–677.

Inouhe, M. Phytochelatins. *Braz. J. Plant Physiol.* **2005,** *17*(1), 65–78.

Kirpichtchikova, T. A.; Manceau, A.; Spadini, L.; Panfili, F.; Marcus, M. A;. Jacquet, T. Speciation and Solubility of Heavy Metals in Contaminated Soil Using X-ray Microfluorescence, EXAFS Spectroscopy, Chemical Extraction, and Thermodynamic Modeling. *Geochim. Cosmochim. Acta* **2006,** *70*(9), 2163–2190.

Martins, L. L.; Mourato, M. P. Effect of Excess Copper on Tomato Plants: Growth Parameters, Enzyme Activities, Chlorophyll, and Mineral Content. *J. Plant Nutr.* **2006,** *29*(12), 2179–2198.

Meharg, A. A. Integrated Tolerance Mechanisms: Constitutive and Adaptive Plant Responses to Elevated Metal Concentrations in the Environment. *Plant Cell Environ.* **1994,** *17*(9), 989–993.

Meharg, A. A. Arsenic and Old Plants. *New Phytol.* **2002,** *156,* 1–8.

Mishra, S.; Srivastava, S.; Tripathi, R. D.; Kumar, R.; Seth, C. S.; Gupta, K. Lead Detoxification by Coontail (*Ceratophyllum demersum* L.) Involves Induction of Phytochelatins and Antioxidant System in Response to its Accumulation. *Chemosphere* **2006,** *65*(6), 1027–1039.

Mohanpuria, P.; Rana, N. K.; Yadav, S. K. Cadmium Induced Oxidative Stress Influence on Glutathione Metabolic Genes of *Camellia sinensis* (L.). O Kuntze. *Environ. Toxicol.* **2007,** *22,* 368–374.

Pichhode, M.; Nikhil, K. Effect of Copper Mining Dust on the Soil and Vegetation in India: A Critical Review. *Int. J. Mod. Sci. Eng. Technol. (IJMSET)* **2015,** *2,* 73–76.

Prasad, M. N. V.; Freitas, H. M. de O. Metal Hyperaccumulation in Plants–Biodiversity Prospecting for Phytoremediation Technology. *Electron. J. Biotechnol.* **2003,** *6*(3), 285–321.

Singh, R.; Gautam, N.; Mishra, A.; Gupta, R. Heavy Metals and Living Systems: An Overview. *Indian J. Pharmacol.* **2011,** *43*(3), 246.

Tsuji, N.; Hirayanagi, N.; Okada, M.; Miyasaka, H.; Hirata, K.; Zenk, M.; Miyamoto, K. Enhancement of Tolerance to Heavy Metals and Oxidative Stress in *Dunaliella tertiolecta* by Zn-Induced Phytochelatin Synthesis. *Biochem. Biophys. Res. Commun.* **2002,** *293*(1), 653–659.

Wuana, R. A.; Okieimen, F. E. Heavy Metals in Contaminated Soils: A Review of Sources, Chemistry, Risks and Best Available Strategies for Remediation. *ISRN Ecol.* **2011**, Article ID 402647, 1–20. http://dx.doi.org/10.5402/2011/402647.

Xiang, C.; Werner, B.; Christensen, E.; Oliver, D. The Biological Functions of Glutathione Revisited in *Arabidopsis* Transgenic Plants with Altered Glutathione Levels. *Plant Physiol.* **2001,** *126*(2), 564–574.

Yadav, S. K. Heavy Metals Toxicity in Plants: An Overview on the Role of Glutathione and Phytochelatins in Heavy Metal Stress Tolerance of Plants. *S. Afr. J. Botany* **2010,** *76*(2), 167–179.

CHAPTER 15

PHYTOCHEMICAL BIOPESTICIDES

OLUMAYOWA VINCENT ORIYOMI

Institute of Ecology and Environmental Studies, Obafemi Awolowo University, Ile-Ife, Osun State, Nigeria, Tel.: +2347031245211, E-mail: yomiyowa@gmail.com.

ORCID: http://orcid.org/0000-0002-2438-6740.

ABSTRACT

Alarming pest infestation leading to food shortage and the corresponding food demand resulting in the indiscriminate application of synthetic pesticides has raised global concerns on food security and environmental safety. Phytochemical biopesticides have been used as repellents, antifeedants, fungicides, herbicides, nematicides, molluscicides, and insecticides among others. Phytochemicals form an interesting group of bioactive compounds which are generally slow in action as plant protectants but safer on the environment and humans as compared to synthetic pesticides. Plant species which belong to families of Solanaceae, Labiatae, Euphorbiaceae, Asteraceae, Meliaceae, and Fabaceae are peculiar among over 2000 plants with secondary metabolites having insecticidal properties. Currently, drawing interests are species of the Araceae family. Plant metabolites (phytochemicals) with most important insecticidal activities are alkaloids, flavonoids, phenols, steroids, and terpenoids. This chapter underlines the unique properties and prospects of phytochemical biopesticides as potential alternatives to synthetic pesticides in the control of agricultural pests.

15.1 INTRODUCTION

World's population has been estimated to surge by 38.57% from 6.134 billion to 8.5 billion inhabitants by 2025 with a significant growth rate in the developing countries (Agrios, 1997). This will inevitably require an additional agricultural production to meet the impending monstrous population growth. Economic history provides us with ample of evidences that agricultural revolution is a veritable ingredient for economic growth especially in developing nations (Izuchukwu, 2011). Agriculture is among the major pillars capable of sustaining any economy. Two-third of today's world population depend on agriculture for livelihood, but nowadays, growth and production of agricultural crops are hampered daily by pests among several other limiting factors (FAO, 2014).

Insect pest is any insect in the wrong place. They are considered pests whenever they are in competition with humans for resources and are present in significant numbers (William and Robert, 1994). Agricultural pest species that damage crops are estimated at 67,000 by Kumar (2015). Insect pests inflict damage on humans, farm animals, and crops. Also, pests damage important agricultural foods as well as their products in godowns, bins, and stores, causing huge physical deterioration and economic losses to stored foods (Oonagh and Paul, 2009). In the world, food availability is adversely affected by insects and pests during growth and post-harvest periods (Kulkarni et al., 2009). Annually, one-fifth of the world's total crop production is damaged by herbivorous insect pests. About 67,000 agricultural pest population has been estimated to be involved in crop damage.

One major factor responsible for pest multiplication is the creation of altered habitats particularly in the tropical and sub-tropical zones, where favorable climate provides a viable environmental atmosphere for a broad range of insect activities and survival (Kfir, 1997). The artificial agroecosystems created fulfill man's needs by providing selected crops with large sizes, high yield, and nutritious value clustered in a confined area. The system satisfies man's demands for agricultural crop production and in the process provides a suitable environment for herbivorous insects (Kerin, 1994). Pests are capable of developing to biotypes capable of beginning new lives and adjust to new situations, for instance, they can become resistant to numerous control measures and agents, thereby escalating the problem of pest infestation. In underdeveloped countries, the menace of pest infestation is further complicated with a rapid annual increase in human population (2.5–3.0%) in comparison to a 1% increase in food production (William and Robert, 1994). Efforts to salvage problems caused by pest infestation have caused the use of pesticides to rise over the years.

Pesticides are defined as natural or synthetic agents capable of killing an unwanted plant or animal pests. They are referred to as substances or mixture of substances intended for preventing, destroying, or controlling pests including vectors of human or animal diseases, harmful species of plants or animals which interfere with production/processing, storage and marketing of food, agricultural commodities, wood and wood products, or animal feeds, or agricultural product that may be administered to animals to control pests inside or outside of their bodies (FAO, 1989). A pesticide is also defined as chemical formulated to combat activities of pests and disease vectors on domestic animals, agricultural crops, and human beings (WHO/UNEP, 1990). The term pesticide includes chemicals applied as growth regulators, defoliants, desiccants, fruit-thinning agents, or chemical agents which are used for preventing premature fall of fruits or substances applied to crops either before or after harvest to prevent deterioration during storage and transport or on animals to control pest infestation and growth retardation. All the definitions stated above show that chemical pesticides (organic) are toxic agents which are used to eliminate or at least reduce insect pest population in other to ensure food availability and security.

Insecticides such as miticides, avicides, defoliants, bactericides, algaecides, piscicides, desiccants, nematicides, herbicides, rodenticides, fungicides, and so on are common examples of pesticides. Unknowingly to some, chemical pesticides have only recently become popular; it was the naturally occurring compounds or extracts that were used as pesticides in ancient times. The earliest pesticides were salt, sulfurous rock, extracts of tobacco, red pepper, and the like. The Napoleonic army was rumored to have applied ground chrysanthemums to combat lice with limited effectiveness. Petroleum oils and other heavy metals were used as natural agents to control pests in the 1940s. They were then replaced for use by heavy synthetic pesticides; the most famous of the synthetic pesticides was dichlorodiphenyltrichloroethane (DDT, $C_{14}H_9Cl_5$). It is noteworthy that pesticides exclude chemicals used as fertilizers, plant and animal nutrients, food additives, and animal drugs. Generally, chemical pesticides are highly toxic, very persistent in the environment, and have residues which are harmful and can contaminate crops, food commodities and also pollute soil and groundwater. According to World Health Organization, the human death toll of about 20,000 people is attributed annually to pesticide poisoning in the third world countries (Casida and Quistad, 2000). Synthetic pesticides adversely affect nontarget organisms such as pollinators, fish, birds, and animals. The indiscriminate and excessive use of synthetic chemicals has resulted in increased resistance to pests. Phytochemicals/biopesticides, on the other hand, are less toxic, least persistent, environment-friendly, and safe to humans and nontarget organisms (Walia et al., 2017). There are interests on phytochemical pesticide due to concerns on a rampant supply of synthetic pesticide and its irreversible impact on the environment and human health at large. Also, its presence in the food web is quite worrisome (Anupam et al., 2012).

According to reports although with developments still in infancy but fast gaining huge attention is the modern approach to pest control involving nanotechnology (science that uses materials having 10^{-9} m size) application. The technology uses nanoparticles (NPs) like mesoporous silica NPs, porous hollow silica NPs, silica NPs, and so on, as nanobiopesticides in biological pest management (Popat et al., 2012). In this process, materials prepared from noble metals such as gold, silver, and platinum or metal oxidase materials (TiO_2, ZnO, AgO, MgO), ceramics, semiconductors, silicates, magnetic materials, lipids, polymers, emulsions, dendrites, and quantum dots are used as NPs. The technology encapsulates bioactive compounds with NPs to form nanobiopesticides used to control pests. NPs possess insecticidal property due to their numerous unique characteristics such as:

1. Extraordinary strength
2. High chemical reactivity
3. High electrical conductivity and optical properties
4. Distinct physical, chemical, and biological properties associated with high atomic strength
5. Specific maintenance of size and shape
6. Size–depth qualities
7. High surface-to-volume ratio
8. High stability
9. An ordered layer of particles arrangement due to hydrogen bonding, dipole forces, hydrophilic and hydrophobic interaction, surface tension, and gravity
10. Slow release and high efficiency on host plant capable of deterring insect attack
11. Higher mobility and lower toxicity
12. High pest specificity and effectiveness
13. High self-assemblage stability, specificity, encapsulation, and biocompatibility (Wang et al., 2009)

15.2 PHYTOCHEMICAL PESTICIDES

Phytochemicals (botanicals) are secondary metabolites which majorly perform the role of defense mechanism and help plants withstand continuous selection pressure from herbivorous predators and other environmental factors (Sarkar and Kshirsagar, 2014). Phytochemical pesticides are naturally slow-acting agents or crop protectants; they are usually safer to the environment as well as to humans than the conventional pesticides with minimal residual effects. Moreover, plant botanicals contain mixtures of biologically active substances which are able to prevent resistance buildup in pests and pathogens. Numerous investigations have established that biological activity is usually distributed in various parts of a plant though the degree of lethality of the active components may vary in these parts (Rajapake and Ratnaseka, 2008). The use of plant botanicals has now been more recommended as a capable substitute for plant protection with minimal negative effects (Isman, 2006). Literature revealed that about 2121 plant species possess pest management properties, out of these, 1005 plant species exhibit insecticidal properties. Among this population, 384 species exhibit antifeedant properties, 297 species show repellent properties while 27 species possess attractant properties and 31 species have growth-inhibiting properties (Gopalakrishnan et al., 2011). At present, the world's botanical pesticides are still at a meager 1% (Anupam et al., 2012).

15.3 ADVANTAGES OF PHYTOCHEMICAL PESTICIDE OVER SYNTHETIC PESTICIDE

Following are the advantages of phytochemical pesticide over synthetic pesticide:

1. Promotes sustainable agriculture: It does not cause a negative effect on crop plants, soil health, and environment. It presents a relatively low risk to beneficial predators and parasites (nontarget organisms).
2. Reduces crop losses: Several plant diseases/plant pathogens can be effectively managed by reducing disease incidence and related losses in the crop plants.
3. Eco-friendly: It does not cause ecological imbalance and fits in suitably in any agro-ecosystem. It is safer to humans and the environment than conventional pesticide as it presents no residue problems and does not persist in the environment.
4. Biodegradable: It rapidly degrades under the exposure of sunlight. It has limited field persistence and a short shelf life. It breaks down rapidly in the environment.
5. Organic farming: It suitably fits in the organic farming system as it is eco-friendly in nature.

6. Cheaper: It is cheaper when compared to synthetic pesticides.
7. Integrated pest management: It is easily included in the framework of integrated pest management routine.
8. Specificity in action: It has a narrow target range and a very specific mode of action.
9. Favorable application period: It has a relatively critical application time and suppresses, rather than eliminate pest population
10. Easy Metabolism: it is easily metabolized by animals receiving sub-lethal doses;
11. Easy Formulation: it has a broad spectrum of activity, and is easy to process and use.

15.4 LIMITATIONS OF PHYTOCHEMICAL BIOPESTICIDES

Following are the limitations of phytochemical biopesticides:

1. Phytochemical biopesticides are easily degraded in the field under high temperature, light, moisture, and pH. Their degradability reduces the availability of their active components.
2. As a result of earlier limitation, frequent application of botanicals is needed. This implies that cost of application will increase. Addition of cheap local materials such as gum arabic, egg white, and so forth, or commercial products and protectants of ultraviolet (UV) rays (e.g., soap water and antioxidants) to extend the residual efficacy of sprayed botanical solution have been suggested (Gahukar, 2010).
3. Operating rules for registration of phytochemical biopesticides are quite stringent and procedures involved are time consuming. The technical formalities prescribed for chemical pesticides are also prescribed for plant products. These procedures need be changed in the future to encourage easy formulations and registration of newer botanicals.
4. Presently, there is an inadequate awareness of the importance and value of patents (regulations provided by government agencies) on the use of phytochemical biopesticides (Gahukar, 2010).
5. Interdisciplinary expertise required for extraction, isolation, separation, purification, structural elucidation, bioassay, regulatory, and other related aspects is still inadequate.
6. Stabilizers, potentiators, UV screens, antioxidants, and other instruments are required to increase stability, shelf life, and residual life

of products; these will help to improve bioefficacy in botanicals in other to suppress resistance development in insects. However, these materials are scares and expensive.

7. Some plant species are indigenous only to a certain region(s). Some plants form a community of biodiversity which are valuable assets for the local people. Most times, plants having insecticidal properties are only abundant in few climatic zones and government protected areas which are un(der) exploited not only for traditional preparations but also for commercial formulations of botanicals. Such plant species are protected by forest rules and regulations against exploitation. These stringent biodiversity protection laws have included many plants in the red list and thus, provision of botanicals has greatly been impeded.
8. Processes involved in isolation, synthesis, and formulation, structural elucidation, bioassay, and others of phytochemicals are long and expensive (Jaglan et al., 1997).

15.5 SELECTION CRITERIA FOR PLANTS SOURCES OF BIOPESTICIDES

Dimetry (2014) prescribed the following criteria for consideration in selecting a plant for botanicals:

1. It should be a perennial plant.
2. The plant should have a broad distribution and be available in large numbers in nature or possibly be grown by agricultural procedures like tissue cultures and genetic engineering. Plant must be easy to replicate or regenerate.
3. Plant parts to be used should be removable: leaves, flowers, fruits, and so forth.
4. Harvesting does not mean total destruction of the plant (always avoid the use of roots or barks).
5. Plants should require small space to thrive and survive. It must be easy to manage and require little water and fertilization.
6. The plants could have additional uses (e.g., medicinal use).
7. The plants should not possess high economic value.
8. Their biologically active components should be effective at a low concentration.

15.6 EFFICACY OF SELECTED PHYTOCHEMICAL BIOPESTICIDES

Researchers have reported the efficacy of several botanicals extracted from plants. Examined below are some of these plants and their phytochemical constituents:

15.6.1 NEEM

Neem tree, scientifically known as *Azadirachta indica* is a good source of phytochemicals and more than 300 bioactive secondary compounds have been isolated from neem. Isolated bioactive chemicals include ketones, limonoids, phenolics, steroids, carotenoids, and enzymes (Rafiq et al., 2012). The chemistry, environmental behavior, and pesticidal effects of neem and neem products have been reported widely (Veitch et al., 2008). Laboratory tests indicated that neem-extract-based insecticides are effective against pest species with agricultural and environmental interests (Koul, 1999). Limonoid, known as tetranortriterpenoid, forms the major group of neem's secondary compounds such as azadirachtin, nimbin, nimbidin, salannin, and so forth (Govidachari et al., 1995). Reports have established that azadirachtin and its compounds possess high insecticidal activity. Neem has many biological properties such as low persistency in nature, low toxicity against nontarget organisms, and systemic action. Azadirachtin has been studied more than any other plant for botanicals and has received greater attention for biopesticide formulation than others because of its bioefficacy against insects (Prakash et al., 2002). Azadirachtin showed antifeedant effects on insects especially those belonging to Lepidoptera order have been found to be most susceptible to azadirachtin as compared to other orders like Coleoptera, Hemiptera, and Homoptera including caterpillars, pink bollworms, leafworms, beetles, gypsy moths, mushroom flies, and so forth, (Mordue and Blackwell, 1993). Azadirachtin influences hormonal coordination in insects which modifies the metamorphosis. It seems to act as "ecdysone blocker" that blocks the release of vital hormones, thereby inhibiting molting in insects and metamorphosis in general (Ascher, 1993). Azadirachtin limits feeding in insects leading to death (Thomson, 1992). Generally, the effects of azadirachtin depend on both dosage and time of application which prevent ecdysis and apolysis that lead to death during molting.

Natural neem has expressed notable anti-insecticidal activity against noctuid moths, leafworm (*Spodoptera litura*), *Peridroma saucia*, *Oncopeltus fasciatus*, leafhopper, *Jacobiasca lybica,* and whitefly (Sharma et al., 2003a, b). This broad range insecticidal activity is aided by neem's phago and oviposition deterrent, repellent, antifeedant, growth depressant, molting depressant, and sterilant properties. Products of neem prolong larval developmental times and prevent larval maturation (Mordue and Blackwell, 1993). Reports of broad insecticidal properties of neem on *Plutella xylostella, Pieris brassicae, Spodoptera littoralis,* and other pests are also well documented (Hasan and Ansari, 2011). High insecticidal activity was also demonstrated by extracts from neem seed kernel under field conditions against insect species of *Orthoptera, Lepidoptera,* and *Coleoptera*. Bioactive products of neem include azadirachtin, nimbinene, salannin, and nimbin. They act as systemic and contact poisons against pests (Koul et al., 1996). Insects differ markedly in their behavioral/physiological responses to azadirachtin/related compounds/neem extracts. Observed differences in physiological responses and toxicity to neem have been observed in *S. littoralis* (Lepidoptera), *O. fasciatus* (Hemiptera), *Schistocerca gregaria* (Orthoptera) (Aerts and Mordue, 1997). Lepidopteran insects show higher sensitivity to azadirachtin than the *Orthopoda*. Summation of neem's antifeedant and toxicity properties increase its efficacy insects. Malformation of *S. littoralis* at various developmental stages by azadirachtins has been confirmed by many authors (Nathan and Kalaivani, 2006). Inter-genus variation in term of effectiveness was also shown by different compounds of neem against Lepidopteran members, *Heliothis virescens* and *Helicoverpa armigera* (Blaney et al., 1990). Reports of interfamily variations of azadirachtin on *Noctuidae* members have been well documented. Inhibition of *S. litura* and *Actebia fennica* were less than other species (Isman, 1993). Nathan et al. (2005) reported growth and antifeedant inhibition activities of various neem products (azadirachtin, deacetylgedunin, salannin, gedunin, 17-hydroxyazadiradione, and deacetylnimbin) against the rice leaf folder and legume pod borer *H. armigera*. Apart from major tetranortriterpenoids (nimbin and salannin) of neem seeds, photo-oxidation products of tetranortriterpenoids such as nimbinolide, isonimbinolide, salanninolide, and isosalanninolide have also demonstrated anti-insect effects against *S. littoralis* (Jarvis et al., 1997). Extracts from neem seed kernel have a profound effect on rice leaf folder and sorghum shootfly *Atherigona soccata*. The effect of neem seed kernel extract (NSKE) was reported for potato tuber moth *Phthorimaea operculella*, *H. armigera*, and *Lampides boeticus* (Irulandi and Balasubramanian, 2000). Azadirachtin is the major active constituent of neem extracts, the effects of neem extracts could be due to the sum or synergy of azadirachtin and other terpenoids present in it (Martinez and Van Emden, 2001). The activity of azadirachtin in neem extracts is high, but non-azadirachtin compounds (e.g., 6-ß-hydroxygedunin or different volatiles from neem) isolated from *A. indica* also seem to be involved in the bioefficacy of neem (Koul et al., 2003).

Purified neem compound/formulation exhibits instability and produces negative effects on natural enemies, its role as a broad-spectrum insecticide at very low concentrations with residual properties and reduced resistance to pests has made these compounds important in insect pest management and commercialization in countries such as the United States, Canada, Mexico, European Union, and New Zealand and in Asian countries, such as India and China. Neem products are the most commercially important of plant species used in insect pest management (Schmutterer, 2002). Examples of commercially available neem products are the Wash Away Louse, Neemix, Neemazal, Tre-san, Neem Gold, Neem-EC, Margosan-O, Thai Neem 111, MiteStop, Picksan Louse Stop, and Neem Excel (Yule and Srinivasan, 2013). Their efficacies have been shown against various pests and insects.

15.6.2 ANNONA

Researches have shown *annonaceae* to be potent elicitors of insecticidal activities. All plant species in this family have toxic compounds such as flavonoids, acetogenins, and alkaloids that confer them insecticidal effects (Grzybowski et al., 2012). In the genus of annona, two species are known to have outstanding insecticidal properties; *Annona muricata* and *Annona squamosa*. The bioactive effects of *Annonaceous acetogenins* (ACGs) have been confirmed against species of insects like *Myzus persicae,* spider mites, mosquito larvae, striped cucumber beetles, melon aphids, Colorado potato beetles, Mexican bean beetles, bean leaf beetles, European corn borers, blowfly larvae, and free-living nematodes (Cólom et al., 2008). Extracts from annonaceous plants have been studied in several groups of agriculturally important insects. There is a similarity in the biological activity of acetogenins to that of limonoid azadirachtin isolated from *A. indica* (Mordue and Nisbet, 2000). Recent reports revealed ACGs are effective against store pests of grains. Extracts of *A. squamosa* and *Annona mucosa* have exhibited toxicity against *Tribolium castaneum* and *Sitophilus zeamais*, respectively (Ribeiro et al., 2013). Isoquinoline alkaloids are also associated with plant protection against herbivorous insect pests. Isoquinoline interacts with neural signal transduction and interfere with neuroreceptors through enzymes involved in neurotransmission and ion-gated channels (Wink, 2000). *A. muricata* and *A. squamosa* have been applied as bioinsecticides to control *Culex quinquefasciatus* and *Aedes albopictus* mosquitoes in Madagascar (Ravaomanarivo et al., 2014). Upon application of the extracts, significant insecticidal effects were observed with the extracts of the two plants compared to induced mortality by deltamethrin, an insecticide of reference. Research has revealed that seeds of *A. squamosal* and *A. muricata* contain a great amount of acetogenins (Das et al., 2007). This group of compounds is referred to as mitochondrial complex I inhibitor. Few alkaloids are associated with *A. muricata* which not only affect mortality of pupal and adult stages of mosquitoes but also reduce reproductive rate of their adults by decreasing their fecundity and egg hatchability (Kaushik and Saini, 2009). Annona products are till date not available commercially and studies have not addressed the commercial use of these products.

15.6.3 PONGAMIA

Pongomia is among the numerous chemicals used to protect plants from pests in modern agriculture (Stepanycheva et al., 2014). It is one of the most interesting subjects of study in recent years with widespread synanthropic and insecticidal activities (Pavela, 2009). The oil of pongamia contains 5–6% flavonoids. Karanjin, a furanoflavonoid compound, is the main constituent of pongomia flavonoid, known for its insecticidal properties (Kumar and Singh, 2002). Isolation of this flavonoid compound from oil and de-fatted oil cakes has been reported by several authors (Susarla et al., 2012). Insecticidal property of Karanjin has been enhanced by structural modifications which convert Karanjin to karanj ketone, karanj ketone oxime esters, and karanj ketone oxime N-O-nonanoate. This modified insecticidal property has been tested on aphid and had a remarkable effect (*Lipaphis erysimi*) (Mondal et al., 2010). In 2014, Stepanycheva et al. revealed that *Pongomia pinnata* oil-based formulated products had aphicidal activity for *M. persicae* adults and larvae. They were found to possess prolonged action and exert negative effects on pest offsprings. Several compounds of pongamia, either oil or extract from methanol/aqueous/chloroform/acetone solvents are biologically active against insect pests. *Pongamia* compounds act as oviposition deterrents, insecticides, repellents, antifeedants, and larvicides (Kumar and Singh, 2002). The extract of *P. pinnata* is toxic against *H. armigera*, *S. litura*, and pests of stored grains (Reena et al., 2012). Karanj oil and Karanj leaf extract have demonstrated insecticidal activities against mustard aphid; *L. erysimi* (Singh, 2007). Karanj extract is a constituent of commercial insecticidal formulations such as Salotrap, Plexin, Karrich,

RD Repelin, and RD9 Repelin used for controlling insect pests. PONEEM is another regulated insecticide formulated from pongam and neem oils. However, compared with neem products, reduced efficacy of Karanj extract in aqueous solutions is a limiting factor for their wide spread acceptability and applications.

15.6.4 JATROPHA

Jatropha curcas, referred to as physic nut, is a tropical plant which belongs to the class of Euphorbiacea native to North America, Africa, and Asia. *J. curcas* is a tropical ubiquitous plant often used for fencing by farmers (Jide-Ojo et al., 2013). The use of *Jatropha* in pest control has been reported by a plethora of researchers around the world (Nash, 2005). Extracts of *Jatropha* possess insecticidal or molluscicidal/anthelminthic activities on agricultural and nonagricultural pests (Musa and Olaniran, 2015). *Jatropha* consist 47% fat and various antinutritional factors such as saponin, phytate, trypsin inhibitor, and cyanogenic glycosides (Rakshit et al., 2008). Many terpenoids are present as secondary metabolites in *Jatropha*. To date, 65 forms of terpenes from *Jatropha* have been formulated (Devappa et al., 2011). Phorbol esters (PEs) are the major toxic constituents of *Jatropha*. Structural property, biological activity, toxicity, medicinal properties, phytochemistry, and pharmacological properties of PEs in *Jatropha* on animals have been fully investigated by researchers (Sabandar et al., 2013). The toxic constituents of PEs present in extracts of *J. curcas* possess molluscicidal, insecticidal, and fungicidal properties (Liu et al., 1997). The PEs contained in *Jatropha* oil were effectively toxic against insect pests of field crops and stored grains such as *Callosobruchus maculatus*, *C. chinensis*, *Clavigralla tomentosicollis*, *S. zeamais*, *Rhyzopertha dominica*, *T. castaneum*, *Oryzaephilus surinamensis*, *L. erysimi*, *Pieris. rapae*, *P. operculella*, *Tetranychus urticae*, *O. fasciatus*, *Coptotermes vastator*, *Amrasca biguttula*, *Aphis gossypii*, and *Aphis fabae* (Adebowale and Adedire, 2006; Silva et al., 2012) by oviposition deterrent, antifeedant, ovicidal, and anti-birth depressants. The PE-enriched fraction of *Jatropha* has been tested against many insect pests such as *Spodoptera. frugiperda*, *C. maculatus*, *Corcyra cephalonica*, *Busseola fusca*, *Sesamia calamistis*, *H. armigera*, and *Manduca sexta* (Khani et al., 2012). Extract from *Jatropha gossypiifolia* showed toxic effects on Lepidopteran pests: *Ostrinia nubilalis*, *B. fusca*, and *S. nonagrioides* (Valencia et al., 2006). Furthermore, PE fraction has shown antifeedant and insecticidal effects against *S. frugiperda and Spodoptera exigua* (Bullangpoti et al., 2012).

15.6.5 WEEDS AS ANTI-INSECTS

Here, it is worth considering the importance of weeds as botanical insecticides. Lantana is an invasive species in the tropical and subtropical zones of the world. Lantana exhibits insecticidal properties on aphids, mites, potato tuber moths, and *Spilosoma obliqua* (Suliman et al., 2003). Parthenium and cyperus were successfully used to minimize *Epilachna* beetle, diamond back moth, and cabbage head caterpillar in vegetables (Prijono et al., 1997). Calotropis was also reportedly active on rice plant hoppers (Prakash et al., 2008).

15.6.6 MEDICINAL HERBS AS PLANT PROTECTANTS

There are reports on the use of medicinally grouped herbs in the control of agriculturally important pests. Herbs such as *Gynandropsis gynandra*, *Vitex*, *Ocimum, Catharanthus roseus*, and *Euphorbia royleana* were effective against caterpillars, *H. armigera*, *Maconellicoccus hirsutus*, mustard aphid, and *Epilachna* beetle (Prakash et al., 2008). Also, *Epilachna* beetle was controlled by herbs such as *Strychnos nux-vomica* and *Solanum xanthocarpum* (Chitra et al., 1991). Plants like *Vernonia amygdalina* and bitter gourd known for their bitter tastes have shown efficacy against flea beetle on okra and coffee leaves (*Leucoptera coffeella*) (Onunkun, 2012). *Passiflora mollissima* referred to as banana passion fruit has been used in food industry to control pests.

15.6.7 SPICES AND CONDIMENTS AS PLANT PROTECTANTS

Reports on domestic botanicals from condiments and spices such as peppers and garlic as sources of botanical pesticides have been well documented (Antonious et al., 2007). Powdered chili pepper, for example, deterred onion fly, *Delia antique*, and *Earias insulana*. Garlic is effective against soft-bodied insects such as aphids, cumin (*Nigella sativa*) and *Epilachna* beetle.

15.6.8 ESSENTIAL OILS

Essential oils (EOs) are mixtures of volatile organic compounds produced as secondary metabolites in plants majorly for defense against pests and pathogens. EOs are majorly extracted from plant families such as Lamiaceae, Myrtaceae, Lauraceae, and Asteraceae. EOs just like other plant botanicals have antifeedant, fumigant, toxicity, repellent, reproduction retardant, and growth-reducing effects on pests (Singh and Singh, 1991). EOs are neurotoxic and interfere with neuromodulator octopamine (Enan, 2005) or ionotropic receptors like GABA-gated ion channels. Zoubiri and Baaliouamer (2014) have reported about 230 plants and EOs with active compounds showing insecticidal activities.

15.6.9 BOTANICAL PESTICIDES FROM HERBAL COMPOST

Together with insecticides derived from leaf and seed extracts of plants, composts from plants have severally been used in insect pest control (Gopalakrishnan et al., 2011). Bio-washes of crude extracts of *Annona*, *Jatropha*, and *Pongamia* vermin composts have killed *H. armigera* and *S. litura*. Compost from maize stover was effective in the control of whiteflies, *Zonocerus variegatus, Podagrica* sp. and *B. tabaci* with high efficacy of 60–80% control. Organic composts, especially the one from maize stover, can be used as an insecticide in organic farms to raise okra. Foliar application of organic composts is effective for controlling pest infestation of *Telfairia occidentalis* (Alao et al., 2011).

15.6.10 MISCELLANEOUS

Plantago, flowers of male *Zea mays*, mahua, *Psoralea corylifolia*, *Lindenbergia grandiflora*, and velvet bean (*Mucuna cochinchinensis*) have all demonstrated degree of insecticidal effects against insect pests of various agricultural crops. Also reported were extracts of tea, *Solanum nigrum*, cassava, *Solanum incanum*, sweet potato, Mexican marigold, Mexican tea, blackjack (*Bidens pilosa*), thorn apple, papaya, and aloe for exhibiting insecticidal effects (Alves et al., 2011).

15.7 SYNERGISM

Biological activities of botanicals enhance combinations of biomolecules. An extensive study was carried out on formulation of PONEEM from pongam and neem oils. Phytochemicals present in PONEEM karanjin and azadirachtin have been used to control *Scirtothrips dorsalis* in chili thrips. They were efficient as feeding deterrent (Packiam and Ignacimuthu, 2013). The phytopesticides was also examined against *S. litura* and *H. armigera*. The study examined different concentrations of the phyto-mixture on oviposition-deterrent activities of the pests (Packiam et al., 2012). A formulation with pongam oil and *Thymus vulgaris/Foeniculum vulgare* showed lower LC_{50} values against diamondback moth (*P. xylostella*) than pongam oil alone indicates the synergism between the botanicals (Pavela, 2012). Combined extract from *Acacia arabica, Bacillus thuringiensis subsp.* kurstaki (Btk), *Nicotiana tabacum, A. squamosa, Eucalyptus globulus, Datura stramonium, Ipomoea carnea, Lantana camara,* and *P. pinnata* was formulated by Rajguru et al. (2011). They investigated the efficacy of the formulated mixture and its synergistic activity against *S. litura* larvae and reported the mixture to be possessing high mortality showing that high effectiveness of the fortified extracts was due to synergistic action. Bioactive extracts from *N. tabacum A. arabica,* and *D. stramonium* have given great results compatible with Btk. Mixture of extracts from neem seed kernel and *Murraya koenigii* leaf was also found to be effective against adult beetles (Radha and Susheela, 2014). The formulated mixture acted as antifeedant with varying degree of toxicity on cowpea weevil as:

NSKE + *M. koenigii* leaf extract > neem > *M. koenigii*.

The use of recombinant DNA technology to enhance the efficacy of biopesticides has been reported by researchers. According to reports, understanding of genes from microorganisms and crop plants has enabled isolation of effective genes against pests and diseases to be controlled (Kumar, 2013). In other cases, fusion proteins are used to design next-generation biopesticides. DNA technology makes use of toxins (though not toxic to higher animals) combined with carrier protein to control pests, the toxins are toxic to insect pests when consumed orally, that is more effective when ingested by predators.

15.8 FUTURE PROSPECTS OF BOTANICAL INSECTICIDES

Evidently, botanical insecticides have plenty benefits over the commonly applied synthetic pesticides with many deleterious effects on humans, animals, environments, and economically important microorganisms. Eco-friendly botanical insecticides probably cannot be expected to completely replace synthetic insecticides within a short time. However, with increasing campaign and advancements in botanical insecticides, the use of botanical insecticides, having numerous benefits will soon outface synthetic pesticides application. Benefits of using botanical insecticides include environment and health safety coupled with the protection of agricultural crops as against synthetic insecticides associated with risk of integrating hazardous residues in food crops. Also, the prospect of botanical insecticides will be appreciated in human and animal protection against medically important vectors or insects (Pavela, 2012).

The future looks bright for botanicals with negative reports on synthetic pesticides associated with environmental risks resulting from their indiscriminate application. These negativities on synthetic pesticides have shifted interest toward botanical pesticides as alternative agents in pest management. Phytochemicals will in the future play vital roles in pest control both in the industrialized and developing countries. Countries rich in viable biodiversity should quickly bioprospect their flora to document their botanicals in order to prevent future biopiracy and establish their sovereignty on botanical pesticides developed from their plants (Dimetry, 2014). Application of botanical biopesticides may require knowledge of insect pests on which the botanicals would be successfully be applied. Also, a correct time of application is essential to ensure the efficacy of the biopesticide (Kumar, 2015). A better understanding of the mode of action of the biopesticides, their effects, regulatory issues that arise on their adoption may help to raise their profile among the public and policy-makers. With this promising future, farmers, research institutes, governments, and all concerned agencies are encouraged to start growing economically important plants reported to be rich in phytochemical biopesticides. Botanical trees may be the next global oil to be explored.

15.9 REGISTRATION AND REGULATIONS OF BOTANICALS

Pesticide registration is the process through which Environmental Protection Agency (EPA) examines the ingredients of a pesticide/botanical, the site or crop on which it is to be used, the amount, frequency, timing of use, and storage and disposal instructions of the plant botanical. Before any botanical can be registered, marketed or used, specific agencies, bodies or authorized ministries empowered by the government of any interested country must ascertain the safety of such botanical for use. A botanical cannot legally be used, sold, or distributed if not registered with EPA in the country. EPA makes online resources, such as the *Pesticide Registration Manual* (blue book) available to assist applicants through the registration process (USEPA, 2014). In the United States, for instance, The Federal Insecticide, Fungicide, and Rodenticide Act requires that EPA evaluates proposed pesticide to assure that its use does not pose risks to the health of humans, environment, biota, and nontarget organisms. This evaluation involves an extensive review of health and safety information of the impending botanical. In Nigeria, the National Agency for Food and Drug Administration and Control (NAFDAC) empowered by Sections 5 and 29 of NAFDAC laws. NAFDAC was itself established by Decree No. 15 of 1993, now encapsulated in the NAFDAC Act, Cap NI Laws of the Federation of Nigeria. NAFDAC mandates include evaluation of pesticides to ensure safe and effective pesticides are available for use by the public. Act No. 19 of 1993 (as amended) specifies that no processed food, drug, cosmetic, drug product, medical device, or water shall be manufactured, advertised, imported, exported, sold, or distributed in Nigeria unless registered in accordance with the provisions of Decree No.15 of 1993. Arising from the law, the Agency has also set various regulations in motion such as Pesticides Registration Regulations, Chemical, and Chemical Products (control, monitoring) Regulations. The latter is still in draft form awaiting approval. Pesticide residues in Nigeria are analyzed and monitored in an International Atomic Energy Agency-accredited laboratory at the NAFDAC Central Laboratory Complex, Oshodi, Lagos.

Pesticides registration is overseen by many units under NAFDAC. The registration of pesticides and agrochemicals is supervised by Veterinary Drugs and Pesticides Unit under Registration and Regulatory Affairs Directorate of NAFDAC. The Chemical Import Control and Chemical Monitoring units of the Narcotics and Controlled Substance Directorate are responsible for controlling agrochemicals and pesticides. NAFDAC has made provisions for a functional database which contains all registered regulated products in Nigeria made available at www.nafdacregistry.net. About 354 pesticides and agrochemicals had been registered in Nigeria as in August 2008. Nigeria is also in support of ECOWAS regional structure and procedures for pesticide registration through the West Africa Committee on Pesticide Registration ratified by ECOWAS council of ministers.

KEYWORDS

- **synthetic pesticides**
- **biopesticides**
- **phytochemicals**
- **future prospects**
- **botanicals**

REFERENCES

Adebowale, K. O.; Adedire, C. O. Chemical Composition and Insecticidal Properties of the Underutilized *Jatropha curcas* Seed Oil. *Afr. J. Biotechnol.* **2006,** *5*(10), 901–906.

Aerts, R. J.; Mordue (Luntz), A. J. Feeding Deterrence and Toxicity of Neem Triterpenoids. *J. Chem. Ecol.* **1997,** *23*(9), 2117–2132.

Agrios, N. G. Control of Plant Diseases. In *Plant Pathology,* 4th ed.; Elsevier, Academic Press: San Diego, California, USA, 1997; 200–216.

Alves, D. S.; Oliviera, D. F.; Carvalho, G. A.; Jr. Santos, H. M.; Carvalho, D. A., Santos, M. A.; de Carvalho, H. W. Plant Extracts as An Alternative to Control *Leucoptera coffeella* (Guérin-Mèneville) (*Lepidoptera*: *Lyonetiidae*). *Neotrop. Entomol.* **2011,** *40*(1), 123–128.

Antonious, G. F.; Meyer, J. E.; Rogers, J. A.; Hu, Y. H. Growing Hot Pepper for Cabbage Looper, *Trichoplusiani* (Hübner) and Spider Mite, *Tetranychus urticae* (Koch) Control. *J. Environ. Sci. Health B.* **2007,** *42*(5), 559–567.

Anupam, G.; Nandita, C.; Goutam, C. Plant Extracts as Potential Mosquito Larvicides. *Indian Journal of Medical Research.* **2012,** *135,* 581–598.

Ascher, K. R. S. Nonconventional Insecticidal Effects of Pesticides Available from the Neem Tree, *Azadirachta indica. Arch. Insect Biochem. Physiol.* **1993,** *22,* 433–449.

Blaney, W. M.; Simmonds, M. S. J.; Ley, S. V.; Anderson, J. C.; Toogood, P. L. Antifeedant Effects of Azadirachtin and Structurally Related Compounds on Lepidopterous Larvae. *Entomol. Exp. Appl.* **1990,** *55,* 149–160.

Bullangpoti. V.; Wajnberg, E.; Feyereisen, P. A. R. Antifeedant Activity of *Jatropha gossypiifolia* and *Melia azedarach* Senescent Leaf Extracts on *Spodoptera frugiperda* (*Lepidoptera*: *Noctuidae*) and their Potential Use as Synergists. *Pest Manage. Sci.* **2012,** *68,* 1255–1264.

Casida, J. E.; Quistad, G. B. Insecticide Targets: Learning to keep up with Resistance and Changing Concepts of Safety. *Agric. Chem. Biotechnol.* **2000,** *43,* 185–191.

Chitra, K. C.; Reddy, P. V. R.; Rao, K. P. Effect of Certain Plant Extracts in the Control of Brinjal Spotted Leaf Beetle, *Henosepilachna vigintioctopunctata* Fabr. *J. Appl. Zool. Res.* **1991,** *2*(1), 37–38.

Cólom, O. A.; Barrachina, I.; Mingol, I. A.; Mass, C. G.; Sanz, P. M.; Neske, A.; Bardon, A. Toxic Effects of *Annonaceous acetogenins* on *Oncopeltus fasciatus*. *J. Pest Sci.* **2008,** *81,* 81–85.

Das, N. G.; Goswami, D.; Rabha, B. Preliminary Evaluation of Mosquito Larvicidal Efficacy of Plant Extracts. *J. Vector Borne Dis.* **2007,** *44,* 145–148.

Devappa, R. K.; Makkar, H. P. S.; Becker, K. Jatropha Diterpenes: A Review. *J. Am. Oil Chemists' Soc.* **2011,** *88,* 301–322.

Dimetry, N. Z. Different Plant Families as Bioresource for Pesticides, In *Advances in Plant Biopesticides*. Singh, D. Ed., Springer: New Delhi, India. 2014, 1–20.

Enan, E. E. Molecular and Pharmacological Analysis of an Octopamine Receptor from American Cockroach and Fruit Fly in Response to Plant Essential Oils. Arch. Insect Biochem. Physiol. **2005,** *59,* 161–171.

Food and Agriculture Organization (FAO). *International Code of Conduct on the Distribution and Use of Pesticides*; Rome, Italy. 1989

Food and Agriculture Organization of the United Nations (FAO). *International Fund for Agricultural Development (IFAD) and World Food Program (WFP). The State of Food*

Insecurity in the World 2014. Strengthening the Enabling Environment for Food Security and Nutrition. Rome, Italy. 2014

Gahukar, R. T. Role and Perspective of Phytochemicals in Pest Management in India. *Current. Science.* **2010,** *98*(7), 897–899.

Gopalakrishnan, S.; Ranga Rao, G. V.; Humayun, P.; Rameshwar, R. V.; Alekhya, G.; Simi, J.; Deepthi, K. S.; Vidya, M.; Srinivas, V.; Mamatha, L.; Rupela, O. Efficacy of Botanical Extracts and Entomopathogens on Control of *Helicoverpa armigera* and *Spodoptera litura*. *Afr. J. Biotechnol.* **2011,** *10*(73), 16667–16673.

Govidachari, T. R.; Narasimhan, N. S.; Suresh, G.; Partho, P. D.; Gopalakrishnan, G.; Kumari, G. N. K. Structure Related Insect Antifeedant and Growth Regulating Activities of Some Liminoids. *J. Chem. Ecol.* **1995,** *21,* 1585–1600.

Grzybowski, A.; Tiboni, M.; da Silva, M. A.; Chitolina, R. F.; Passos, M.; Fontana, J. D. The Combined Action of Phytolarvicides for the Control of Dengue Fever Vector, *Aedes aegypti*. *Rev. Bras. Farmacogn.* **2012,** *22*(3), 549–557.

Hasan, F.; Ansari, M. S. Toxic Effects of Neem-Based Insecticides on Pieris brassicae (Linn.). *Crop Protection.* **2011,** *30,* 502–507.

Irulandi, S.; Balasubramanian, G. Report on the Effect of Botanicals against *Megalurothrips distalis* (Karny) (*Thripidae*: *Thysanoptera*) and *Lampides boeticus* Linn. (*Lycaenidae*: *Lepidoptera*) on Greengram. *Insect Environ.* **2000,** *5*(4), 175–176.

Isman, M. B. Growth Inhibitory and Antifeedant Effects of Azadirachtin on Six *Noctuids* of Regional Economic Importance. *Pesticide Science*. **1993,** *38,* 57–63.

Isman, M. B. Botanical Insecticides, Deterrents and Repellents in Modern Agriculture and Increasingly Regulated World. *Ann. Rev. Entomol.* **2006,** *51,* 45–66.

Izuchukwu, O. O. Analysis of the Contribution of Agricultural Sector on the Nigerian Economic Development. *World Rev. Bus. Res.* **2011,** *1*(1), 191–200.

Jaglan, M. S.; Khokhar, K. S.; Malik, M. S.; Taya, J. S. Standardization of Method of Extraction of Bioactive Components from Different Plants of Insecticidal Properties. *Indian J. Agric. Sci.* **1997,** *31,* 167–173.

Jarvis, A. P.; Johnson, S.; Morgan, E. D.; Simmonds, M. S. J.; Blaney, W. M. Photoxidation of Nimbin and Salannin, Tertranortriterpenoids from the Neem Tree (*Azadirachta indica*). *J. Chem. Ecol.* **1997,** *23*(12), 2841–2860.

Jide-Ojo, C. C.; Guingula, D. T.; Ojo, O. O. Extracts of *Jatropha curcas* L. Exhibit Significant Insecticidal and Grain Protectant Effects against Maize Weevi, *Sitophilius zeamais* (Coleoptera:Curculionidae). *J. Stored Prod. Post-harvest Res.* **2013,** *4*(3), 44–50.

Kaushik, R.; Saini, P. Growth Inhibiting Effects of Annona squamosa Leaf Extract on Vector Mosquitoes. *J. Exp. Zool.* **2009,** *12,* 395–398.

Kerin, J. In *Opening Address,* Proceedings of the 6th International Working Conference on Stored-product Protection, Canberra, *Australia*. 17–23 April **1994,** Volume 1. http://spiru.cgahr.ksu.edu/proj/iwcspp/iwcspp6.html (accessed January 23, 2018).

Kfir, R. Natural Control of the Cereal Stemborers *Busseola fusca* and *Chilo partellus* in South Africa. *Insect Sci. Appl.* **1997,** *17*(1), 61–67.

Khani, M.; Awang, R. M.; Omar, D.; Rahmani, M. Bioactivity Effect of *Piper nigrum* L. and *Jatropha curcas* L. Extracts against *Corcyra cephalonica* (Stainton). *Agrotechnology* **2012,** *2*(1), 1–6.

Koul, O. Insect Growth Regulating and Antifeedant Effects of Neem Extracts and zadirachtin on Two Aphid Species of Ornamental Plants. *J. Biosci.* **1999,** *1,* 85–90.

Koul, O.; Shankar, J. S.; Kapil, R. S. The Effect of Neem Allelochemicals on Nutritional Physiology of Larval *Spodoptera litura*. *Entomol. Exp. Appl.* **1996,** *79,* 43–50.

Koul, O.; Multani, J. S.; Singh, G.; Daniewski, W. M.; Berlozecki, S. 6-Beta-hydroxygedunin from *Azadirachta indica*; Its Potentiation Effects with Some Nonazadirachtin Limonoids in Neem against *Lepidopteran* Larvae. *J. Agric. Food Chem.* **2003,** *51,* 2937–2942.

Kulkarni, J.; Kapse, N.; Kulkarni, O. K. Plant Based Pesticides for Control of *Helicoverpa armigera* on *cucumis*. *Asian Agri-History*. **2009,** *13*(4), 327–332.

Kumar, M.; Singh, R. Potential of *Pongamia glabravent* as an Insecticide of Plant Origin. *Biol. Agric. Hortic.* **2002,** *20,* 29–50.

Kumar, S. The Role of Biopesticides in Sustainably Feeding the Nine Billion Global Populations. *J. Biofert. Biopestici.* **2013,** *4*(2), 1–3.

Kumar, S. Biopesticide: An Environment Friendly Pest Management Strategy. *J. Biofert. Biopestici*. **2015,** *6,* (1), 1–3.

Liu, S. Y.; Sporer, F.; Wink, M.; Jouurdane, J.; Henning, R.; Li, Y. L.; Ruppel, A. Anthraquinones in *Rheum palmatum* and *Rumex dentatus* (*Polygonaceae*) and Phorbol Esters in *Jatropha. curcas* (*Euphorbiaceae*) with Molluscicidal Activity against the Schistosome Vector Snails *Oncomelania, Biomphalaria* and *Bulinus*. *Trop. Med. Int. Health.* **1997,** *2,* 179–188.

Martinez, S. S.; Van Emden, H. F. Growth Disruption, Abnormalities and Mortality of *Spodoptera littoralis* (Boisduval) (*Lepidoptera*: *Noctuidae*) Caused by Azadirachtin. *Neotroprical Entomol.* **2001,** *30,* 113–125.

Mondal, A.; Walia, S.; Shrivastava, C.; Kumar, B.; Kumar, J. Synthesis and Insecticidal Activity of Karanj Ketone Oxime and its Ester Derivatives against the Mustard Aphid (*Lipaphis erysimi*). *Pestic. Res. J.* **2010,** *22*(1), 39–43.

Mordue, A. J.; Blackwell, A. Azadirachtin : An Update. *J.Insect Physiol.* **1993,** *39,* 903–924.

Mordue, A. J.; Nisbet, A. J. Azadirachtin from the Neem Tree, *Azadirachta indica*: its Action against Insects. *Entomol.Soc. Braz.* **2000,** *29,* 615–632.

Musa, A. K.; Olaniran, J. O. Studies on the Efficacy of *Jatropha curcas* L. Seed Oil on Adult Mortality and Emergence of Seed Beetle, *Callosobruchus maculatus* (F.) (Coleoptera: Chrysomelidae) in Cowpea. *Int. J. Phytofuels Allied Sci.* **2015,** *4*(1), 1–12.

Nash, J. M. *Crop Preservation and Storage in Cool Temperate Climates*; Pergamon Press: Oxford, 2005; pp 54–57.

Nathan, S. S.; Kalaivani, K. Combined Effects of Azadirachtin and Nucleopolyhedrovirus (SpltNPV) on *Spodoptera littoralis Fabricius* (*Lepidoptera: Noctuidae*) larvae. Biol. Control. **2006,** *39,* 96–104.

Nathan, S. S.; Kalaivani, K.; Murugan, K.; Paul G. C. Efficacy of Neem Limonoids on *Cnaphalocrocis medinalis* (Guenée) (*Lepidoptera*: *Pyralidae*) the Rice Leaffolder. *Crop Protection*. **2005,** *24,* 760–763.

Onunkun, O. Evaluation of Aqueous Extracts of Five Plants in the Control of Flea Beetles on Okra (*Abelmoschus esculentus* (L.) Moench). *J. Biopest.* **2012,** *5,* 62–67.

Oonagh, M. B.; Paul, A. V. N. Insect Pests and their Management. In *Biology Control Laboratory, Division of Entemology;* Erskine, W., Muehlbauer, F.J., Sarker, A., Sharma, B, Eds.; Indian Agricultural Research Institute. Publisher: CABI, New Delhi, 2009; pp 282–305.

Packiam, S. M.; Ignacimuthu, S. Effect of Botanical Pesticide Formulations against the Chilli Trips (*Scirtothrips dorsalis* Hood) on Peanut Ecosystem. *Int. J. Nat. Appl. Sci.* **2013,** *2*(1), 1–5.

Packiam, S. M.; Anbalagan, V.; Ignacimuthu, S.; Vendan, S. E. Formulation of a Novel Phytopesticide PONNEEM and its Potentiality to Control Generalist Herbivorous *Lepidopteran* Insect Pests, *Spodoptera litura* (*Fabricius*) and *Helicoverpa armigera* (Hubner) (*Lepidoptera*: *Noctuidae*). *Asian Pac. J. Trop. Dis.* **2012,** *2*(2), 720–723.

Pavela, R. Effectiveness of some botanical insecticides against *Spodoptera littoralis* Boisduvala (Lepidoptera: Noctudiae), Myzus persicae Sulzer (Hemiptera: Aphididae) and Tetranychus urticae Koch (Acari: Tetranychidae)," *Plant Protection Sci.* **2009,** *45*(4), 161–167.

Pavela, R. Efficacy of Three Newly Developed Botanical Insecticides Based on Pongam Oil against *Plutella xylostella* L. Larvae. *J. Biopest.* **2012,** *5*(1), 62–70.

Popat, A.; Liu, J.; Hu, Q.; Kennedy, M.; Peters, B.; Lu, G. Q. M.; Qiao, S. Z. Adsorption and Release of Biocides with Mesoporous Silica Nanoparticles. *Nanoscale.* **2012,** *4*(3), 970–975.

Prakash, G.; Bhojwani, S. S.; Srivastava, A. K. Production of Azadirachtin from Plant Tissue Culture-State of the Art and Culture Prospects, Biotechnol. *Bioprocess Eng.* **2002,** *7,* 185–193.

Prakash, A.; Rao, J.; Nandagopal, V. Future of Botanical Pesticides in Rice, Wheat, Pulses and Vegetables Pest Management. *J. Biopestic.* **2008,** *1*(2), 154–169.

Prijono, D.; Gani, M. S.; Syahputra, E. Insecticidal Activity of Annonaceous Seed Extracts against *Crocidolomia binotalis* Zeller (*Lepidoptera*: *Pyralidae*). *Bull. Plant Pests Dis.* **1997,** *9,* 1–6.

Radha, R.; Susheela, P. Efficacy of Plant Extracts on the Toxicity, Ovipositional Deterrence and Damage Assessment of the Cowpea Weevil, *Callosobruchus maculatus* (*Coleoptera: Bruchidae*). *J. Entomol. Zool. Stud.* **2014,** *2*(3), 16–20.

Rafiq, M.; Dahot, M. U.; Naqvi, S. H.; Mali, M.; Ali, N. Efficacy of Neem (*Azadirachta indica* A. Juss) Callus and Cells Suspension Extracts against Three Lepidopteron Insects of Cotton. *J. Med. Plants Res.* **2012,** 6(40), 5344–5349.

Rajapake, R. H. S.; Ratnaseka, D. Pesticidal Potential of Some Selected Tropical Plant Extracts against *Callosobruchus maculatus* (F.) and *Callosobruchus chinensis* L. *Trop. Agric. Res. Ext.* **2008,** *11,* 69–71.

Rajguru, M.; Sharma, A. N.; Banerjee, S. Assessment of Plant Extracts Fortified with *Bacillus thuringiensis* (*Bacillales*: *Bacillaceae*) for Management of *Spodoptera litura* (*Lepidoptera*: *Noctuidae*). *Int. J. Trop. Insect Sci.* **2011,** *31*(1–2), 92–97.

Rakshit, K. D.; Darukeshwara, J.; Rathina, R. K.; Narasimhamurthy, K.; Saibaba, P.; Bhagya, S. Toxicity Studies of Detoxified *Jatropha curcas M*eal (*Jatropha curcas*) in Rats. *Food Chem. Toxicol.* **2008,** *46,* 3621–3625.

Ravaomanarivo, R. H. L.; Razafindraleva, H. A.; Raharimalala, F. N.; Rasoahantaveloniaina, B.; Ravelonandro, P. H.; Mavingui, P. Efficacy of seed extracts of *Annona squamosa* and *Annona muricata* (*Annonaceae*) for the control of *Aedes albopictus* and *Culex quinquefasciatus* (*Culicidae*). *Asian Pac. J. Trop. Biomed.* **2014,** *4*(10), 787–795.

Reena; Singh, R.; Sinha, B. K. Evaluation of *Pongamia pinnata* Seed Extracts as an Insecticide against American Bollworm *Helicoverpa armigera* (Hubner). *Int. J. Agric. Sci.* **2012,** *4*(6), 257–261.

Ribeiro, L. P.; Vendramim, J. D.; Bicalho, K. U.; Andrade, M. S.; Fernandes, J. B.; Moral, R. A.; Demétrio, C. G. B. *Annona mucosa* Jacq. (*Annonaceae*), A promising Source of Bioactive Compounds against *Sitophilus zeamais* Mots. (*Coleoptera*: *Curculionidae*). *J. Stored Prod. Res.* **2013,** *55,* 6–14.

Sabandar, C. W.; Ahmat, N.; Jaafar, F. M.; Sahidin, I. Medicinal Property, Phytochemistry and Pharmacology of Several Jatropha species (*Euphorbiaceae*), A Review. *Phytochem.* **2013,** *85,* 7–29.

Sarkar, M.; Kshirsagar, R. Botanical Pesticides: Current Challenges and Reverse Pharmacological Approach for Future Discoveries. *J. Biofertil. Biopestici.* **2014,** *5*(2), 1–2.

Schmutterer, H. *The Neem Tree,* 2nd ed.; Neem Foundation: Mumbai, 2002; p 893.

Sharma, P. R.; Sharma, O. P.; Saxena, B. P. Effect of Neem Gold on Haemocytes of Tobacco Armyworm, *Spodoptera littoralis* (*Fabricius*) (*Lepidoptera*; *Noctuidae*). *Curr. Sci.* **2003a,** *84,* 690–695.

Sharma, V.; Walia, S.; Kumar, J.; Nair, M. G.; Parmar, B. S. An Efficient Method for the Purification and Characterization of Nematicidal Azadirachtins A, B and H using MPLC and ESIMS. *J. Agric. Food Chem.* **2003b,** *51,* 3966–3972.

Silva, G. N.; Faroni, L. R. A.; Sousa, A. H.; Freitas, R. S. Bioactivity of *Jatropha curcas* L. to Insect Pests of Stored Products. *J. Stored Prod. Res.* **2012,** *48,* 111–113.

Singh, D.; Singh, A. K. Repellent and Insecticidal Properties of Essential Oils against Housefly *Musca domestica* L. *Insect Sci. Appl.* **1991,** *12*(4), 487–491.

Singh, Y. P. Efficacy of Plant Extracts against Mustard Aphid, *Lipaphis erysimi* on Mustard. *Ind. J. Plant Prot.* **2007,** *35*(1), 116–117.

Stepanycheva, E. A.; Petrova, M. O.; Chermenskaya,T. D.; Pavela, R. Prospects for the Use of Pongamia pinnata Oil-Based Products against the Green Peach Aphid Myzus persicae (Sulzer) (Hemiptera: Aphididae). *Psyche.* **2014,** Article ID 705397, 1–5. http://dx.doi.org/10.1155/2014/705397

Suliman, R., Saker, I.; Namora, D. In *Importance of Plant Extracts in Managing Aphis fabae,* The Eighth Arab Congress of Plant Protection, Omar Al-Mukhtar University, Oct 12–14, 2003; Khateeb, N.A., Ed.; El-Beida City, Libya.

Thomson, W. T. Agricultural Chemicals, In *Insecticides;* Thomson Publications: Fresno, CA. 1992.

U. S. Environmental Protection Agency. Office of Pesticide Programs, Web Page FIFRA. **2014,** http://www.epa.gov/pesticides/bluebook/FIFRA.pdf (accessed September 28).

Valencia, A.; Frérot, B.; Guénego, H.; Múnera, D. F.; Grossi De Sá, M. F.; Calatayud, P. A. Effect of *Jatropha gossypiifolia* Leaf Extracts on Three Lepidoptera Species. *Rev. Colomb. Entomol.* **2006,** *32*(1), 45–48.

Veitch, G. E.; Boyer, A.; Ley, S. V. The Azadirachtin Story. *Angew. Chem. Int. Ed.* **2008,** 47, 9402–9429.

Walia, S.; Saha, S.; Tripathi, V.; Sharma, K. K. Phytochemical Biopesticides: Some Recent Developments. *Phytochem. Rev.* **2017,** 1–19.

Wang, H.; Wang, J.; Choi, D.; Tang, Z.; Wu, H.; Lin, Y. EQCM Immunoassay for Phosphorylated Acetylcholinesterase as a Biomarker for Organophosphate Exposures Based on Selective Zirconia Adsorption and Enzyme-Catalytic Precipitation. *Biosens. Bioelectron.* **2009,** *24,* 2377–2383.

WHO/UNEP. *Public Health Impact of Pesticides Use in Agriculture*; Switzerland, Geneva, 1990.

William, H. L.; Robert, L. M. *Introduction to Insect Pest Management;* 3rd ed., A Wiley-Interscience Publication: John Wiley and Sons, Incorpooration, New York, 1994.

Wink, M. Interference of Alkaloids with Neuroreceptors and Ion Channels. In *Bioactive Natural Products;* Rahman X. A. (Ed) Elsevier: Amsterdam, Netherlands. **2000,** 3–129.

Yule, S.; Srinivasan, R. Evaluation of Bio-Pesticides against Legume Pod Borer, *Maruca vitrata* Fabricius (*Lepidoptera*: *Pyralidae*), In Laboratory and Field Conditions in Thailand. *J. Asia-Pac. Entomol.* **2013,** *16,* 357–360.

Zoubiri, S.; Baaliouamer, A. Potentiality of Plants as Source of Insecticide Principles. *J. Saudi Chem. Soc.* **2014,** *18*(6), 925–936.

CHAPTER 16

A SUSTAINABLE APPROACH IN INTEGRATED PEST MANAGEMENT: ROLE OF PHYTOMOLECULES AS BIOPESTICIDE

RAKESH KUMAR GUPTA[1], PREM PRAKASH KUSHWAHA[2], and SHASHANK KUMAR[2,*]

[1]*School of Environment and Earth Science, Environmental Science and Technology, Central University of Punjab, Bathinda, Punjab 151001, India, Mob.: +919335647413*

[2]*Department of Biochemistry and Microbial Sciences, School of Basic and Applied Sciences, Central University of Punjab, Bathinda, Punjab 151001, India*

Corresponding author. E-mail: shashankbiochemau@gmail.com, shashank.kumar@cupb.edu.in

**ORCID: https://orcid.org/0000-0002-9622-0512*

ABSTRACT

Though the use of pesticides has offered significant economic benefits by enhancing the food production and the prevention of vector-borne diseases, evidence suggests that their use has adversely affected the health of human populations and the environment. In the search for eco-friendly solutions to control the insect pest and environmental management, the great interest in plants and their chemo-biodiversity as a potential source of phytochemicals for biopesticides has increased over the time. Plants are a rich source of bioactive molecules for biopesticides. These substances have been exploited as commercial products and may play an important role in an integrated pest management as a benefit of humankind and suitable for environmental protection. For a successful application of phytochemical-based biopesticides limited a broad range of criteria such as biological, environmental, commercial, and regulatory must be satisfied. Plant products are compatible with several other biopesticides and synthetic pesticides. They are therefore recommended for large-scale application in pest control and sustainable environment. There is thus an urgent need to organize sustainable natural sources, develop quality control, adopt standardization strategies, and modify regulatory mechanisms.

16.1 INTRODUCTION

An estimate of the global crop losses due to pest has declined from 13.6% in post-green revolution era to 10.8% toward the beginning of this century while in India follows the same trend from 23.3 to 15.7% at present (Dhaliwal et al., 2015). Thus, the worldwide food production is adversely affected by these pests during the crop growth, harvest, and storage (Kulkarni et al., 2009). Although the synthetic chemical method has effective tools in modern crop management to control the pest and diseases. The extensive use of pesticides effectively control insect pest and led to increase the agricultural output. Ideally, a pesticide must be destructive to the targeted pests, but not to nontarget species, including man (Aktar et al., 2009). However, the synthetic pesticides are highly toxic, recalcitrant, and longtime persistent in the environment. It contaminated crops, food commodities, and their toxic residues accumulated in food, water, air, and soil. Unfortunately, the widespread use of these chemical has led to many negative consequences (Pavela, 2008). Besides, the use of plant-based biopesticides offers an attractive alternative to manage the insect pests and diseases in an eco-friendly way. Because phytochemical-based biopesticides are natural, renewable, readily biodegradable, non-pollutive, nontoxic, easily available, and relatively cost-effective. Besides these attributes high specificity to target pests, and pose no or less hazard to the environment or to human health, slow resistance development, and less residual activity environment. Owing to the above attributes, the role of biopesticides is considered as a potent and reliable tool in integrated pest management programme (IPM) to manage insect pests. Thus, these increase attention to search out plants-based natural insecticidal products (Pirali-Kheirabadi and da Silva, 2010).

It may contribute potential substitute to currently used insect control agents. Plants constitute a rich source of plant-based bioactive chemicals (Qin et al., 2010). Plant-derived insecticides contain natural active biological compound which act as a deterrents or repellents (Islam et al., 2009), fumigants (Choi et al., 2006), insecticides (Tang et al., 2007), antifeedants (González-Coloma et al., 2006), and may the influence some other biological parameters such as growth rate (Nathan et al., 2008), life duration, and reproduction (Isikber et al., 2006). These compounds belong to various groups of chemicals such as alkaloids, rotenoids and pyrethrins, steroids, terpenoids, phenolics, and essential oils have been reported for their insecticidal properties (Shaalan et al., 2005). Most of them are secondary metabolites that are known for their insecticidal properties (Lopez et al., 2008) and in many cases plants have been used as home remedies to kill or repel insects (Kim et al., 2010). The novel research on the interactions between plants and insects pest has clearly shown the potential use of plant-based metabolites for this purpose (Kamaraj et al., 2010).

To investigate the suitable alternatives to traditional insecticides, phytochemical-based biopesticides have been widely scrutinized. With the objective of contributing to these studies, there were many plants species that have been tested and evaluated against a diverse group of insect pests in the laboratory as well as field conditions, particularly for insecticidal activity. Research on insecticidal activity of various plants and plant materials against different insect has been conducted and has yielded positive results (Khaliq et al., 2014; Radha, 2014; Yohannes, 2014). This has revealed in terms of toxicity, mortality, inhibition, suppression of oviposition repellency and reduces the reproduction potentiality. This chapter focuses on the plant-based pesticide product and its activity against the economically important insect pests. The aim of this chapter is to contribute an overview of the plant's origin biological active compounds that have been reported to possess insecticidal activity against insect pest.

In this regard, plants being considered as an alternative source of insect control agents owing to constitute a rich source of plant-driven bioactive chemicals (Kim et al., 2003). Yet only a few phytochemicals are currently used in agriculture, and there are few promises for the commercial advancement of new biopesticides products. Several factors appear to limit the success of plant-driven biopesticide, most notably regulatory barriers and the availability of competing products of microbial-based biofertilizers that are cost-effective and relatively safe compared with their predecessors. The significance of these plant genetic resources, as potential insecticides become evident when looking at the context of an increasing number of insects, showing resistance against conventional insecticides (Adeyemi, 2010).

However, threat and problems allied with the use of chemicals lead to increasingly rigorous environmental regulation of pesticides (Pavela et al., 2010). There is thus a need to develop safer, more eco-friendly, and efficient substitute that has the potential to replace conventional pesticides and are suitable to use (Tapondjou et al., 2005). In this context, screening of plant-based natural products has received much attention of researchers around the world (Kebede et al., 2010). Keeping all these facts in mind, an emerging challenge in the new millennium is to produce more and more food from keeping the environment safe and sustainable IPM.

16.2 CONCEPT OF BIOPESTICIDES FROM PLANTS-BASED GREEN COMPOUND

Phytochemicals (botanicals) are plant-based natural occurring products of biological active compound as potential sources of new green biopesticides over the conventional synthetic pesticides (Table 16.1). They are also called natural insecticides or biopesticides. The term phytochemical-based biopesticide embraced a wide diversity of biologically active chemical. In general, these active ingredients extracts/isolated from different parts of the plants such as leaves, roots, barks, fruits, seeds (Altemimi et al., 2017). These botanicals products from plants classified as either primary or secondary plant metabolites. There are several medicinal and aromatic plants that have the ability to synthesise and produce numerous secondary metabolites which are known for their insecticidal properties (Lopez et al., 2008). These compounds belong to various groups of chemicals such as alkaloids, rotenoids and pyrethrins, steroids, terpenoids, phenolics, and essential oils have been reported for their insecticidal properties (Shaalan et al., 2005). These plant-based active constituents act in various way including insecticides (kill to adults, ova, and larvae), insect repellents, antifeedants, molluscicides, fungicides, and phytotoxins (Okwute, 2012). Few of the secondary metabolites alter the behavior and life cycle of insect's pests which are called as semiochemicals. In addition, currently, essential oil which is a mixture of volatile compounds accumulated in seeds, flowers, and leaves are among the best-known substances evaluated against insects (Pitasawat et al., 2007). Various conventional use of phytochemicals have been reported such as nicotine from *Nicotiana tabacum,* rotenone from *Lonchocarpus* sp., derris dust from *Derris elliptica,* and pyrethrum from *Chrysanthemum cinerariiaefolium* (El-Wakeil, 2013).

TABLE 16.1 Phytochemical-based Insecticide Used to Control Different Insect Pests.

Plant	Scientific name	Family	Active principle	Plant parts used	Insect pests
Neem	*Azadirachta indica*	Meliaceae	Azadirachtin	Seeds and leaves	Aphids, whiteflies, leafhoppers, psyllids, scales, mites and thrips, armyworms, cutworms, stem borers, bollworms, leaf miners, lepidoptera
Pyrethrum	*Chrysanthemum cinerariifolium*	Asteraceae	Pyrethrin	Dried flowers	Caterpillars, aphids, bugs, cabbage worms, beetles, leafhoppers, spider mites
Sabadilla	*Schoenocaulon officinale*	Liliaceae	Cevadine and vertridine	Seeds	Grasshoppers, codling moths, armyworms, cabbage loopers, squash bugs, aphids
Ryanodine	*Ryania speciosa*	Flacourtaceae	Ryanoids	Woody stems	Codling moths, potato aphids, onion thrips, corn earworms
Tobacco	*Nicotiana tobaccum and Nicotiana rustica*	Solanaceae	Nicotine	Plants leaves	Aphids, thrips, caterpillars
Rotenone	*Derris eliptica and Lonchocarpus* spp.	Fabaceae	Rotenone, related isoflavones	Roots	Bugs, aphids, potato beetles, spider mites, carpenter ants

16.3 CONVENTIONAL BOTANICALS: AZADIRACHTIN, NICOTINE, ROTENONES, SABADILLA, AND PYRETHRUM AND THEIR MODE OF ACTION

16.3.1 AZADIRACHTIN: MODE OF ACTION

Neem, *Azadirachta indica* is evergreen, tall, and fast-growing plants belonging to Meliaceae family, native to Indian subcontinent (Bhattacharyya et al., 2007; Lokanadhan et al., 2012). It has medicinal and pesticidal properties that have been used from the ancient time at least before 2500 years (Bhattacharyya et al., 2007). Various part of neem plants such as the seeds, bark, and leaves contain active compounds with justifying medicinal properties such as antiseptic, anti-inflammatory, antiviral, antipyretic, antifungal uses, and anti-ulcer. At present, neem plant is recognized as a natural and eco-friendly product which has much to offer in solving global agricultural, environmental, and public health problems. There are hundreds of active compound that have driven from neem tree used to manufacture a number of valuable products. Azadirachtin is the main bioactive ingredient used to manufacture biopesticides. Neem oil and seed extracts and other active ingredients known to possess as insect growth regulators with the addition to germicidal and antibacterial properties which are used to protect and control bacteria, fungi, nematode, and different kinds of other insect pests. Neem insecticides and their other product are very helpful in plant protection and management (Lokanadhan et al., 2012).

The active compound of neem acts at different levels and in various ways (Lokanadhan et al., 2012). Azadirachtin, a well-studied compound acts as antifeedant, antiperistaltic, oviposition deterrent, growth regulator, and affect juvenile hormone (Bhattacharyya et al., 2007; Lokanadhan et al., 2012). It has been reported that azadirachtin significantly affects the Lepidopteran group of pest as antifeedants (<1–50 ppm, depending upon species) while Hemiptera, Homoptera, and Coleoptera, are less affected to azadirachtin behaviorally with up to 100% antifeedants. Azadirachtin active compound affects the synthesis and release of ecdysteroids (molting hormone). These lead to the disruption of the endocrine hormonal system controlling growth and mounting process. This regulates the release of eclosion hormone which controls the motor programme of molting. It has an insecticidal effect on severely reduced growth which causes abnormal and delayed molts resulting in death before the molt. It targets the reproductive organ led to alteration to ecdysteroid and juvenile hormone resulting in the reduction of viable egg and their progeny. Other physiological effect such as cellular processes through affecting the blockage of cell division, inhibition of the digestive enzyme, protein synthesis, and losses of muscle tone in muscles cells. (Lokanadhan et al., 2012).

16.3.2 NICOTINE: MODE OF ACTION

Nicotine and nornicotine an alkaloid obtained from *N. tabacum* and *Nicotiana rustica* belong to the members of the *Solanaceae* (Walia et al., 2014; Ononuju et al., 2016). It is well-known botanical insecticide. Other nicotine analogs compound are nornicotine and anabasine obtained from the plants belong to the family Chenopodiaceae have also possessed insecticidal properties (Ononuju et al., 2016). Nicotine is active against piercing and sap-sucking insects such as aphids, whiteflies, thrips, leafhoppers, and mites.

Nicotine and nornicotine compounds are extremely lethal and fast-acting nerve toxins agonistic to acetylcholine. The synthetic compound of nicotine such as imidacloprid, thiocloprid, nitempiram, acetamiprid, and thiamethoxam are less toxic. They are binding to acetylcholine receptors in the nervous system causing synaptic blocking and resulting in the failure of the central nervous (Ononuju et al., 2016).

16.3.3 ROTENONES: MODE OF ACTION

It is a naturally occurring isoflavonoid with insecticidal, acaricidal, and piscicidal properties (Walia et al., 2014). It is obtained from the plant roots of species of *Derris* (*D. elliptica, D. involuta*) and *Lonchocarpus*. Subsequently, rotenone has been isolated from several members of the other plant family such as *Tephrosia virginiana* (Hoary pea), *Tephrosia vogelii*, *Pachyrhizus erosus* (Mexican yambean, Jicama), *Sphenostylis stenocarpa* (African yam bean), *Mundulea sericea* (cork bush), *Piscidia piscipula* (Florida fish poison tree) *Dalbergia* spp. (African blackwood), and *Millettia laurenti*. (Ononuju et al., 2016). It is a selective, nonspecific and has been extensively used as insecticide, for household, gardens, and for insect control such as lice and tick. It is potent poison for fish and used for eradication as part of water body management. Rotenone is slightly soluble in water and is used either as a dust or in an oil/kerosene solution. It exerts its toxic action by acting as a general inhibitor of cellular respiration. (Walia et al., 2014).

Rotenone is a lipophilic, isoflavonoid compound, and a strong toxic to insects and aquatic lives such as fish but moderately toxic to birds and mammals (Ononuju et al., 2016). This plant-derived chemical reportedly acts by electron transport inhibition at cytochrome b, denying cells to utilize tissue oxygen, with cell death eventually ensuing (Enyiukwu et al., 2014). The mechanism of this action is linked to the inhibition of the transfer of electrons from iron-sulfur centers in complex 1 to ubiquinone in the mitochondria. This spills into interference with nicotinamide adenine dinucleotide during the creation of energy in the form of cellular adenosine triphosphate (ATP). Therefore, build a backup of electrons within the mitochondrial matrix which leads to a reduction in cellular oxygen to radical, and inducing a reactive oxygen species which then damages deoxyribonucleic acid and other components of the mitochondria (Ononuju et al., 2016).

16.3.4 SABADILLA: MODE OF ACTION

Sabadilla (*Schoenocaulon officinale*) is alkaloid producing plants belonging to the family Liliaceae contain many seeds-derived alkaloids—cevadine and its close relative veratridine. These alkaloids with alkaline yield cevacine (cevine) and protocevacine (cevadillin) which have been reported as the active principles of the extracts (Kupchan et al., 1953). The insecticidal properties of sabadilla come from hydrolysis, the alkaloid fraction, which constitutes 3–6% of the extract. Two most important compound such as veratridine and cevadine have been extracted and identified, the former being more potent insecticidal (Walia et al., 2014).

The hydrolytic isolate is more toxic then the former and both act by disrupting neuron cell membrane of nerve activity, symptomized by paralysis and death of susceptible organisms. The mechanism of the sabadilla poisoning is binding to sodium channels, which regulate to nerve excitability resulting in paralysis in insects. Its mode of action is likely to that of the pyrethroids and acts through disruption of nerve cell membranes causing loss of nerve function, an increase in the duration of the action potential, repetitive firing, and a depolarization of the nerve membrane potential due to effects on the sodium channel (Walia et al., 2014; Ononuju et al., 2016). Sabadilla alkaloids are labile and break down rapidly in sunlight. These are less toxic to mammals than other insecticides and are therefore safe to use (Walia et al., 2014).

16.3.5 PYRETHRUM: MODE OF ACTION

Pyrethrum, the most widely used traditional botanical insecticide on the market (Veer and Gopalakrishnan, 2016; Walia et al., 2014). It is highly insecticidal in nature and effective against flying insects such as houseflies and mosquitoes. This crop was extensively grown in considerably large commercial quantities in Kenya, Tanzania, Rwanda, Japan, and Ecuador (Schleier and Peterson, 2011). It is obtained by crushing dried flowers of African daisies belonging to the family of Asteraceae such as *Chrysanthemum*. spp., *Pyrethrum*. spp., and *Tanacetum*. spp. (Walia et al., 2014). This plant species produces an insecticidal compound named, oleoresin that can be extracted with organic solvents and contains six major pyrethrin compounds such as pyrethrin I and II, jasmolin I and II, and cinerin I and II. The toxins, namely pyrethrins, cinerins, and jasmolins, have some unusual insecticidal properties (Arnason and Scott, 2012).

After the exposure of this compound, it acts both on the central nervous system and the peripheral nervous system. After exposure of pyrethrins in affected organisms generally presents symptoms of hyperexcitability, prostration, convulsions, and finally death. It disrupted the membrane pumps that participate in calcium ion-dependent ATPase, and calcium/magnesium ion-dependent ATPase in different biological contexts on different receptors like GABA-gated, and voltage sensitive chloride and calcium channels, and peripheral benzodiazepine receptors (Schleier and Peterson, 2011). It acts on sodium ions and voltage-gated sodium channels, disallows the closing of these channels which result in convulsions and paralysis. The rapid action of pyrethrins is called knockdown effect. However, it has low toxicity to vertebrates but has significant toxicity for no targeted species, especially aquatic organism likely to fish and invertebrates. Like most other natural pesticides, pyrethrins have limited stability to sunlight, air, and atmospheric moisture and reduce stability under field conditions, consider the risks related to its use (Ntalli and Menkissoglu-Spiroudi, 2011). Owing to it instability, the market for natural pyrethrum declined while synthetic pyrethroids have become major commercial product. Thus, successful use of traditional natural pyrethrin is now showing revival due to new bioactive phytochemicals and extractives as possible source of pest control methods (Walia et al., 2014).

16.4 PHYTOCHEMICAL-BASED GREEN PESTICIDE AND INTEGRATED PEST MANAGEMENT (IPM) STRATEGIES

Insect pest and diseases cause substantial agricultural losses through direct and indirect damage (Shukla et al., 2016). We are experiencing a rapid control over the last 50 years on single control agents, particularly chemical pesticides. These synthetic pesticides have increasing difficulties and complications in managing these pests resulting in control failures, resistance in target species, environmental degradation, and contamination of food commodities. It has been reported that assurance of single tactics seriously detracts the sustainability and environment (Koul and Cuperus, 2007). However, different control strategies based on physical barriers, pesticides, biotic agents, and host–plant resistances have been used to control these pests and disease (Shukla et al., 2016).

But none of these strategies can effectively control the pest and diseases owing to their limitation which do not make them ideal controlling agent. At present, we need to implement a management system to deal with these pests. It is a well-established fact that IPM has its own potential, issues, and challenges (Dhaliwal et al., 2004); however, IPM practices control the damage to the environment which is an essential component of sustainable agriculture and environment. Therefore, one of the goals would be the deployment of green chemistry-based IPM practices (Kennedy and Sutton, 2000). Phytochemical-based green pesticides are desirable because the technology could control the pest without affecting the environment. This idea was to support the IPM pattern from centralizing on insect pest management approach depend on pesticide management to a system strategies primarily on plant-driven chemicals.

Botanical insecticides have long been offered an attractive alternative to synthetic pesticides for pest management (Isman, 2006; Khanan et al., 2006). Hence, botanical pesticides are natural, eco-friendly, cost-effective, target specific and less persistent and biodegradable. There are a number of native plants species that have been evaluated against a range of insect pests and diseases on various crops. Their efficacy is more efficient against a number of different pests compared to chemicals that give consistent results under practical conditions, under laboratory, greenhouse, semi-field, field conditions, and in different environments. Botanical pesticides act as a synergistic component in IPM strategies. The IPM is necessary for environmental sustainability to control the insect pests and various diseases (Koul and Cuperus, 2007). This suggests that IPM programmes should represent "a sustainable approach to control pests combining chemical, physical, biological, and cultural practice to ensure favorable economic, ecological, and sociological consequences" (Kennedy and Sutton, 2000). Development of a new strategy for managing insect pests is necessary for sustainable productivity and profitability of agriculture owing to pose substantial threats to the production, quality, and yields of agricultural commodities (Koul and Cuperus, 2007).

16.4.1 MAIN ADVANTAGES OF USING PHYTOCHEMICAL IN IPM

The application of plant-driven insecticide in IPM offers several advantages over synthetic chemical pesticides. As many native plants have adapted the phytochemical in response to the combined selection pressure of phytopathogens, insects, nematodes, and effective against diseases (Dhaliwal and Koul, 2011). Botanical biopesticide is naturally occurring from indigenous plant sources, easily available, cost-effective, and easily accessible. It is potent in very small quantities; generally, affect the selective insect pest and closely related organisms. It is often less persistent, often decompose quickly in the environment, avoiding the pollution leading to the less hazardous environment as well as farmers and consumers. There are harmful effects on plant growth, seed viability and other plant's physiologically process.

16.5 CURRENT RESEARCH AND COMMERCIALIZATION CHALLENGES

The uses of natural plant-based insecticidal products in sustainable agriculture have been increasing globally. It has been a considerable practice happening in the world for finding solutions for economically important pest control through botanicals. Everybody wants to have quick results for saving cost, time, and energy. However, in developing countries, the expenditure on research and development, technological facilities, and expertise are lacking. The potential insecticidal values of plant products are not being properly harnessed and research and development in this area are lacking behind. Thus, most of the research is incomplete and not significant because of its design have limited goals. If plant-based products are to be successful and competitive it must develop and adopt the four major strategies such as organize the resource, develop quality control, adopt standardization strategies, and modify regulatory constraints. This section tries to elucidations of all the necessary steps needed to conduct research and development in this area to impose statutory regulations on ensuring the quality, safety, efficacy, and commercial distribution of such products.

There is a need for large-scale utilization and advances in research of botanicals to maintain the standards of quality and safety of the products. The government and non-governmental organizations are expected to initiate political and financial support needed to establish the infrastructure and to encourage the necessary research and development in this area and impose regulations for commercial production. To enhance the commercialized utilization and efficacy of botanicals pesticides, there should be a developed synergist such as piperonyl butoxide for crop protection. Once a new bioactivity is identified in a plant, simultaneously, the commercialization of that plant-based product, raw material sourcing such as cultivation and propagation of any wild species remains to be a great challenge. The consumption of plant-based insecticide is widespread and increasing. The chief source of raw material is native plant from the wild which is causing reduction of genetic diversity and damage to their habitat. Thus, local farming is a feasible substitute that offers the enabling ground to overcome challenges of discrepancy in plant materials. Conventional plant breeding and genetically modified crops may improve both agronomic and insecticidal traits. There has been significant progress in the research in the biotechnological field. Attention should be paid to develop the awareness, offering training programme, promote improved processing, formulation, and marketing of plant-based pesticides.

ACKNOWLEDGMENT

All the authors acknowledge the necessary infrastructure facilities provided by the Central University of Punjab, Punjab, India.

KEYWORDS

- **pests**
- **biopesticides**
- **insecticides**
- **plant-derived chemicals**
- **sabadilla**

REFERENCES

Adeyemi, M. H. The Potential of Secondary Metabolites in Plant Material as Deterents Against Insect Pests: A Review. *Afr. J. Pure Appl. Chem.* **2010,** *4*(11), 243–246.

Aktar, W.; Sengupta, D.; Chowdhury, A. Impact of Pesticides Use in Agriculture: Their Benefits and Hazards. *Interdiscip. Toxicol.* **2009,** *2*(1), 1–12.

Altemimi, A.; Lakhssassi, N.; Baharlouei, A.; Watson, D. G.; Lightfoot, D. A. Phytochemicals: Extraction, Isolation, and Identification of Bioactive Compounds from Plant Extracts. *Plants (Basel)* **2017,** *6*(4), 1–23.

Arnason, J. T.; Sims, S. R.; Scott, I. M. Natural Products from Plants as Insecticides. *Phytochem Pharmacog; Encyclopedia of Life Support Systems.* **2012,** 1–8.

Bhattacharyya, N.; Chutia, M.; Sarma, S. Neem (*Azadirachta indica* A. Juss), a Potent Biopesticide and Medicinal Plant: A Review. *J. Plant Sci.* **2007,** *2*(3), 251–259.

Choi, W. S.; Park, B. S.; Lee, Y. H.; Yoon, H. Y.; Lee, S. E. Fumigant Toxicities of Essential Oils and Monoterpenes Against *Lycoriella mali* Adults. *Crop Prot.* **2006,** *25*(4), 398–401.

Dhaliwal, G. S.; Jindal, V.; Mohindru, B. Crop Losses Due to Insect Pests: Global and Indian Scenario. *Indian J. Entomol.* **2015,** *77*(2), 165–168.

Dhaliwal, G. S.; Koul, O. *Biopesticides and Pest Management: Conventional and Biotechnological Approaches;* Kalyani Publishers: India, 2011.

Dhaliwal, G.S.; Koul, O.; Arora, R. Integrated pest management: Retrospect and Prospects. In *Integrated pest management: potential, constraints and challenges*. Koul, O.; Dhaliwal, G. S.; Cuperus, G. W.; Eds.; CABI Publishing: Wallingford, UK. 2004. P. 14.

El-Wakeil, N. E. Botanical Pesticides and their Mode of Action. *Gesunde Pflanz.* **2013,** *65*(4), 125–149.

Enyiukwu, D. N.; Awurum, A. N.; Ononuju, C. C.; Nwaneri, J. A. Significance of Characterization of Secondary Metabolites from Extracts of Higher Plants in Plant Disease Management. *Int. J Adv. Agric. Res.* **2014,** *2*, 8–28.

González-Coloma, A.; Martín-Benito, D.; Mohamed, N.; Garcia-Vallejo, M. C.; Soria, A. C. Antifeedant Effects and Chemical Composition of Essential Oils from Different Populations of *Lavandula luisieri* L. *Biochem. Syst. Ecol.* **2006,** *34*(8), 609–616.

Isikber, A. A.; Alma, M. H.; Kanat, M.; Karci, A Fumigant Toxicity of Essential oils from *Laurus nobilis* and *Rosmarinus officinalis* Against all Life Stages of Tribolium Confusum. *Phytoparasitica* **2006,** *34*(2), 167–177.

Islam, M. S.; Hasan, M. M.; Xiong, W.; Zhang, S. C.; Lei, C. L. Fumigant and Repellent Activities of Essential Oil From *Coriandrum sativum* (L.) (Apiaceae) Against Red Flour Beetle *Tribolium castaneum* (Herbst)(Coleoptera: Tenebrionidae). *J. Pest Sci.* **2009,** *82*(2), 171–177.

Isman, M. B. Botanical Insecticides, Deterrents, and Repellents in Modern Agriculture and an Increasingly Regulated World. *Annu. Rev. Entomol.* **2006,** *51,* 45–66.

Kamaraj, C.; Rahuman, A. A.; Mahapatra, A.; Bagavan, A.; Elango, G. Insecticidal and Larvicidal Activities of Medicinal Plant Extracts Against Mosquitoes. *Parasitol Res.* **2010,** *107*(6), 1337–1349.

Kebede, Y.; Gebre-Michael, T.; Balkew, M. Laboratory and Field Evaluation of Neem (*Azadirachta indica* A. Juss) and Chinaberry (*Melia azedarach* L.) Oils as Repellents Against Phlebotomus Orientalis and P. Bergeroti (Diptera: Psychodidae) in Ethiopia. *Acta Trop.* **2010,** *113*(2), 145–150.

Kennedy, G. G; Sutton, T. B. Emerging Technologies for Integrated Pest Management. *Insect. Sci. Applic.* **2000,** *20*(3), 233–234.

Khaliq, A.; Nawaz, A.; Ahmad, M. H.; Sagheer, M. Assessment of Insecticidal Potential of Medicinal Plant Extracts for Control of Maize Weevil, *Sitophilus zeamais* Motschulsky (Coleoptera: Curculionidae).*Basic Res. J. Agric. Sci. Rev.* **2014,** *3*(11), 100–104.

Khanam, L. M.; Talukder, D.; Hye, M. A. Toxic and Repellent Action of Sugarcane Bagasse-Based Lignin Against Some Stored Grain Insect Pests. *Uni J Zoo, Rajshahi Uni.* **2006,** *25,* 27–30.

Kim, S. I.; Park, C.; Ohh, M. H.; Cho, H. C.; Ahn, Y. J. Contact and Fumigant Activities of Aromatic Plant Extracts and Essential Oils Against *Lasioderma serricorne* (Coleoptera: Anobiidae). *J. Stored Prod. Res.* **2003,** *39*(1), 11–19.

Kim, S. I.; Yoon, J. S.; Jung, J. W.; Hong, K. B.; Ahn, Y. J.; Kwon, H. W. Toxicity and Repellency of Origanum Essential Oil and its Components Against *Tribolium castaneum* (Coleoptera: Tenebrionidae) Adults. *J. Asia-Pac. Entomol.* **2010,** *13*(4), 369–373.

Koul, O.; Cuperus, G. W. *Ecologically Based Integrated Pest Management;* CABI: U.K., 2007.

Kulkarni, J.; Kapse, N.; Kulnarni, D. Plant Based Pesticide for Control of Helicoverpa Armigera on *Cucumis sativus*. *Asian Agri. Hist.* **2009,** *13*(4), 327–332.

Kupchan, S. M.; Lavie, D.; Deliwala, C. V.; Andoh, B. Y. A. Schoenocaulon Alkaloids. I. Active Principles of Schoenocaulon officinale. Cevacine and Protocevine[1,2]. *J. Am. Chem. Soc.* **1953,** *75*(22), 5519–5524.

Lokanadhan, S.; Muthukrishnan, P.; Jeyaraman, S. Neem Products and their Agricultural Applications. *J. Biopestic.* **2012,** *5,* 72–76.

Lopez, M. D.; Jordán, M. J.; Pascual-Villalobos, M. J. Toxic Compounds in Essential Oils of Coriander, Caraway and Basil Active Against Stored Rice Pests. *J. Stored Prod. Res.* **2008,** *44*(3), 273–278.

Nathan, S. S.; Hisham, A.; Jayakumar, G. Larvicidal and Growth Inhibition of the Malaria Vector Anopheles Stephensi by Triterpenes from *Dysoxylum malabaricum* and *Dysoxylum beddomei*. *Fitoterapia* **2008,** *79*(2), 106–111.

Ntalli, N. G.; Menkissoglu-Spiroudi, U. Pesticides of Botanical Origin: A Promising Tool in Plant Protection. In *Pesticides-Formulations;* Fate, E., Stoytcheva, M., Eds.; InTech: U.K. 2011; pp 1–24.

Okwute, S. K. Plants as Potential Sources of Pesticidal Agents: A Review. In *Pesticides-Advances in Chemical and Botanical Pesticides;* Soundararajan, R. P., Ed.; InTech: U.K., 2012, pp 207–232.

Ononuju, D. E. C.; Awurum, A. N.; Nwaneri J. A. Modes of Action of Potential Phyto-Pesticides from Tropical Plants in Plant Health Management. *IOSR J. Pharm.* **2016,** *6,* 1–17.

Pavela, R. Larvicidal effects of various Euro-Asiatic plants against Culex quinquefasciatus Say larvae (Diptera: Culicidae).*Parasitol. Res.* **2008,** *102*(3), 555–559.

Pavela, R.; Sajfrtová, M.; Sovová, H.; Bárnet, M.; Karban, J. The Insecticidal Activity of *Tanacetum parthenium* (L.) Schultz Bip. Extracts Obtained by Supercritical Fluid Extraction and Hydrodistillation. *Ind. Crops Prod.* **2010,** *31*(3), 449–454.

Pirali-Kheirabadi, K.; da Silva, J. A. T. Lavandula Angustifolia Essential oil as a Novel and Promising Natural Candidate for Tick (Rhipicephalus (Boophilus) Annulatus) Control. *Exp. Parasitol.* **2010,** *126*(2), 184–186.

Pitasawat, B.; Champakaew, D.; Choochote, W.; Jitpakdi, A.; Chaithong, U.; Kanjanapothi, D.; Chaiyasit, D. Aromatic Plant-Derived Essential Oil: An Alternative Larvicide for Mosquito Control. *Fitoterapia* **2007,** *78*(3), 205–210.

Qin, W.; Huang, S.; Li, C.; Chen, S.; Peng, Z. Biological Activity of the Essential Oil from the Leaves of *Piper sarmentosum Roxb.*(Piperaceae) and its Chemical Constituents on *Brontispa longissima* (Gestro) (Coleoptera: Hispidae).*Pestic. Biochem. Physiol.* **2010,** *96* (3), 132–139.

Radha, R. Toxicity of Three Plant Extracts Against Bean Weevil, *Callosobruchus maculatus* (F.) and Maize Weevil, Sitophilus zeamais Motsch. *Int. J. Curr. Res.* **2014,** *6*(04), 6105–6109.

Schleier III, J. J.; Peterson, R. K. Pyrethrins and Pyrethroid Insecticides. *Green Trends in Insect Control* **2011,** *1,* 94–131.

Shaalan, E. A. S.; Canyon, D.; Younes, M. W. F.; Abdel-Wahab, H.; Mansour, A. H. A Review of Botanical Phytochemicals with Mosquitocidal Potential. *Environ. Int.* **2005,** *31*(8), 1149–1166.

Shukla, A. K.; Upadhyay, S. K.; Mishra, M.; Saurabh, S.; Singh, R.; Singh, H.; Thakur, N.; Rai, P.; Pandey, P.; Hans, A. L.; Srivastava, S. Expression of an Insecticidal Fern Protein in Cotton Protects Against Whitefly. *Nat. Biotechnol.* **2016,** *34*(10), 1046–1051.

Tang, G. W.; Yang, C. J.; Xie, L. D. Extraction of *Trigonella foenum-graecum* L. by supercritical fluid CO_2 and its contact toxicity to *Rhyzopertha dominica* (Fabricius) (Coleoptera: Bostrichidae). *J. Pest Sci.* **2007,** *80*(3), 151–157.

Tapondjou, A. L.; Adler, C.; Fontem, D. A.; Bouda, H.; Reichmuth, C. H. Bioactivities of Cymol and Essential Oils of *Cupressus sempervirens* and *Eucalyptus saligna* against *Sitophilus zeamais* Motschulsky and *Tribolium confusum* du Val. *J Stored Prod Res.* **2005,** *41*(1), 91–102.

Veer, V.; Gopalakrishnan, R. *Herbal Insecticides, Repellents and Biomedicines: Effectiveness and Commercialization;* Springer: India, 2016;

Walia, S.; Saha, S.; Rana, V. S. Phytochemical Pesticides. In *Advances in Plant Biopesticides;* Singh, D., Ed.; Springer: India, 2014; pp 295–322.

Yohannes, A.; Asayew, G.; Melaku, G.; Derbew, M.; Kedir, S.; Raja, N. Evaluation of Certain Plant Leaf Powders and Aqueous Extracts Against Maize Weevil, *Sitophilus zeamais* Motsch. (Coleoptera: Curculionidae). *Asian J. Agric. Sci.* **2014,** *6*(3), 83–88.

CHAPTER 17

ESSENTIAL OILS IN PEST CONTROL AND DISEASE MANAGEMENT

ARVIND SAROJ[1,*], ATUL KUMAR SRIVASTAVA[1], ASHISH KUMAR NAYAK[2], C. S. CHANOTIYA[3], and A. SAMAD[1]

[1]*Department of Plant Pathology, Central Institute of Medicinal and Aromatic Plants, Lucknow, India*

[2]*Department of Microbial Genomics and Diagnostic Laboratory, Regional Plant Resource Centre, Bhubaneswar, India*

[3]*Department of Analytical Chemistry, Central Institute of Medicinal and Aromatic Plants, Lucknow, India*

[*]*Corresponding author. E-mail: amicro27@gmail.com*
[*]*ORCID: https://orcid.org/0000-0002-6083-5291*

ABSTRACT

Plant pathogens damage agriculture products to a large extent resulting in poor crop yield and quality. The well-followed practice to curb plant diseases are mostly involved with the application of conventional fungicides (synthetic chemical). However, their continuous and uncontrolled use has emerged as a big challenge for humans due to its hazardous effect on the environment. This can also lead to the development of resistance to plant pathogens. Green chemistry-based approaches have revolutionized the development of new strategies to curb plant diseases. Natural products mainly essential oils (EOs) have the potential to replace conventional fungicides to some extent. The current chapter aims to discuss the role of EO as biopesticide against plant pathogens (pests and fungal diseases).

17.1 INTRODUCTION: ESSENTIAL OILS (EOs) IN SUSTAINABLE AGRICULTURE

Around the 19th century, Bordeaux mixture as a first chemical fungicide was used to treat pathogen causing downy mildew of grapes. Since then, many conventional fungicides were developed in order to minimize substantial crops damage. As a result, excessive use of conventional fungicides has completely changed the scenario by now. Moreover, uncontrolled use of these chemicals for many decades resulted in several adverse effects to the environment, soil fertility, and human health. This also leads to the development of resistant and more destructive plant pathogens. Therefore, demand and necessity of eco-friendly and biopesticides is the foremost need of modern agriculture.

Biopesticides are derived from natural materials such as plants and microorganisms. For example, L-carvone, Citronellol, p-menthane-3, 8-diol, verbenone (terpenoids class), and methyl eugenol (phenylpropanoid class) are considered biopesticides. There are 299 registered biopesticides active ingredients and 1401 active biopesticides product registrations were registered in The United States Environmental Protection Agency (https://www.epa.gov/ingredients-used-pesticide-products/biopesticide-active-ingredients). Essential oils (Eos) are well documented as natural biopesticides and also proven their effectiveness against various plant pathogens (Pragadheesh et al., 2013a; Maia et al., 2014; Saroj et al., 2015; Ma et al., 2016). Owing to the complexity of oil composition, pathogens may develop resistance slowly.

EOs are produced by plants mainly using two biochemical pathways isopentenyl diphosphate pathway and its isomer dimethylallyl diphosphate pathway (Rehman et al., 2016). EO has been used not only in perfumery, cosmetics, detergents, pharmacology, fine chemistry, and food production industries but also contributing in ethnobotanical medicines since ancient time (Bakkali et al., 2008; Regnault-Roger et al., 2012). Besides this, EO is also well documented as multiple toxic, fumigant, repellent, pesticidal properties, ovicidal, larvicidal (Freitas et al., 2010), and antifeedant activities (Pavela, 2011).

A mixture of compound produced by plants can be divided into primary and secondary metabolites. Primary metabolites are important for the survival of the plant but secondary metabolites do not have a direct impact on the survivability of the plants. EOs are the type of secondary metabolite extracted from an aromatic plant through different hydrodistillation methods. Valgimigli (2012) defined EOs as concentrated hydrophobic liquids having many types of volatile compounds which produce aroma. Terpenes are the main component of the EO, a collection of ethereal lipophilic compounds in a liquid form, obtained from aromatic plants using different hydro or steam distillation techniques (Shah et al., 2012; Garcia et al., 2012 and Amorati et al., 2013). EOs are named after "the oil of the plant they extracted from" but some people have objection or get confused with the other nonvolatile edible vegetable oils such as corn oil, soya oil, and so forth. EOs are produced from all plant organs of aromatic herbs such as buds, leaves, flowers, stems, seeds, twigs, roots, wood, fruits (Andrade et al., 2014). Plant store EOs mainly in glandular trichomes though other oil-bearing glands are also present such as secretory cells, cavities, canals, and epidermis cells (Valgimigli, 2012).

17.2 JOURNEY OF EO

Evidence of EO use was recorded from Lascaux in the form of cave paintings, located in the Dordogne region of France. These cave paintings are first clear evidence of human understanding regarding knowledge of EO-bearing plants and its healing properties. In the 16th century, first time Paracelsus von Hohenheim coined the term "Quinta essential" (EO) as an effective component of drug (Guenther, 1950).

Since ancient time Egyptians use "Kyphi," as herbal medicine, incense, and perfume, made up of 16 different ingredients. They do not have any cleaning agent for body and hairs so used EO as cleaning alternatives like soaps and shampoo. The knowledge of EO recorded in Greece between 400 and 500 BCE which is adapted from the Egyptians. The Greek physician Hippocrates (460–377 B. C. E.) is known as "Father of Medicine," given perfume fumigation and recognized the effect of 300 plants, includes thyme, marjoram, saffron, peppermint, and cumin. The EOs during the ancient time was used in the production of wines, aromatic, breath-refreshing gums, and in the food industry. French used aromatic plants such as rosemary, chamomile, lemon, and thyme in the field of cosmetics and in perfume formation. They also used EOs in the body creams also (Valgimigli, 2012). In China during the period of Huang Ti, aromatic oil uses come in human knowledge. Huang Ti wrote a medicinal-based book "The Yellow Emperor's Book of Internal Medicine" in which he explained the use of EO. Even today, this book is used for the medical purposes in eastern medicine. Romans use EO abundantly for applying essence in their bodies, clothes, and bedding. Roman physicians' spread the knowledge of EOs through books written by Galen and Hypocrites, the texts of this book were later translated into different languages such as Arabic, Persian, and some other as well. The process of EOs extraction through distillation was discovered by Ali-Ibn Sana. The term "Aromatherapie" was first time used by French Chemist René-Maurice Gattefossé while exploring the medicinal properties of EOs. His book "Aromatherapie" was published in 1928, discussed medicinal properties of EOs and their healing potential. Likewise in India, Ayurveda is well known as the traditional therapy based on plant parts and its extracts. Ayurveda used plants as medicine in the treatment of many chronic and acute diseases since 3000 years and EOs for its healing property.

It is assumed that the extraction of EOs using the distillation method began in Egypt, Persia, and India during middle ages (Guenther, 1948). However, later on, extraction of EOs through liquid carbon dioxide, low or high-pressure distillation, steam distillations was discovered as the knowledge of EOs increases. For perfumery, extraction of EOs using lipophilic solvents and supercritical carbon dioxide are found to be the best extraction processes. Although steam distillation is preferred when the EO is used for antimicrobial, pesticidal activities, and pharmaceutical uses as well as for the flavor and preservatives in the food. Recent understanding regarding the composition of EOs and its components such as the detection of hydrocarbons and terpenes lays the foundation of advanced current distillation techniques (Başer and Buchbauer, 2010).

Presently in our daily life, EOs directly or indirectly gets benefited due to its role in medicine, flavor, and cosmetic industries. Depending on the chemical composition of EO resulted in many biological activities such as bactericidal, fungicidal, and pesticidal. Recent research revealed that terpenoids and phenolic compounds are highly toxic to pests and microorganism makes EO more effective in repelling the harmful insects and microorganism (Valgimigli, 2012). Some of the EOs also possess antimicrobial effect including bergamot (*Citrus aurantium* bergamia), black pepper (*Piper nigrum*), cinnamon (*Cinnamomum cassia*), eucalyptus (*Eucalyptus globulus*), orange (*Citrus aurantium* dulcis), rosemary (*Rosmarinus officinalis*), ginger (*Zingiber officinale*), lavender (*Lavandula officinalis*), and lemongrass (*Cymbopogon schoenanthus*) (Andrade et al., 2014). The EOs are well documented for bactericidal, fungicidal, and insecticidal activities (Amorati et al., 2013; Yanishlieva et al., 2006; Bakkali et al., 2008; Valgimigli, 2012; Pragadheesh et al., 2013a, 2013b and Saroj et al., 2015). Some plants of EO importance were presented in Table 17.1.

TABLE 17.1 Essential Oils (EOs) are Derived from Various Parts of Plants.

Plant parts	Name of the plants
Leaves	Basil, bay leaf, cinnamon, eucalyptus, lemon grass, melaleuca, oregano, patchouli, peppermint, pine, rosemary, spearmint, tea tree, wintergreen thyme, palmarosa, citronella, petitgrain
Flowers	Chamomile, clary sage, clove, geranium, hyssop, jasmine, lavender, manuka, marjoram, orange, rose, neroli
Peel	Bergamot, grapefruit, lemon, lime, orange, tangerine
Seeds	Almond, anise, celery, cumin, nutmeg
Wood	Camphor, cedar, rosewood, sandalwood
Berries	Allspice, juniper
Bark	Cassia, cinnamon
Resins	Frankincense, myrrh
Rhizome	Ginger
Root	Valerian, vetiver

17.3 COMPOSITION OF EOS

EOs are normally mixtures of more than 200 components mainly terpenes or derivatives of phenolic compounds. The chemical and structural differences between components of EOs are minimal. On the basis of nature of the compound, it can be classified into volatile and nonvolatile component. More than 90–95% of the EO comprises volatile compounds, primarily monoterpene and sesquiterpene hydrocarbons as well as their oxygenated derivatives along with alcohols, aliphatic aldehydes, and esters. A nonvolatile component comprises about 1–10% of the EO, containing hydrocarbons, fatty acids, carotenoids, sterols, flavonoids, and waxes. Most of the hydrocarbons found in the EO are present as isoprene (Fig. 17.1), which act as a unit of terpenes. Terpenes are the cyclic molecule having the chemical formula $C_{10}H_{16}$.

Limonene, camphene, pinene, methyl chavicol, geraniol, and so forth are the example of terpenes and used as anti-inflammatory, bactericidal, antiviral, antifungal, and antiseptic agent. Terpenes are classified into monoterpenes, sesquiterpenes, and diterpenes. Monoterpenes are a class of terpenes that consist of two isoprene units and present in the form of either acyclic or contain rings. When two isoprene units join head to tail, the result is a monoterpene, when three joins, it is sesquiterpenes, and four linked isoprene units are diterpenes. Terpenes are described below for more information:

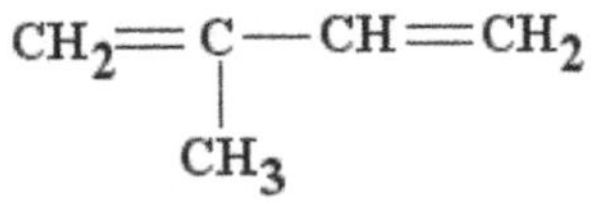

FIGURE 17.1 Structure of isoprene

17.3.1 MONOTERPENES

The molecular formula of monoterpenes is $C_{10}H_{16}$ and made up of two isoprene units, widely distributed in nature with more than 400 natural monoterpenes (Fig. 17.2). Oxidation or biochemical modification of monoterpenes produces the derivative of monoterpenes such as alcohols, ketones, and carboxylic acids that are known as monoterpenoids. Monoterpenes are known for its analgesic, bactericidal, expectorant, and stimulant properties.

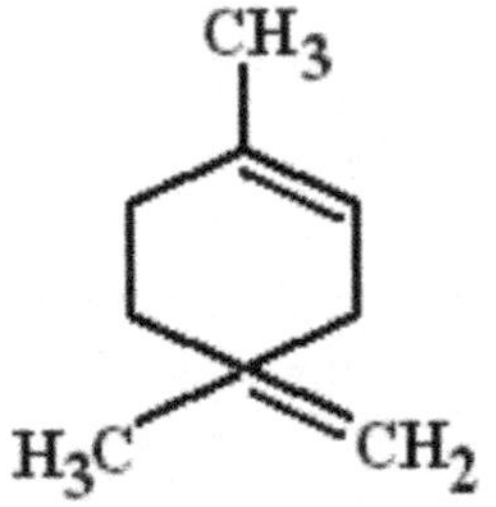

FIGURE 17.2 Structure of limonene (monoterpene).

Moreover, besides being linear derivatives (geraniol, citronellol), the monoterpenes can be cyclic molecules (menthol—monocyclic; camphor—bicyclic; pinenes—α and β). Borneol and camphor are two general monoterpenes used for various purposes. Borneol, isolated from pine oil, is used as a deodorant and disinfectant. Camphor is used as a counterirritant, expectorant, anesthetic, and antipruritic among many other uses. Thujone is a type of monoterpene which act as a toxic agent found in *Artemisia absinthium* (wormwood) from which the liqueur, absinthe, is made.

17.3.2 SESQUITERPENES

Sesquiterpenes are a class of terpenes made up of three isoprene units. The molecular formula of sesquiterpene is $C_{15}H_{24}$. Sesquiterpenes are biogenetically derived from farnesyl pyrophosphate and like monoterpenes, sesquiterpenes may be acyclic or contain rings, including many unique combinations. Biochemical modifications such as oxidation or rearrangement produce the related sesquiterpenoids. They are anti-inflammatory, analgesic, antiseptic, anti-allergic, and antimicrobial in nature. Those sesquiterpenes which are having structural features such as α, β-unsaturated-γ-lactones, showing better biological activities. Beta-caryophyllene in basil and black pepper, Farnesene in chamomile and lavender are the common examples of sesquiterpene (Fig. 17.3).

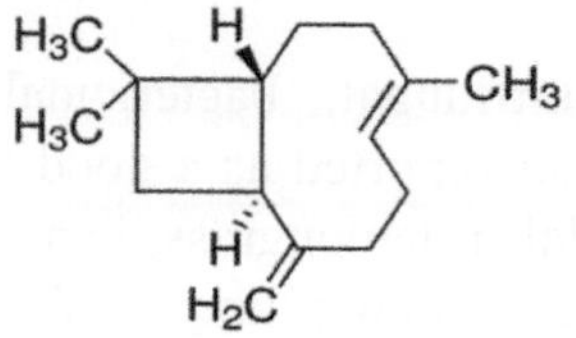

Beta-caryophyllene

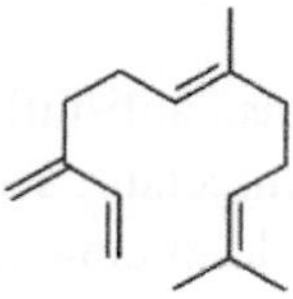

Farnesene

FIGURE 17.3 Structures of sesquiterpenes.

17.3.3 *DITERPENES*

Diterpenes are a class of terpene, made up of four isoprene unit with the molecular formula of $C_{20}H_{32}$. About 2500 natural diterpenes are reported so far. They are biosynthesized by plants, animals, and fungi through the HMG-CoA reductase pathway, with geranylgeranyl pyrophosphate being a primary intermediate. Diterpenes form the basis for biologically important compounds such as retinol, phytol, and retinal. They are known to exhibit antimicrobial and anti-inflammatory property with expectorant, hypotensive, and hormonal balancers. The biosynthesis occurs in plastids and interestingly mixtures of monoterpenes and diterpenes are the major constituents of plant resins. In a similar manner to monoterpenes, diterpenes arise from metabolism of geranyl pyrophosphate (GGPP).

Besides terpenes, alcohols, aldehydes, esters, ketones, and lactones are also present in the EO.

17.3.4 *ALCOHOLS*

Alcohols are compound have a hydroxyl group, present naturally either as a free compound or in combined with a terpenes/ester. When terpenes are attached to an oxygen atom, and a hydrogen atom, the result is an alcohol. When the terpene is monoterpene, the resulting alcohol is called a monoterpenol. Alcohols have a very low or totally absent toxic reaction in the body or on the skin. Therefore, they are considered safe to use. They mainly used individually as antiseptic, bactericidal, antiviral, and germicidal agent. Geraniol in geranium, linalool is in *Ocimum* and *Lippia* is an example of terpineol.

17.3.5 ALDEHYDES

It functions as anti-inflammatory, antifungal, bactericidal, antiviral, antiseptic, disinfectant, sedative and also reported as a good insecticidal. Cinnamaldehyde in cinnamon, citronellal in lemongrass, lemon balm, and citrus eucalyptus and citral in lemon is a good example of an aldehydic present in EO.

17.3.6 ESTERS

Esters are formed through the reaction of alcohols with acids. Esters are the main source of balancing, pleasant, and soothing effects in EOs. Because of the presence of alcohol, they are effective antibacterial and antifungal agents. Medicinally, esters are reported as a sedative, with a balancing act on the nervous system. Geranyl formate in geranium and linalyl acetate in lavender is the best example of ester present in EO.

17.3.7 KETONES

EOs containing ketones are useful in wound healing and encouraging the formation of scar tissues. Ketones are generally toxic such as thujone found in sage, tansy, and thuja. Aromatic nontoxic ketones are jasmone in jasmine oil, carvone in spearmint, and menthone in peppermint oil. Ketones are also having some medicinal properties like anti-catarrhal, expectorant, healing, and cell proliferant.

17.3.8 LACTONES

Lactones particularly known for their anti-inflammatory action play a role in the reduction of prostaglandin synthesis and expectorant actions. The lactones are present in nature in the form of saturated or unsaturated gamma and delta-lactones. A number of substrates have been utilized to demonstrate the microbial formation of lactones. Oleic acid, ricinoleic acid, castor oil gamma keto-acid are some example of lactones.

17.4 BIOACTIVITY OF EOs

The indiscriminate use of antimicrobial agents has resulted in the emergence of a number of drug-resistant bacteria and fungi. To overcome the increasing resistance of pathogenic microorganism and insects, more effective agents with a novel mode of action must be developed. Recently, rigorous research in the field of EOs and extracts of certain plant materials have the potential to replace synthetic pesticides against certain plant pathogens including pest, fungal, and bacterial diseases. EOs derived from several plant families especially Lamiaceae (*Ocimum* spp.), Myrtaceae (*Syzygium* spp.), Lauraceae (*Cinnamomum camphora*), and Asteraceae (*Tagetes patula*) have been reported to have antimicrobial and pesticidal properties (Table 17.2–17.4).

17.4.1 ANTIFUNGAL ACTIVITY

EOs are composed of a number of different components such as aromatic phenols, terpenes, oxides, ethers, alcohols, esters, aldehydes, and ketones in different composition or combinations (Bakkali et al., 2008). Some of the components remain present in very high concentration while some in very low concentration. The antifungal efficacy of EO is mainly either attributed to the overall synergistic effects of all the major and minor compounds or to the bioactivity of the major compounds (Mishra et al., 2013; Saroj et al., 2015). The chemical composition may vary according to the method of EO extraction, the age of the plant, time of harvest, ecological and geographical variations. Hence, before large-scale application, the chemical standardization of EO must be endorsed. As it is well known that ergosterol is specific to the fungal cell membrane and is its major sterol component responsible for maintaining the cell function and integrity. One of the important mechanisms of EO is the reduction in ergosterol synthesis in fungal cells. Some studies have shown that EOs have the potency to cause a considerable reduction in the quantity of ergosterol in the fungal cell membrane (Pinto et al., 2009). The primary action mechanism of azole antifungal drugs is the interruption of sterol biosynthetic pathways resulting in reduced ergosterol biosynthesis

TABLE 17.2 EOs as Antifungal Agents Against a Wide Range of Post-Harvest Fungi.

S/ No.	Plant for essential oil (EO) isolation	Against storage fungi	Method	Used observation	References
1	*Brassica nigra* (S) Brassicaceae	*Aspergillus niger* *Aspergillus ochraceous* *Penicillium citrinum*	Vapor phase and direct contact	100% growth Inhibition at 4 μL/mL concentration in direct contact method and at 47/μL air concentration in vapor phase	Mejia-Garibay et al. (2015)
2	*Mentha arvensis* (AP) Lamiaceae	*Aspergillus fumigatus* *Aspergillus flavus* *A. niger* *Penicillium oxalicum* *Rhizopus* spp. *Curvularia* spp. *Mucor* spp.	In vivo volatile assay wheat seeds	100% protection at 600 ppm except A.f.	Varma and Dubey (2001)
3	*Chenopodium ambrosioides* (L) Amaranthaceae	*A. glucans* *A. niger* *A. flavus* *A. ochraceous*	Poisoned food technique	100% growth inhibition at 0.3% concentration	Jardim et al. (2008)
4	*Cicuta virosa* (F) Apiaceae	*A. ochraceous* *A. niger* *A. flavus* *Alternaria alternata*	Poisoned food technique	100% protection at 300 ppm	Tian et al. (2011)
5	*Cinnamomum jensenianum* (Ba) Lauraceae	*A. flavus*	Poisoned food technique	MIC at 8 μL/mL concentration	Tian et al. (2012)

TABLE 17.2 *(Continued)*

S/ No.	Plant for essential oil (EO) isolation	Against storage fungi	Method	Used observation	References
6	*Cuminum cyminum* (S) Apiaceae	*A. alternata* *Penicillium citrinum* *Aspergillus unguis* *A. flavus* *A. niger* *Curvularia lunata* *Aspergillus nidulans* *Mucor* spp	Poisoned food technique	100% growth inhibition at 0.6 μL/mL concentration except R.s.	Kedia et al. (2014)
7	*Cympopogon citratus* (AP) Poaceae	*A. niger* *Botrytis cinerea*	Dilution method	100% growth inhibition at 500	Tzortzakis and Economakis (2007)
8	*Cymbopogon martini* (L) Poaceae	*A. fumigates* *A. flavus* *A. niger* *Fusarium* spp. *Penicillium* spp.	Dilution by broth method	100% growth inhibition at 0.5 μL/mL concentration	Mishra et al. (2015)
9	*Foeniculum vulgare* (S) Apiaceae	*A. fumigates*	Dilution by broth method	MIC at 10 μg/L concentration	Roby et al. (2013)
10	*Laurus nobilis* (L) Lauraceae	*Botrytis cinerea* *Penicillium digitatum*	Poisoned food technique	At 1000 μg/mL concentrated 100% growth inhibition of B.C. and M.l. but 71% inhibition to P.d.	Corato et al. (2010)

TABLE 17.2 *(Continued)*

S/ No.	Plant for essential oil (EO) isolation	Against storage fungi	Method	Used observation	References
11	*Lippia rugosa* (L) Lamiaceae	*A. flavus*	Agar medium assay	MIC at 1000 ppm	Tatsadjieu et al. (2009)
12	*Mentha spicata* (AP) Lamiaceae	*A. alternata* *A. terreus* *A.flavus* *A. niger* *C. lunata* *A. glutans* *A. nidulans* *Mucor* spp.	Poisoned food technique	100% growth inhibition at 1.0 µL/mL concentration except A.lu. and A.t.	Kedia et al. (2014)
13	*Ocimum sanctum* (AP) Lamiaceae	*Rhizoctonia solani and Choanephora cucurbitarum*	Poisoned food technique	1200 and 900 ppm respectively	Kumar et al. (2010)
14	*Ocimum sanctum* (L) Lamiaceae	*C. cucurbitarum* and *R. solani*	Poisoned food technique	MIC at 730 and 1200 ppm	Pragadheesh et al. (2013b)
15	*Rosmarinus officinalis* (L) Lamiaceae	*A. fumigatus* *A. alternata* *A. flavus* *A. niger* *Mucor* spp.	Contact assay	100% growth inhibition at 1.5 µL/mL concentration except A.a and C.c.	Prakash et al. (2015)
16	*Satureja hortensis* (AP) Lamiaceae	*A. flavus*	Agar dilution method	MIC at 500 ppm	Omidbeygi et al. (2007)

TABLE 17.2 *(Continued)*

S/ No.	Plant for essential oil (EO) isolation	Against storage fungi	Method	Used observation	References
17	*Syzygium cumini* (L)	*R. solani and C. cucurbitarum*	Poison food method and volatile phase	MIC at 1200 ppm	Pinto et al. (2009)
18	*Syzygium aromaticum* (B) Myrtaceae	*A. flavus* *A. fumigatus* *A. niger*	Broth dilution method	100% inhibition at 0.64 μL/mL concentration	Pinto et al. (2009)
19	*Tagetes patula* (Fl) Asteraceae	*Penicillium digitatum* *Botrytis cinerea*	Poisoned food method	MIC for B.c. at 10 μL/mL and for P.d. at 1.85 μL/mL concentration	Romagnoli et al. (2005)
20	*Thymus pulegioides* (AP) Lamiaceae	*A. flavus* *A. fumigatus* *A. niger*	Broth dilution method	100% inhibition at 0.32 μL/mL concentration	Pinto et al. (2006)
21	*Trachyspermum ammi* (F) Apiaceae	*Aspergillus glucans* *A. alternata* *A. flavus* *A. niger* *A. terreus* *C. lunata* *Penicillium citrinum* *A. unguis* *A. nidulans* *Mucor* spp.	Poisoned food method	100% growth inhibition at 0.8 μL/mL concentration	Kedia et al. (2015)

TABLE 17.2 *(Continued)*

S/ No.	Plant for essential oil (EO) isolation	Against storage fungi	Method	Used observation	References
22	*Zataria multiflora* (AP) Lamiaceae	*A. flavus*	Liquid agar dilution method	MIC at 400 ppm	Gandomi et al. (2009)
23	*Cinnamomum camphora* (L) Lauraceae	*C. cucurbitarum*	Poisoned food method	MIC at 1200 ppm	Pragadheesh et al. (2013a)
24	*Ocimum basilicum* (L) Lamiaceae	*R. solani and C. cucurbitarum*	Poisoned food method	MIC at 1200 ppm	Padalia et al. (2014)

Plant part: AP=aerial part; B=bud; Ba=Bark; F=Fruit; Fl=flower; L=leaf; S=seed. MIC=Minimum inhibitory concentration.

TABLE 17.3 Some Commercial Plant Health Products from plant Natural Products used as Fungicide.

Botanical source	Product	Main bioactive components	Mode of action	Examples of trade names	References
Azadirachta indica A. Juss	neem (neem oil, medium, polarity extracts)	Azadirachtin, dihydroazadirachtin, variety of triterpenoids (nimbin, salannin, and others)	Moulting inhibitors (ecdysone antagonists), antifeedant/ repellent, physical smothering, and desiccation	Ecozin, azatrol EC, agroneem, trilogy	Copping and Duke (2007)
Cassia tora L., cassia obtusifolia	Cinnamaldehyde	Cinnamaldehyde	Disruption of the fungal membranes, repellent and attractant	Vertigo, Cinnacure	Dayan et al. (2009)
Reynoutria sachalinensis (Fr. Schm) Nakai	Extract of giant knotweed	Physcion, emodin	Induction of SAR (phenolic phytoalexines)	Milsana, Regalia	Regnault-Roger (2012)
Macleaya cordata R. Br.	Pink plume poppy extract	Anguinarine chloride, alkaloids, and chelerythrine chloride	Induction of SAR (phenolic phytoalexines)	Qwel	Regnault-Roger (2012)
Trigonella foenum-graecum L.	Stifénia	Unknown	Stimulation of plant defence	Stifénia	Regnault-Roger (2012)
Plant-derived acid	Citric acida	Citric acid	Not identified with Certainty	Sharp shooter, Repellex	Copping and Duke (2007)
Simmondsia californica Nutt., *Salvia* chinensis Link	jojoba essential oil (EO)	straight-chain wax esters	suffocation (eggs and immature life stages), repellent, blocking access to oxygen	Detur, Erasem, Eco E-Rase, Permatrol, ERase	Dayan et al. (2009)
Capsicum spp. (Capsicum frutescens Mill)	Capsicum oleoresin	Capsaicin	Neurotoxic, repellent	Hot pepper wax insect repellent, hot pepper wax	Copping and Duke (2007)
Thymus vulgaris *Thymus* spp.	Thyme EO	thymol, carvacrol	Neurotoxic, interference with GABA-gated chloride channels	Proud 3, Organic Yard Insect Killer, Promax	Fischer et al. (2013)
Rosmarinus officinalis	Rosemary EO	1,8-cineole (borneol, camphor, monoterpenoids)	Octopamine antagonists; membrane disruptors, others	Ecotrol, Sporan	Isman and Machial (2006)

TABLE 17.4 List of Active Substance from Different Plants and its Mode of Action Against Microorganisms, Weeds, and Insects.

Source	Active substance	MoA	References
Target: bacteria and fungi			
Cassia plants (*Cassia tora* L.)	Cinnamaldehyde	Unknown	Brown (2013)
Allium crops (garlic and onion)	Diallylsulphide	Unknown	Davis (2007)
Laminaria digitata	Laminarin	Host plant defense Induction	Aziz et al. (2003)
Oudemansiella mucida	Oudemansin	Inhibitor of mitochondrial electron transport (complex III)	Akita (2009)
Target: Insect			
Azadirachta indica	Azadirachtin	Unknown	López and Pascual-Villalobos (2010)
Capsicum spp.	Capsaicin	Nervous system dysfunction	USEPA (1992)
Mentha spicata var. *crispa* (Lamiaceae) *Carumcarvi* L. (Apiaceae)	Carvone	Repellent	López and Pascual-Villalobos (2010)
Allium crops (garlic and onion)	Diallylsulphide	Repellent	USEPA (2010)
Estragon and conifer Trees	Estragole	Repellent	USEPA (2001)
Corymbia citriodora	*p*-Menthane-3,8-diol	Repellent	Elmhalli et al. (2009)
Nicotiana tabacum L.	Nicotine	Nicotinic acetylcholine receptor (nAChR) Agonists	Shi et al. (2006)
Chrysanthemum cinerariaefolium and *Chrysanthemum coccineum*	Pyrethrin I and II	Sodium channel modulators	Casida (2011)
Tropical plants in the genus *Derris*, *Lonchocarpus* or *Tephrosia*	Rotenone	Mitochondrial complex I electron transport inhibitors	Chauvin et al. (2001)
Saccharopolyspora spinosa and *Saccharopolyspora Pogona*	Spinosyns	Nicotinic, acetylcholine receptor (nAChR) allosteric activator	Kirst et al. (1991)

(Mishra et al., 2015). Further, the studies of *Cuminum cyminum, Mentha spicata, Trachyspermum ammi*, and *Cinnamomum jensenianum.* EOs have a clear evidence of reduced ergosterol biosynthesis due to EO treatment on *Aspergillus flavus* cells (Kedia et al., 2014). Being lipophilic in nature, the EOs targets the plasma membrane (Fig. 17.4) and the membranous organelles of the fungal cell by either crossing or accumulating in the cell membrane. This results in interaction with the enzymes and proteins therein, disturb cell permeability by producing a flux of protons toward the cell exterior which ultimately disrupts the fungal cell organization and causes cell death (Kelly et al., 1995). The effects included membrane swelling, change in fluidity, and increased passive flux of protons. The releases of ions are not based on their size and/or formation of holes in the membrane. However, the EO accumulates in the plasma membrane, causes increased membrane bilayer disorder and ion leakage. These effects cause a disturbance in the osmotic balance of the cell, making its membrane-associated proteins inefficient leading to inhibition of cell growth. Some of the well-known EO components namely thymol, carvacrol, eugenol, and other phenolic components have been reported to disrupt cell membrane by dissipating H^+ and K^+ ion gradients causing leakage of vital cellular constituents which results in water imbalance, depletion of intracellular ATP concentration, and finally cell death (Mejia-Garibay et al., 2015).

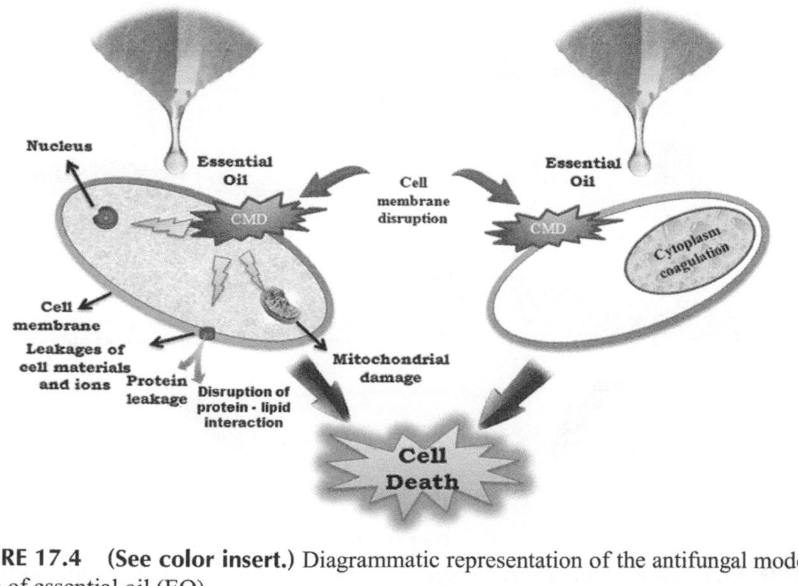

FIGURE 17.4 (See color insert.) Diagrammatic representation of the antifungal mode of action of essential oil (EO).

17.4.2 PESTICIDAL ACTIVITY

The compound of plant EO has been known as a traditional source of pesticide, which controls/reduce the number of harmful insects from the environment. Industries develop a large number of EO-based commercial products including pesticide for human being. Secondary metabolites play an important role in plant-insect interaction, work as insecticidal, antifeedant, and repellent activity (Bernays and Chapman 1994). The physiological action of EO on insects is not much clearer in knowledge but the action of EO or it's compound cause symptoms that suggest a neurotoxic mode of action (Coats et al., 1991; Kostyukovsky et al., 2002). Monoterpene (like linalool, citronellal) effect on ion transport system of insect nervous system to release acetylcholine esterase (Re et al., 2000). Octopamine-1 and octopamine-2 are two class of receptor; behave as a neurotransmitter or neurohormone work on a biological system of insect (Evans, 1980; Hollingworth et al., 1984; Evans, 1981). Interrupting the functioning of octopamine results in total crash of the nervous system of insects (Fig. 17.5). Therefore, an octopaminergic system of insects represents a biorational target for insect control.

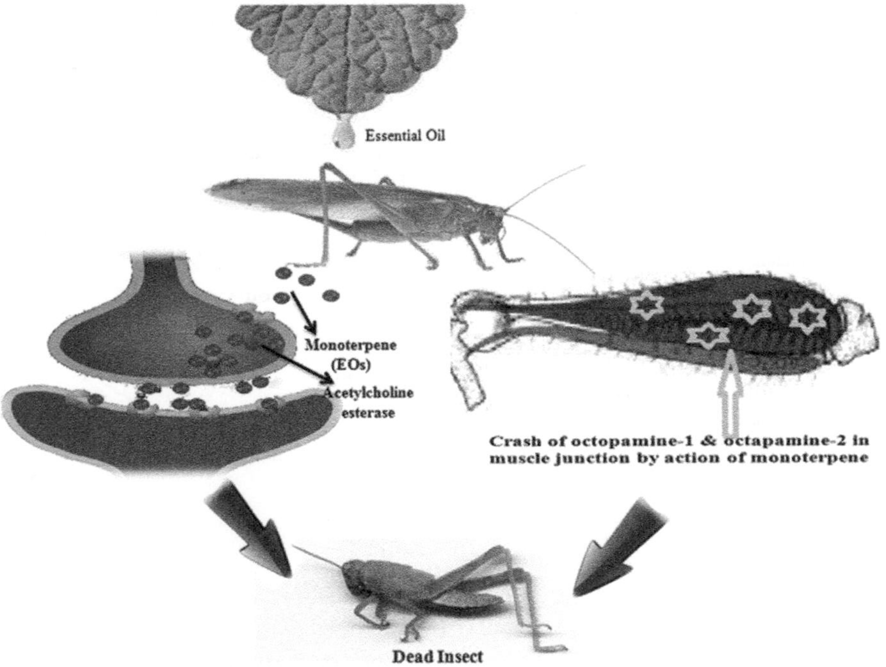

FIGURE 17.5 (See color insert.) Target sites in insects as a possible neurotransmitter-mediated toxic action of essential oils.

17.5 ROLE OF EOS IN DISEASE MANAGEMENT

EO as biological control has been advanced and now an alternative to synthetic fungicides and considerable success in laboratory and pilot scale tests have been realized utilizing antagonistic microorganisms to control crops diseases. EOs are also considered as a promising alternative with many having antifungal properties (Hammer et al., 2003). Several antagonistic fungi and bacteria have been isolated and shown to have a broad spectrum of activity against a number of pathogens on different varieties of fruits. Recently, an interest has been shown in combining microbial biocontrol agents with other chemical components to increase their activity against phytopathogens (Droby et al., 1998). Application of EO is a very attractive method for controlling plant diseases.

EOs and their different components are gaining increasing interest because of their relatively safe status, their wide acceptance by consumers, and their exploitation for potential multi-purpose functional use (Ormancey et al., 2001). EOs have been used successfully in combination with a variety of treatments, such as antimicrobial agents, mild heat, and salt compounds (Karatzas et al., 2000).

Production of EOs by plants is believed to be predominantly a defense mechanism against pathogens and pests. EOs are made up of many different volatile compounds that contribute in its composition quite often varies between species (Mishra and Dubey, 1994). It is difficult to associate the antimicrobial activity with single compounds or classes of compounds. It seems that the insecticidal and antimicrobial effects are the result of many compounds acting synergistically (Bagamboula et al., 2004). After application of EOs, the chances of development of resistant races of fungi/insects get reduced. Currently, the management of necrotrophic fungi infecting tomatoes is controlled by the use of protectant fungicides such as mancozeb and chlorothalonil or systemic fungicides in the strobilurin class (Diver et al., 1999). However, studies carried out by many research groups revealed that EOs are other sustainable disease management option. EO of spearmint is associated with a number of antifungal properties. Spearmint has been studied and found to be potential against necrotrophic phytopathogens. Consequently, EOs are found to be more effective against many gram-positive and gram-negative bacteria. Spearmint has an inhibitory effect against *Staphylococcus aureus*, *Klebsiella sp.*, *Escherichia coli*, and *Pseudomonas aeruginosa.*

EOs from "alecrim-pimenta" (*Lippia sidoides* Cham.), wild basil (*Ocimum gratissimum* L.), lemongrass (*Cymbopogon citratus* Stapf) and "cidrao" (*Lippia citriodora* Kunth) inhibited the germination and mycelial growth of *Colletotrichum gloeosporioides* conidia (Souza Júnior, 2009). Thyme, eucalyptus citriodora, citronella, and neem oils showed a direct effect on *Phakopsora pachyrhizi*, because they reduce Asian soybean rust severity. Some of the EOs are commercialized with different names such as orange EOs on wheat seeds (Stülp et al., 2011) and neem EOs on rice seeds.

17.5.1 CURRENT SCENARIO OF EO AS BIOPESTICIDE

Natural products such as repellent EOs are becoming increasingly popular because of their low toxicity and customer approval. Therefore, the market of EO will have the strongest growth of all the botanical pesticides markets in coming years. Similarly, the antimicrobial potential of *Ocimum* spp. against *E. coli*, *Bacillus subtilis*, *Staphylococcus* spp makes it potential to be commercialized at large scale. However, studies conducted by many research groups revealed that *Ocimum canum* and *Ocimum sanctum* have been reported as the most effective bactericide among the studied *Ocimum* EOs. Bozin et al. (2006) reported that the antibacterial activity of *Ocimum basilicum* against 13 human pathogenic bacteria and find that the minimum inhibitory concentration ranges 8–30 μL/mL. Atanda et al. (2007) investigated the ability of sweet basil (*O. basilicum*) in the growth control of aflatoxigenic fungus *Aspergillus parasiticus*.

17.5.2 EMERGING PROSPECT OF EO

A long list of plant-derived products as potential pesticides exists and this list will keep counting in the future. Consequently, resistance against EOs may develop slowly because of its complex composition and more than single target sites. Antifungal activity of the EO has been established due to induction of changes in cell wall composition, cell lysis, cytoplasm coagulation, and plasma membrane disruption (Knobloch et al., 1989; Pragadheesh et al., 2013a) in the phytopathogens. Though, in order to exploit these products to their full extent safety issue must be addressed.

EO, which showed fungistatic activity served as a better commercial option for the management of damping-off diseases as compared to fungicidal oils. As soil harbors natural microflora including bacteria and fungi. These microfloras are required for the plant growth promotion. If treated with fungicidal oils, it can also disturb the natural microflora of that particular area leading to poor plant growth. Research on action mechanism of EO may help to select suitable EO or combination of EOs which will be used to identify resistance/susceptibility status of the target pest/pathogen. Such studies allow a more targeted approach, further adapted for the selection of EO, also providing more sites to be explored. Combination of piperonyl butoxide with other EO components such as eugenol and thymol may increase the activity of these compounds to different sorts of arthropods (Yadav et al., 2009; Rossi and Palacios, 2013). Studies on detoxification pathways may also lead to an advantageous way to analyze kinds of EOs that can be used on pesticide-resistant insects, similarly in chemotherapy treatment of cancers where over express drug metabolizing enzymes are targeted using pro-drugs. Additionally, it may be possible to increase the toxicity of EOs, such as that of *Mintostachy verticillate*, further by inducing the expression of detoxification enzymes.

Futuristic approach to make EOs more effective against a range of pests and plant pathogens lies in its synergistic combinations. Combination of EO may lead to activating multiple mechanisms to inhibit pathogens, eventually resolve the problem of pathogens resistance development nature. Synergism between carvacrol and some hydrocarbons monoterpenes (such as α-pinene, camphene, myrcene, α-terpinene, and p-cymene) that typically showed low antimicrobial properties has been observed (Moreno et al., 2007). However, the ability of hydrocarbons to interact with cell membrane facilitates the penetration of carvacrol into the cell (Jaenson et al., 2006; Moreno et al., 2007, McAllister and Adams, 2010).

17.6 FUTURE PERSPECTIVES AND CONCLUSIONS

Prolong uncontrolled use of chemical pesticides for many decades resulted in several adverse effects to the environment, soil fertility, and human health. Therefore, sustainable development in agriculture is the foremost need of the current global scenario to sustain the growing population, especially in developing countries. In the on-going search to find out alternatives, EOs showing the promising potential to establish EO-based products against specific pests in a number of ways. For many of such products still needed to prove efficacy, safety, and modes of action to identify its limitations such as minimal residual activity with advances in fields such as slow-release technology (nanocoating of EO). Molecular-based studies may enhance the understanding of the identification of targets and detoxification pathways, which ultimately leads to ensuring product safety and effectiveness.

Allowing EOs, compounds/combinations to be used on the same specific modes of action which are used by existing synthetics in general activity that target similar pathways. EOs and their components applied singly or in specific combinations, are effective against a range of important arthropod pests and plant pathogens.

To commercialize EO-based pesticides generally face three obstacles to be overcome: (i) availability of natural resources; (ii) the need for chemical standardization, mode of action, toxicity and quality control; and (iii) difficulties in the registration of such products. Although most of the EOs are found to be nontoxic to mammals and not persist in the environment for too long these properties may play an important role to ease its commercialization (Isman, 1999; Isman, 2000).

KEYWORDS

- **plant pathogens**
- **essential oils**
- **pest control**
- **disease management**
- **botanicals**

REFERENCES

Akita, H. Recent Advances in the Syntheses of Biologically Active Natural Products using Biocatalyst. *Heterocycles* **2009,** *78,* 1667–1713.

Amorati, R.; Foti, M. C.; Valgimigli, L. Antioxidant Activity of Essential Oils. *J. Agric. Food Chem.* **2013,** *61,* 10835–10847.

Andrade, B. F.; Barbosa, L. N.; Probst, I. Antimicrobial Activity of Essential Oils. *J. Essent. Oil Res.* **2014,** *26,* 34–40.

Atanda, O. O.; Akpan, I.; Oluwafemi, F. The Potential of Some Spice Essential Oils in the Control of *A. Parasiticus* CFR 223 and Aflatoxin Production. *Food Control* **2007,** *18,* 601–607.

Aziz, A.; Poinssot, B.; Daire, X.; Adrian, M.; Bezier, A.; Lambert, B.; Joubert, J. M.; Pugin, A. Laminarin Elicits Defense Responses in Grapevine and Induces Protection Against *Botrytis cinerea* and *Plasmopara viticola. Mol. Plant Microbe Interact.* **2003.** *16,* 1118–1128.

Bagamboula, C. F.; Uyttendaele, M.; Debevere, J. Inhibitory Effect of Thyme and Basil Essential Oils, Carvacrol, Thymol, Estragol, linalool and *p*-cymene Towards *Shigella sonnei* and *S. flexneri. Food Microbiol.* **2004,** *21,* 33–42.

Bakkali, F.; Averbeck, S.; Averbeck, D.; Idaomar, M. Biological Effects of Essential Oils – A Review. *Food and Chemical Toxicology*. **2008,** *46,* 446–475.

Başer, K. H. C.; Buchbauer, G. *Handbook of Essential Oils: Science: Technology, and Applications;* CRC Press, Taylor & Francis Group: New York, 2010.

Bernays, E. A.; Chapman, R. F. *Host-Plant Selection by Phytophagous Insects;* Chapman & Hall: New York, 1994.

Bozin, B.; Mimica-Dukic, N.; Simin, N.; Anackov, G. Characterization of the Volatile Composition of Essential Oils of Some Lamiaceae Spices and the Antimicrobial and Antioxidant Activities of the Entire Oils. *J. Agric. Food Chem.* **2006,** *54,* 1822–1828.

Brown, A. E. Mode of Action of insecticides and Related Pest Control Chemicals for Production Agriculture, Ornamentals and Turf. Pesticide Information Leaflet No. 43. University of Maryland, USA, 2013, 1–13. http://pesticide.umd.edu/uploads/1/3/5/6/13565116/pil43_modeofaction-agornamturf_2005-2013.pdf (accessed November 3, 2017).

Casida, J. E. Curious About Pesticide Action. *J. Agric. Food Chem.* **2011,** *59,* 2762–2769.

Chauvin, C.; De Oliveira, F.; Ronot, X.; Mousseau, M.; Leverve, X.; Fontaine, E. Rotenone Inhibits the Mitochondrial Permeability Transition-Induced Cell Death in U937 and KB cells. *J. Biol. Chem.* **2001,** *276,* 41394–41398.

Coats, J. R.; Karr, L. L.; Drewes, C. D. Toxicity and Neurotoxic Effects of Monoterpenoids: In Insects and Earthworms. In *Naturally Occurring Pest Bioregulators;* Hedin, P. A. Ed.; ACS Symposium Series: Washington, DC, 1991; *449* (20), pp 305–316.

Copping, L. G.; Duke, S. O. Natural Products that have been used commercially as crop Protection Agents. *Pest Manage. Sci.* **2007,** *63,* 524–554.

Corato, U.; Maccioni, O.; Trupo, M., Sanzo, G. Use of Essential Oil of *Laurus nobilis* Obtained by Means of a Supercritical Carbon Dioxide Technique Against Post Harvest Spoilage Fungi. *Crop Prot.* **2010,** *29,* 142–147.

Davis, R. M.; Hao, J. J.; Romberg, M. K.; Nunez, J. J.; Smith, R. F. Efficacy of Germination Stimulants of Sclerotia of *Sclerotium cepivorum* for Management of White Rot of Garlic. *Plant Dis.* **2007,** *91,* 204–208.

Dayan, F. E.; Cantrell, C. L.; Duke, S. O. Natural Products in Crop Protection. *Bioorg. Med. Chem.* **2009,** *17,* 4022–4034.

Diver, S.; Kuepper, G.; Born, H. Organic Tomato Production. *ATTRA* **1999,** *800,* 1–24.

Droby, S. L.; Cohen, A.; Daus, M. E.; Wisniewski, B. W. Commercial testing of Aspire: A Yeast Preparation for the Biological Control of Postharvest Decay of Citrus. *Biol. Control* **1998,** *12,* 97–101.

Elmhalli, F. H.; Palsson, K.; Orberg, J.; Jaenson, T. G. Acaricidal Effects of *Corymbia citriodora* oil Containing Para-menthane-3,8-diol Against Nymphs of *Ixodes ricinus* (*Acari*: *Ixodidae*). *Exp. Appl. Acarol.* **2009,** *48,* 251–262.

Evans, P. D. Biogenic Amines in the Insect Nervous System. *Adv. Insect Physiol.* **1980,** *15,* 317–473.

Evans, P. D. Multiple Receptor Types for Octopamine in the Locust. *J. Physiol.* **1981,** *318,* 99–122.

Fischer, D.; Imholt, C.; Pelz, H. J.; Wink, M.; Prokope, A.; Jacoba, J. The Repelling Effect of Plant Secondary Metabolites on Water Voles. *Arvicola amphibious*. *Pest Manage. Sci.* **2013,** *69,* 437–443.

Freitas, F. P.; Freitas, S. P.; Lemos, G. C.; Vieira, I. J.; Gravina, G. A.; Lemos, F. J. Comparative Larvicidal Activity of Essential Oils from Three Medicinal Plants Against *Aedes Aegypti* L. *Chem. Biodiversity*. **2010,** *7,* 2801–2807.

Gandomi, H.; Misaghi, A.; Basti, A. A.; Bokaei, S.; Khosravi, A.; Abbasifar, A.; Javan, A. J. Effect of *Zataria multiflora* Boiss. Essential Oil on Growth and Aflatoxin Formation by *Aspergillus flavus* in Culture Media and Cheese. *Food and Chemical Toxicology.* **2009,** *47,* 2397–2400.

Garcia, L. C.; Tonon, R. V.; Hubinger, M. D. Effect of Homogenization Pressure and Oil Load on the Emulsion Properties and the Oil Retention of Microencapsulated Basil Essential Oil (*Ocimum basilicum* L.). *Drying Technol. Int. J.* **2012,** *30,* 1413–1421.

Guenther, E. The Essential Oil. D. Van Nostrand Company: New York, Inc., 1948.

Guenther, E. The Essential Oil. D. Van Nostrand: New York, 1950; Vol. 4.

Hammer, K. A.; Carson, C. F.; Riley, T. V.; Antifungal Activity of the Components of *Melaleuca alternifolia* (tea tree) Oil. *J. Appl. Microbiol.* **2003,** *95,* 853–860.

Hollingworth, R. M.; Johnstone, E. M.; Wright, N. Aspects of the Biochemistry and Toxicology of Octopamine in Arthropods. In *Pesticide Synthesis through Rational Approaches;* Magee, P. S., Kohn, G. K., Menn, J. J. Eds.; 1984, *255,* 103–125.

Isman, M. B. *Pestic. Outlook.* **1999,** *10,* 68–72.

Isman, M. B. Plant Essential Oils for Pest and Disease Management. *Crop Prot.* **2000,** *19,* 603–608.

Isman, M. B.; Machial, C. M. Pesticides Based on Plant Essential Oils: From Traditional Practice to Commercialization. In *Naturally Occuring Bioactive Compounds;* Rai, M. Carpinella, M. C., Eds.; Elsevier: Amsterdam Netherland, 2006; pp 29–44.

Jaenson, T. G.; Garboui, S.; Palsson, K. Repellency of Oils of Lemon Eucalyptus, Geranium, and Lavender and the Mosquito Repellent MyggA Natural to *Ixodes ricinus* (Acari: Ixodidae) in the Laboratory and Field. *J. Med. Entomol.* **2006,** *43,* 731–736.

Jardim, C. M.; Jham, G. N.; Dhingra, O. D.; Freire, M. M. Composition and Antifungal Activity of the Essential Oil of the Brazilian *Chenopodium ambrosioides* L. *J. Chem. Ecol.* **2008,** *34,* 1213–1218.

Karatzas, A. K.; Bennik, M. H.; Smid, E. J.; Kets, E. P. Combined Action of S-carvone and Mild Heat Treatment on *Listeria monocytogenes* Scott A. *J. Appl. Microbiol.* **2000,** *89,* 296–301.

Kedia, A.; Prakash, B.; Mishra, P. K.; Chanotiya, C. S.; Dubey, N. K. Antifungal, Antiaflatoxigenic, and *Insecticidal* Efficacy of *Spearmint* (*Mentha spicata* L.) Essential Oil. *Int. Biodeterior. Biodegrad.* **2014,** *89,* 29–36.

Kedia, A.; Prakash, B.; Mishra, P. K.; Dwivedy, A. K.; Dubey, N. K. *Trachyspermum ammi* L. Essential Oil as Plant Based Preservative in Food System. *Indust. Crops Prod.* **2015,** *69,*104–109.

Kelly, S. L.; Lamb, D. C.; Corran, A. J.; Baldwin, B. C.; Kelly, D. E. Mode of Action and Resistance to Azole Antifungals Associated with the Formation of 14 alpha-methylergosta-8,24(28)-dien-3 beta,6 alpha-diol. *Biochem. Biophys. Res. Commun.* **1995,** *207,* 910–915.

Kirst, H. A.; Michel, K. H.; Martin, J. W.; Creemer, L. C.; Chio, E. H.; Yao, R. C.; Nakatsukasa, W. M.; Boeck, L. D.; Occolowitz, J. L.; Paschal, J. W. et al. A83543A-D, Unique Fermentation-Derived Tetracyclic Macrolides. *Tetrahedron Lett.* **1991,** *32,* 4839–4842.

Knobloch, K.; Pauli, P.; Iberl, B.; Weigand, H.; Weiss, N. Antibacterial and Antifungal Properties of Essential Oil Components. *J. Essent. Oil. Res.* **1989,** *1,* 119–128.

Kostyukovsky, M.; Rafaeli, A.; Gileadi, C.; Demchenko, N.; Shaaya, E. Activation of Octopaminergic Receptors by Essential Oil Constituents Isolated from Aromatic Plants: Possible Mode of Action Against Insect Pests. *Pest Manage. Sci.* **2002,** *58,* 1101–1106.

Kumar, A.; Shukla, R.; Singh, P.; Dubey, N. K. Chemical Composition, Antifungal and Antiaflatoxigenic Activities of *Ocimum sanctum* L. Essential Oil and its Safety Assessment as Plant Based Antimicrobial. *Food Chem. Toxicol.* **2010,** *48,* 539–543.

López, M. D.; Pascual-Villalobos, M. J. Mode of Inhibition of Acetylcholinesterase by Monoterpenoids and Implications for Pest Control. *Ind. Crops Prod.* **2010,** *31,* 284–288.

Ma, B.-X.; Ban X.-Q.; He, J.-S.; Huang, B.; Wang, Y.-W.; et al. Antifungal Activity of *Ziziphora clinopodioides* Lam. Essential Oil Against *Sclerotinia sclerotiorum* on Rapeseed Plants (*Brassica campestris* L.). *Crop Prot.* **2016,** *89,* 289–295.

Maia, A. J.; Oliveira, J. S. B.; Schwan-Estrada, K. R. F.; Faria, C. M. R.; Batista, B. N. The Control of Isariopsis Leaf Spot and Downy Mildew in Grapevine cv. Isabel with the Essential Oil of Lemon Grass and the Activity of Defensive Enzymes in Response to the Essential Oil. *Crop Prot.* **2014,** *63,* 57–67.

McAllister, J. C.; Adams, M. F. Mode of Action for Natural Products Isolated from Essential Oils of Two Trees is Different from Available Mosquito Adulticides. *J. Med. Entomol.* **2010,** *47,* 1123–1126.

Mejia-Garibay, B.; Palou, E.; Lopez-Malo, A. Composition, Diffusion, and Antifungal Activity of Black Mustard (*Brassica nigra*) Essential Oil when Applied by Direct Addition or Vapor Phase Contact. *J. Food Prot.* **2015,** *4,* 843–848.

Mishra, A. K.; Dubey, N. K. Evaluation of Some Essential Oils for Their Toxicity Against Fungi Causing Deterioration of Stored Food Commodities. *Appl. Environ. Microbiol.* **1994,** *60,* 1101–1105.

Mishra, P. K.; Singh, P.; Prakash, B.; Kedia, A.; Dubey, N. K.; Chanotiya, C. S. Assessing Essential Oil Components as Plant-Based Preservatives Against Fungi that Deteriorate Herbal Raw Materials. *Int. Biodeterior. Biodegrad.* **2013,** *80,* 16–21.

Mishra, P. K.; Kedia, A.; Dubey, N. K. Chemically Characterized *Cymbopogon martinii* (Roxb.) Wats. Essential Oil for Shelf Life Enhancer of Herbal Raw Materials Based on Antifungal, Antiaflatoxigenic, Antioxidant Activity, and Favorable Safety Profile. *Plant Biosyst. Int. J. Dealing All Aspects Plant Biol.* **2015,** *50,* 1313–1322.

Moreno, P. R. H.; Lima, M. E. L.; Sobral, M.; Young, M. C. M.; Cordeiro, I.; Apel, M. A.; Limberger, R. P.; Henriques, A. T. Essential Oil Composition of Fruit Colour Varieties of Eugenia Brasiliensis Lam. *Sci. Agric.* **2007,** *64,* 428–432.

Omidbeygi, M.; Barzegar, M.; Hamidi, Z.; Naghdibadi, H. Antifungal Activity of Thyme, Summer Savory and Clove Essential Oils Against *Aspergillus flavus* in Liquid Medium and Tomato Paste. *Food Control* **2007,** *18,* 1518–1523.

Ormancey, X.; Sisalli, S.; Coutiere, P. Formulation of Essential Oils in Functional Perfumery. *Parfums Cosmet. Actual.* **2001,** *157,* 30–40.

Padalia, R. C.; Verma, R. S.; Chauhan, A.; Goswami, P.; Chanotiya, C. S.;Saroj, A.; Samad, A.; Khaliq, A. Compositional Variability and Antifungal Potentials of *Ocimum basilicum*, *O. tenuiflorum*, *O. gratissimum* and *O. kilimandscharicum* Essential Oils Against *Rhizoctonia solani* and *Choanephora cucurbitarum*. Nat. Prod. Commun. **2014,** *9,* 1507–1510.

Pavela, R. Insecticidal and Repellent Activity of Selected Essential Oils Against of the *Pollen beetle*, *Meligathes aeneus* (Fabricius) Adults. *Ind. Crops Prod.* **2011,** *34,* 888–892.

Pinto, E.; Pina-Vaz, C.; Salgueiro, L.; Goncalves, M. J.; Costa-de-Oliveira, S.; Cavaleiro, C.; Palmeira, A.; Rodrigues, A.; Martinez-de-Oliveira, J. Antifungal Activity of the Essential Oil of *Thymus pulegioides* on *Candida*, *Aspergillus* and Dermatophyte Species. *J. Med. Microbiol.* **2006,** *55,* 1367–1373.

Pinto, E.; Vale-Silva, L.; Cavaleiro, C.; Salgueiro, L. Antifungal Activity of the Clove Essential oil from *Syzygium aromaticum* on *Candida*, *Aspergillus* and Dermatophyte Species. *J. Med. Microbiol.* **2009,** *58,* 1454–1462.

Pragadheesh, V. S.; Saroj, A.; Yadav, A.; Chanotiya, C. S.; Alam, M.; Samad, A.; Chemical Characterization and Antifungal Activity of *Cinnamomum camphora* Essential Oil. *Ind. Crops Prod.* **2013a,** *49,* 628–633.

Pragadheesh, V. S.; Saroj, A.; Yadav, A.; Samad, A.; Chanotiya, C. S. Compositions, Enantiomer Characterization and Antifungal Activity of two *Ocimum* Essential Oils. *Ind. Crops Prod.* **2013b,** *50,* 333–337.

Prakash, B.; Kedia, A.; Mishra, P. K.; Dwivedy, A. K.; Dubey, N. K. Assessment of Chemically Characterized *Rosmarinus officinalis* L. Essential Oil and its Major Compounds as Plant-Based Preservative in Food System Based on their Efficacy Against Food-Borne Moulds and Aflatoxin Secretion and as Antioxidant. *Int. J. Food Sci. Technol.* **2015,** *50,* 1792–1798.

Re, L.; Barocci, S.; Sonnino, S.; Mencarelli, A.; Vivani, C.; Paolucci, G.; Scarpantonio, A.; Rinaldi, L.; Mosca, E. Linalool Modifies the Nicotinic Receptor-Ion Channel Kinetics at the Mouse Neuromuscular Junction. *Pharmacol. Res.* **2000,** *42,* 177–181.

Regnault-Roger, C. Trends for Commercialisation of Biocontrol Agent (Biopesticide) Products. In *Plant Defence: Biological Control, Progress in Biological Control;* Mérillon, J. M., Ramawat, K. G., Eds.; Springer: Dordrecht Netherland, 2012; Vol. 12, pp 139–160.

Regnault-Roger, C. et al. Essential Oils in Insect Control: Low-Risk Products in a High-Stakes World. *Annu. Rev. Entomol.* **2012,** *57,* 405–424.

Rehman, R.; Hanif, M. A.; Mushtaq, Z.; Al-Sadi, A. M. Biosynthesis of Essential Oils in Aromatic Plants: A Review. **2016,** *32,* 117–160.

Roby, M. H. H.; Sarhan, M. A.; Selim, K. A.; Khalel, K. I. Antioxidant and Antimicrobial Activities of Essential Oil and Extracts of Fennel (*Foeniculum vulgare* L.) and Chamomile (*Matricaria chamomilla* L.). *Ind. Crops Prod.* **2013,** *44,* 437–445.

Romagnoli, C.; Bruni, R.; Andreotti, E.; Rai, M. K.; Vicentini, C. B.; Mares, D. Chemical Characterization and Antifungal Activity of Essential Oil of Capitula from Wild Indian *Tagetes patula* L. *Protoplasma* **2005,** *225,* 57–65.

Rossi, Y. E.; Palacios, S. M. Fumigant Toxicity of Citrus *Sinensis* Essential Oil on *Musca domestica* L. Adults in the Absence and Presence of a P450 Inhibitor. *Acta Trop.* **2013,** *127,* 33–37.

Saroj, A.; Pragadheesh, V. S.; Palanivelu., Yadav; A., Singh; S. C., Samad; A., Negi; A. S., Chanotiya, C. S. Anti-Phytopathogenic Activity of *Syzygium cumini* Essential Oil, Hydrocarbon Fractions and its Novel Constituents. *Ind. Crops Prod.* **2015,** *74,* 337–335.

Shah, B.; Davidson, P. M.; Zhong, Q. Encapsulation of Eugenol using Maillard-Type Conjugates to form Transparent and Heat Stable Nanoscale Dispersions. *LWT - Food Sci. Technol.* **2012,** *49,* 139–148.

Shi, Q. M.; Li, C. J.; Zhang, F. S. Nicotine Synthesis in *Nicotiana tabacum* L. Induced by Mechanical Wounding is Regulated by Auxin. *J. Exp. Bot.* **2006,** *57,* 2899–2907.

Souza Júnior, I. T. Fungitoxic Essential Oils Effect on *Colletotrichum gloeosporioides*, Isolated from the Yellow Passion Fruit. *Biotemas* **2009,** *22,* 77–83.

Stülp, J. L. et al. Action Essential Oil Orange in Different Concentrations and Chemical Fungicide Thiram + Carboxim on the Germination and Disease in Wheat Seeds (*Triticumaestivum*). *Cad. Agroecologia* **2011,** *6,* 1–4.

Tatsadjieu, N. L.; Dongmo, P. J.; Ngassoum, M. B.; Etoa, F. X.; Mbofung, C. M. F. Investigations on the Essential Oil of *Lippia rugosa* from Cameroon for its Potential use as Antifungal Agent Against *Aspergillus flavus* Link ex. Fries. *Food Control* **2009,** *20,* 161–166.

Tian, J.; Ban, X.; Zeng, H.; He, J.; Huang, B.; Wang, Y. Chemical Composition and Antifungal Activity of Essential Oil from *Cicuta virosa* L. var. Latisecta Celak. *Int. J. Food Microbiol.* **2011,** *145,* 464–470.

Tian, J.; Huang, B., Luo, X., Zeng, H., Ban, X., He, J., Wang, Y. The Control of *Aspergillus flavus* with *Cinnamomum jensenianum* Hand.-Mazz Essential Oil and its Potential use as a Food Preservative. *Food Chem.* **2012,** *130,* 520–527.
Tzortzakis, N. G.; Economakis, C. D. Antifungal Activity of Lemongrass (*Cympopogon citratus* L.) Essential Oil Against Key Postharvest Pathogens. *Innovative Food Sci. Emerging Technol.* **2007,** *8,* 253–258.
USEPA. Reregistration Eligibility Document (RED): Capsaicin, United States Environmental Protection Agency, 1992. http://www.epa.gov (accessed November 3, 2017).
USEPA. 4-Allyl anisole. Biopesticides Registration Action Document, United States Environmental Protection Agency, 2001. http://www.epa.gov (accessed November 3, 2017).
USEPA. Garlic oil: Proposed Registration Review Final Decision. Case **4007,** United States Environmental Protection Agency, 2010. http://www.epa.gov (accessed November 3, 2017).
Valgimigli, L. *Essential Oils as Natural Food Additives: Composition, Applcations, Antioxidant and Antimicrobial Properties;* Nova Science Publishers, Inc.: New York, 2012; *1,* 173–265.
Varma, J.; Dubey, N. K. Efficacy of Essential Oils of *Caesulia axillaris* and *Mentha arvensis* Against Some Storage Pests Causing Biodeterioration of Food Commodities. *Int. J. Food Microbiol.* **2001,** *68,* 207–710.
Yadav, S.; Mittal, P. K.; Saxena, P. N.; Singh, R. K. Effect of Synergist Piperonyl Butoxide (PBO) on the Toxicity of Some Essential Oils Against Mosquito Larvae. *J. Commun. Dis.* **2009,** *41,* 33–38.
Yanishlieva, N. V.; Marinova, E.; Pokorny, J. Natural Antioxidants from Herbs and Spices. *Eur. J. Lipid Sci. Technol.* **2006,** *108,* 776–793.

CHAPTER 18

INHIBITION OF MILD STEEL CORROSION IN ACIDIC MEDIA BY PHYTOCHEMICALS

BASU MAAN DAAS

Department of Chemistry, Netaji Subhash Mahavidyalaya, Udaipur, Tripura, India, Tel.: +917005115828, E-mail: basu.maandaas@visva-bharati.ac.in

ORCID: https://or-cid.org/0000-0003-2861-1914

ABSTRACT

The chapter deals with the phenomenon of corrosion of mild steel, its causes, consequences, and inhibition by means of phytochemicals. Corrosion is a major hazard in the application of metals in various fields and its inhibition is to be addressed for rapid and smooth progress in civil, industrial, transport, and other sectors. In this chapter, the inhibition of corrosion of mild steel by means of chemicals extracted from plants is elaborately discussed. This chapter is going to be very useful for researchers who are working or planning to work in the field of corrosion inhibition by phytochemicals because many organic corrosion inhibitors are toxic in nature and there is a constant search for non-toxic inhibitors. In this chapter, the major achievements in the inhibition of corrosion of mild steel till recent years are compiled and discussed. The electrochemistry and mechanism of corrosion of mild steel in acidic media and its inhibition by green phytochemicals are discussed in this chapter.

18.1 INTRODUCTION

Roman philosopher, Pliny (23–79 AD) wrote about corrosion of iron in an essay named *Ferrum Corrumpitar* (Ahmad, 2016). Corrosion is to eat away or be eaten away gradually, especially by chemical action (Webster's Dictionary). Corrosion is the process of corroding or being corroded (Oxford and Cambridge Dictionaries). Corrosion is deterioration of a metal because of a reaction with the environment (NACE Corrosion Basics). The word *corrosion* comes from the Latin words—*rodere* means gnawing and *corrodere* means gnawing to pieces.

Corrosion has been a major hazard since ancient times when metals were first used. Corrosion affects the microstructure, mechanical properties and the physical appearance of the metal. Corrosion is a continuous hazard for buildings, bridges, oil pipelines, water supply lines, toilets and bathrooms, chemical and industrial plants, and so on. Corroded electrical contacts can catch fire due to short circuit and corroded medical implants may lead to blood poisoning and tetanus as well as other problems. Furthermore, corrosion continuously damages arts and sculptures around the world. Corrosion also damages the storage containers used for safe disposal of radioactive waste for tens of thousands of years which can be or is a severe concern (The Electrochemical Society).

Steel is a major ingredient in the progress of modern civilization. It is invariably used in the construction of instruments, machines, engines, buildings, roadways, bridges, highways, factories, industries, and the list is too long to be mentioned in details here. In short, to think of progress and development without the varied applications of steel in its various forms is impossible as far as our latest research, discoveries, and inventions are concerned. So, if steel gets corroded due to atmospheric influences, which is a severe concern, then the progress of mankind gets jerked and retarded. This is the reason why inhibition of steel corrosion is of prime importance for mankind and researchers are toiling hard in the laboratories to find viable solutions to address this phenomenon.

18.1.1 CORROSION TYPES

Broadly, corrosion can be classified as the following depending on the causes, that is, environment, material, or chemical reaction and effects (Chigondo and Chigondo, 2016).

- *Uniform corrosion* damages and thins out the whole metal surface.
- *Galvanic corrosion* takes place with an electrolyte with metals having different values of electrical potentials.

- *Pitting corrosion* damages particular parts of the metal surface forming holes or pits which act as the anode, while the undamaged metal surface the cathode.
- *Stress corrosion* cracking takes place due to stress and corrosive environment. Corrosion fatigue takes place due to the combination of cyclic stress and corrosion.
- *Intergranular corrosion* takes place onto the granular boundaries of a metal.
- *Crevice corrosion* takes place due to the trapping of corrosive liquid between the gaps in the metal.
- *Filiform corrosion* takes place on a metal surface coated with a thin organic film.
- *Erosion corrosion* takes place due to the movement of corrosive liquids on a metal surface.
- *Fretting corrosion* takes place due to the combination of corrosion and fretting of metal.

18.1.2 CORROSION ELECTROCHEMISTRY

Most metals generally occur in nature as compounds, such as oxides, sulfides, silicates, or carbonates, barring aside very few metals that occur in native form. Extraction of a metal from ore involves reduction, while the oxidation of metal is commonly called corrosion where metals tend to lose electrons to oxygen or other oxidizing agents in air or water. The most common kinds of corrosion result from electrochemical reactions which occur when water or moisture gets trapped between two electrical contacts (Fig. 18.1), having a voltage between them, generate an accidental electrolytic cell (The Electrochemical Society).

The process of corrosion of mild steel in the presence of moisture illustrated the preceding diagram shows that when an oxide-free metal surface gets exposed to moisture, iron is oxidized to positively charged metal ions yielding electrons which can freely move through the mild steel structure up to the surface of the metal. Two electrochemical regions are generated. At the cathodic region, these free electrons cause reduction of atmospheric oxygen into water, while at the anodic region, the oxidized iron reacts with oxygen and water to create rust, thus corroding the surface (Toussaint, 2015). These residual electrons provide a negative charge on the metal surface, thus increasing the potential difference between the metal and adjacent solution. Hike in this potential difference facilitates deposition of dissolved metal ions from the solution back onto the metal surface till a point of equilibrium when the opposing rates of dissolution and deposition become equal (Chatterjee et al., 1991). Once this steady state is achieved, the potential is called *reversible potential* and by this time a very small amount of metal gets dissolved into the adjacent moisture. Potential of a metal in the solution remains positive but lower than the *reversible potential.*

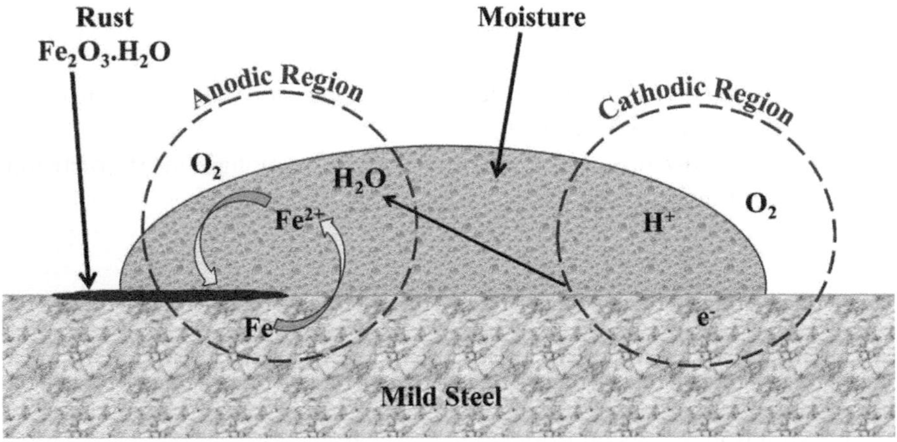

FIGURE 18.1 Process of corrosion of mild steel in the presence of moisture

Source: Modified from Toussaint (2015).

In acid media, the corrosion is expedited; in the presence of acidic solution, hydrogen ions are adsorbed on the metal surface from the solution and electrons react with them to produce hydrogen gas (Fig. 18.2). Sustained passage of metal ions into solution phase leads to corrosion of the metal surface.

The anodic dissolution of mild steel in HA occurs as,

$$Fe + A^- \rightarrow (FeA^-)_{ads}$$

$$(FeA^-)_{ads} \rightarrow (FeA)_{ads} + e^-$$

$$(FeA^-)_{ads} \rightarrow (FeA^+)_{ads} + e^-$$

$$(FeA^+)_{ads} \rightarrow Fe^{2+} + A^-$$

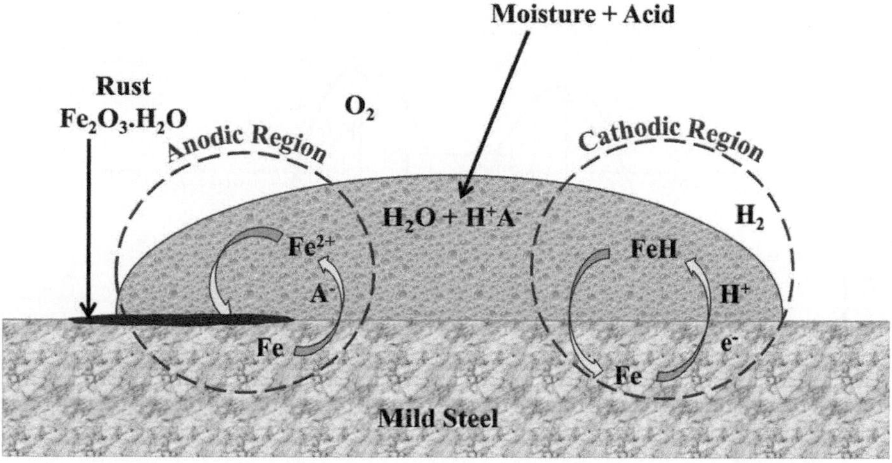

FIGURE 18.2 Process of corrosion of mild steel in the presence of moisture and acid

Source: Modified from Toussaint (2015).

The cathodic hydrogen evolution in HA occurs as,

$$Fe + H^+ \rightarrow (FeH^+)_{ads}$$

$$(FeH^+)_{ads} + e^- \rightarrow (FeH)_{ads}$$

$$(FeH)_{ads} + H^+ + e^- \rightarrow Fe + H_2$$ (Shahid, 2011)

18.2 CORROSION INHIBITION

Corrosion inhibitors are used to combat the damage due to corrosion (Corrosionpedia). Corrosion inhibition is more economical, practical, and convenient than cathodic protection in controlling corrosion on a metal surface in an aqueous environment (Solomon and Umoren, 2015).

In fact, corrosion is a natural phenomenon that is thermodynamically favored. Metals, barring aside the noble metals, have a tendency to be in compounds (Toussaint, 2015). The uncombined metal is thermodynamically unstable and with some assistance transform into some or other form of a compound. The corrosion thus is a very favorable phenomenon in case of exposed metal surfaces. Therefore, the role of corrosion inhibitors is to somehow resist this thermodynamically favorable process by increasing the activation energy required to perform the transformation reaction (Fig. 18.3). This is done by causing hindrance to the anodic and/or cathodic reactions and slowing them so that corrosion is inhibited.

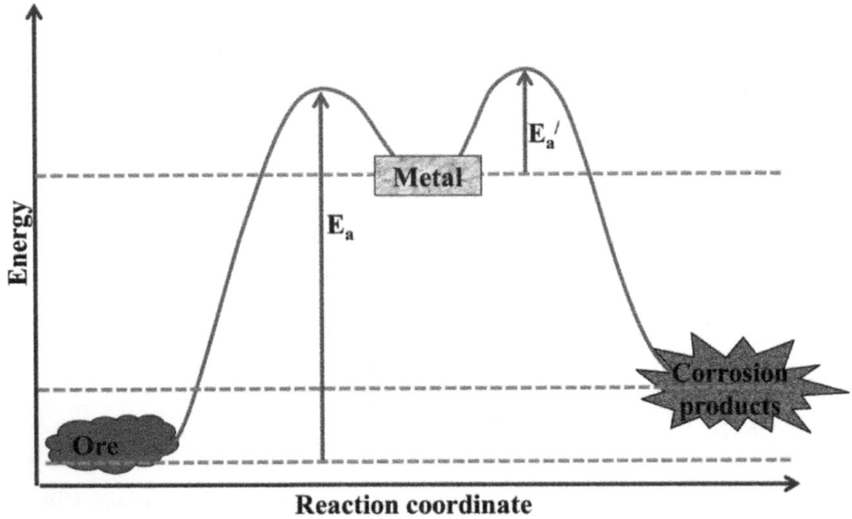

FIGURE 18.3 Energy states of metal in various forms.

Source: Modified from Toussaint (2015).

Corrosion inhibitors perform by any of the following ways (Toussaint, 2015):

- Hindering the anodic and/or cathodic region reactions by raising polarization behavior therein
- Hindering ionic diffusion to the metal surfaces
- Raising electrical resistance of the metal surfaces
- Blocking the metal surfaces and/or the adjacent corrosive environment from coming into direct contact with each other
- Getting adsorbed on to the metal surfaces to form a resistant layer between the metal surfaces and the adjacent corrosive environment

The most common trend to inhibit corrosion of iron-containing materials has been painting one or two coats of zinc compound containing material over the metal surfaces. However, zinc compounds are by themselves hazardous toward mankind and environment alike. Zinc compounds are harmful to both mankind and environment if their percentage in the composition of the corrosion prevention materials is more than mere 2.5% of the total amount. Zinc can locally jeopardize aquatic environment as it gets accumulated in aquatic fauna and subsequently poison them and also those who eat them (Toussaint, 2015; Scottish Environment Protection Agency, 2008). Thus, the use of such near primitive methods to inhibit has to be discarded for the betterment of the society at large.

Corrosion inhibitors actually inhibit the metal dissolution and acid consumption by getting adsorbed on the metal surface (Chigondo and Chigondo, 2016). Organic compounds containing nitrogen can effectively inhibit corrosion of steel in acidic media by adsorption of the organic inhibitors on the metal surface (Chatterjee et al., 1991; Elachouri et al., 1995; Mernari et al., 1998; Elkadi et al., 2000; Bentiss et al., 2000; Elkanouni et al., 1996; Walker, 1975; Kertit and Hammouti, 1996; Bentiss et al., 1999).

Organic corrosion inhibitors are generally toxic in nature and this toxicity is the main reason of an urgent need to identify nontoxic alternatives to inhibit corrosion of mild steel in acidic media for smooth and rapid development in diverse sectors.

18.2.1 ORGANICVERSUSINORGANICCORROSIONINHIBITORS

Generally, the functioning of the two chemically different types of inhibitors is primarily diverse in approach.

The chemical characteristics of organic and inorganic corrosion inhibitors are dissimilar and thus the way they act on the metal surfaces in a totally dissimilar manner to inhibit the corrosion of the metal surfaces (Vishnudevan and Thangavel, 2007).

The organic corrosion inhibitors have high molecular mass with heteroatoms, unsaturation, and aromaticity. They generally act on the metal surfaces by prominent adsorption on to the surfaces, thus forming a corrosion-resistant coating on them reducing the chances of corrosion. These normally prevent the intensity of corrosion of the metal surfaces by a combination of the following ways (Toussaint, 2015).

- Facilitating adhesion of the coating which is termed as *an interfacial activity*
- Forming insoluble complex salts on to the anodic defect sites which is termed as an *anodic activity*
- Assisting formation of precipitate by making the cathodic sites more alkaline which is termed as *cathodic activity*
- Diminishing permeability of the metal surfaces to the adjacent corrosive environment which is termed as *cathodic barrier activity*
- Growing a hydrophobic coating on the metal surfaces which is termed as *cathodic adsorption activity*

The adsorption of corrosion inhibitors on the metal surfaces is substitutive adsorption between the inhibitor in the aqueous solution, Org_{aq} and the water molecules adsorbed on the metal surfaces, H_2O_{ads}.

$$Orga_q + nH_2O_{ads} \Leftrightarrow Org_{ads} + nH_2O_{aq}$$

Here n, the size ratio, is the number of water molecules replaced by each inhibitor molecule (Bastidas, 2000). Organic corrosion inhibitors have cathodic and anodic and adsorption actions and the total efficiency of corrosion inhibitor is equal to a summation of all the factors mentioned.

$$\mathcal{E} = \sum [f_{ia} + f_{aa} + f_{ca} + f_{cba} + f_{caa}]$$

However, on the other hand, inorganic corrosion inhibitors are salts of some metals such as Ca, Ba, Sr, Mo, or Al and amphoteric elements that can react both as an acid as well as a base; they generally have cathodic actions or anodic actions only, although in some cases they can even react with the metal surfaces to scavenge corrosive ions (Kumar, 2014).

Again, if toxicity is considered then both the organic and inorganic corrosion inhibitors are toxic in nature toward mankind and the environment. Although the toxicity of inorganic corrosion inhibitors is appreciable, the organic corrosion inhibitors are far more toxic.

Thus, the emphasis on the naturally occurring phytochemical approach towards inhibition of corrosion of metal surfaces such as mild steel, aluminum, and so forth, in recent years is predictable since to resist the hazard of corrosion of metal surfaces, we are automatically getting exposed to poisonous chemical substances.

18.2.2 ADVANTAGES AND DISADVANTAGES OF ORGANIC AND INORGANIC CORROSION INHIBITORS

Organic corrosion inhibitors are normally more effective in inhibiting corrosion of metal surfaces than their inorganic competitors. Organic corrosion inhibitors are found to act on the metal surfaces by means of adsorption on to the surfaces. On the contrary, the inorganic corrosion inhibitors are generally found to act through anodic passivation but this is highly debatable in case of high concentration of chloride ions (Vishnudevan and Thangavel, 2007). This is because in organic corrosion inhibitors, the presence of conjugated or single double bonds owing to the presence of π-electrons facilitates chelating with the metal ions, thus favoring pulling away of the metal component from the metal surfaces. This naturally corrodes away the metal from the exposed surface. Thus, bigger inhibitor molecules decorated with such functional groups that can form chelate compounds in the organic corrosion inhibitors are instrumental in pulling away metal from the metal surfaces.

Another advantage of organic corrosion inhibitors is that they do not react with the metal surfaces as they form an adsorbed hydrophobic coating over the surfaces, while their inorganic counterparts may react with the surfaces and this may change the chemical and physical characteristics of the metals.

The disadvantage of organic corrosion inhibitors compared to inorganic ones is that the organic inhibitors are generally more toxic to human beings and environment. However, it is not that the inorganic corrosion inhibitors are harmless and nontoxic, inorganic corrosion inhibitors containing chromate (CrO_4^{2-}) and/or nitrate (NO_3^-) and/or nitrite (NO_2^-) ions are highly toxic toward both human beings and the environment, while those containing zinc and/or barium salts are highly toxic toward the environment (Toussaint, 2015).

18.3 MILD STEEL AND ITS CORROSION

Mild steel is the most common form of steel used owing to relatively low cost and properties suitable for the varied form of applications (Singh et al., 2016). Mild steel is tough, ductile, and malleable with superb tensile strength. It is extensively used as an engineering material in this modern era. In fact, the invention of steel is a huge factor in the development of mankind. However, its low corrosion resistance, especially in the acidic environment, is a hurdle to be addressed for smooth application of steel in progress and development (Alaneme et al., 2016a).

18.3.1 STEEL CATEGORIES

Steel can be prepared in various forms. It is an alloy of iron and carbon and accounts for 90% of total steel production. Steel is classified into three groups, based on their carbon content.

1. Low-carbon or mild steels (carbon <0.3%)
2. Medium-carbon steels (carbon = 0.3–0.6%)
3. High-carbon steels (carbon >0.6%)

18.3.2 MILD STEEL CORROSION

Most organic corrosion inhibitors have at least one polar unit with atoms of nitrogen (N), sulfur (S), oxygen (O), and in some cases phosphorous (P). It has been reported that the inhibition efficiency decreases in the order to O<N<S<P. The polar unit is regarded as the reaction center for the chemisorption process. Furthermore, the size, orientation, shape, and electric charge on the molecule determine the degree of adsorption and hence the effectiveness of inhibitor. On the other hand, iron is well known for its coordination affinity to heteroatom-bearing ligands (Singh and Quraishi, 2010).

18.4 MILD STEEL CORROSION INHIBITION BY PHYTOCHEMICALS

A comprehensive list of the recent research and findings in the application of phytochemicals in inhibiting corrosion of mild steel are illustrated in Table 18.1.

18.5 MECHANISM OF CORROSION INHIBITION BY PHYTOCHEMICALS

Inhibition of corrosion is attributed to the adsorption of inhibitor phytochemicals at the metal/solution interface, thus forming a protective film. The rate of adsorption is usually rapid, and hence, the reactive metal surface is shielded from the acid solutions (Chao et al., 1981). The adsorption of inhibitor phytochemicals depends on the chemical structure, molecular size, nature of metal surface, and charge distribution over the inhibitor. Adsorption of inhibitor phytochemicals occurs through the replacement of solvent molecules from the metal surface. It is seen that all the phytochemicals contain basic polar functional groups that facilitate adsorption on the metal/solution interface. Higher the adsorption, higher is the inhibition of corrosion of mild steel or any other metal as the case may be. Phytochemicals bearing polar electronegative functional groups as well as a planar structure can get adsorbed easily and cover the metal surface effectively. Moreover, organic inhibitors contain lone pair of electrons in functional groups and π-electrons in conjugated double or triple bonds and have the ability to supply electrons through π-orbitals that can facilitate adsorption of the inhibitor molecules on to the metal surfaces to inhibit corrosion of the metal surface by forming a protective coating on them (Vishnudevan and Thangavel, 2007; Yadav et al., 2016). In short, the size

TABLE 18.1 Recent Findings World Over.

Green inhibitor	Scientific name	Phytochemicals present	Work cited
African oil bean roots extract	*Pentaclethra macrophylla*	Tannins, alkaloids, nitrogen bases, carbohydrates, amino acids, and proteins	Nnanna et al. (2016)
Aloe vera extract	*Aloe barbadensis*	Mannose-6-phosphate	Shah and Agarwal (2014), Montemor (2016)
Anise herb extract	*Pimpinella anisum*	Conjugated double bonds and benzene rings, and alkoxy, ether, and carbonic groups in anethol and chavicol	Khamis and Alandis (2002)
Arjuna bark extract	*Terminalia arjuna*	Hydroxyl group in b-sitosterol	Singh et al. (2012)
Bamboo leaf extract	*Gigantochloa manggong*	Flavonoids and phenolic acids, such as chlorogenic acid, caffeic acid, ferulic acid, p-coumaric acid, orientin, homoorientin, vitexin, and isovitexin	Khan et al. (2015), Quraishi et al. (2010)
Banana peel extract	*Musa sapientum*	Oxo, amino, and hydroxyl groups in gallocatechin and dopamine	Eddy and Ebenso (2008), Singh et al. (2012), Gunavathy and Murugavel (2013)
Barley extract	*Hordeum vulgare*	Benzene rings and hydroxyl and carbonic groups flavonoids such as isovitexin 7-*O*-β-[6-*O*-(*E*)-*p*-coumaroyl]glucoside (6-coumaroylsaponarin), isovitexin 7-*O*-β-[6′-*O*-(*E*)-feruloyl] glucoside, isoorientin 7-*O*-β-[6‴-*O*-(*E*)-feruloyl]glucoside, and tricin 7-*O*-β-glucoside	Saadawy (2014)
Bitter orange extract	*Citrus aurantium*	Carbonyl and hydroxyl groups in threonine	Singh et al. (2012)
Bitter kola seed extract	*Garcinia kola*	Amino and carboxylic groups in 15 fatty and 18 amino acids	Eleyinmi et al. (2006), Okafor et al. (2007)
Black cumin herb extract	*Nigella sativa*	Double bonds and hydroxyl and ether groups in saponin	Khamis and Alandis (2002)
Black pepper extract	*Piper nigrum fem. Piperaceae*	Carbonyl, tertiary amino, alkoxyl groups in piperine and its isomers	Gorgani et al. (2017), Quraishi et al. (2009)
Black plum extract	*Syzygium cumini*	Carbonyl, hydroxyl, and carbonic groups in ellagic acid, gallic acid, quercetin, and cafeic acid	Singh et al. (2012)

TABLE 18.1 *(Continued)*

Green inhibitor	Scientific name	Phytochemicals present	Work cited
Blue-green algae extract	*Spirulina platensis*	Amino and carboxylic groups in acids and carbohydrates	de Oliveira et al. (1999), Babadzhanov et al. (2004), Alvarenga et al. (2011)
Brahmi leaf extract	*Bacopa monnieri*	Hydroxyl and carbonic groups in bacoside a	Singh et al. (2012)
Brazilian rosewood plant extract	*Aniba rosaeodora*	Anibine as the major alkaloid	Chevaliera et al. (2014)
Ceylon spinach extract	*Basella alba*	Alkaloids, pseudo tannins, chorogenic acid, anthocyanin, steroidal glycosides, flavonoids, and coumarin	Vimala et al. (2016)
Coffee plum bark extract	*Flacourtia jangomas*	Hydroxyl, phenolic, ketone, and amine in tannin and flavonoids	Sisodia and Hasan (2013)
Common wormwood plant extract	*Artemisia mesatlantica*	Carbonic, hydroxyl, and alkyl groups and bicyclic rings in β-thujone, camphor, 1,8-cineole, and α-thujone	Boumhara et al. (2015), Boumhara et al. (2014)
Coriander herb extract	*Coriandrum sativum*	Benzene rings, conjugated double bonds and hydroxyl, ether and carbonyl groups in linalool, terpinine, piene, coumarins, phthalides, and phenolic acids.	Khamis and Alandis (2002)
Corn oil		Carbonyl group	Abbasov et al. (2013)
Cotula leaf extract	*Cotula coronopifolia*	Tertiary and secondary amino, oxo groups in anagyrine and cytosine	Raja and Sethuraman (2008a), Singh et al. (2012)
Curry leaf extract	*Murraya koenigii*	Carbonyl, secondary amino and carbonic groups in murrafoline-i, pyrayafoline-d, and mahabinine-a	Singh et al. (2012)
Curry leaf extract	*Murraya koenigii*	Monoterpene hydrocarbons (pinene, camphene, myrcene, and limonene) and monoterpene-derived alcohols: linalool, terpinene-4-ol, nerol, and geraniol, also their acetates with at least one functional polar group	Sharmila et al. (2010)
Custard apple extract	*Annona squamosa*	Liriodenine, oleuropein, and oxoanalobine	Lebrini et al. (2010), Singh et al. (2012)

TABLE 18.1 *(Continued)*

Green inhibitor	Scientific name	Phytochemicals present	Work cited
Davana plant extract	Asteraceae	Monoterpenes, sesquiterpenes, furan rings, bicyclic compounds, isoprenologs, longipinanes, cubebane-type sesquiterpenoids, aristolanes, and bourbonane	Zhigzhitzhapova et al. (2016)
Desert germander extract	*Teucrium oliverianum*	Neo-clerodane diterpenoids and their derivatives	Al-Yahya et al. (2002), Al-Otaibi et al. (2014)
Devil pepper extract	*Rauvolfia serpentina*	Reserpine, ajmalicine, ajmaline, isoajmaline, ajmalinine, chandrine	Raja and Sethuraman (2008a), Singh et al. (2012)
Drumstick leaf extract	*Moringa oleifera*	Amino and carboxylic groups in arginine	Singh et al. (2012)
False daisy extract	*Eclipta alba*	Hydroxyl, alkoxyl, and ketoxy groups in wedelolactone	Shyamala and Arulanantham (2009), Singh et al. (2012)
Fenugreek seed extract	*Trigonella foenum-graecum*	Carboxylic, amino, tertiary amino, and sulfide groups in methionine and choline	Noor (2007), Singh et al. (2012)
Garden cress herb extract	*Lepidium sativum*	Benzene rings, double bonds, and secondary amino, hydroxyl, sulfonate, sulfide, and ether groups in benzyl glucosinolate	Khamis and Alandis (2002)
Golden rain tree leaf extract	*Cassia fistula*	A range of carboxylic, amino, carbonic, and hydroxyl groups	Omotosho et al. (2017)
Gum exudate	*Khaya senegalensis*, *Albizia ferruginea*	Myrcene, camphene, alpha-thujene/origanene, nopinen/pseudopinen, 4(10)-thujene (bicyclo[3.1.0]hexane), alpha-campholena, 2,6-dimethyl hepta-1,5-diene, nerolidol isobutyrate, limonene/cajepetene, verbenol, cis-verbenol, myrtenol, carvacrol, diisopropenyl-1-methyl-1-vinyl cyclohexane, o-menth-8-ene-4-methanol, 7-hexadecenal, 2-methylene cholestan-3-ol, and 5 alpha-pregnane-12,20-dione	Ameh (2015)
Guvar bean extract	*Cyamopsis tetragonoloba*	3-epikatonic acid 7-o-beta-(2-rhamnosyl-glucosyl) myricetin, ash, astragalin, caffeic acid, and chlorogenic acid	Subhashini et al. (2010), Singh et al. (2012)
Hairy fig leaf extract	*Ficus hispida*	Hydroxyl group and double bonds in stigmasterol	Muthukrishnan et al. (2015)

TABLE 18.1 *(Continued)*

Green inhibitor	Scientific name	Phytochemicals present	Work cited
Henna extract	*Anvillea garcinii*	Germacranolide	Abdel-Sattar and McPhail (2000), Al-Otaibi et al. (2014)
Henna leaf extract	*Lawsonia*	Oxo and hydroxyl groups in lawsone (2-hydroxy-1,4-naphtho quinone) and tannin	El-etre et al. (2005), Singh et al. (2012), Montemor (2016)
Hibiscus herb extract	*Hibiscus sabdariffa*	Carboxylic, carbonic, and hydroxyl groups in hibiscus, malic acid, citric acid and tartaric acid	Khamis and Alandis (2002), Mak et al. (2013)
Hop bush extract	*Dodonaea viscosa*	Dihydroxy, dimethyl, and other substituted catechols, which are postulated as pyrolysate derivatives of the anti-spasmodic flavonoids quercetin, rutin, kaempferol, and sakuranetin	Leelavathi and Rajalakshmi (2013)
Indian bael extract	*Aegle marmelos*	Carbonic and tertiary amino groups, skimmianine	Singh et al. (2012)
Jatropha leaf extract	*Jatropha curcas*	Carbohydrates, cardiac glycosides, keller kilani, kedde, borntragers, monosaccharide, reducing sugar, saponins, and falvonoids	Mshelia et al. (2017)
Kalmegh leaf extract	*Andrographis paniculata*	Carbonyl, hydroxyl, and carbonic groups in andrographolide	Singh et al. (2012)
Kuchla seed extract	*Strychnos nux-vomica*	Oxo and tertiary amino groups in brucine	Singh et al. (2012)
Leadwood tree extract	*Terminalia catappa*	Hydroxyl, carbonic, alkoxyl, and tertiary amino groups in saponin, tannin, phlobatanin, anthraquinone, cardiac glycosides, flavanoid, terpene, and alkaloid	Eddy et al. (2009)
Long pepper extract	*Piper longum*	Tertiary amino, oxo, carbonic, and hydroxyl groups in piperine, piplartine, and rutin.	Singh et al. (2012)
Marine red alga extract	*Kappaphycus alvarezii*	Phenolic, carboxylic, and amino groups and conjugated double bonds in phycocolloids, fatty acids, carrageenan, lectins, hema-glutannin, and carotenoids	Kamal and Sethuraman (2013)

TABLE 18.1 *(Continued)*

Green inhibitor	Scientific name	Phytochemicals present	Work cited
Mayweed extract	*Tripleurospermum auriculatum*	Unsaturated fatty acids and sterols	Al-Otaibi et al. (2014)
Moraceae extract	*Ficus asperifolia*	Alkaloids, flavonoids, saponins, tannins anthraquinones, and reducing sugars	Fadare et al. (2016)
Morroccan medicinal plant extract	*Salvia aucheri mesatlantica*	Carbonic, hydroxyl, and alkyl groups and benzene rings in α-thujone, β-thujone, α-pinene, β-pinene, p-cymene, and many other components	El ouadi et al. (2014)
Muell leaf extract	*Acalypha torta*	Fused benzene rings and O-heteroatoms in the rings in polyphenols, terpenoids, and plant sterols	Krishnegowda et al. (2013), Adesina et al. (2000), Montemor (2016)
Napier grass extract	*Pennisetum purpureum*	Crude protein, organic matter, and acid detergent lignin	Alaneme et al. (2016b)
Neem seed extract	*Azadirachta indica*	Azadirachtin, monosaccharide, reducing sugar, tannins, saponins, kedde, keller kilan, cardiac glycosides, and carbohydrates	Okafor et al. (2010), Mshelia et al. (2017), Manickam et al. (2016), Sharma et al. (2010)
Ochrosia oppositifolia bark and leaf extract	*Ochrosia oppositifolia*	Carbonyl, secondary amino and alkyl groups in isoreserpiline	Raja et al. (2013)
Olive leaf extract	*Olea europaea*	Ester, hydroxyl, and carbonic groups in oleuropein and hydroxytyrosol	El-etre (2007), Singh et al. (2012), Montemor (2016)
Olive leaf extract	*Osmanthus fragrans*	Carbonic and alkoxyl groups in flavonoids, ascorbic acid, and gallic acid	Li et al. (2012), Muthukrishnan et al. (2015)
Pongam tree extract	*Pongamia pinnata*	Carbonyl, hydroxyl, and carbonic groups in karanjin, pongapine, kanjone, and pongaglabrone	Singh et al. (2012)
Red tasselflower extract	*Emilia sonchifolia*	Carbonic, hydroxyl, and alkoxyl groups in amino acids, flavonoids, quinones, carbohydrates, cardio glycosides, saponins, tannins, fats, and oils	Onuegbu et al. (2013)

TABLE 18.1 *(Continued)*

Green inhibitor	Scientific name	Phytochemicals present	Work cited
Red-leafed pulai leaf extract	*Alstonia angustifolia*	Tertiary amino groups in alstogustine and 19-epialstogustine	Raja et al. (2013)
Retama leaf extract	*Retama raetam*	Tertiary and secondary amino, oxo groups in anagyrine and cytosine	Raja and Sethuraman (2008b), Singh et al. (2012)
Sacred fig extract	*Ficus religiosa*	Hydroxyl group in lanosterol	Singh et al. (2012)
Safflower extract	*Carthemus tinctorius*	Unsaturated fatty acids, flavanoids and their glycosides, adenosine, adenine, uridine, thymine, uracil, roseoside, acetylenic and aromatic glycosides.	Zhou et al. (2008), Al-Otaibi et al. (2014)
Sagebrush extract	*Artemisia sieberi*	Flavanoids, terpenoids, and their glycosides	Marco et al. (1993), Al-Otaibi et al. (2014)
Saudi henna extract	*Cassia italica*	Coumarins, carotenoids, flavonoids, anthraquinones, sterols, and triterpenes	Kazmi et al. (1994), Al-Otaibi et al. (2014)
Soursop leaves extract	*Annona muricata*	6-hydroxyundulatine and other alkaloids	Iroha and Chidiebere (2017), Vimala et al. (2012)
Taily weed extract	*Ochradenus baccatus*	Flavanoids and their glycosides	Barakat et al. (1991), Al-Otaibi et al. (2014)
Thyme herb extract	*Thymus vulgaris*	Benzene rings, bicycle rings, double bonds, and hydroxyl and alkyl groups in thymol, p-cymene, borneol, nerol, and carvacrol.	Khamis and Alandis (2002)
Winged prickly ash leaf extract	*Zanthoxylum armatum*	Carbonic, alkoxyl, hydroxyl, alkyl, ester, phenyl, and carboxylic groups, double bonds and benzene rings in methoxyanthraquinone, hydroxyanthraquinone, diphenyl alatumoic dimethyl ester, salicylic acid, methoxysalicylic acid, zanthoxylumflavone xyloside, and b-sitosterol-b-d-glucoside	Gunasekaran and Chauhan (2004), Akhtar et al. (2009)
Wormwood leaf extract	*Artemisia herba-alba*	Tertiary and secondary amino, oxo groups in anagyrine and cytosine	Raja and Sethuraman (2008b), Singh et al. (2012)

of corrosion inhibitor molecules, the substituent groups linked to them, the functional hetero adsorption atoms present in them, the extent of conjugated bonds, and any presence of aromaticity play a vital role in determining the efficiency and effectiveness of the corrosion inhibitors (El-Naggar, 2007).

18.6 CONCLUSION

Phytochemicals are a good alternative as corrosion inhibitors because these are naturally occurring and comparatively very less toxic barring a few examples. These environment-friendly compounds can provide a better option in tackling the major hazard of corrosion of mild steel in acidic media. The R&D around the globe is constantly at work in identifying better phytochemical inhibitors of corrosion of mild steel in acidic media.

KEYWORDS

- **mild steel corrosion**
- **organic corrosion**
- **inorganic corrosion**
- **adsorption**
- **corrosion inhibitors**

REFERENCES

Abbasov, V. M.; Abd El-Lateef, H. M.; Aliyeva, L. I.; Qasimov, E. E.; Ismayilov, I. T.; Khalaf, M. M. A Study of the Corrosion Inhibition of Mild Steel C1018 in CO_2-Saturated Brine Using Some Novel Surfactants Based on Corn Oil. *Egypt. J. Pet.* **2013,** *22,* 451–470.

Abdel-Sattar, E.; McPhail, A. T.; Cis-Parthenolid-9-One from *Anvillea garcinii*. *J. Nat. Prod.* **2000,** *63*(11), 1587–1589.

Adesina, S. K.; Idowu, O.; Ogundaini, A. O.; Oladimeji, H.; Olugbade, T. A.; Onawunmi, G. O.; Pais, M. Antimicrobial Constituents of the Leaves of *Acalypha wilkesiana* and *Acalypha hispida*. *Phytother. Res.* **2000,** *14,* 371–374.

Ahmad, Z. *Principles of Corrosion Engineering and Corrosion Control*, 1st ed.; Butterworth-Heinemann, Elsevier: Amsterdam, 2006; pp 1–8.

Akhtar, N.; Ali, M.; Alam, M. S. Chemical Constituents from the Seeds of *Zanthoxylum alatum*. *J. Asian Nat. Prod. Res.* **2009,** *11*(1), 91–95.

Alaneme, K. K.; Olusegun, S. J.; Adelowo, O. T. Corrosion Inhibition and Adsorption Mechanism Studies of *Hunteria umbellata* Seed Husk Extracts on Mild Steel Immersed in Acidic Solutions. *Alexandria Eng. J.* **2016a,** *55*(1), 673–681.

Alaneme, K. K.; Olusegun, S. J.; Alo, A. W. Corrosion Inhibitory Properties of Elephant Grass (*Pennisetum purpureum*) Extract: Effect on Mild Steel Corrosion in 1 M HCl Solution. *Alexandria Eng. J.* **2016b,** *55,* 1069–1076.

Al-Otaibi, M. S.; Al-Mayouf, A. M.; Khan, M.; Mousa, A. A.; Al-Mazroa, S. A.; Alkhathlan, H. Z. Corrosion Inhibitory Action of Some Plant Extracts on the Corrosion of Mild Steel in Acidic Media. *Arabian J. Chem.* **2014,** *7,* 340–346.

Alvarenga, R. R.; Rodrigues, P. B.; Cantarelli, V. D.; Zangeronimo, M. G.; da Silva, J. W., Jr.; da Silva, L. R.; dos Santos, L. M.; Pereira, L. J. Energy Values and Chemical Composition of Spirulina (*Spirulina platensis*) Evaluated with Broilers. *Rev. Bras. Zootec.* **2011,** *40*(5), 992–996.

Al-Yahya, M. A.; El-Feraly, F. S.; Dunbar, D. C.; Muhammad, I. *neo*-Clerodane Diterpenoids from *Teucrium oliverianum* and Structure Revision of Teucrolin E. *Phytochemistry* **2002,** *59*(4), 409–414.

Ameh, P. O. A Comparative Study of the Inhibitory Effect of Gum Exudates from *Khaya senegalensis* and *Albizia ferruginea* on the Corrosion of Mild Steel in Hydrochloric Acid Medium. *Int. J. Met.* **2015,** Article ID 824873, 1–13.

Babadzhanov, A. S.; Abdusamatova, N.; Yusupova, F. M.; Faizullaeva, N.; Mezhlumyan, L. G.; Malikova, M. K. *Chem. Nat. Compd.* **2004,** *40*(3), 276–279.

Barakat, H. H.; El-Mousallamy, A. M. D.; Souleman, A. M. A.; Awadalla, S. Flavonoids of *Ochradenus baccatus*. *Phytochemistry* **1991,** *30,* 3777–3779.

Bastidas, J. M.; Polo, J. L.; Cano, C.; Torres, C. L. Tributylamine as Corrosion Inhibitor for Mild Steel in Hydrochloric Acid. *J. Mater. Sci.* **2000,** *35,* 2637–2642.

Bentiss, F.; Lagrenee, M.; Traisnel, M.; Hornez, J. C. The Corrosion Inhibition of Mild Steel in Acidic Media by a New Triazole Derivative. *Corros. Sci.* **1999,** *41*(4), 789–803.

Bentiss, F.; Traisnel, M.; Lagrenee, M. The Substituted 1,3,4-Oxadiazoles: A New Class of Corrosion Inhibitors of Mild Steel in Acidic Media. *Corros. Sci.* **2000,** *42*(1), 127–146.

Boumhara, K.; Bentiss, F.; Tabyaoui, M.; Costa, J.; Desjobert, J.-M.; Bellaouchou, A.; Guenbour, A.; Hammouti, B.; Al-Deyab, S. S. Use of Artemisia Mesatlantica Essential Oil as Green Corrosion Inhibitor for Mild Steel in 1 M Hydrochloric Acid Solution. *Int. J. Electrochem. Sci.* **2014,** *9,* 1187–1206.

Boumhara, K.; Tabyaoui, M.; Jama, C.; Bentiss, F. Artemisia Mesatlantica Essential Oil as Green Inhibitor for Carbon Steel Corrosion in 1M HCl Solution Electrochemical and XPS Investigations. *J. Ind. Eng. Chem. Res.* **2015,** *29,* 146–155.

Chao, C. Y.; Lin, L. F.; Macdonald, D. D. A Point Defect Model for Anodic Passive Films. *J. Electrochem. Soc.* **1981,** *128*(6), 1187–1194.

Chatterjee, P.; Benerjee, M. K.; Mukherjee, K. P. Synergistic Inhibition of Inorganic Anions with Pyridine-Derivatives for Steel in Hydrochloric-Acid. *Indian J. Technol.* **1991,** *29*(4), 191.

Chevaliera, M; Robert, F.; Amusant, N.; Traisnel, M.; Roosa, C.; Lebrini, M. Enhanced Corrosion Resistance of Mild Steel in 1 M Hydrochloric Acid Solution by Alkaloids Extract from *Aniba rosaeodora* Plant: Electrochemical, Phytochemical and XPS Studies. *Electrochim. Acta* **2014,** *131,* 96–105.

Chigondo, M; Chigondo, F. Recent Natural Corrosion Inhibitors for Mild Steel: An Overview. *J. Chem.* **2016,** Article ID 6208937, 1–7.

The Electrochemical Society. Corrosion and Corrosion Prevention. [Online]. http://www.electrochem.org/corrosion-science (accessed Dec 10, 2017).

Corrosionpedia. Corrosion. [Online]. https://www.corrosionpedia.com/definition/2/corrosion (accessed Dec 10, 2017).

de Oliveira, M. A. C. L.; Monteiro, M. P. C.; Robbs, P. G.; Leite, S. G. F. Growth and Chemical Composition of *Spirulina maxima* and *Spirulina platensis* Biomass at Different Temperatures. *Aquacult. Int.* **1999,** *7*(4), 261–275.

Eddy, N. O.; Ebenso, E. E. Adsorption and Inhibitive Properties of Ethanol Extracts of *Musa sapientum* Peels as a Green Corrosion Inhibitor for Mild Steel in H_2SO_4. *Afr. J. Pure Appl. Chem.* **2008,** *2,* 46–54.

Eddy, N. O.; Ekwumemgbo, P. A.; Mamza, P. A. P. Ethanol Extract of *Terminalia catappa* as a Green Inhibitor for the Corrosion of Mild Steel in H_2SO_4. *Green Chem. Lett. Rev.* **2009,** *2*(4), 223–231.

El ouadi, Y.; Bouyanzer, A.; Majidi, L.; Paolini, J.; Desjobert, J. M.; Costa, J.; Chetouani, A.; Hammouti, B. *Salvia officinalis* Essential Oil and the Extract as Green Corrosion Inhibitor of Mild Steel in Hydrochloric Acid. *J. Chem. Pharm. Res.* **2014,** *6*(7), 1401–1416.

Elachouri, M.; Hajji, M. S.; Kertit, S.; Essassi, E. M.; Salem, M.; Coudert, R. Some Surfactants in the Series of 2-(alkyldimethylammonio) Alkanol Bromides as Inhibitors of the Corrosion of Iron in Acid Chloride Solution. *Corros. Sci.* **1995,** *37*(3), 381–389.

El-Etre, A. Y.; Abdallah, M.; El-Tantawy, Z. E. Corrosion Inhibition of Some Metals Using Lawsonia Extract. *Corros. Sci.* **2005,** *47,* 385–395.

El-Etre, A. Y. Inhibition of Acid Corrosion of Carbon Steel Using Aqueous Extract of Olive Leaves. *J. Colloid Interface Sci.* **2007,** *314*(2), 578–583.

Eleyinmi, A. F., Bressler, D. C.; Amoo, I. A.; Sporns, P.; Oshodi, A. A. Chemical Composition of Bitter Cola (*Garcinia kola*) Seed and Hulls. *Pol. J. Food Nutr. Sci.* **2006,** *15*(56), 395–400.

Elkadi, L.; Mernari, B.; Traisnel, M.; Bentiss, F.; Lagrenee, M. The Inhibition Action of 3,6-bis(2-methoxyphenyl)-1,2-dihydro-1,2,4,5-tetrazine on the Corrosion of Mild Steel in Acidic Media. *Corros. Sci.* **2000,** *42*(4), 703–719.

Elkanouni, A.; Kertit, S.; Srhiri, A.; Bachir, A. B Triazoles as Inhibitors of Corrosion and Hydrogen Surface Blistering for the Armco Iron in Acid Chloride Solution. *Bull. Electrochem.* **1996,** *12*(9), 517–522.

El-Naggar, M. M. Corrosion Inhibition of Mild Steel in Acidic Medium by Some Sulfa Drugs Compounds. *Corros. Sci.* **2007,** *49,* 2226–2236.

Fadare, O. O.; Okoronkwo, A. E.; Olasehinde, E. F. Assessment of Anti-Corrosion Potentials of Extract of *Ficus asperifolia*-Miq (*Moraceae*) on Mild Steel in Acidic Medium. *Afr. J. Pure Appl. Chem.* **2016,** *10*(1), 8–22.

Gorgani, L.; Mohammadi, M.; Najafpour, G. D.; Nikzad, M. Piperine—the Bioactive Compound of Black Pepper: From Isolation to Medicinal Formulations. *Compr. Rev. Food Sci. Food Saf.* **2017,** *16,* 124–140.

Gunasekaran, G; Chauhan, L. R. Eco Friendly Inhibitor for Corrosion Inhibition of Mild Steel in Phosphoric Acid Medium. *Electrochim. Acta* **2004,** *49,* 4387–4395.

Gunavathy, N; Murugavel, S. C. Corrosion Inhibition Study of Bract Extract of *Musa acuminata* Inflorescence on Mild Steel in Hydrochloric Acid Medium. *IOSR J. Appl. Chem.* **2013,** *5*(2), 29–35.

Iroha, N. B.; Chidiebere, M. A. Evaluation of the Inhibitive Effect of *Annona muricata* L Leaves Extract on Low-Carbon Steel Corrosion in Acidic Media. *Int. J. Mater. Chem.* **2017,** *7*(3), 47–54.

Kamal C.; Sethuraman, M. G. *Kappaphycus alvarezii*—a Marine Red Alga as a Green Inhibitor for Acid Corrosion of Mild Steel. *Mater. Corros.* **2013,** *64*(9999), 1–9.

Kazmi, M. H., Malik, A., Hameed, S., Akhta, N.; Noor Ali, S. An Anthraquinone Derivative from Cassia Italic. *Phytochemistry* **1994,** *36*(3), 761–763.

Kertit, S.; Hammouti, B. Corrosion Inhibition of Iron in 1M HCl by 1-Phenyl-5-mercapto-1,2,3,4-tetrazole. *Appl. Surf. Sci.* **1996,** *93*(1), 59–66.

Khamis, E.; Alandis, N. M. Herbs as New Type of Green Inhibitors for Acidic Corrosion of Steel. *Materialwiss. Werkstofftech.* **2002,** *33,* 550–554.

Khan, G.; Newaz, K. M. S.; Basirun, W. J.; Ali, H. B. M.; Faraj, F. L.; Khan, G. M. Application of Natural Product Extracts as Green Corrosion Inhibitors for Metals and Alloys in Acid Pickling Processes—a Review. *Int. J. Electrochem. Sci.* **2015,** *10,* 6120–6134.

Krishnegowda, P. M.; Venkatesha, V. T.; Krishnegowda, P. K. M.; Shivayogiraju, S. B. *Acalypha torta* Leaf Extract as Green Corrosion Inhibitor for Mild Steel in Hydrochloric Acid Solution. *Ind. Eng. Chem. Res.* **2013,** *52,* 722–728.

Kumar, N. A Study on Corrosion Inhibition of is 2062 e 250 b Mild Steel in Trichloroacetic Acid. Ph.D. Dissertation, Hemchandracharya North Gujarat University, Patan, India, 2014.

Lebrini, M.; Robert, F.; Roos, C. Inhibition Effect of Alkaloids Extract from *Annona squamosa* Plant on the Corrosion of c38 Steel in Normal Hydrochloric Acid Medium. *Int. J. Electrochem. Sci.* **2010,** *5*(11), 1698–1712.

Leelavathi, S.; Rajalakshmi, R. *Dodonaea viscosa* (L.) Leaves Extract as Acid Corrosion Inhibitor for Mild Steel—a Green Approach. *J. Mater. Environ. Sci.* **2013,** *4*(5), 625–638.

Li, L.; Zhang, X.; Lei, J.; He, J.; Zhang, S.; Pan, F. Adsorption and Corrosion Inhibition of *Osmanthus fragran* Leaves Extract on Carbon Steel. *Corros. Sci.* **2012,** *63,* 82–90.

Mak, Y. W.; Chuah, L. O.; Ahmad, R.; Bhat, R. Antioxidant and Antibacterial Activities of Hibiscus (*Hibiscus rosa-sinensis* L.) and *Cassia* (*Senna bicapsularis* L.) Flower Extracts. *J. King Saud Univ.* **2013,** *25,* 275–282.

Manickam, M.; Sivakumar, D.; Thirumalairaj, B.; Jaganathan, M. Corrosion Inhibition of Mild Steel in 1 mol l^{-1} HCl Using Gum Exudates of *Azadirachta indica*. *Adv. Phys. Chem.* **2016,** *2016,* Article ID 5987528, 1–12.

Marco, J. A.; Sanz-Cervera, J. F.; Sancenon, F.; Jakupovica, J.; Rustaiyanta, A.; Mohamadit, F. Oplopanone Derivatives Monoterpene Glycosides from *Artemisia sieberi*. *Pytochemistry* **1993,** *34*(4), 1061–1065.

Mernari, B.; El Attari, H.; Traisnel, M.; Bentiss, F.; Larenee, M. Inhibiting Effects of 3,5-bis(n-pyridyl)-4-amino-1,2,4-triazoles on the Corrosion for Mild Steel in 1 M HCl Medium. *Corros. Sci.* **1998,** *40*(2–3), 391–399.

Montemor, M. F. Fostering Green Inhibitors for Corrosion Prevention. In *Active Protective Coatings;* Hughes, A., Mol, J., Zheludkevich, M., Buchheit, R., Eds.; Springer: Dordrecht, 2016; Vol. 233, pp 107–113.

Mshelia, A. D.; Aji, I. S.; Yawas, D. S. Comparative Analysis of *Jatropha curcas* and Neem Leaves Extracts as Corrosion Inhibitors on Mild Steel. *Faculty Eng. Sem. Series, Univ. Maiduguri* **2017,** *8,* 106–113.

Muthukrishnan, P; Prakash, P.; Jeyaprabha, B.; Shankar, K. Stigmasterol Extracted from *Ficus hispida* Leaves. *Arabian J. Chem.* [Online early access]. DOI: 10.1016/j.arabjc.2015.09.005. Published Online: September 28, 2015. http:// www.sciencedirect.com (accessed Dec 10, 2017).

Nnanna, L.; Nnanna, G.; Nnakaife, J.; Ekekwe, N.; Eti, P. Aqueous Extracts of *Pentaclethra macrophylla Bentham* Roots as Eco-Friendly Corrosion Inhibition for Mild Steel in 0.5 M KOH Medium. *Int. J. Mater. Chem.* **2016,** *6*(1), 12–18.

Noor, E. A. Temperature Effects on the Corrosion Inhibition of Mild Steel in Acidic Solutions by Aqueous Extract of *Fenugreek* Leaves. *Int. J. Electrochem. Sci.* **2007,** *2,* 996–1017.

Okafor, P. C.; Osabor, V. I.; Ebenso, E. E. Eco-Friendly Corrosion Inhibitors: Inhibitive Action of Ethanol Extracts of *Garcinia kola* for the Corrosion of Mild Steel in H_2SO_4 Solutions. *Pigm. Resin Technol.* **2007,** *36*(5), 299–305.

Okafor, P. C.; Ebenso, E. E.; Ekpe, U. J. *Azadirachta indica* Extracts as Corrosion Inhibitor for Mild Steel in Acid Medium. *Int. J. Electrochem. Sci.* **2010,** *5,* 978–993.

Omotosho, O. A.; Okeniyi, J.; Loto, C.; Ogbiye, S. *Cassia fistula* Leaf-Extract Effect on Corrosion-Inhibition of Stainless-Steel in 0.5 M HCl. *Proceedings of 3rd Pan American Materials Congress,* San Diego, USA, Feb. 27–March 2, 2017.

Onuegbu, T. U.; Umoh, E. T.; Ehiedu, C. N. *Emilia sonchifolia* Extract as Green Corrosion Inhibitor for Mild Steel in Acid Medium Using Weight Loss Method. *J. Nat. Sci. Res.* **2013,** *3*(9), 52–55.

Quraishi, M. A.; Yadav, D. K.; Ahamad, I. Green Approach to Corrosion Inhibition by Black Pepper Extract in Hydrochloric Acid Solution. *Open Corros. J.* **2009,** *2,* 56–60.

Quraishi, M. A.; Singh, A.; Singh, V. K.; Yadav, D. K.; Singh, A. K. Aromatic Triazoles as Corrosion Inhibitors for Mild Steel in Acidic Environments. *Mater. Chem. Phy.* **2010,** *122,* 114–122.

Raja, P. B.; Sethuraman, M. G. Natural Products as Corrosion Inhibitor for Metals in Corrosive Media—a Review. *Mater. Lett.* **2008a,** *62*(1), 113–116.

Raja, P. B.; Sethuraman, M. G. Inhibitive Effect of Black Pepper Extract on the Sulphuric Acid Corrosion of Mild Steel. *Mater. Lett.* **2008b,** *62,* 2977–2979.

Raja, P. B.; Qureshi, A. K.; Rahim, A. A.; Awang, K.; Mukhtar, M. R.; Osman, H. Indole alkaloids of *Alstonia angustifolia* var. *latifoliaas* Green Inhibitor for Mild Steel Corrosion in 1 M HCl Media. *J. Mater. Eng. Perform.* **2013,** *22*(4), 1072–1078.

Saadawy, M. An Important World Crop—Barley—as a New Green Inhibitor for Acid Corrosion of Steel. *Anti-Corros. Method. Mater.* **2014,** *62*(4), 220–228.

Scottish Environment Protection Agency. Environmental Quality Standards for Trace Metals in the Aquatic Environment. [Online] 2008. https:// www.sepa.org.uk/media/163220/trace_metals_aquatic_environment.pdf (accessed Dec 10, 2017).

Shah, P; Agarwal, S. Aloe-Vera —a Green Corrosion Inhibitor. *Int. J. Res. Appl. Sci. Eng. Tech.* **2014,** *2*(V), 14–17.

Shahid, M. Corrosion Protection with Eco-Friendly Inhibitors. *Adv. Nat. Sci.: Nanosci. Nanotechnol.* **2011,** *2,* 1–6.

Sharma, S. K.; Mudhoo, A.; Jain, G.; Sharma, J. Corrosion Inhibition and Adsorption Properties of *Azadirachta indica* Mature Leaves Extract as Green Inhibitor for Mild Steel in HNO_3. *Green Chem. Lett. Rev.* **2010,** *3*(1), 7–15.

Sharmila, A.; Prema, A. A.; Sahayaraj, P. A. Influence of *Murraya koenigii* (curry leaves) Extract on the Corrosion Inhibition of Carbon Steel in HCl Solution. *Rasayan J. Chem.* **2010,** *3*(1), 74–81.

Shyamala, M.; Arulanantham, A. *Eclipta alba* as Corrosion Pickling Inhibitor on Mild Steel in Hydrochloric Acid. *J. Mater. Sci. Technol.* **2009,** *25*(5), 633–636.

Singh, A. K.; Quraishi M. A. Corrosion Inhibition of Carbon Steel in HCl Solution by Some Plant Extracts. *Corros. Sci.* **2010,** *52*(1), 152–160.

Singh, A.; Ebenso, E. E.; Quraishi, M. A. Corrosion Inhibition of Carbon Steel in HCl Solution by Some Plant Extracts. *Int. J. Corros.* **2012,** *2012,* Article ID 897430, 1–20.

Singh, D. K.; Kumar, S.; Udayabhanu, G.; John, R. P. 4(N,N dimethylamino) Benzaldehyde Nicotinic Hydrazone as Corrosion Inhibitor for Mild Steel in 1M HCl Solution: An Experimental and Theoretical Study. *J. Mol. Liq.* **2016,** *216,* 738–746.

Sisodia, P; Hasan, S. K. Corrosion Inhibition of Mild Steel by Phytochemicals in Acidic Media. *J. Corros. Sci. Eng.* **2013,** *16*(25), 1–9.

Solomon, M. M.; Umoren, S. A. Enhanced Corrosion Inhibition Effect of Polypropylene Glycol in the Presence of Iodide Ions at Mild Steel/Sulphuric Acid Interface. *J. Environ. Chem. Eng.* **2015,** *3*(3), 1812–1826.

Subhashini, S.; Rajalakshmi, R.; Prithiba, A.; Mathina, A. Corrosion Mitigating Effect of *Cyamopsis tetragonaloba* Seed Extract on Mild Steel in Acid Medium. *E-J. Chem.* **2010,** *7*(4), 1133–1137.

Toussaint, A. Use of Organic and Inorganic Corrosion Inhibitors in High Performance Coatings. *Proceedings of Eastern Coatings Show*, Atlantic City, New Jersey, USA, June 1–4, 2015 [Online]. https://www.halox.com/news/ files/Toussaint-ECS.pdf (accessed Dec 10, 2017).

Vimala, J. R.; Leema, R. A.; Raja, S. A Study on the Phytochemical Analysis and Corrosion Inhibition on Mild Steel. *Der Chemica Sinica* **2012,** *3*(3), 582–588.

Vimala, J. R.; Priyadharshini P.; Prasanthi, R. H. *Basella alba* L. Extract as Corrosion Inhibitor for Mild Steel in Acid Medium. *World J. Pharm. Pharm. Sci.* **2016,** *5*(3), 1704–1713.

Vishnudevan, M.; Thangavel, K. A Comparative Study of Inorganic Versus Organic Corrosion Inhibitors for Mitigation of Steel in Chloride Contaminated Alkaline Solution. *Indian J. Chem. Technol.* **2007,** *14*(1), 22–28.

Walker, R. Triazole, Benzotriazole and Naphthotriazole as Corrosion Inhibitors for Copper. *Corros. Sci.* **1975,** *31*(3), 97–100.

Yadav, M.; Gope, L.; Kumari, N.; Yadav, P. Corrosion Inhibition Performance of Pyranopyrazole Derivatives for Mild Steel in HCl Solution: Gravimetric, Electrochemical and DFT Studies. *J. Mol. Liq.* **2016,** *216,* 78–86.

Zhigzhitzhapova, S. V.; Radnaeva, L. D.; Gao, Q.; Chen, S.; Zhang, F. Chemical Composition of Volatile Organic Compounds of *Artemisia vulgaris* L. (*Asteraceae*) from the Qinghai—Tibet Plateau. *Ind. Crops Prod.* **2016,** *83,* 462–469.

Zhou, Y.-Z.; Chen, H.; Qiao, L.; Lu, X.; Hua, H.-M.; Pei, Y.-H. Five New Aromatic Glycosides from *Carthamus tinctorius*. *Helvetica* **2008,** *91*(7), 1277–1285.

PART IV
Recent Advances

CHAPTER 19

NOVEL TERPENOIDS AS ANTICANCER STEM CELL AGENTS

REBATI MALIK[1], SANTOSH KUMAR MAURYA[1], PREM PRAKASH KUSHWAHA[1], PUSHPENDRA SINGH[2], and SHASHANK KUMAR[1,*]

[1]*School of Basic and Applied Sciences, Department of Biochemistry and Microbial Sciences, Central University of Punjab, Bathinda, Punjab 151001, India*

[2]*National Institute of Pathology, New Delhi, India*

[*]*Corresponding author. E-mail: shashankbiochemau@gmail.com; shashank.kumar@cupb.edu.in, Mob.: +91 9335647413*
[*]*ORCID: https://orcid.org/0000-0002-9622-0512*

ABSTRACT

Tumor tissue has some small subpopulation of cells known as cancer stem cells (CSCs). These populations are capable of self-renewal, differentiation, and have the unique property to evade radiotherapy and chemotherapy. This subpopulation of cells is the major cause of resistance to current cancer treatments. It is also reported that CSCs are associated with relapse in cancer patients. Compared to the differentiated tumor cells, CSCs have some important distinguishing feature that confers chemoresistance in these cells. Different proteins such as Bcl2, CXCR4, carbonic anhydrase 2, MTH1, CHK1, and VEGFR2 have been reported to be involved in cancer cell stemness. Nowadays, natural products are popular remedies against various diseases including cancer. These products have been reported for their low/nontoxicity and cost-effectiveness. In the present chapter, we have discussed the phytochemistry, natural, synthetic pathways and pharmacological activities of terpenoids with special references to cancer cell stemness and anti-cancer property. Furthermore, we also performed in silico studies to identify potent terpenoids active against a protein involved in cancer cell stemness.

19.1 INTRODUCTION

Terpenoids are the biggest class of naturally occurring compounds derived from five-carbon isoprene units. They are produced by plants and also known as isoprenoids. Majority of the terpenoids protect plants from abiotic and biotic stress. Plants commonly use terpenoids in their development and growth. Terpenoids have a crucial role in plant physiology such as hormone regulation and chlorophyll pigment development. Several terpenoids are being used by pharmaceutical, chemical, and food industries. Systematic and genomic biology is exploring the potential of terpenoids with their high value in microbes and plants. Scientists are giving attention to developing terpenoids as a pest control agent. Literature shows the various benefits of a terpenoid. Thus, terpenoid biosynthesis pathways should be explored in more depth (Tholl, 2015).

Biosynthesis of terpenoids depends on the flux of precursors. The first step of terpenoid biosynthesis is formation of the five-carbon (C5) units which undergoes through the mevalonate or methylerythritol phosphate (MEP) pathway to generate terpenes. Terpenoids can be classified as hemiterpenes (C5), monoterpenes (C10), sesquiterpenes (C15), diterpenes (C20), sesquiterpenes (C25), triterpenes (C30), tetraterpenes (C40) and polyterpenes on the basis of C5 unit (Ashour et al., 2010; Martin et al., 2003). Terpene synthase (dimethylallyl diphosphate diphosphate-lyase) is the key enzyme for terpene synthesis. The enzyme requires Mg^{2+} or Mn^{2+} as a cofactor (Silver and Fall, 1995; Wildermuth and Fall, 1996). It produces isoprene and pyrophosphate from dimethylallyl pyrophosphate (DMAPP) (Fig. 19.1). Plants and many of the prokaryotes are known to produce isoprenes (Kuzma et al., 1995). Cytosolic mevalonic acid (MVA) and plastidial MEP pathway generate the key precursor (isopentenyl pyrophosphate (IPP) and DMAPP) of terpenoids (Fig. 19.2).

MVA pathway synthesizes cytosolic precursor sesquiterpenoids, polyprenols, phytosterols, brassinosteroids, and triterpenoids. Ubiquinones and polyprenols are the two important precursors for the synthesis of mitochondrial terpenoids (Tholl, 2006). The first step of the mevalonic acid pathway starts with the condensation of the acetyl-CoA with another acetyl-CoA in the presence of acetoacetyl-CoA thiolase (Fig. 19.3). Acetoacetyl-CoA condenses with another acetyl-CoA to form 3-hydroxy-3-methylglutaryl-CoA (HMG-CoA) with the help of HMG-CoA synthase. These reactions are followed by different steps involving HMG-CoA reductase, mevalonate-5-kinase, mevalonate pyrophosphate decarboxylase, and isopentenyl pyrophosphate isomerase enzyme resulting in the formation of DMAPP. On the other hand, the MEP pathway is initiated with the reaction of pyruvate and glyceraldehyde 3-phosphate (Fig. 19.4). Different enzymes of the pathway work in a sequential step to form (E)-4-Hydroxy-3-methyl-but-2-enyl pyrophosphate (HMB-PP) as the end product of the pathway. Another enzyme called IspH finally converts the HMBPP to the IPP and DMAPP.

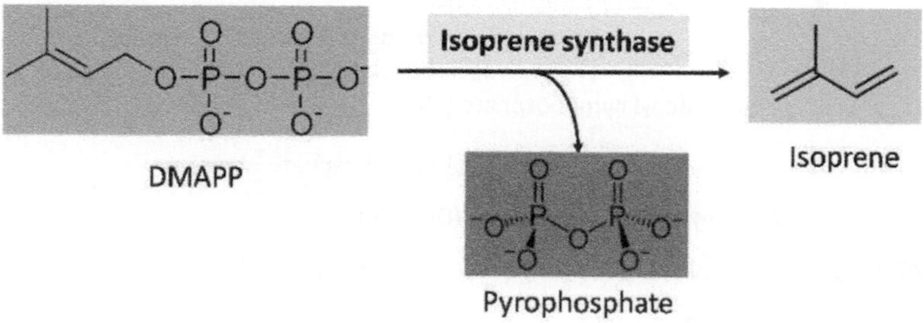

FIGURE 19.1 Isoprene synthesis from dimethylallyl pyrophosphate and isoprene synthase.

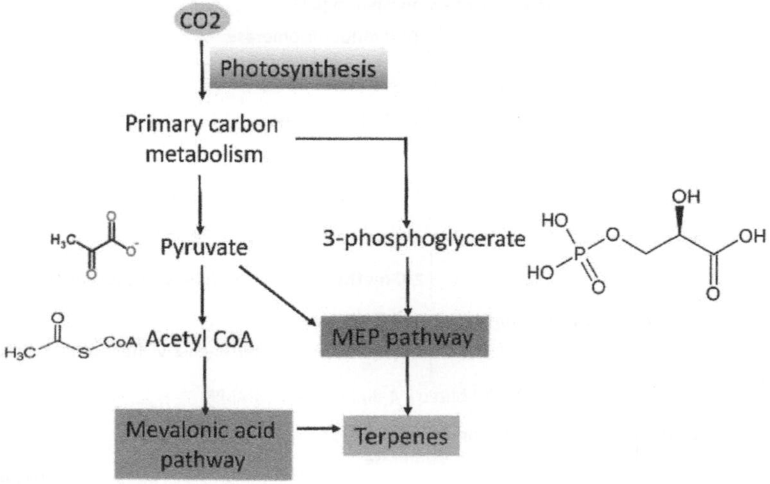

FIGURE 19.2 Common pathway involved in terpene biosynthesis.

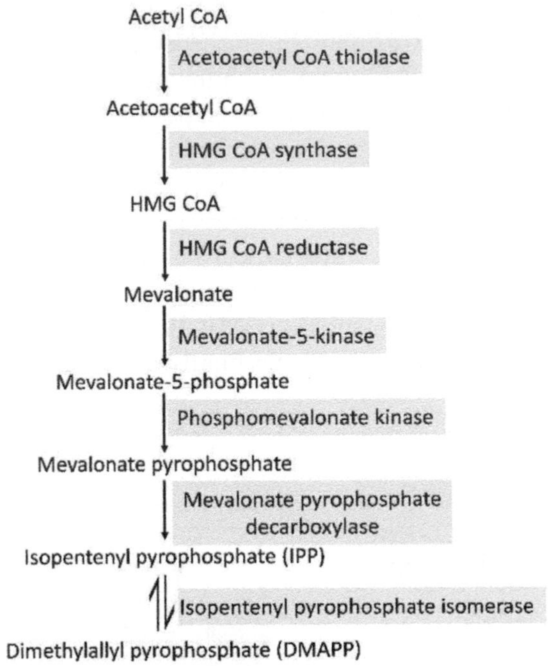

FIGURE 19.3 Step involved in the mevalonic acid pathway.

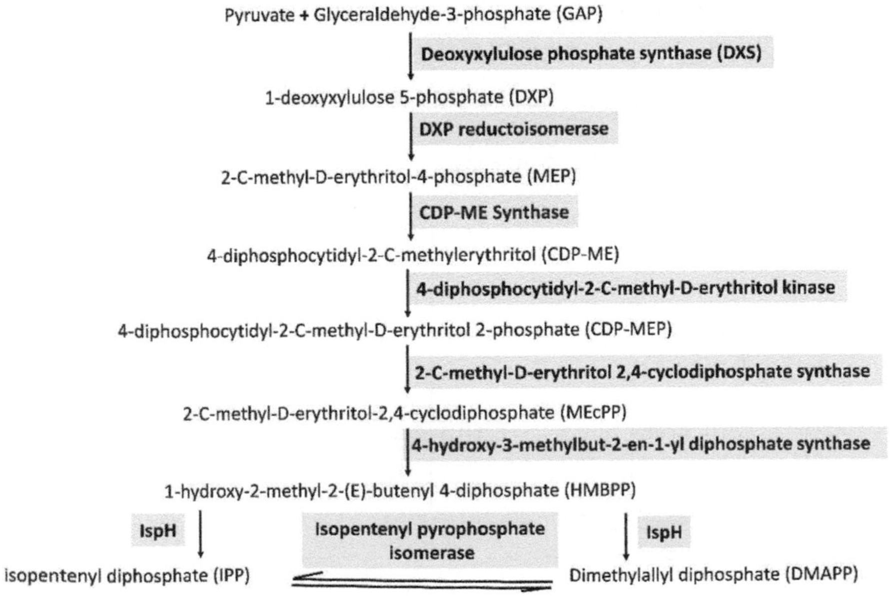

FIGURE 19.4 Steps involved in methylerythritol phosphate pathway.

Hemiterpene (C5), the simplest class of terpenes is mostly found in oil. There are around 100 hemiterpene aglycones known. Mostly, they are water-insoluble, but some of them contain sugar group and are water-soluble. Isoprene is a very common and extremely known hemiterpene. Chlorinated hemiterpenes such as utililactone and epiutililactone have been reported in *Prinsepia utilis* leaves. Monoterpene is a type of hydrocarbon comprised of two condensed isoprene units (C5). It is an ingredient of fragrant oils obtained from leaves of the different plant. It is a monocyclic monoterpene such as limonene that has remarkable chemopreventive/chemotherapeutic potential against multiple types of cancer (Sun, 2007). Limonene is known to induce apoptosis and can modulate polyamine metabolism in colon cancer. Limonene treatment showed increased Bax/Bcl2 ratio with upregulation of cleaved caspase-3, caspase-9, poly ADP ribose polymerase, and cytochrome C. It has been reported that patients fed with limonene conferred a striking effect in tumor regression. Monoterpene limonene has very low toxicity and does not report any mutagenic, carcinogenic or nephrotoxic risk to humans (Vigushin et al., 1998). A hydroxylated form of limonene, Perillyl alcohol showed inhibition of azoxymethane-induced rat colon carcinogenesis (Reddy et al., 1997). Carvacrol downregulates cyclin B1 expression, arrests G2/M phase of cell cycle and initiates apoptosis in HCT116 and LoVo cancer cell lines (Fan et al., 2015). Carvacrol also showed anti-invasive potential via decreasing matrix metalloprotease-2 and matrix metalloprotease-9 expression. Sesquiterpenes are a cluster of 15 carbon compounds resulting from the assembly of three isoprenoids (C5) units. Sesquiterpene lactones are kept at the top position in pharmacological studies and have an unusual anticancer activity (Orofino et al., 2012). Sesquiterpene lactones, namely isobutyroplenolin and arnicolide D, zerumbone, isolated from *Centipede minima* and *Zingiber zerumbet* respectively, showed proliferation inhibition and induction of apoptosis (Huang et al., 2014; Murakami et al., 2004). Four isoprene units or two terpene units form diterpenes. Andrographolide diterpene lactones isolated from *Andrographis paniculata* showed cytotoxic properties in different cancers such as breast, melanoma, lung, and leukemia cell lines (Nanduri et al., 2004). Pseudolaric acid B is another diterpene isolated from the root bark of *Pseudolarix kaempferi* that showed antiproliferative potential in different cancers (Pan et al., 1990). Triterpenoids such as saponins, betulinic acid, and phytosterols are well known for their biological activities. Betulinic acid showed antiproliferative potential and induced apoptosis in colon cancer cell (Rzeski et al., 2006). Another triterpenoid oleanolic acid comprises antiinflammatory and cytotoxicity efficacy against various types of colon cancer cell lines (Li et al., 2002). Glycyrrhizic acid or glycyrrhizin from the licorice root extracts can inhibit N-acetyltransferase enzyme (Chung et al., 2000). Carotenoids and lycopenes are some other terpenoids having the anticancer potential (Scolastici et al., 2007).

19.2 CANCER STEM CELLS (CSCS)

In a malignant tumor, there is some subpopulation of CSCs. Many overacting and abnormal signaling pathways contribute to the survival of cancer stem cells (CSCs). CSCs are capable of differentiation, self-renewal and generation of heterogeneous tumors in a different type of cancer. There are two models which explain heterogeneity within the tumor: the clonal evolution model and cancer stem cell model. Clonal evolution model is also known as a stochastic model. According to this model, every cell can develop into cancer cell through successive mutations (Merlo et al., 2006). CSC model is also known as hierarchical model. CSCs are always placed at the top in this model (Reya et al., 2001). According to CSC model, only CSCs have the property of tumor formation within the tumor (Sottoriva et al., 2010). In 2014, a new model was purposed which creates a bridge between these models and this model is now called plasticity model. According to this model, CSC has property to change into non-CSC cell and vice versa (Tetteh et al., 2015). Like normal stem cells, all the properties of CSCs are regulated by their specific niche. CSCs present different types of markers on their surface like oct4, CD44, aldehyde dehydrogenase 1 (ALDH1), CD24, CD29, CD90, CD133, epithelial-specific antigen, and so forth. Expression of this marker is tissue type-specific or tumor subtype-specific (Ajani et al., 2015). Expression of these markers depends on singling pathways. These pathways are interconnected to each other, and these interwoven networks of signaling meditator feed into one another. In breast CSC-like cells, JAK/STAT including IFNK, IFNGR, IL6, STAT1, and the activated form of STAT3 are highly upregulated and promote cancer stemness (Stine and Matunis, 2013). Aberrant Hedgehog signaling (overexpression of Gli1, SHH, and PATCHED1) in CSCs is documented into basal cell carcinoma, multiple myeloma, glioblastoma, chronic myeloid leukemia and colon cancer (Peacock et al., 2007). Aberrant Wnt signaling (upregulation of β-catenin and downregulation of APC, GSK-3β) show stemness properties in different types of CSCs (breast, gastric and colorectal cancer) (Lindvall et al., 2006). A higher level of Notch signaling genes notch1, notch3, jag1, jag2, and Notch target gene hes1, are documented in several types of cancers stem cells (pancreatic, blood and breast) (Ranganathan et al., 2011). Similarly, overexpression of NF-kβ signaling pathway has been reported in chronic lymphocytic leukemia and multiple myeloma (Zhao et al., 2012). Stemness of cancer is also regulated by their microenvironment or niche (Junttila and de Sauvage, 2013). Chronic inflammation is one the major factors influencing the metastatic property of CSCs (Grivennikov et al., 2010). CSCs have multidrug resistance (MDR) property, for example, exposure of temozolomide against glioblastoma expand the stem cell pool and increase the overexpression of markers such as Oct4 and Nestin (Abubaker et al., 2013). Hypoxia also induces stemness in different type of CSCs (Axelson et al., 2005).

19.3 PHYTOCHEMICALS AND CSC

Among anticancer drugs, 50% are natural products or their derivatives extracted from plants and seeds. Many phytoextracts are used as an anticancer drug, for example, gamma-tocotrienol which is extracted from palm oil, polysaccharide peptide obtained from mushroom, inhibits tumor formation capacity of CSCs (Luk et al., 2011). Triterpenes present in many fruits (stop the self-renewal power of CSC of liver cell (Lee et al., 2011). Genistein which is an isoflavone, has antiproliferative effect on different types of cancer (Hewitt and Singletary, 2003). Brassicaceae (watercress and broccoli) extracts contain isothiocyanates such as phenethyl isothiocyanates and sulforaphane that target the proliferation, stemness, metastatic potential in colorectal cancer (Table 19.1). Curcumin (dietary polyphenol) is a chemopreventive agent in a variety of cancers (breast, liver, prostate, hematological, gastrointestinal and colorectal cancer) inhibits metastasis (Kunnumakkara et al., 2008), growth and self-renewable (Kakarala et al., 2010) properties of CSCs. Epigallocatechin-3-gallate (EGCG), a type of catechin synthesized by green tea, is a polyphenolic constituent of green tea having the potency for apoptosis and inhibits growth of various cancers through different mechanisms (Jung and Ellis, 2001). Retinoic acid derived from vitamin A, differentiates CSCs or depletes their formation by regulating Notch signaling (Moreb et al., 2005). Selenoproteins are biologically active form of selenium and act as anticarcinogenic nutrients.

TABLE 19.1 Cancer Stem Cell Signaling Targets by Phytochemicals.

Phytochemicals	Targeted signaling	References
Cyclopamine, Sulforaphane	Hedgehog signaling	Oh et al., 2016
Epigallocatechin-3-gallate (EGCG), Vitamin D, Curcumin	Wnt signaling	
Retinoic acid, Curcumin	Notch signaling	
Selenium, Sulforaphane	RTKs signaling	
Genistein, Quercetin	mTOR signaling	

19.4 TERPENOIDS AND CSCS

In China, a special type of timber tree named *Albizia julibrissin* is distributed (Pharmacopoeia committee of China, 2015). The stem bark of this plant is used as medicine (Ikeda et al., 1997). The oleanane-type triterpenoids are main constituents (Zou et al., 2000). Oleanane-type triterpenoid is made up of acetic acid glycan and monoterpenoid glycosyl. Some triterpenoid saponins have cytotoxic and anti-angiogenic activity against cancer cell line (Liang et al., 2005). In recent times, ten new oleanane-type triterpenoid saponins and six triterpenoid saponins have been identified (Zheng et al., 2010).

Hinokitiol shows the anti-CSC effect on glioma cancer. It is a compound of aromatic tropolone derived from *Chamaecyparis taiwanensis* (Shih et al., 2013). Besides the anti-CSC effect, it has antimicrobial, anti-inflammatory effects (Shih et al., 2014). It has been shown that hinokitiol increases antioxidant enzymes in CSCs and exerts anticancer effect (Huang et al., 2015b). Hinokitiol suppresses the phosphorylation of mitogen-activated protein kinase signaling and inhibits migration of cancer melanoma cells (Huang et al., 2015a). In breast cancer, hinokitiol reduces the vasculogenic mimicry activity by stimulating epidermal growth factor receptor (Tu et al., 2016).

Retinoic acid derived from vitamin A, plays an important role in limiting the synthesis of ALDH and performs negative feedback effect (Moreb et al., 2005). It was reported that exogenous addition of retinoic acid suppresses ALDH activity in the cancer cell. This negative feedback of ALDH renders it sensitive to 4-hydroperoxycyclophosphamide (4-HC). 4-HC is a derivative of cyclophosphamide and an aldehyde substrate of ALDH (Moreb et al., 2007). All-trans-retinoic acid (ATRA) induces cell differentiation in malignant tumor type, including breast cancer (Sutton et al., 1997). Retinoic acid (RA) targets the CSCs and is less toxic to normal cell, thus more conventional in chemotherapy (Garattini et al., 2007). It has been shown that retinoic acid receptors (RARs) bind to retinoid X receptors (RXRs) present as a heterodimer (RAR/RXR) to the RAR response element at the promoter of the target gene. Once the RAR interacts with the RA ligand and binds to RXR, it takes conformational changes to recruit the coactivator and dissociate the corepressor, leading to the start of transcription of the target gene. There are three forms of RARs present in a cell, RARα, RARβ, and RARγ. Among them, the loss of RARβ expression is significantly correlated with the tumor-forming capacity and RA-resistant property (Tang and Gudas, 2011). ATRA directs the breast cancer cells though RARβ-TET2-miR-200c-PKCζ signaling pathway (Shimono et al., 2009). *Ailanthus triphysa,* a therapeutic agent locally named Yom-Pa, is a deciduous tree distributed over Asia and Australia. The dichloromethane and dichloromethane-methanol extracts of the stem and its bark, show a good inhibition of cancer cell line (Kundu and Luskar, 2010). *Amoora rohituka* is a medicinal plant, a member of Meliaceae family and grows in India, Sri Lanka, Malaysia, Indonesia, China, and Bangladesh. Many plants extracts comprises triterpenoids, diterpenoids, limonoid, glycosides and alkaloids and are used in the treatment of tumor, liver disease, and abdominal complaints (Ghani, 2003). Petroleum ether extracted from *A. rohituka* causes the death of pancreatic cancer cells (PANC-1, Mia-Paca2, Capan1, and MFC-7) (Chan et al., 2011). A synthetic triterpenoid, methyl 2-cyano-3,12-dioxooleana-1,9 (11) dien-28-oate, induces apoptosis and inhibits telomerase activity in PANC-1 and Mica-Paca2 cells (Deeb et al., 2012). Cucurbitacin B, a tetracyclin terpenoid extracted from *Trichosanthes kirllowii,* inhibits JAK2, STAT3, and STAT5, increases p21, and induces apoptosis of pancreatic cancer. Gemcitabine affects the K-Ras mutant pancreatic cancer cell and reduces the size of pancreatic tumor xenografts (Abbassi et al., 2009). AMR-MeoAc is a monoacetate of a triterpene amooranin extracted from *A. rohituka* stem bark, inhibits oncogenic K-Ras through ERK, Akt, and survivin in HPAF-II cells of pancreatic cancer (Rabi and Venkatanarasimhan, 2014). Aphanin, a triterpene, was extracted through column chromatography for the first time from the stem of *A. rohituka,* and inhibits cell proliferation, induces G0-G1 cell cycle arrest and promotes apoptosis with a dynamic change in Bax/Bcl-2 retio in lung cancer A549 cells. Aphanin inhibits the proliferation with G0-G1 cell cycle arrest, induces apoptosis by inhibition of K-Ras, STAT3, Akt, cyclin D1, c-Myc, and activates the caspase cascade of pancreatic cancer (Rabi et al., 2007).

Tingenone is cytotoxic against many cancer types including breast cancer (Gomes et al., 2011). The tingenin b (22β-hydroxytingenone) has antibacterial (Maregesi et al., 2010), antiparasitic (de Sousa et al., 2015) and anticancer activity (Bavovada et al., 1990). Tingenin b induces a cytotoxic effect and apoptosis in breast CSCs (MCF-7). Cytotoxic effect of tingenin b against any type of cancer still remains unidentified. Tingenin b has cytotoxic activity by inducing apoptosis which is caused by mitochondrial injury. Even endoplasmic reticulum is also involved in inducing apoptosis in breast CSCs (in vitro) (Karakas et al., 2015).

LANGDU derived from *Euphorbia prolifera* Buch.-Ham found in southest China is a herbal medicine and used to treat cancer and inflammation (Li et al., 2008). The myrsinol diterpene extracted from *E. prolifera* Buch.-Ham inhibits the proliferation of tumor cells (Li et al., 2011). P-glycoprotein exports a verity of the cytotoxic drug from the cytoplasm and cell membrane to body fluids and provides MRD (Hennessy and Spiers, 2007). Overexpression of P-gp reduces intracellular concentration of drugs and protects cancer cells from cytotoxicity (Eichhorn and Efferth, 2012). A variety of diterpenes extracted from Euphorbia species, including LANGDU, inhibits P-gp-dependent efflux and reverse MDR of the breast cancer cell line (Corea et al., 2004).

A sesquiterpene lactone named parthenolide (PTL), extracted from the shoots of *Tanacetum parthenium* (Stojakowska and Kisiel, 1997), has shown anticancer and anti-inflammatory activities (Wiedhopf et al., 1973). PTL is the first small molecule selected against CSCs. PTL targets specific signaling pathways and kills cancer cells at their roots. In 1973, it was found that PTL has antitumor and anti-inflammatory effect by targeting of NF-kB signaling pathways (Bork et al., 1997). Thus, PTL is often purchased as a pharmacological NF-kB inhibitor. In 2005, the molecular mechanism of its anticancer properties through epigenetic regulations was found. Thus, PTL is also used as an epigenetic-based chemoprevention technique (Gopal et al., 2007).

We performed an in silico study to find out active terpenoids (Fig. 19.5) against cancer stem cell signaling pathway proteins Bcl2, CXCR4, CHK1, MTH1, VEGFR2, and Carbonic anhydrase 2. These proteins are mainly involved in cancer cell stemness initiation and progression. Various offline and online tools were used for docking study (protein, ligand, and structure preparation). The best dock score of various terpenoids is shown in Figures 19.6–19.11. Schematic representation of the different type of interactions (hydrogen bonds and hydrophobic interactions) among lead compounds and targeted proteins was developed using LigPlot+v.1.4.5 and results are depicted in Figure 19.12. We also predicted ADME/T and drug-likeness properties by using PreADMET server. The result of these parameters is shown in Tables 19.2 and 19.3.

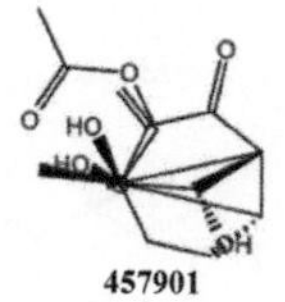

457901

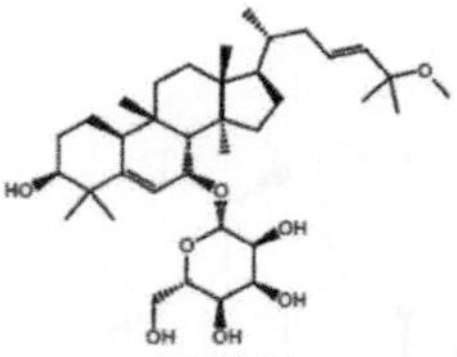

44555454

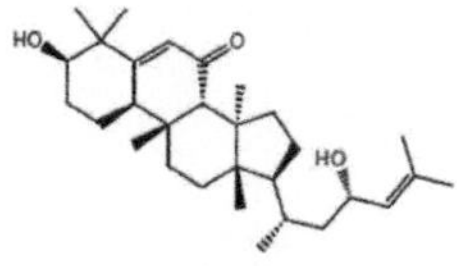

46912852

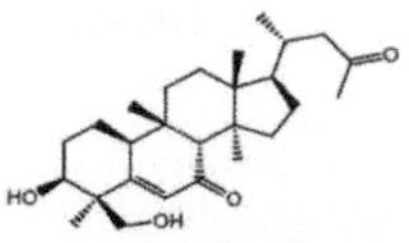

52947048

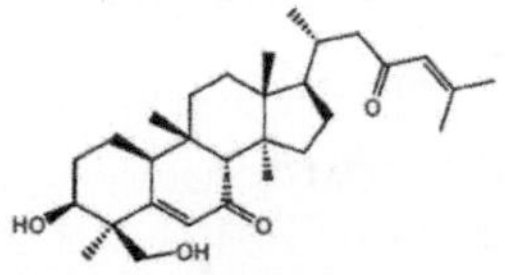

52947022

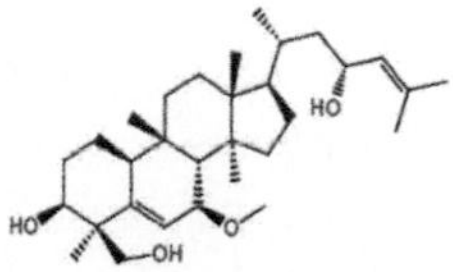

44607277

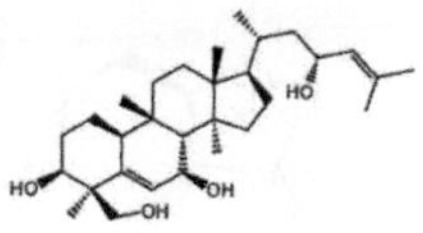

44607276

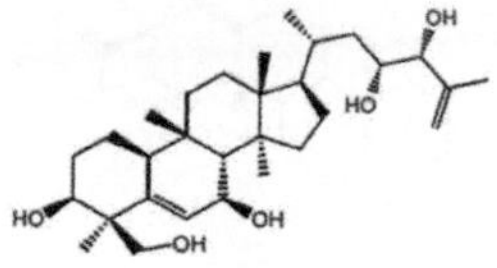

44607275

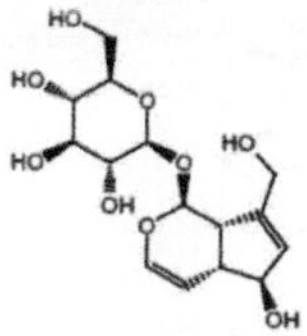

91458

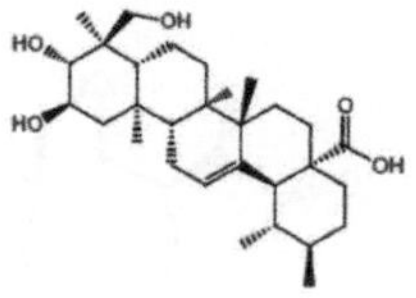

119034

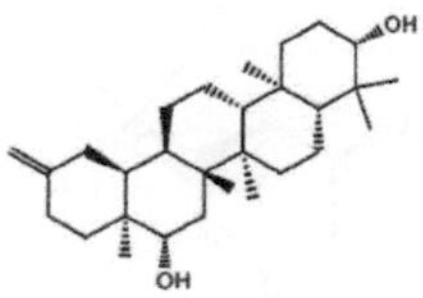

470259

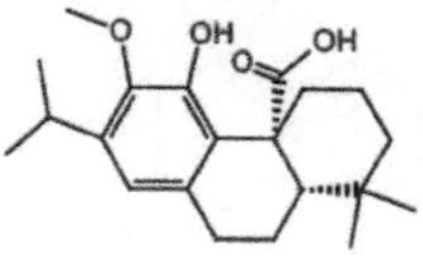

9974918

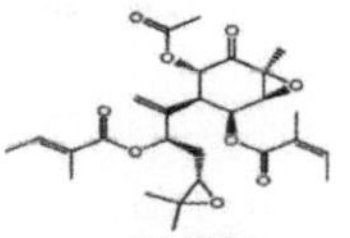

46186621

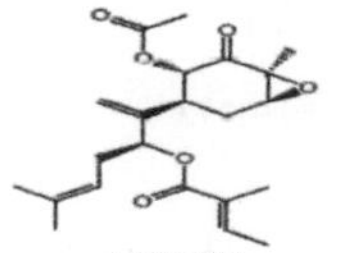

46186620

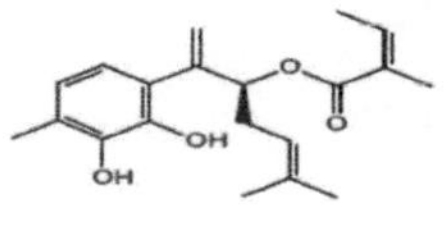

46186371

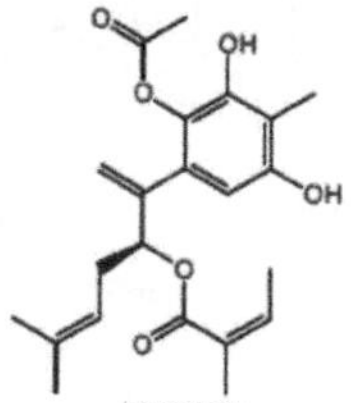

46186370

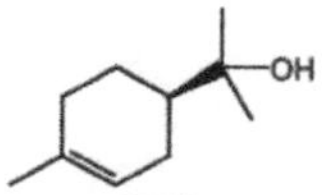

17100

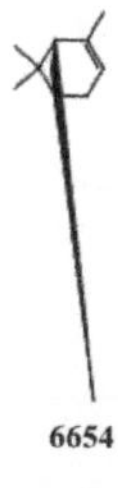

6654

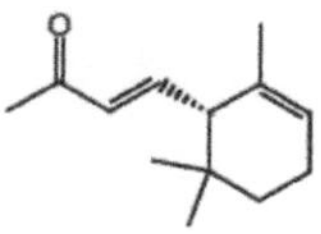

5282108

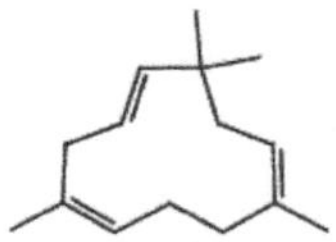

5281520

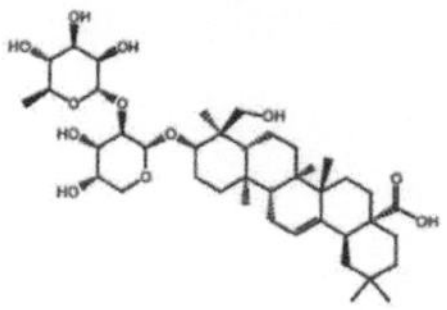

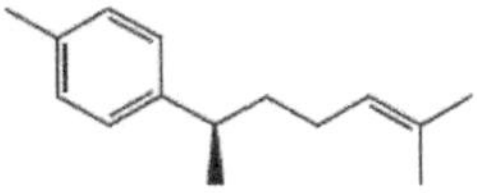

442360

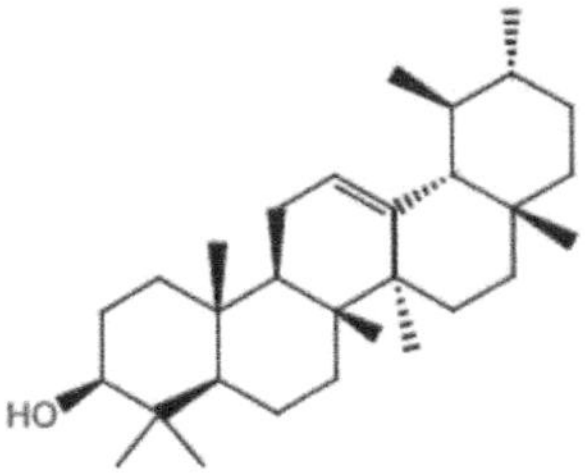

73170

73296

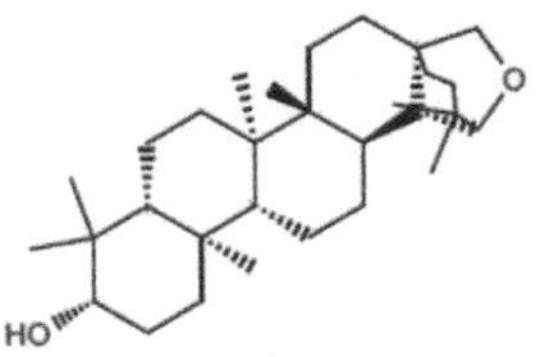

11954143

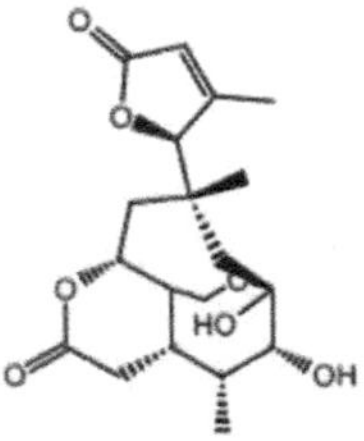

15432541

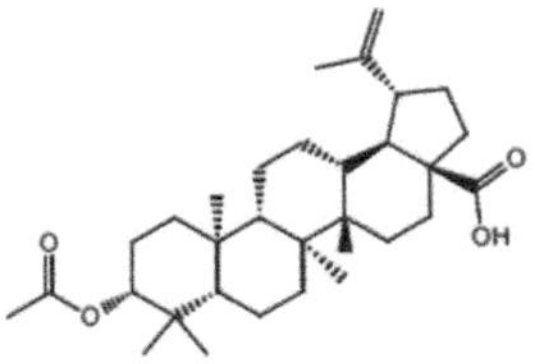

289984

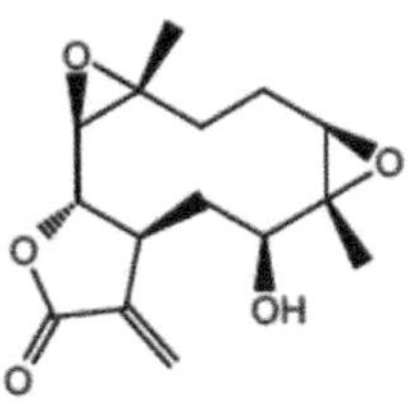

500219

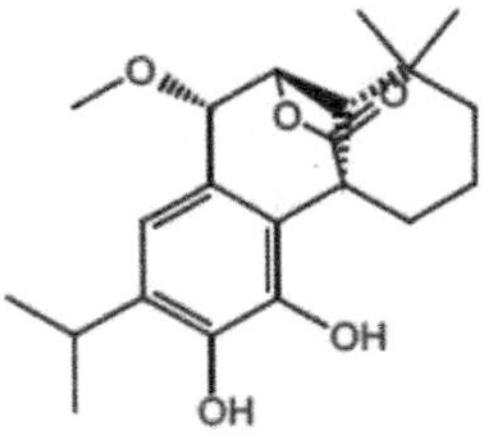

455262

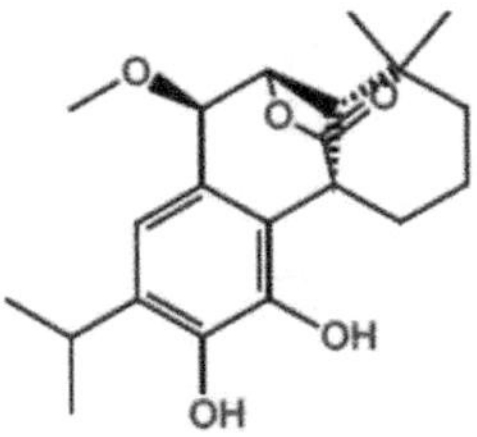

9950773

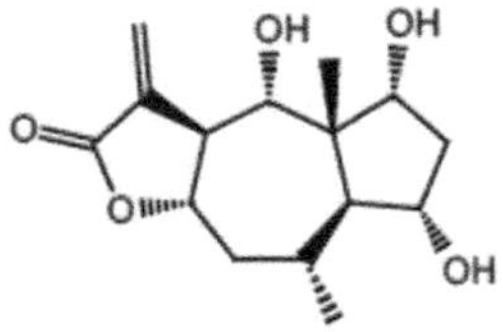

16401759

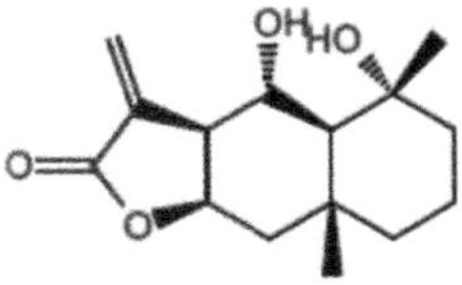

10445633

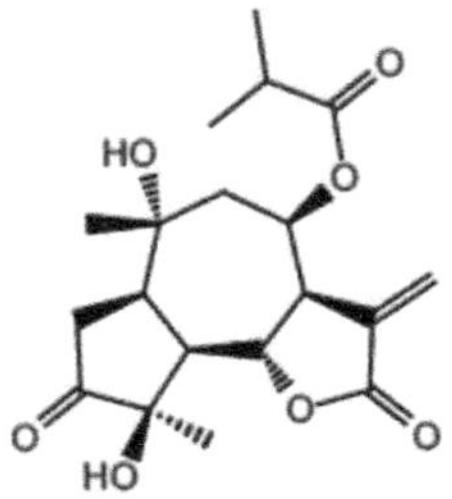

11474040

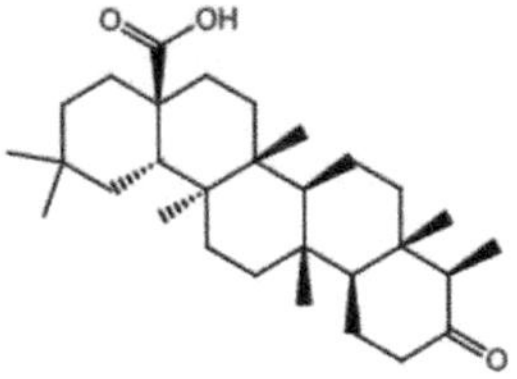

469744

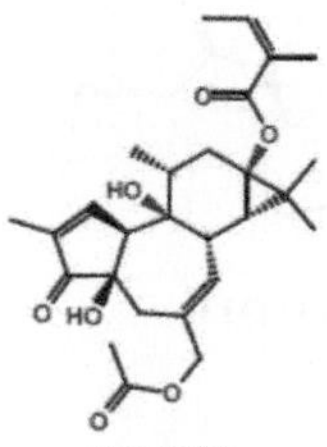

6444377

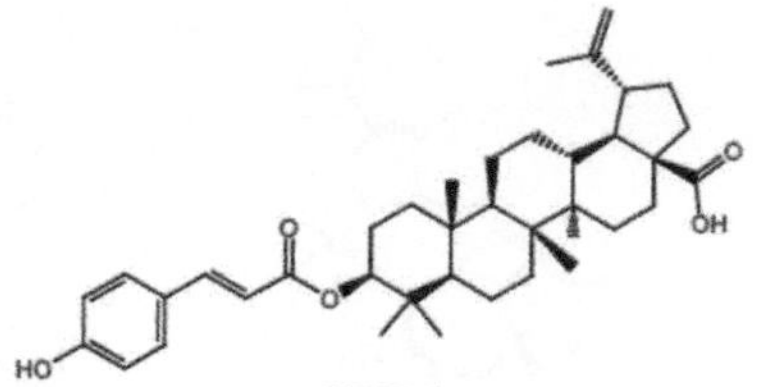

6479753

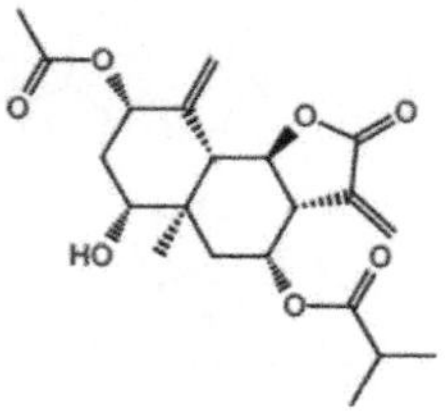

9977821

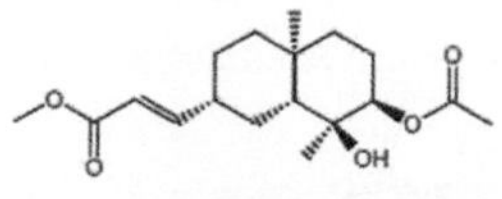

11120895

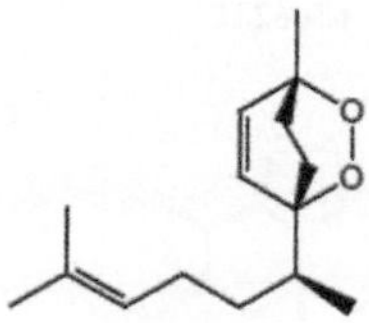

10014355

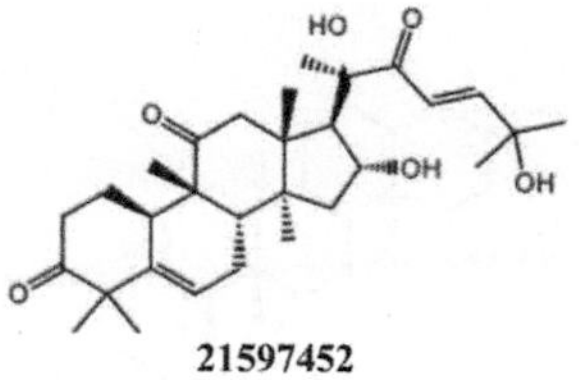

21597452

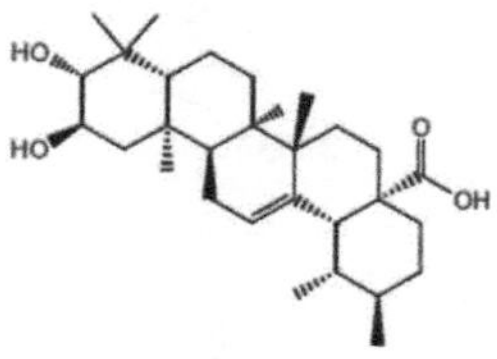

5318379

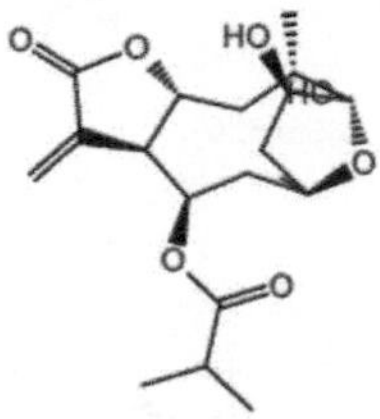

636756

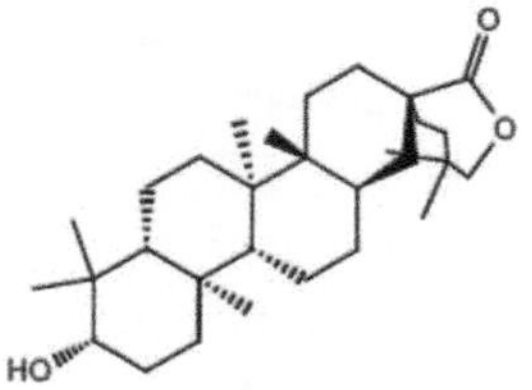

12305935

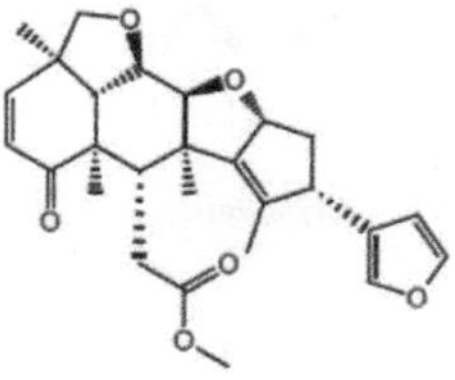

159573

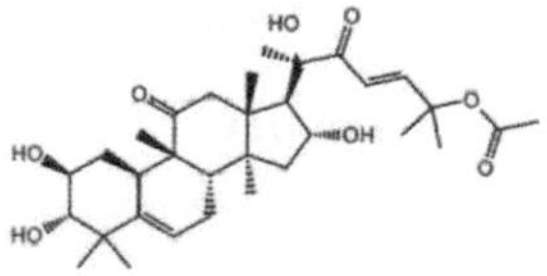

14165733

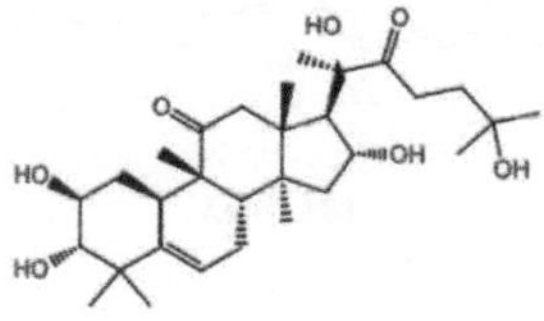

72421

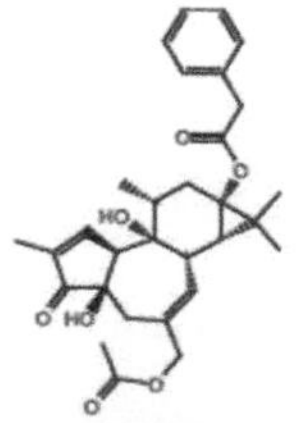

3034821

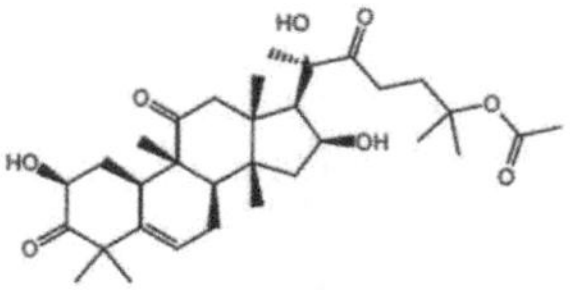

588303

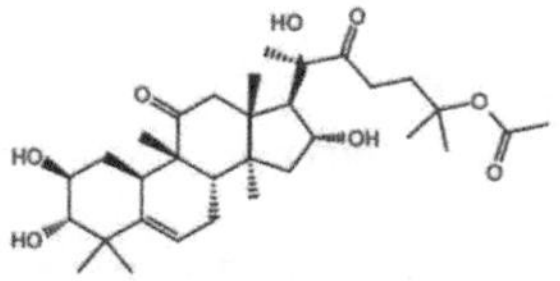

181183

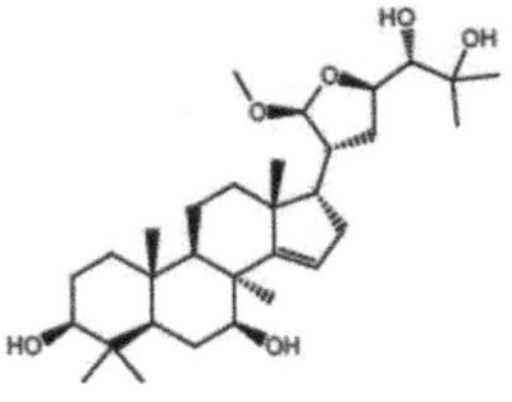

5319791

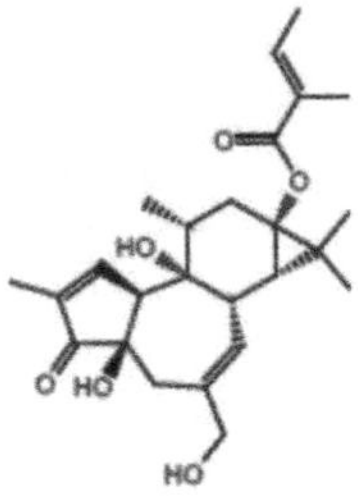

6506231

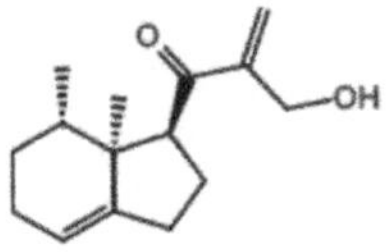

10243131

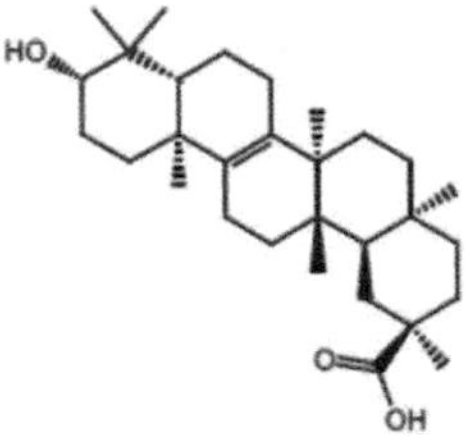

472768

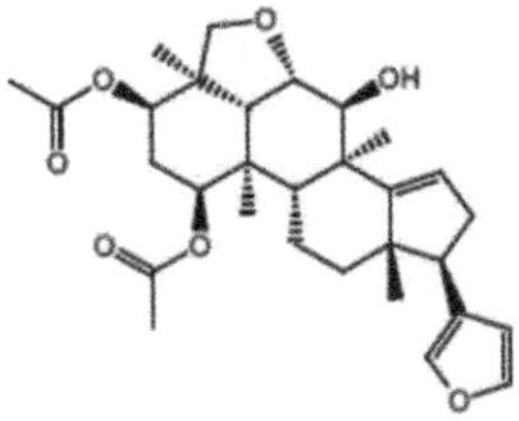

44566526

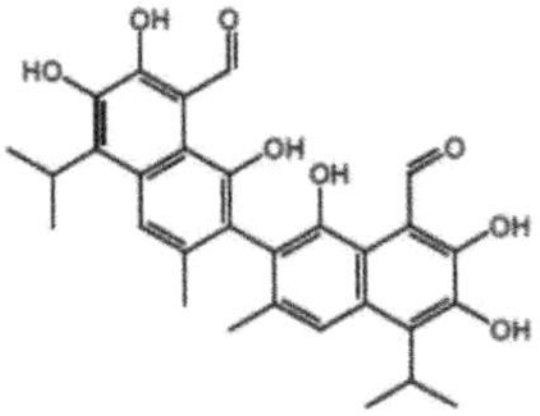

3503

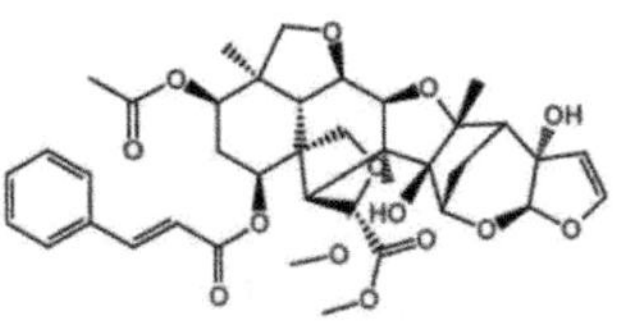

10327653

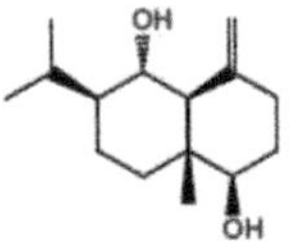

10466743

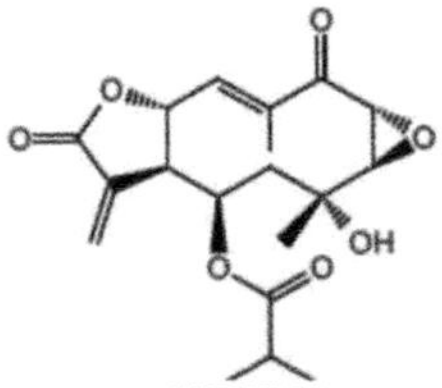

44566960

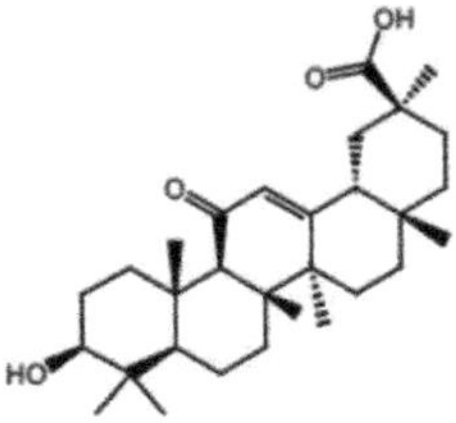

10114

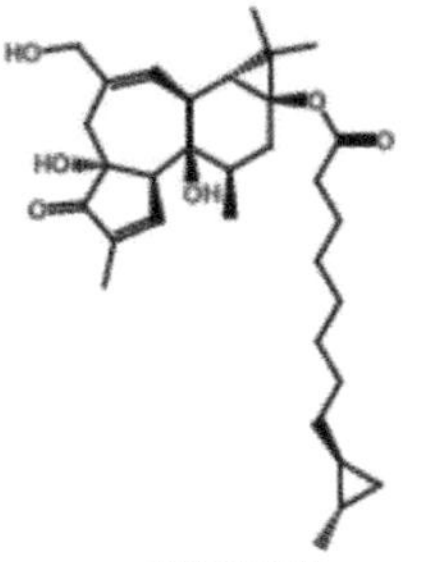

10369667

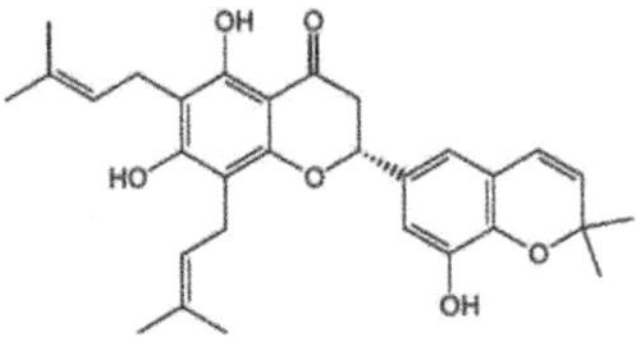

42607999

FIGURE 19.5 Structure and PubChem-IDs of the terpenoid used in the present study.

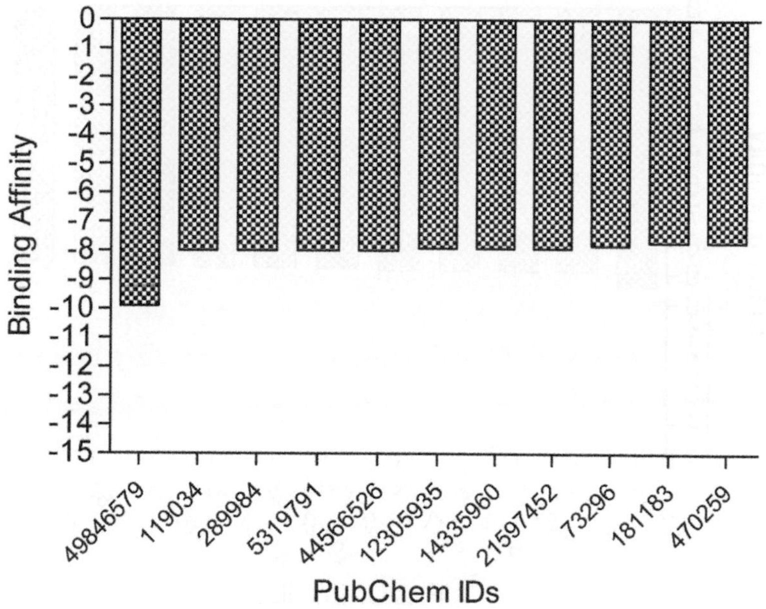

FIGURE 19.6 Dock score of terpenoids with Bcl2 protein and standard inhibitor.

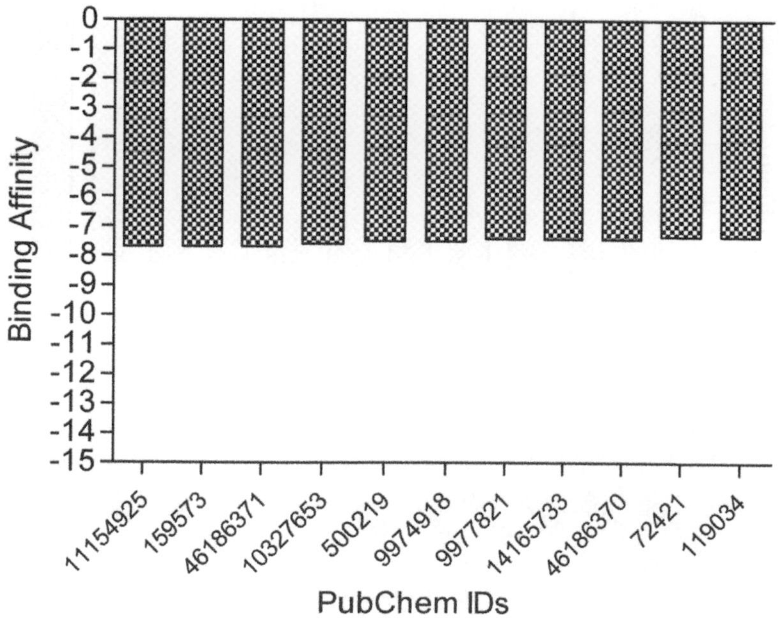

FIGURE 19.7 Dock score of terpenoids with VEGFR2 protein and standard inhibitor.

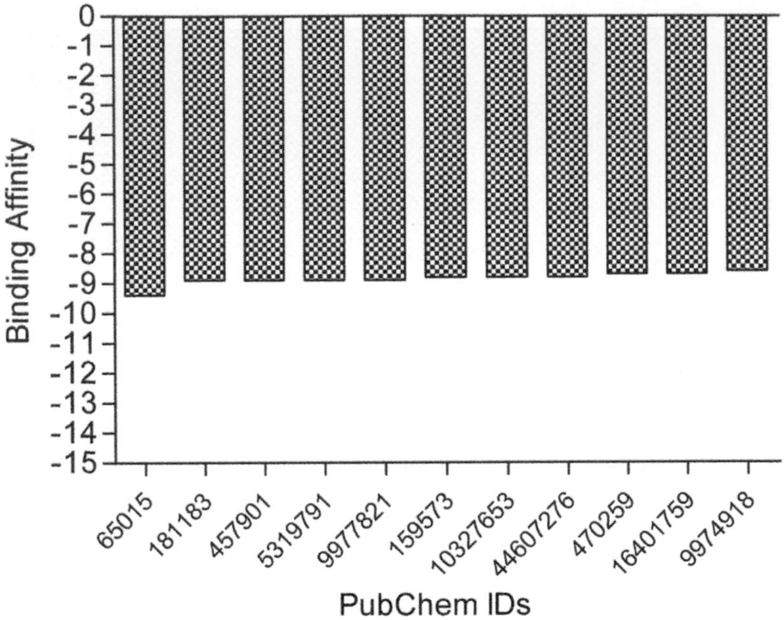

FIGURE 19.8 Dock score of terpenoids with CXCR4 protein and standard inhibitor.

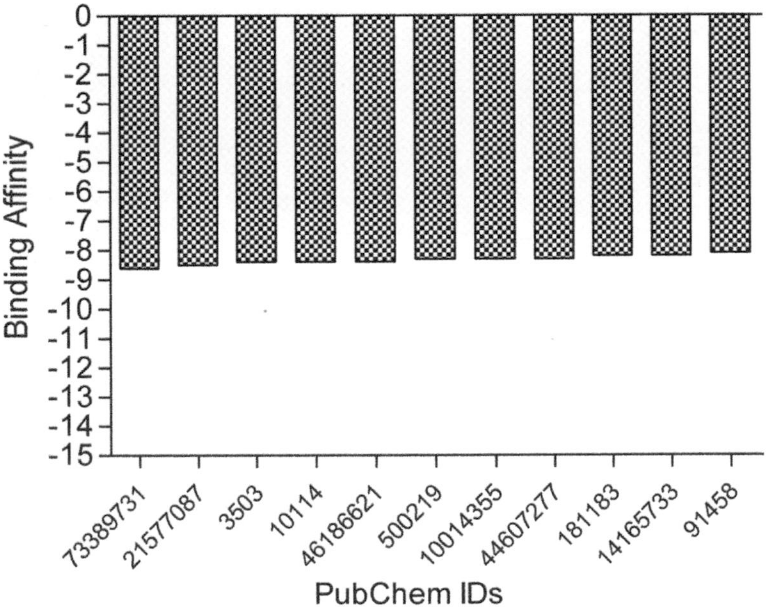

FIGURE 19.9 Dock score of terpenoids with MTH1 protein and standard inhibitor.

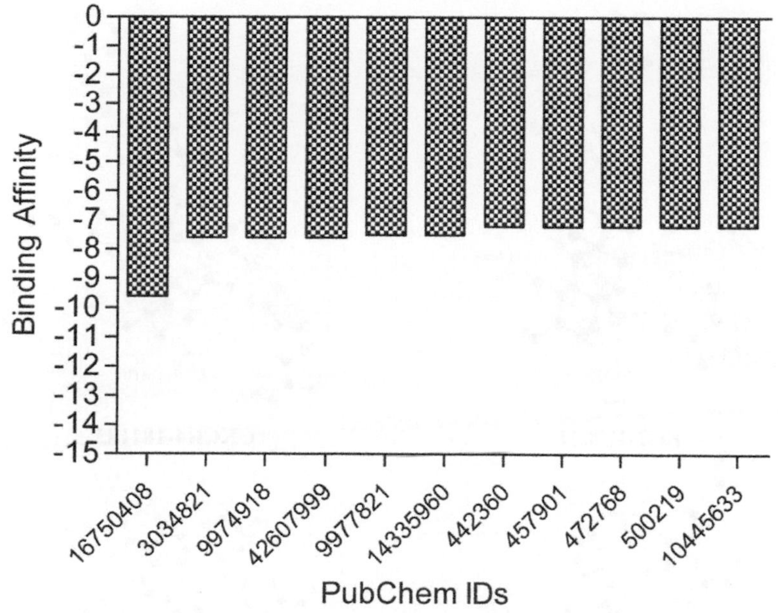

FIGURE 19.10 Dock score of terpenoids with CHK1 protein and standard inhibitor.

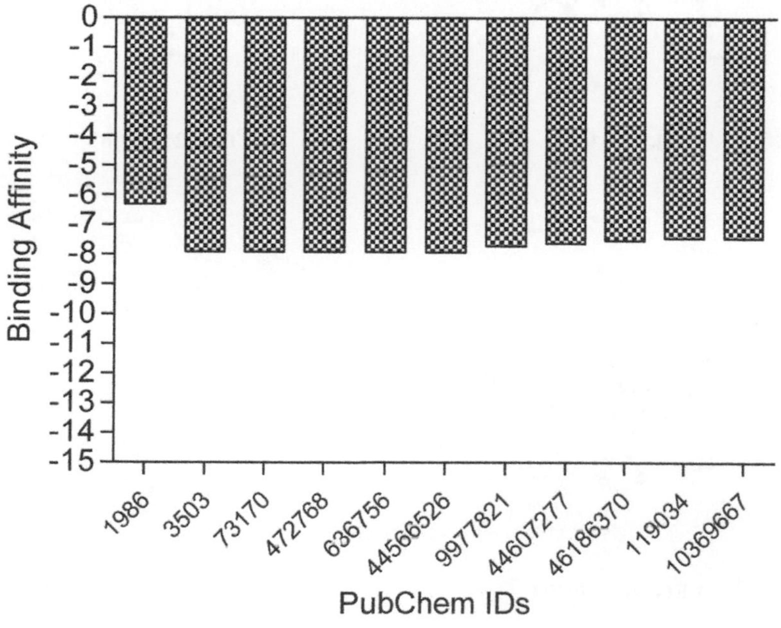

FIGURE 19.11 Dock score of terpenoids with Carbonic anhydrase 2 protein and standard inhibitor.

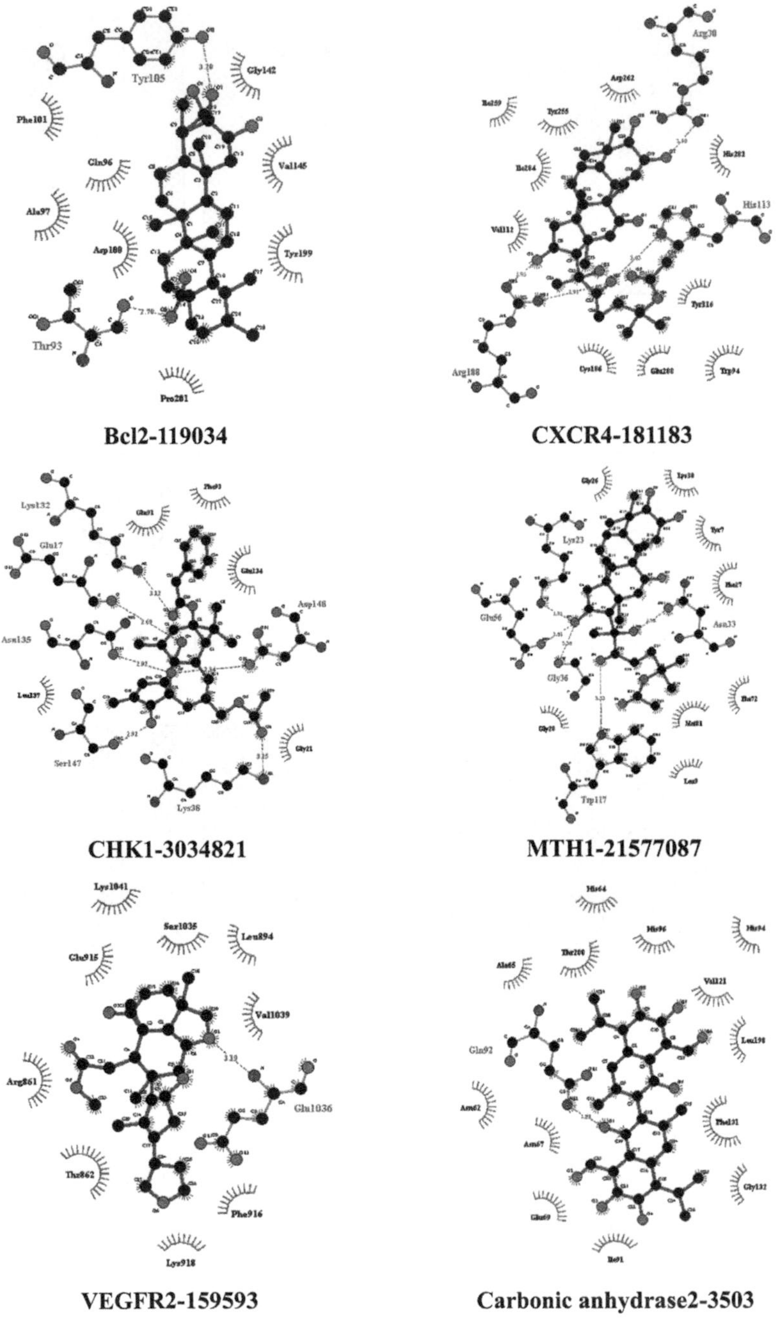

FIGURE 19.12 (See color insert.) LigPlot of lead terpenoids with Bcl2, VEGFR2, CXCR4, MTH1, CHK1 and Carbonic anhydrase 2 proteins.

TABLE 19.2 ADME Properties of the Terpenoid used in the Present Study.

PubChem ID	BBB	Caco2	Pgp-inhibition	HIA	MDCK	PPB
3503	1.24369	20.7934	Inhibitor	85.10669	0.0434204*	100
6654	5.5333	23.6322	Inhibitor	100	304.815	100
10,114	2.21347	21.5166	Inhibitor	96.71404	0.0467336	98.14341
17,100	5.11925	50.8083	None	100	191.284	23.41631
72,421	0.0742244	19.4817	Inhibitor	76.45951	0.0507847	55.11564
73,170	20.9638	47.1744	Inhibitor	100	1.43045*	100
73,296	0.0911556	20.6726	Inhibitor	59.91227	0.0434156*	87.67771
91,458	0.0545602	9.93766	None	20.68248	0.532271	25.22242
119,034	0.628392	20.9771	Inhibitor	91.23933	0.0434811	96.45518
159,573	0.304079	36.7279	None	98.82558	4.73654	86.62276
181,183	0.0720654	19.9336	Inhibitor	84.01712	0.044098	59.79623
289,984	3.04333	23.6383	Inhibitor	97.99076	0.0435672*	100
442,360	14.5943	23.4036*	Inhibitor	100	63.7385*	100
455,262	2.68366	21.5394	Inhibitor	92.96128	197.161	93.0993
457,901	0.0383007	21.1051	None	82.10811	0.934989	60.86894
469,744	5.05936	22.2889	Inhibitor	97.76701	0.110106*	100
470,259	13.7696	31.1248	Inhibitor	94.40467	0.204598*	100
472,768	8.48839	21.8826	Inhibitor	95.99632	0.0498201*	100
500,219	0.528504	22.827	None	91.83539	7.32962	55.9652
588,303	0.0398137	20.0244	Inhibitor	88.70174	0.0440033	58.48968
636,756	0.557916	21.4232	None	84.48824	2.73672	69.58589
3,034,821	0.0282505	21.9967	Inhibitor	95.66251	0.165431	86.8339
5,281,520	14.2219	23.633	Inhibitor	100	60.6852*	100
5,282,108	1.73523	53.0214	Inhibitor	100	305.112	99.46857
5,318,379	2.78849	21.2642	Inhibitor	94.27844	0.0435056	99.22454
5,319,791	0.821186	22.7052	Inhibitor	87.92062	0.043855	85.97652
6,444,377	0.0573358	20.8179	None	94.40623	0.22335	86.39517
6,479,753	7.62409	23.176	Inhibitor	96.72772	0.0434161*	100
6,506,231	0.2271	18.9858	Inhibitor	90.54322	1.83684	87.60205
9,950,773	2.68366	21.5394	Inhibitor	92.96128	197.161	93.0993
9,974,918	1.83781	21.2963	Inhibitor	96.14894	108.741	93.92846
9,977,821	0.0104038	13.4916	Inhibitor	92.77509	13.1789	72.44668

TABLE 19.2 *(Continued)*

PubChem ID	BBB	Caco2	Pgp-inhibition	HIA	MDCK	PPB
10,014,355	6.81085	23.3109	Inhibitor	100	11.2712	100
10,243,131	2.7124	6.45265	None	95.30722	152.927	100
10,327,653	0.0426706	25.8336	None	92.10519	0.0435758*	46.44425
10,369,667	2.03623	21.7023	Inhibitor	92.28835	0.0515458	94.03352
10,445,633	0.626686	20.5558	None	89.9543	11.8002	66.75749
10,466,743	5.13469	22.7531	None	90.6887	82.1451	100
11,120,895	0.0699499	22.3454	Inhibitor	94.52302	34.0304	87.77617
11,474,040	0.0120793	17.7412	None	80.57817	0.798585	47.01546
11,954,143	17.4	53.2259	Inhibitor	97.8963	0.044665	100
12,305,935	11.5378	31.7521	Inhibitor	96.01623	0.0435947	100
14,165,733	0.0766897	19.9277	Inhibitor	85.70879	0.0440213	65.90702
15,432,541	0.373606	19.2105	None	84.75231	0.979548	43.39387
16,401,759	0.278196	21.1146*	None	80.01777	1.15224	53.06102
21,597,452	0.139588	20.3242	Inhibitor	91.81901	0.0486388	80.47152
44,555,454	0.488299	22.3963	Inhibitor	85.86073	0.0434181*	92.61243
44,566,526	0.0162074	29.1051	Inhibitor	97.58165	0.0930119	87.8218
44,566,960	0.22473	14.5047	None	88.89729	3.00037	68.63116
44,607,275	1.49938	20.8858	Inhibitor	83.90136	0.0452909	100
44,607,276	4.42918	21.514	Inhibitor	89.39868	0.0453023	100
44,607,277	5.40051	24.188	Inhibitor	92.65427	0.0460208	100
46,186,370	1.87206	24.0539	Inhibitor	94.19949	7.27395	95.43168
46,186,371	5.71784	28.9288	Inhibitor	93.38052	50.5665	100
46,186,620	0.0513656	45.4987	Inhibitor	98.23901	12.0251	88.83777
46,186,621	0.383625	37.7897	Inhibitor	94.83327	0.0536684	83.19236
46,912,852	8.55914	27.1709	Inhibitor	94.61309	0.0484552	100
52,947,022	4.03427	22.1689	Inhibitor	94.51553	0.045275	96.43383
52,947,048	0.937266	21.3756	Inhibitor	93.89857	0.227083	93.25572
426,077,999	6.17967	17.5039	Inhibitor	93.74117	0.0434744*	98.37829

Human Intestinal Absorption (HIA), Carcino Rat (Caco-2), Plasma Binding Protein (PPB), Madin-Darby Canine Kidney cells (MDCK), Pgp inhibition (Pgp-I) and Blood Brain Barrier (BBB) penetration, BBB^+: penetrable to Blood-Brain Barrier; BBB^-: not penetrable to Blood Brain Barrier).

TABLE 19.3 Drug Likeness and Toxicity Profile of the Terpenoid used in the Present Study.

PubChem id	Drug-likeness		Toxicity		
	CMC like Rule	**Rule of Five**	**Ames test**	**hERG inhibition**	**Carcino Rat**
3503	Not qualified	Violated	Mutagen	Medium risk	Positive
6654	Not qualified	Suitable	Mutagen	Medium risk	Positive
10,114	Not qualified	Suitable	Non-mutagen	Low risk	Positive
17,100	Not qualified	Suitable	Mutagen	Low risk	Negative
72,421	Not qualified	Suitable	Non-mutagen	Ambiguous	Positive
73,170	Not qualified	Suitable	Non-mutagen	Low risk	Positive
73,296	Not qualified	Violated	Mutagen	Ambiguous	Negative
91,458	Not qualified	Suitable	Mutagen	Low risk	Negative
119,034	Not qualified	Suitable	Non-mutagen	Low risk	Positive
159,573	Qualified	Suitable	Mutagen	Medium risk	Positive
181,183	Not qualified	Suitable	Non-mutagen	Ambiguous	Positive
289,984	Not qualified	Suitable	Mutagen	Low risk	Positive
442,360	Qualified	Suitable	Mutagen	Medium risk	Positive
455,262	Qualified	Suitable	Non-mutagen	Low risk	Positive
457,901	Qualified	Suitable	Mutagen	Ambiguous	Positive
469,744	Not qualified	Suitable	Non-mutagen	Low risk	Positive
470,259	Not qualified	Suitable	Mutagen	Low risk	Positive
472,768	Not qualified	Suitable	Non-mutagen	Low risk	Positive
500,219	Qualified	Suitable	Mutagen	Low risk	Negative
588,303	Not qualified	Suitable	Mon-mutagen	Ambiguous	Positive
636,756	Qualified	Suitable	Mutagen	Low risk	Positive
3,034,821	Not qualified	Suitable	Non-mutagen	Ambiguous	Positive
5,281,520	Qualified	Suitable	Non-mutagen	Medium risk	Positive
5,282,108	Qualified	Suitable	Mutagen	Low risk	Negative
5,318,379	Not qualified	Suitable	Non-mutagen	Low risk	Positive
5,319,791	Not qualified	Suitable	Non-mutagen	Low risk	Positive
6,444,377	Qualified	Suitable	Non-mutagen	Low risk	Positive
6,479,753	Not qualified	Violated	Mutagen	Medium risk	Positive
6,506,231	Qualified	Suitable	Non-mutagen	Low risk	Positive
9,950,773	Qualified	Suitable	Non-mutagen	Low risk	Positive

TABLE 19.3 *(Continued)*

PubChem id	Drug-likeness		Toxicity		
	CMC like Rule	Rule of Five	Ames test	hERG inhibition	Carcino Rat
9,974,918	Qualified	Suitable	Mutagen	Low risk	Negative
9,977,821	Qualified	Suitable	Mutagen	Low risk	Positive
10,014,355	Failed	Suitable	Mutagen	Low risk	Positive
10,243,131	Qualified	Suitable	Mutagen	Low risk	Negative
10,327,653	Not qualified	Violated	Non-mutagen	Low risk	Positive
10,369,667	Not qualified	Suitable	Non-mutagen	Low risk	Positive
10,445,633	Qualified	Suitable	Mutagen	Low risk	Positive
10,466,743	Qualified	Suitable	Mutagen	Low risk	Negative
11,120,895	Qualified	Suitable	Non-mutagen	Low risk	Positive
11,474,040	Qualified	Suitable	Mutagen	Low risk	Positive
11,954,143	Not qualified	Suitable	Non-mutagen	Low risk	Positive
12,305,935	Not qualified	Suitable	Non-mutagen	Low risk	Positive
14,165,733	Not qualified	Suitable	Non-mutagen	Ambiguous	Positive
15,432,541	Qualified	Suitable	Non-mutagen	Low risk	Positive
16,401,759	Qualified	Suitable	Mutagen	Low risk	Negative
21,597,452	Not qualified	Suitable	Non-mutagen	Ambiguous	Positive
42,607,999	Not qualified	Suitable	Non-mutagen	Medium risk	Negative
44,555,454	Not qualified	Suitable	Non-mutagen	Low risk	Negative
44,566,526	Not qualified	Suitable	Mutagen	Medium risk	Positive
44,566,960	Qualified	Suitable	Mutagen	Low risk	Negative
44,607,275	Not qualified	Suitable	Mutagen	Ambiguous	Negative
44,607,276	Not qualified	Suitable	Non-mutagen	Low risk	Positive
44,607,277	Not qualified	Suitable	Non-mutagen	Low risk	Positive
46,186,370	Qualified	Suitable	Non-mutagen	Medium risk	Positive
46,186,371	Qualified	Suitable	Non-mutagen	Medium risk	Positive
46,186,620	Qualified	Suitable	Non-mutagen	Low risk	Positive
46,186,621	Not qualified	Suitable	Non-mutagen	Low risk	Positive
46,912,852	Not qualified	Suitable	Non-mutagen	Low risk	Positive
52,947,022	Not qualified	Suitable	Non-mutagen	Low risk	Positive
52,947,048	Not qualified	Suitable	Non-mutagen	Low risk	Positive

ACKNOWLEDGMENT

Shashank Kumar acknowledges Central University of Punjab, Bathinda and University Grants Commission, India for providing the necessary infrastructure facility and financial support in the form of UGC-BSR Research Start-Up-Grant, GP: 87 [No. F.30–372/2017 (BSR)] respectively. PPK acknowledges financial support from University Grants Commission, India in the form of CSIR-UGC Junior Research fellowship. Rebati Malik and Santosh Kumar Maurya acknowledge Central University of Punjab, Bathinda, India for providing necessary infrastructure facility.

KEYWORDS

- **terpenoids**
- **anticancer**
- **stem cell**
- **phytochemicals**
- **cytotoxicity**

REFERENCES

Abubaker, K.; Latifi, A.; Luwor, R.; Nazaretian, S.; Zhu, H.; Quinn, M. A.; Thompson, E. W.; Findlay, J. K.; Ahmed, N. Short-Term Single Treatment of Chemotherapy Results in the Enrichment of Ovarian Cancer Stem Cell-Like Cells Leading to an Increased Tumor Burden. *Mol. Cancer* **2013**, *12*, 24.

Ajani, A.; Song, S.; Hochster, S.; Steinberg, B. Cancer Stem Cells: The Promise and the Potential. *Semin. Oncol.* **2015**, *42*(1), 3–17.

Ashour, M.; Wink, M.; Gershenzon, J. Biochemistry of Terpenoids: Monoterpenes, Sesquiterpenes and Diterpenes. In *Annual Plant Reviews;* Wink, M., Ed.; Wiley: New York, 2010; Vol. 40, pp 258–303.

Axelson, H.; Fredlund, E.; Ovenberger, M.; Landberg, G.; Påhlman, S. Hypoxiainduced Dedifferentiation of Tumor Cells–A Mechanism Behind Heterogeneity and Aggressiveness of Solid Tumors. *Semin. Cell Dev. Biol.* **2005**,*16*, 554–563.

Bavovada, R.; Blasko, G.; Shieh, H. L.; Pezzuto, J. M.; Cordell, G. A. Spectral Assignment and Cytotoxicity of 22-Hydroxytingenone from *Glyptopetalum sclerocarpum. Planta Med.* **1990**, *56,* 380–382.

Bork, P. M.; Schmitz, M. L.; Kuhnt, M.; Escher, C.; Heinrich, M. Sesquiterpene Lactone Containing Mexican Indian Medicinal Plants and Pure Sesquiterpene Lactones as Potent Inhibitors of Transcription Factor NF-kB. *FEBS Lett.* **1997**, *402*(1), 85–90.

Chan, L. L.; George, S.; Ahmed, I.; Gosangari, S. L.; Abbasi, A.; Cunningham, B. T.; Watkin, K. L. Cytotoxicity Effects of *Amoora rohituka* and Chittagonga on Breast and Pancreatic Cancer Cells. *Evid. Based Complement Altern. Med.* **2011**, *2011,* 860605.

Chung, J. G.; Chang, H. L.; Lin, W. C.; Wang, H. H.; Yeh, C. C.; Hung, C. F.; Li, Y. C. Inhibition of N-Acetyltransferase Activity and DNA-2-Aminofluorene Adducts by Glycyrrhizic Acid in Human Colon Tumour. *Food Chem. Toxicol.* **2000,** *38,* 163–172.

Corea, G.; Fattorusso, E.; Lanzotti, V.; Motti, R.; Simon, P. N.; Dumontet, C.; Di Pietro A. Structure-Activity Relationships for Euphocharacins A-L, a New Series of Jatrophane Diterpenes, as Inhibitors of Cancer Cell P-Glycoprotein. *Planta Med.* **2004**, *70*(7), 657–665.

de Sousa, L. R.; Wu, H.; Nebo, L.; Fernandes, J. B.; da Silva, M. F.; Kiefer, W.; Schirmeister, T.; Vieira, P. C. Natural Products as Inhibitors of Recombinant Cathepsin L of *Leishmania mexicana*. *Exp. Parasitol.* **2015**, *156,* 42–48.

Deeb, D.; Gao, X.; Liu, Y.; Kim, S. H.; Pindolia, K. R.; Arbab, A. S.; Gautam, S. C. Inhibition of Cell Proliferation and Induction of Apoptosis by Oleanane Triterpenoid (CDDO-Me) in Cancer Cells is Associated with the Suppression of hTERT Gene Expression and its Telomerase Activity. Biochem. *Biophys. Res. Commun.* **2012**, *422,* 561–567.

Eichhorn, T.; Efferth, T. P-Glycoprotein and its Inhibition in Tumors by Phytochemicals Derived from Chinese Herbs. *J. Ethnopharmacol.* **2012**, *141,* 557–570.

Fan, K.; Li, X.; Cao, Y.; Qi, H.; Li, L.; Zhang, Q.; Sun, H. Carvacrol Inhibits Proliferation and Induces Apoptosis in Human Colon Cancer Cells. *Anti-Cancer Drugs* **2015**, *26*(8), 813–823.

Garattini, E.; Gianni, M.; Terao, M. Cytodifferentiation by Retinoids, a Novel Therapeutic Option in Oncology: Rational Combinations with Other Therapeutic Agents. *Vitam. Horm.* **2007**, *75,* 301–354.

Ghani, A. *Medicinal Plants of Bangladesh with Chemical Constituents and uses,* 2nd ed.; Asiatic Society of Bangladesh: Dhaka, 2003.

Gomes, J. P.; Cardoso, C. R.; Varanda, E. A.; Molina, J. M.; Fernandez, M. F.; Olea, N.; Vilegas, W. Antitumoral, Mutagenic and (Anti) Estrogenic Activities of Tingenone and Pristimerin. *Rev. Bras. Farmacogn.* **2011**, *21,* 963–971.

Gopal, Y. N.; Arora, T. S.; Van Dyke, M. W. Parthenolide Specifically Depletes Histone Deacetylase 1 Protein and Induces Cell Death Through Ataxia Telangiectasia Mutated. *Chem. Biol.* **2007**, *14,* 813–823.

Grivennikov, S. I.; Greten, F. R.; Karin, M. Immunity, Inflammation, and Cancer. *Cell.* **2010**, *140,* 883–899.

Hennessy, M.; Spiers, J. P. A Primer on the Mechanics of P-Glycoprotein the Multidrug Transporter. *Pharmacol. Res.* **2007**, *55*(1), 1–15.

Hewitt, A. L.; Singletary, K. W. Soy Extract Inhibits Mammary Adenocarcinoma Growth in a Syngeneic Mouse Model. *Cancer Lett.* **2003**, *192,* 133–143.

Huang, X.; Awano, Y.; Maeda, E.; Asada, Y.; Takemoto, H.; Watanabe, T.; Kojima-Yuasa, A.; Kobayashi, Y. Cytotoxic Activity of Two Natural Sesquiterpene Lactones, Isobutyroylplenolin and Arnicolide D, on Human Colon Cancer Cell Line HT-29. *Nat. Prod. Res.* **2014**, *28*(12), 914–916.

Huang, C. H.; Lu, S. H.; Chang, C. C.; Thomas, P. A.; Jayakumar, T.; Sheu, J. R. Hinokitiol, a Tropolone Derivative, Inhibits Mouse Melanoma (B16-F10) Cell Migration and in Vivo Tumor Formation. *Eur. J. Pharmacol.* **2015a**, *746,* 148–157.

Huang, C. H.; Jayakumar, T.; Chang, C. C.; Fong, T. H.; Lu, S. H.; Thomas, P. A.; Choy, C. S.; Sheu, J. R. Hinokitiol Exerts Anticancer Activity Through Downregulation of MMPs

9/2 and Enhancement of Catalase and SOD Enzymes: In Vivo Augmentation of Lung Histoarchitecture. *Molecules* **2015b**, *20,* 17720–17734.

Ikeda, T.; Fujiwara, S.; Araki, K.; Kinjo, J.; Nohara, T.; Miyoshi, T. Cytotoxic Glycosides from *Albizia julibrissin*. *J. Nat. Prod.* **1997**, *60,* 102–107.

Jung, Y. D.; Ellis, L. M. Inhibition of Tumor Invasion and Angiogenesis by Epigallactocatechin Gallate (EGCG), a Major Component of Green Tea. *Int. J. Exp. Pathol.* **2001**, *82,* 309–316.

Junttila, M. R.; de Sauvage, F. J. Influence of Tumour Micro-Environment Heterogeneity on Therapeutic Response. *Nature* **2013**, *501,* 346–354.

Kakarala, M.; Brenner, D. E.; Korkaya, H.; Cheng, C.; Tazi, K.; Ginestier, C.; Liu, S.; Dontu, G.; Wicha, M. S. Targeting Breast Stem Cells with the Cancer Preventive Compounds Curcumin and Piperine. *Breast Cancer Res. Treat.* **2010**, *122,* 777–785.

Karakas, D.; Cevatemre, B.; Aztopal, N.; Ari, F.; Yilmaz, V. T.; Ulukaya, E. Addition of Niclosamide to Palladium (II) Saccharinate Complex of Terpyridine Results in Enhanced Cytotoxic Activity Inducing Apoptosis on Cancer Stem Cells of Breast Cancer. *Bioorg. Med. Chem.* **2015**, *23,* 5580–5586.

Kundu, P.; Laskar, S. A Brief Resume on the Genus *Ailanthus*: Chemical and Pharmacological Aspects. *Phytochem. Rev.* **2010**, *9,* 379–412.

Kunnumakkara, A. B.; Anand, P.; Aggarwal, B. B. Curcumin inhibits proliferation, invasion, angiogenesis and metastasis of different cancers through interaction with multiple cell signaling proteins. *Cancer Lett.* **2008**, *269,* 199–225.

Kuzma, J.; Nemecek-Marshall, M.; Pollock, W. H.; Fall, R. Bacteria Produce the Volatile Hydrocarbon Isoprene. *Curr. Microbiol.* **1995**, *30*(2), 97–103.

Lee, T. K.; Castilho, A.; Cheung, V. C.; Tang, K. H.; Ma, S.; Ng, I. O. Lupeol Targets Liver Tumor-Initiating Cells Through Phosphatase and Tensin Homolog Modulation. *Hepatology* **2011**, *53,* 160–170.

Li, J.; Guo, W. J.; Yang, Q. Y. Effects of Ursolic Acid and Oleanolic Acid on Human Colon Carcinoma Cell Line HCT15. *World J. Gastroenterol.* **2002,** *8*(3), 493–495.

Li, W.; Cai, X.; Hu, Z.; Wang, Y. Advances on Researches of Medicinal Plants in *Euphorbia* L. *Chin. Wild Plant Resour.* **2008**, *27*(5), 1–9.

Li, J.; Zhao, W.; Deng, L.; Li, X. R. Components of Myrsinane-Type Diterpenes from Euphorbia Prolifera. *Zhejiang Da Xue Xue Bao Yi Xue Ban*. **2011**, *40*(4), 380–383.

Liang, H.; Tong, W. Y.; Zhao, Y. Y.; Cui, J. R.; Tu, G. An Antitumor Compound Julibroside J28 from *Albizia julibrissin*. *Bioorg. Med. Chem. Lett.* **2005**, *15,* 4493–4495.

Lindvall, C.; Evans, N. C.; Zylstra, C. R.; Li, Y.; Alexander C. M.; Williams, B. O. The Wnt Signaling Receptor Lrp5 is Required for Mammary Ductal Stem Cell Activity and Wnt1-Induced Tumorigenesis. *J. Biol. Chem.* **2006**, *281,* 35081–35087.

Luk, S. U.; Yap, W. N.; Chiu, Y. T.; Lee, D. T.; Ma, S.; Lee, T. K.; Vasireddy, R. S.; Wong, Y. C.; Ching, Y. P.; Nelson, C.; Yap, Y. L.; Ling, M. T. Gamma-Tocotrienol as an Effective Agent in Targeting Prostate Cancer Stem Cell-Like Population. *Int. J. Cancer*. **2011**, *128,* 2182–2191.

Maregesi, S. M.; Hermans, N.; Dhooghe, L.; Cimanga, K.; Ferreira, D.; Pannecouque, C.; Vanden Berghe, D. A.; Cos, P.; Maes, L.; Vlietinck, A. J.; Apers, S.; Pieters, L. Phytochemical and Biological Investigations of *Elaeodendron schlechteranum*. *J. Ethnopharmacol.* **2010**, *129,* 319–326.

Martin, V. J. J.; Pitera, D. J.; Withers, S. T.; Newman, J. D.; Keasling, J. D. Engineering a Mevalonate Pathway in *Escherichia coli* for Production of Terpenoids. *Nat. Biotechnol.* **2003**, *21*(7), 796–802.

Merlo, L. M. F.; Pepper, J. W.; Reid, B. J.; Maley, C. C. Cancer as an Evolutionary and Ecological Process. *Nat. Rev. Cancer*. **2006**, *6,* 924–935.

Moreb, J. S.; Gabr, A.; Vartikar, G. R.; Gowda, S.; Jucali, J. R.; Mohuczy, D. Retinoic Acid Downregulates Aldehyde Dehydrogenase and Increases Cytotoxicity of 4-Hydroperoxycyclophosphamide and Acetaldehyde. *J. Pharmacol. Exp. Ther*. **2005**, *312,* 339–345.

Moreb, J. S.; Mohuczy, D.; Ostmark, B.; Zucali, J. R. RNA-Imediated Knockdown of Aldehyde Dehydrogenase Class-1A1 and Class-3A1 is Specific and Reveals that Each Contributes Equally to the Resistance Against 4-Hydroperoxycyclophosphamide. *Cancer Chemother. Pharmacol*. **2007**, *59,* 127–136.

Murakami, A.; Miyamoto, M.; Ohigashi, H. Zerumbone, an Anti-Inflammatory Phytochemical, Induces Expression of Proinflammatory Cytokine Genes in Human Colon Adenocarcinoma Cell Lines. *BioFactors* (Oxford, England), **2004**, *21*(1–4), 95–101.

Nanduri, S.; Nyavanandi, V. K.; Thunuguntla, S. S. R.; Kasu, S.; Pallerla, M. K.; Sai Ram, P.; Rajagopal, S.; Kumar, R. A.; Ramanujam, R.; Babu, J. M.; Vyas, K.; Devi, S.; Reddy, G. O.; Akella, V. Synthesis and Structure–Activity Relationships of Andrographolide Analogues as Novel Cytotoxic Agents. *Bioorg. Med. Chem. Lett*. **2004**, *14*(18), 4711–4717.

Oh, J.; Hlatky, L.; Jeong, Y. S.; Kim, D. Therapeutic Effectiveness of Anticancer Phytochemicals on Cancer Stem Cells. *Toxins* **2016**, *8*(7), 199.

Orofino, K. M. R.; Grootjans, S.; Biavatti, M. W.; Vandenabeele, P.; D'Herde, K. Sesquiterpene Lactones as Drugs with Multiple Targets in Cancer Treatment. *Anti-Cancer Drugs*. **2012,** *23*(9), 1–14.

Pan, D. J.; Li, Z. L.; Hu, C. Q.; Chen, K.; Chang, J. J.; Lee, K. H. The Cytotoxic Principles of *Pseudolarix kaempferi*: Pseudolaric Acid-A and -B and Related Derivatives. *Planta Medica.***1990,** *56*(4), 383–385.

Peacock, C. D; Wang, Q; Gesell, G. S.; Corcoran-Schwartz, I. M.; Jones, E.; Kim, J.; Devereux, W. L.; Rhodes, J. T.; Huff, C. A.; Breachy, P. A.; Watkins, D. N.; Matsui, W. Hedgehog Signaling Maintains a Tumor Stem Cell Compartment in Multiple Myeloma. *Proc. Natl. Acad. Sci. U S A*. **2007**, *104,* 4048–4053.

Pharmacopoeia Committee of China. *Chinese Pharmacopoeia 2015;* Chemical Industry Press: Beijing, 2015.

Rabi, T.; Venkatanarasimhan, M. Novel Synthetic Oleanane Triterpenoid AMR-MeOAc Inhibits K-Ras Through ERK, Akt and Survivin in Pancreatic Cancer Cells. *Phytomedicine* **2014**, *21,* 491–496.

Rabi, T.; Wang, L.; Banerjee, S. Novel Triterpenoid 25-Hydroxy-3Oxoolean-12-en-28-Oic Acid Induces Growth Arrest and Apoptosis in Breast Cancer Cells. *Breast Cancer Res. Treat*. **2007**, *101,* 27–36.

Ranganathan, P; Weaver, K. L.; Capobianco, A. J. Notch Signalling in Solid Tumours: a Little Bit of Everything But Not All the Time. *Nat. Rev. Cancer.* **2011**, *11,* 338–351.

Reddy, B. S.; Wang, C. X.; Samaha, H.; Lubet, R.; Steele, V. E.; Kelloff, G. J.; Rao, C. V. Chemoprevention of Colon Carcinogenesis by Dietary Perillyl Alcohol. *Cancer Res*. **1997**, *57*(3), 420–425.

Reya, T.; Morrison, S. J.; Clarke, M. F.; Weissman, I. L. Stem Cells, Cancer, and Cancer Stem Cells. *Nature* **2001**, *414,* 105–111.

Rzeski, W.; Stepulak, A.; Szymański, M.; Sifringer, M.; Kaczor, J.; Wejksza, K.; Zdzisińska, B.; Kandefer-Szerszeń, M. Betulinic Acid Decreases Expression of Bcl-2 and Cyclin D1, Inhibits Proliferation, Migration and Induces Apoptosis in Cancer Cells. *Naunyn Schmiedebergs Arch. Pharmacol*. **2006**, *374*(1), 11–20.

Scolastici, C.; de Lima, R. O. A.; Barbisan, L. F.; Ferreira, A. L.; Ribeiro, D. A.; Salvadori, D. M. F. Lycopene Activity Against Chemically Induced DNA Damage in Chinese Hamster Ovary Cells. *Toxicol. In Vitro* **2007**, *21*(5), 840–845.

Shih, Y. H.; Chang, K. W.; Hsia, S. M.; Yu, C. C.; Fuh, L. J.; Chi, T. Y.; Shieh, T. M. In Vitro Antimicrobial and Anticancer Potential of Hinokitiol Against Oral Pathogens and Oral Cancer Cell Lines. *Microbiol. Res.* **2013**, *168,* 254–262.

Shih, Y. H.; Lin, D. J.; Chang, K. W.; Hsia, S. M.; Ko, S. Y.; Lee, S. Y.; Hsue, S. S.; Wang, T. H.; Chen, Y. L.; Shieh, T. M. Evaluation Physical Characteristics and Comparison Antimicrobial and Anti-Inflammation Potentials of Dental Root Canal Sealers Containing Hinokitiol in Vitro. *PLoS One* **2014**, *9,* e94941.

Shimono, Y.; Zabala, M.; Cho, R. W.; Lobo, N.; Dalerba, P.; Qian, D.; Diehn, M.; Liu, H.; Panula, S. P.; Chiao, E.; Dirbas, F. M.; Somlo, G.; Pera, R. A.; Lao, K.; Clarke, M. E. Downregulation of miRNA-200c Links Breast Cancer Stem Cells with Normal Stem Cells. *Cell.* **2009**, *138,* 592–603.

Silver, G. M.; Fall, R. Characterization of Aspen Isoprene Synthase, an Enzyme Responsible for Leaf Isoprene Emission to the Atmosphere. *J. Biol. Chem.* **1995**, *270*(22), 13010–13016.

Sottoriva, A.; Sloot, P. M. A.; Medema, J. P.; Vermeulen, L. Exploring Cancer Stem Cell Niche Directed Tumor Growth. *Cell Cycle* **2010**, *9,* 1472–1479.

Stine, R. R.; Matunis, E. L. JAK-STAT Signaling in Stem Cells. *Adv. Exp. Med. Biol.* **2013**, *786,* 247–267.

Stojakowska, A.; Kisiel, W. Production of Parthenolide in Organ Cultures of Feverfew. *Plant Cell Tissue Organ. Cult.* **1997**, *47,* 159–162.

Sun, J. D-Limonene: Safety and Clinical Applications. *Altern. Med. Rev.* **2007**, *12*(3), 259–264.

Sutton, L. M.; Warmuth, M. A.; Petros, W. P.; Winer, E. P. Pharmacokinetics and Clinical Impact of All-Trans Retinoic Acid in Metastatic Breast Cancer: A Phase II Trial. *Cancer Chemother. Pharmacol.* **1997**, *40,* 335–341.

Tang, X.-H.; Gudas, L. J. Retinoids, Retinoic Acid Receptors, and Cancer. *Annu. Rev. Pathol. Mech. Dis.* **2011**, *6,* 345–364.

Tetteh, P. W.; Farin, H. F.; Clevers, H. Plasticity Within Stem Cell Hierarchies in Mammalian Epithelia. *Trends Cell Biol.* **2015**, *25,* 100–108.

Tholl, D. Terpene Synthases and the Regulation, Diversity and Biological Roles of Terpene Metabolism. *Curr. Opin. Plant Biol.* **2006**, *9*(3), 297–304.

Tholl, D. Biosynthesis and Biological Functions of Terpenoids in Plants. In *Advances in Biochemical Engineering/Biotechnology;* Schrader, J., Bohlmann, J., Eds.; Springer International Publishing: Switzerland, 2015; Vol. 148, pp 63–106.

Tu, D. G.; Yu, Y.; Lee, C. H.; Kuo, Y. L.; Lu, Y. C.; Tu, C. W.; Chang, W. W. Hinokitiol Inhibits Vasculogenic Mimicry Activity of Breast Cancer Stem/Progenitor Cells Through Proteasome-Mediated Degradation of Epidermal Growth Factor Receptor. *Oncol. Lett.* **2016**, *11,* 2934–2940.

Vigushin, D. M.; Poon, G. K.; Boddy, A.; English, J.; Halbert, G. W.; Pagonis, C.; Jarman, M.; Coombes, R. C. Phase I and Pharmacokinetic Study of D-Limonene in Patients with Advanced Cancer. *Cancer Chemother. Pharmacol.* **1998**, *42*(2), 111–117.

Wiedhopf, R. M.; Young, M.; Bianchi, E.; Cole, J. R. Tumor Inhibitory Agent from *Magnolia grandiflora* (Magnoliaceae). I. Parthenolide. *J. Pharm. Sci.* **1973**, *62,* 345.

Wildermuth, M. C.; Fall, R. Light-Dependent Isoprene Emission (Characterization of a Thylakoid-Bound Isoprene Synthase in Salix Discolor Chloroplasts). *Plant Physiol.* **1996**, *112*(1), 171–182.

Zhao, C.; Xiu, Y.; Ashton, J.; Xing, L.; Morita, Y.; Jarden, C. T.; Boyce, B. F. Noncanonical NF-kappa B Signaling Regulates Hematopoietic Stem Cell Self-Renewal and Microenvironment Interactions. *Stem Cells* **2012**, *30,* 709–718.

Zheng, L.; Zheng, J.; Zhang, Q. Y.; Wang, B.; Zhao, Y. Y.; Wu, L. J. Three New Oleanane Triterpenoid Saponins Acetylated with Monoterpenoid Acid from *Albizia julibrissin*. *Fitoterapia* **2010**, *81,* 859–863.

Zou, K.; Cui, J. R.; Zhao, Y. Y.; Zhang, R. Y.; Zheng, J. H. A Cytotoxic Saponin with Two Monoterpenoids from *Albizia julibrissin*. *Chin. Chem. Lett.* **2000,** *11,* 39–42.

CHAPTER 20

EVALUATION OF THE PHYTOHEMAGGLUTININS ACTIVITIES OF ECHINACEA SPECIES IN ONTOGENESIS

SERGEY V. POSPELOV

Department of Agriculture and Agrochemistry, Faculty Agrotechnology and Ecology, Poltava State Agrarian Academy, 1/3 Skovorody St., Poltava 36003, Ukraine, Tel.: +380951213218

E-mail: sergii.pospielov@pdaa.edu.ua
ORCID: https://orcid.org/0000-0003-0433-2996

ABSTRACT

It is established that purple coneflower (*Echinacea purpurea* (L.) Moench) and pale purple coneflower (*Echinacea pallida* [Nutt.] Nutt.) contains specific protein compound—lectins, which have the ability to reversibly interact with carbohydrates and exhibit high biological activity at the cellular and organism levels. An original methodology of hemagglutination activity of *Echinacea* extracts evaluation was developed. The study of the dynamics of lectin activity showed that in the *E. purpurea* high level of hemagglutinins was found in roots with rhizomes, stems, both forming an open inflorescences. It has been established that during the vegetation of *E. pallida* the highest level of phytolectins observed in leaves—twice as much higher as in roots with rhizomes. In the genesis period, hemagglutination activity of herb extracts was higher than roots with rhizomes extracts. *Echinacea* overground mass considered as important raw materials for preparative isolation of lectins.

20.1 INTRODUCTION

Species of the *Echinacea* (*Echinacea* Moench, family: Asteraceae) are used in many countries of the world as raw materials in the preparation of immunostimulating, anti-inflammatory, and antiseptic effects due to its unique chemical composition (Bauer and Wagner, 1990; Miller, 2004). This is typical for Ukraine and all CIS countries, where *Echinacea* is actively studied and widely used, especially in connection with the creation of new products and drugs for the elimination of the consequences of the chernobyl accident (Dubinska, 1998; Dreval et al., 2003).

In the Poltava State Agrarian Academy (Ukraine), as a result of 25 years of systematic researches, the genus *Echinacea* species were collected and studied; a varieties of *Echinacea purpurea* (*Zirka Mykoly Vavilova*) and *Echinacea pallida* (*Krasunya prerii*) were selected; the largest plantation cultivation in the CIS was organized, which is capable of providing all consumers with eco-friendly raw materials of the highest quality; the new technologies for growing *Echinacea* as medical raw material, feed for livestock, melliferous plant for beekeeping were developed and patented (Pospelov and Samorodov, 2009).

20.2 ANALYSIS OF PREVIOUS STUDIES

In connection with an in-depth study of the chemical composition (Samorodov et al., 1996) and clarification of the nature of the immunostimulating properties of *Echinacea* lectins—biologically active substances of a protein nature that have properties to selectively and reversibly interact with carbohydrates and carbohydrate-containing polymers, deserve attention, which gives them a number of unique properties (Lutsik et al., 1981).

There are data about the search for lectins in the seeds of *Echinacea augustifolia* DC among other 167 plant species of the North American flora (Hardman et al., 1983). The authors used human erythrocytes (processed and non-processed with enzymes) for this purpose, but no agglutinating activity of the extracts was found.

A systematic search for *E. purpurea* lectins was conducted in Ukraine (Pospelov and Samorodov, 1996) and Lithuania (Kondrotas et al., 1996). In the studies, the employees of the Kaunas Medical Academy, the hemagglutinating activity of the *E. purpurea* extracts (it was not specified which part of the plant) with the human erythrocytes of all four groups, rabbit, pig, mouse, and frog has been estimated. At the same time, weak activity was registered when interacting with the blood cells of human B(III) blood group and mouse blood cells. Earlier, in our experiments (Pospelov and Samorodov, 1996) the extraction of roots, leaves, stems, inflorescences, and fruits with buffered saline in raw material ratios extragent 1:5 and 1:10, was carried out. In all cases, negative results were obtained.

Several other data were received by the employees of the Taras Shevchenko National University of Kyiv (Pohorila et al., 1997). Water-salt extracts of roots and stems of 10-day-old seedlings, as well as stems, leaves, non-blossoming inflorescences, and plant seeds of the second year of vegetation, did not interact with human erythrocytes. At the same time, extracts of roots and inflorescences showed specific activity. The authors found that the albumin fraction showed no activity, while the globulin and gliadin fractions of the proteins reacted with extracts of stems, non-blossoming inflorescences, leaves, flowering inflorescences and roots (by the degree of activity decrease). A positive reaction was obtained in almost all variants with the use of rat erythrocytes, which indicates the specificity of the *Echinacea* lectin receptors.

20.3 MATERIALS AND METHODS

As a plant raw material, the aboveground and underground parts of the *E. purpurea* (L.) Moench (Figs. 20.1 and 20.2) and *E. pallida* (Nutt.) Nutt. (Figs. 20.3 and 20.4) were used. Evaluation of lectin activity was carried out by setting the hemagglutination reaction in immunological plates (Lutsik et al., 1981). For this, 0.05 ml of physiological solution or buffer mixtures were added to each well of the plate, then 0.05 ml of extract was added and the series of successive two-fold dilutions were prepared. After that, 0.05 ml of a 2% suspension of washed red blood cells was added to each well and the plate was left at 25°C for 2 h. The evaluation was carried out visually on a five-point scale (Golynskaya et al., 1992):

- 3 points—sharply expressed agglutination. Erythrocytes in the form of a thin film more or less evenly distributed at the bottom of the well;
- 2 points—moderate agglutination. Erythrocytes diverge on the bottom of the well at a distance of more than 2 mm in diameter, forming a ring with sharply expressed granularity at the edges;
- 1 point—weak agglutination. Erythrocytes diverge on the bottom of the hole at a distance of less than 2 mm, forming a ring or disk;

- 0.5 point—minimal agglutination. A small clearance appears in the center of the aggregate of erythrocytes, which have settled on the bottom of the well;
- 0 point—no agglutination. Erythrocytes accumulate in the center of the well.

After a visual assessment of the agglutination in each well of the dilution series, the sum was counted in all wells where the reaction was determined. Thus, the maximum activity in eight wells can be $8 \times 3.0 = 24$ points.

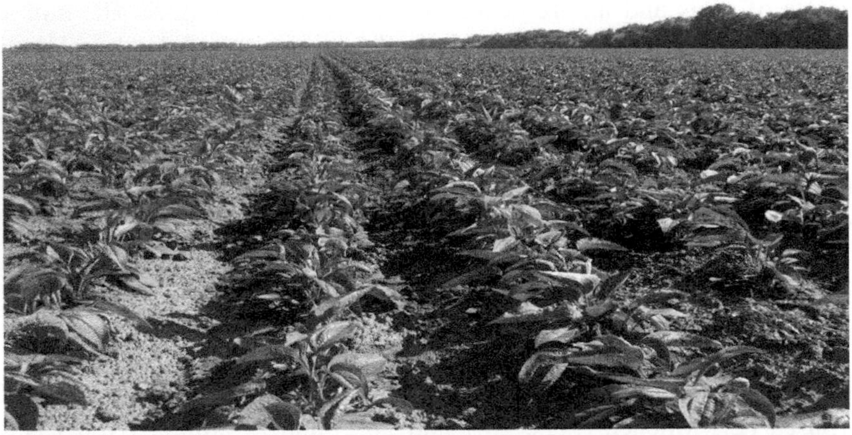

FIGURE 20.1 *Echinacea purpurea* of the first year of vegetation.

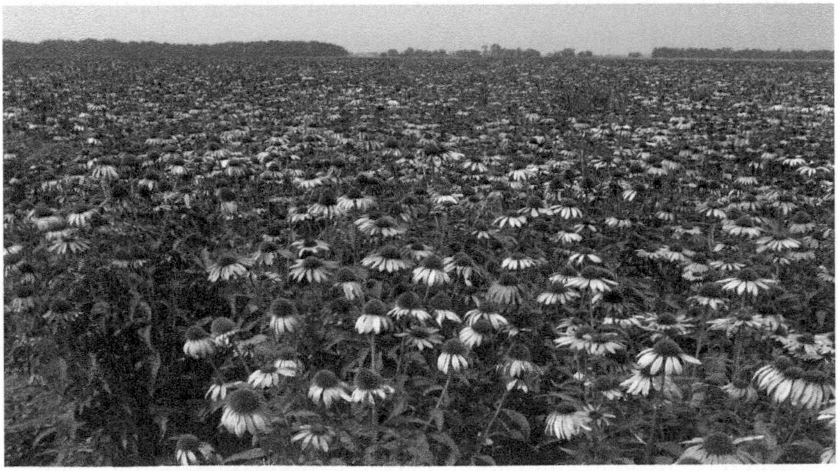

FIGURE 20.2 *E. purpurea* of the second year of vegetation.

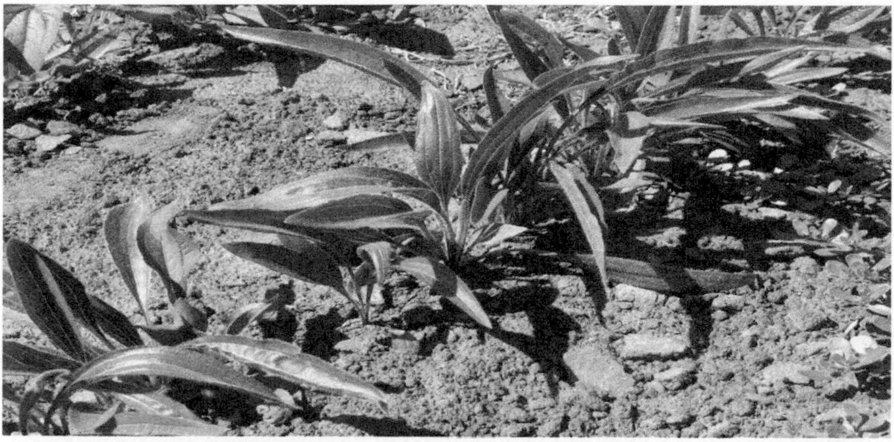

FIGURE 20.3 *Echinacea pallida* of the first year of vegetation.

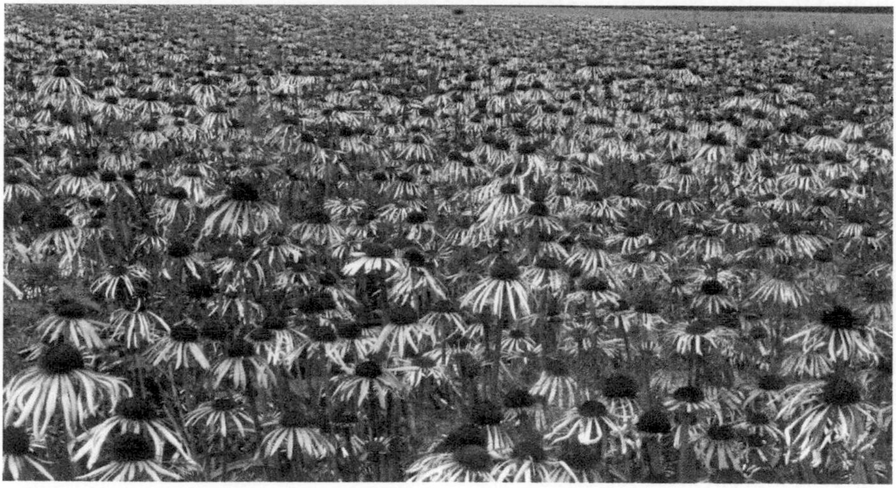

FIGURE 20.4 *E. pallida* of the second year of vegetation.

Carbohydrate specificity was determined according to the method developed by us earlier (Golynskaya et al., 1992). The preparation of lectins with a constant titer (1:4) was placed in immunological plates, mixed with equal volumes of carbohydrates in the series of their successive two-fold dilutions. The system had been incubated for 1 h at room temperature, after which a volume, equal to the initial volume of lectins, of 2% suspension of triply washed red blood cells was put into each well and left for 1–2 h at a temperature of 25°C. Similarly, the hemagglutination reaction with lectins was carried out without the addition of an inhibitory carbohydrate. To estimate the specificity, the sum of the activity of the lectins without the carbohydrate inhibitor was calculated, then with the carbohydrate, and the affinity of lectins to carbohydrates was determined by the difference. In this case, the larger the difference, the higher the specificity.

The statistical evaluation according to Student's t-test was carried out using the analysis package in the Excel program.

20.4 DEVELOPMENT OF METHODS FOR DETERMINING THE ACTIVITY OF LECTINS

The ambiguity of the obtained data stimulated us to improve the technique for determining the activity of *Echinacea* lectins. It is known that fruits and seeds of plants contain the maximum amount of lectins (Lutsik et al., 1981). We studied the activity of fruit extracts after their fractionation. It was determined by us step by step in the process of the stepwise low-temperature ethanol fractionation up to 20, 35, 50, and 76% the final concentration (Pospelov, 1998).

We found that the optimal conditions for fractionation were saturation of the extract with ethanol to 20% final concentration, bringing the solution to pH 8.0, cooling and centrifugation (Table 20.1). The resulting sediment showed high activity in the reaction with erythrocytes of different human blood groups in the ABO system: with the first O(I) group it was 16 points, A(II)—15 points, and AB(IV)—11 points.

TABLE 20.1 Hemagglutinating Activity of the Fruit Extract of *Echinacea purpurea* at the Different Stages of Ethanol Fractionation.

Stages of fractionation	Activity, points
Extraction with physiological solution	0,0
Sediment after 20% saturation, pH = 3.0	14,0±0,9
Sediment after 20% saturation, pH = 8.0	22,0±1,2
Supernatant at 20% saturation	0,0
Sediment after 35% saturation	0,0
Supernatant at 35% saturation	0,0
Sediment after 50% saturation	0,0
Supernatant at 50% saturation	0,0
Sediment after 76% saturation	0,0
Supernatant at 76% saturation	0,0

According to the described method by Golynskaya et al. (1992), we evaluated the interaction of partially purified lectins of leaves, stems, and rhizomes with roots of *E. purpurea* with carbohydrates arabinose, glucose, galactite, xylose, galactose, and fructose. At the same time, inhibition of the agglutination reaction was practically not observed.

Antonjuk and Rybak (2002) isolated and received lectins *of E. purpurea* with a high degree of purification, studied their carbohydrate specificity. The authors concluded that lectins of *Echinacea* can be attributed to the group of mannose-specific ones, although they differ from lectins of monocotyledonous and dicotyledonous, in particular, legume family, which also belong to this group. The yield of the purified product is 133 mg/kg of air dry raw material.

In our experiments, we used physiological saline as an extractant, and the further evaluation was carried out with using a phosphate-citrate buffer mixture on the basis of physiological saline (Table 20.2). The results indicate that *Echinacea* lectins show their activity in the acidic zone in our experiments at pH = 4.0–4.4. In this case, certain regularities can be traced. When extracting protein compounds from the stem, complete and partial lysis at pH = 4.0–4.2 and a well-defined location of red blood cells in the wells of the plate at pH = 4.4 are observed. When extracting protein compounds from the rhizomes, the lysis was only at pH = 4.0. At the same time, the lectins of the leaves were well defined in the acidic zone (pH = 4.0–4.4).

TABLE 20.2 Dependence of Hemagglutinating Activity of Lectins on pH of the Solution.

Terms of determination	Activity, points		
	Leaves	Stem	Rhizome
Physiological saline + PCBM, pH = 4.0	9,0±0,7	L.comp.	Lysis
Physiological saline + PCBM, pH = 4.2	9,0±0,6	L. part.	3,0±0,3
Physiological saline + PCBM, pH = 4.4	5,5±0,2	7,5±0,3	1,5±0,1
Physiological saline + PCBM, pH = 4.6	0,0	0,0	0,0
Physiological saline + PCBM, pH = 4.8	0,0	0,0	0,0
Physiological saline + PCBM, pH = 5,0	0,0	0,0	0,0
Physiological saline + PCBM, pH = 6.0	0,0	0,0	0,0
Physiological saline + PCBM, pH = 7.0	0,0	0,0	0,0
Physiological saline + PCBM, pH = 8.0	0,0	0,0	0,0

Note: L. comp.—lysis is complete; L. part.—lysis is partial.

Evaluation of the results visually in scores allows you to quickly, objectively, and accurately determine the intensity of the hemagglutination reaction. The well-known Ukrainian lectinologist, Yevgenia Golynskaya, widely applied this method in her studies, popularized it in every possible way and considered it more accurate than the titre estimation (Golynskaya et al., 1992). In addition, the obtained data can be compared and statistically estimated, which is also very important. Table 20.3 shows the data of the activity evaluation by the agglutination titer and in scores. The agglutinating activity of the extracts of the *E. purpurea* inflorescence varies from 4.5 to 6.0 in the experiment, while at the same time it is 1:8–1:16 by the agglutination titer. *E. pallida* extracts have a high activity—20.5–24.0 points and a titer—1:256. Evaluation of the results of the experiment on the agglutination titer does not allow to carry out statistical calculations, at the same time, as the estimation in points allows to compare experiment variants and to make judgments about the reliability of the obtained data.

TABLE 20.3 *Echinacea* Lectin Activity and Their Statistical Evaluation.

Variants	Inflorescences of Echinacea purpurea		Inflorescences of Echinacea pallida	
	Titer evaluation	Evaluation in points	Titer evaluation	Evaluation in points
Repetitions of the experiment: 1	1:8	4,5	1:256	20,5
2	1:16	6,0	1:256	21,0
3	1:16	5,0	1:256	22,0
4	1:8	4,5	1:256	24,0
Average	–	5,0	–	21,9
Dispersion	–	0,5	–	2,39
$t_{0.01}$ (theor.)= 3,18*				
$t_{0.01}$ (act.) = 17,47				

*The difference is reliable if the value of $t_{0.01}$ (actual) is more than $t_{0.01}$ (theoretical).

Thus, it can be concluded, that the use of a phosphate-citrate buffer mixture with pH = 4.4, prepared on the basis of physiological saline should be considered as the optimal conditions for assessing the lectin activity of *Echinacea* extracts (Pospelov, 2012).

20.5 ACTIVITY OF LECTINS AND THEIR DYNAMICS IN *ECHINACEA PURPUREA*

An analysis of the available literature showed us that, despite the established fact of the presence of lectins in *E. purpurea*, many aspects remain poorly understood. In Table 20.4 we summarize data on the detection of lectins in different parts and organs of *Echinacea* and the method of their evaluation. It can be concluded that the results of the research are ambiguous, and the authors themselves find them difficult to interpret. So, the employees of the Taras Shevchenko National University of Kyiv (Pohorila et al., 1997) found that lectins in extracts of leaves, stems, and achenes are not determined with the help of human erythrocytes but roots and inflorescences gave a positive reaction. At the same time, according to (Antonjuk and Rybak, 2002), human erythrocytes do not react to lectins contained in the root system of *Echinacea*. The situation is similar for the extracts of achenes in our studies, lectin activity was registered (Pospelov, 1998; Pospelov et al., 2001), but according to the data of the Kiev authors (Pohorila et al., 1997), it was not noted.

At the same time, certain regularities can be traced. Due to the presence of the receptors of a certain type, the erythrocytes of animals (rat, mouse, and rabbit) are more suitable for determining the activity of *Echinacea* lectins. Human erythrocytes are more unstable and do not always give a positive reaction, which may be associated with the technique, the conditions of their storage, the preparation, and quality of the raw materials, and so forth. It should be noted that the authors (Kondrotas et al., 1999; Antonjuk and Rybak, 2002) are unambiguous in their opinion that the erythrocytes of the human blood group B(III) react more specifically to lectins of *Echinacea*. However, a more detailed research of carbohydrate specificity (Antonyuk and Rybak, 2002) does not give us the right to state this definitively yet.

TABLE 20.4 Results of the Study of the Activity of *E. purpurea* Lectins.

Object of study	Receptors (erythrocytes of human or animal)	Positive (+) or negative (−) reaction	References
Roots	Human O(I)	+	Pohorila et al. (1997) Antonjuk and Rybak (2002)
	Human A(II)	+	
	Human B(III)	+	
	Mouse	+	
	Human	−	
	Rabbit	+	
Inflorescences	Human O(I)	+	Pohorila et al. (1997)
	Human A(II)	+	
	Human B(III)	+	
	Mouse	+	
Leaves	Human O(I)	−	Pohorila et al. (1997) Antonjuk and Rybak (2002)
	Human A(II)	−	
	Human B(III)	−	
	Mouse	+	
	Human	−	
	Rabbit	+	

TABLE 20.4 *(Continued)*

Object of study	Receptors (erythrocytes of human or animal)	Positive (+) or negative (−) reaction	References
Stems	Human O(I)	−	Pohorila et al. (1997)
	Human A(II)	−	
	Human B(III)	−	
	Mouse	+	
Fruits	Human O(I)	−	Pohorila et al. (1997) Pospelov (1998) Antonjuk and Rybak (2002)
	Human A(II)	−	
	Human B(III)	−	
	Mouse	+	
	Human O(I)	+	
	Human A(II)	+	
	Human AB(IV)	+	
	Human	−	
	Rabbit	+	
Extract of Echinacea*	Human O(I)	−	Kondrotas et al. (1999)
	Human A(II)	−	
	Human B(III)	+	
	Human AB(IV)	−	
	Rabbit	−	
	Guinea pig	−	
	Mouse	+	
	Frog	−	

*—not specified from which part of the plant.

The absence of system data on the dynamics of lectin accumulation at different stages of the ontogenesis of *E. purpurea* prompted us to study this issue (Pospelov and Pospelova, 2012). Figure 20.5 shows the evaluation of the activity of lectins in extracts from different parts and organs of the *E. purpurea* of the first year of vegetation. There is a general tendency of a high level of hemagglutinating activity of extracts of blossoming inflorescences, as well as rhizomes with roots and stems (from 4 to 8 units). The average level was characteristic of the leafstalks of the leaves and of the developing inflorescences (from 2 to 6 units) and in the leaf blades, the activity level of the lectins did not exceed 0.5 units. At the end of the first year of vegetation, there is a slight decrease in the activity of phytolectins.

A more detailed analysis of the lectin activity in the leaves made it possible to reveal certain regularities (Fig. 20.6). If in the leaf blades of all the studied leaves the activity of lectins was minimal during the vegetative period (0.5 points) then in the leafstalks their level increased several times, especially in the rosette leaves (3.0–4.5 points). This leads to a thought that the leaf blade is the main place of the biosynthesis of lectins, which are then transported through the vascular system of the leafstalks. Considering the fact that *E. purpurea* contains a significant amount of polysaccharides (Samorodov et al., 1996) as well as the ability of lectins to reversibly bind to carbohydrates, the transport of lectin-polysaccharide complex is quite possible.

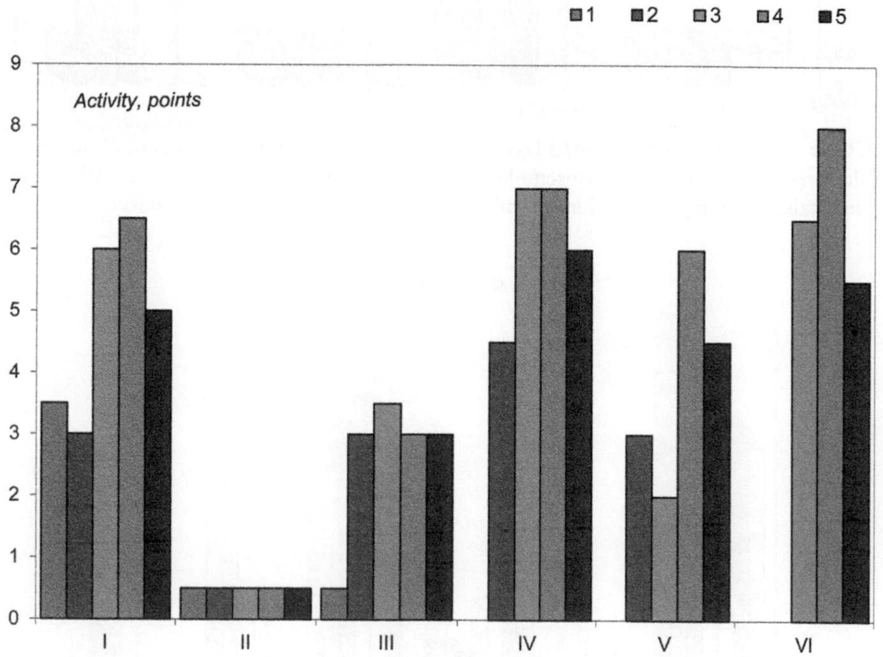

FIGURE 20.5 (See color insert.) Dynamics of activity of lectins of *E. purpurea* of the first year of vegetation. I—root system; II—leaf blade; III—leafstalk; IV—stems; V—not blossoming inflorescences; VI—blossoming inflorescences. Sampling time: 1 June; 2 July; 3 August; 4 September; 5 October.

The study of the dynamics of the activity of lectins in parts and organs of the *E. purpurea* of the second year of vegetation makes it possible to draw the following conclusions (Fig. 20.7). Hemagglutinating activity of extracts of leaf blades and leafstalks was low, in the range of 0.5–3.5 points. In a wider range, it changed in developing inflorescences (0.5–5.0 points). Stably high activity of lectins was in the roots with rhizomes, stems, and blossoming inflorescences (5.5–9.0 points).

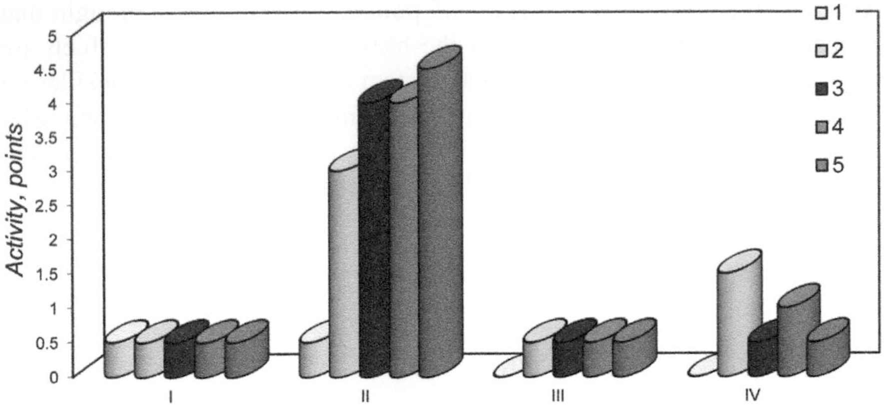

FIGURE 20.6 (See color insert.) Dynamics of activity of lectins in leaves of *E. purpurea* of the first year of vegetation. Rosette leaves: I-blade; II-leafstalk; Stem leaves: III- blade; IV-leafstalk. Sampling time: 1-June; 2-July; 3-August; 4-September; 5-October.

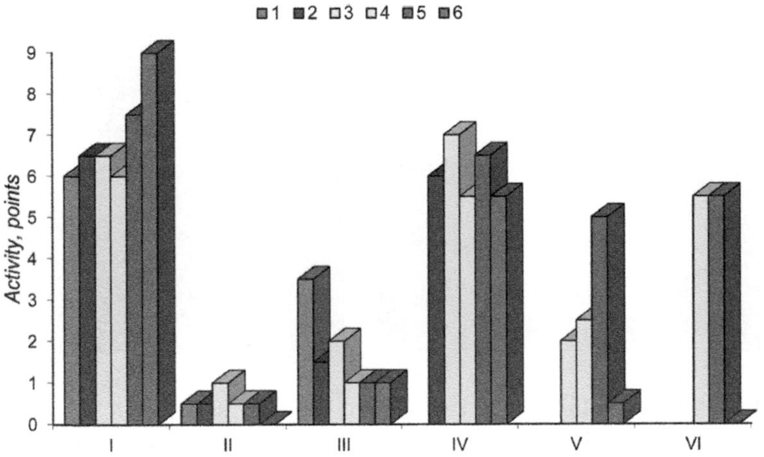

FIGURE 20.7 Dynamics of activity of lectins of *E. purpurea* of the second year of vegetation. I—rhizome with roots; II—leaf blade; III—leafstalk; IV—stems; V—not blossoming inflorescences; VI—blossoming inflorescences. Sampling time: 1—renewal of vegetation; 2—regrowth; 3—formation of inflorescences; 4—flowering; 5—fruit formation; 6—ripening of fruits.

Figure 20.8 presents data on the evaluation of hemagglutinating activity of *Echinacea* leaves. It can be concluded that in *Echinacea* of the second year of vegetation, rosette leaves are the main place of the synthesis of lectins—their activity in plates increased from April to June (0.5–1.5 points) and decreased to zero at the end of vegetation (Fig. 20.8, I). In the leafstalks, hemagglutinating activity was the highest at the beginning of the growing season—3.5 points and in the subsequent samples, it was 1.5–2.0 points (Fig. 20.8, II). In the stem leaves, lectins were not detected (Fig. 20.8, III and IV). Only in August, there was little activity in leaf blades. However, it would be a mistake to talk about their absence. More likely, our methods are not sensitive enough to detect the activity of phytolectins.

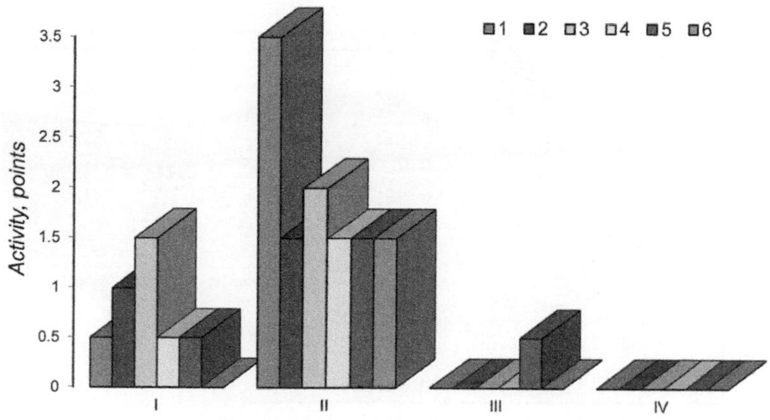

FIGURE 20.8 (See color insert.) Dynamics of activity of lectins in leaves of *E. purpurea* of generative period of ontogenesis. Rosette leaves: I—blades; II—stems; Stem leaves: III—blade; IV—leafstalk; Sampling time: 1—renewal of vegetation; 2—regrowth; 3—formation of inflorescences; 4—flowering; 5—fruit formation; 6—ripening of fruits.

20.6 ACTIVITY OF LECTINS AND THEIR DYNAMICS IN *ECHINACEA PALLIDA*

The protein complex of *E. pallida* was not studied enough, which served us as a basis for studying lectins in its samples. If there is information about the presence of lectins in *E. purpurea*, then we have not found such information for *E. pallida*. In this connection, the purpose of the present studies was to study the activity of lectins in different parts and organs of *E. pallida* during ontogenesis (Pospelov, 2013).

For 3 years we had been conducting systematic take samples of *E. pallida* of the first year of vegetation. The results of their analysis are shown in Figure 20.9. The evaluation of the activity of lectins in leaf blades (Fig. 20.9, II) shows a sufficiently high level during the entire growing season. In young blades, activity averaged 12.0 points, with time it increased and in October reached 16.0 points. An analogous regularity was also characteristic of leafstalks (Fig. 20.9, III). In July, the agglutination activity was minimal—9.0 points and at the end of the vegetation, it increased to 17.0 points. Determination of activity in the underground part showed that in young rhizomes with roots lectins were not detected, and only in October their content was estimated at 2.0 points.

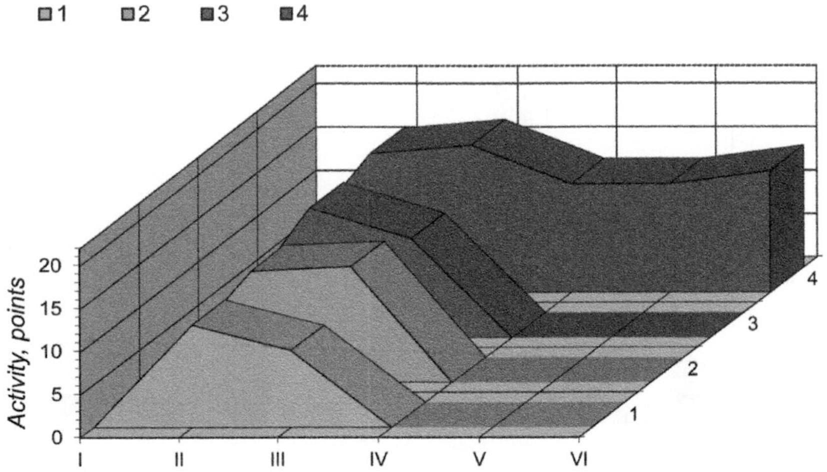

FIGURE 20.9 (See color insert.) Dynamics of activity of lectins of *E. pallida* of the first year of vegetation. I—root system; II—leaf blade; III—leafstalk; IV—stems; V—not blossoming inflorescences; VI—blossoming inflorescences. Sampling time: 1 July; 2 August; 3 September; 4 October.

For *E. pallida* transition to the generative period of ontogenesis, as a rule, occurs in the second year of vegetation (Samorodov and Pospelov, 1999). At the same time, in the conditions of Poltava region, a small number of plants blossomed at the end of the first year, in October. We used them for our research. It should be noted that the activity of lectins in stems and developing inflorescences was relatively high—12.5 points. An even higher level was noted in the blossoming baskets—14.0 points (Fig. 20.9).

The obtained data allow to draw a conclusion that in plants of the first year of vegetation, the leaves act as the main place of synthesis and localization of lectins in the plant. Young rhizomes with roots only accumulate phytolectins to a small extent at the end of vegetation, they apparently enter the stems and inflorescences together with other necessary substances and subsequently localize there. Thus, the overground mass at the end of the growing season accumulates a significant amount of lectins and is of interest as a source of raw materials of these specific protein compounds.

We also determined the presence of lectins in the samples of *E. pallida* of the second year of vegetation. The study of the dynamics of their activity has been carried out by us for 3 years, indicates a greater accumulation in the overground part in comparison with the rhizomes and roots. Figure 20.10 shows the change in the activity of lectins in the rosette leaves of *E. pallida.* During the period of regrowth—the beginning of flowering (May–June) the agglutinating activity of extracts of leaf blades was 5.5–6.0 points. Later it increased to 21.0–24.0 points. Similarly, the activity of lectins in the leafstalks also changed. If in the May samples it was 7.0 points, then in June to September, at the level of 18.0–24.0 points. This leads to a thought that in May to June lectins are actively synthesized in leaves and through the leafstalks are transported to other parts of the plant. In the subsequent (July to August) simultaneously with the synthesis, processes of agglutinin accumulation in the leaves takes place.

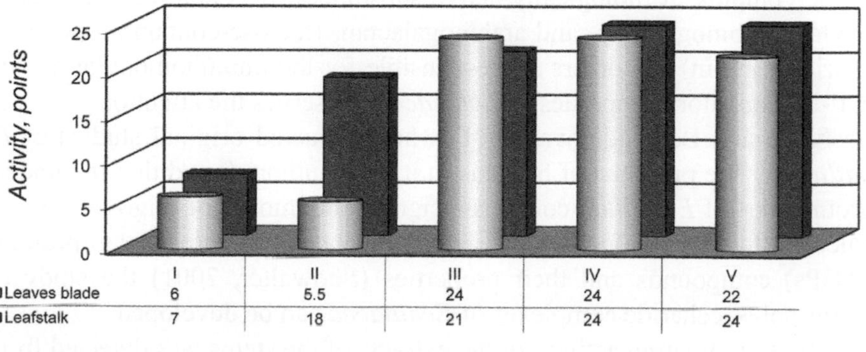

FIGURE 20.10 (See color insert.) Dynamics of activity of lectins in rosette leaves of *E. pallida* of the second year of vegetation. Sampling time: I—regrowth; II—formation of inflorescences; III—flowering; IV—fruit formation; V—ripening of fruits.

Similar regularities are also characteristic for stem leaves (Fig. 20.11). In spring, during the growth, the activity of lectins was 9.5 points in leaf blades and 10.0 in leafstalks. From the beginning of flowering to the end of vegetation, the agglutinating activity of the extracts increased from 18.0–19.5 points to 21.0–24 points. It is known that a specific feature of lectins is the ability of reversibly and specifically bind to carbohydrate ligands, which makes it possible to move agglutinins through the plant (Lutsik et al., 1981; Ignatov, 1997). It is highly possible that the polysaccharide complex of *Echinacea* can not only perform a transport function in relation to lectins but also bind to them, accumulating in parts and organs of the plant.

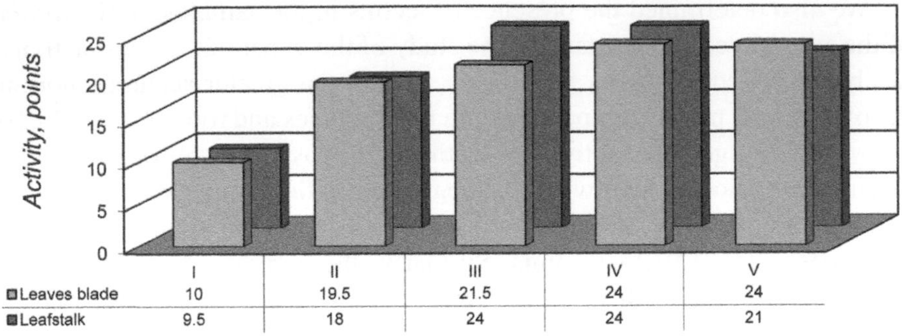

FIGURE 20.11 (See color insert.) Dynamics of activity of lectins in stem leaves of *E. pallida* of the second year of vegetation. Sampling time: I–regrowth; II–formation of inflorescences; III–flowering; IV–fruit formation; V–ripening of fruits.

For *Echinacea* species, the polysaccharide complex is an important link in the complex of biologically active substances. It is believed that heteroxylan, arabinogalactan, and arabinogalactan, fructose-containing polysaccharides (inulin) and others are responsible for the immunomodulating and anti-inflammatory properties of *Echinacea*. Deserves the attention works of Vasfilova and Bagautdinova (2011) who conducted original studies of *E. pallida* for the presence of fructans in it. The authors found that the underground part of *E. pallida* contains a significant amount of oligo- and polyfructans. In connection with the recently isolated arabinogalactan-proteins (AGPs) compounds and their properties (Showalter, 2001) the study of lectin-polysaccharide complexes of *Echinacea* can be developed.

The agglutinating activity of the extracts of the stems was detected from the moment of their formation (Fig. 20.12). In May, activity was minimal (12.0 points), later it increased and reached its maximum at the end of vegetation (20.0–21.0 points).

Interesting regularities were revealed when studying the dynamics of lectin activity of inflorescences (Fig. 20.13). In *Echinacea*, inflorescences, located on the main shoot, begin to blossom first, and then on lateral shoots. In the conditions of Ukraine, *E. pallida* massively blooms in June, but separate inflorescences can be formed until August. It was found that the activity of lectins in the forming baskets in June is maximal and is 19.5 points, in inflorescences, which were formed in July—14.0 points, and in August— it was not detected. The opposite relationship was noted by us when assessing the level of activity of phytolectins in flowering inflorescences. In the baskets selected in June, lectins were not detected and the activity of lectins in the blossoming inflorescences (July) was 21.5 points. During the period of fruit formation (August) agglutination activity reached a maximum of 24 points. It should be noted that when determining the activity of phytolectins in fruits, extracted from baskets in August and September, it did not exceed 4.5 points. Thus, the physiological role of lectins in stems and inflorescences is still unclear, when the maximum number of lectins accumulates at the end of vegetation, while the aboveground mass actually dies.

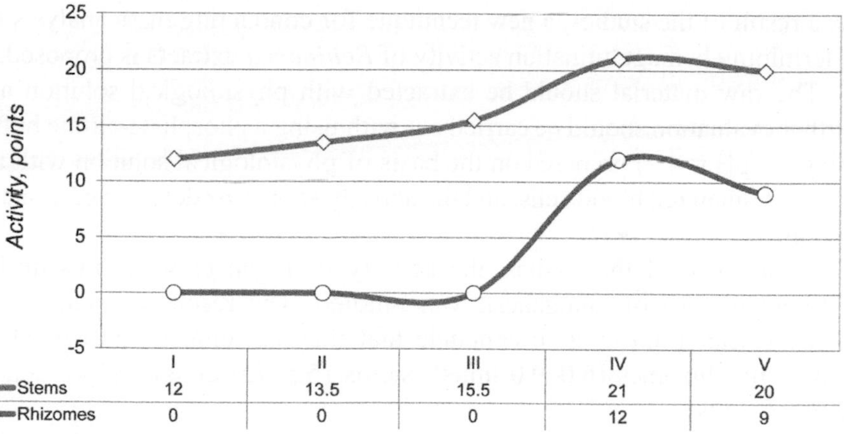

FIGURE 20.12 (See color insert.) Dynamics of activity of lectins in stems and rhizomes of *E. pallida* of the second year of vegetation. Sampling time: I—regrowth; II—formation of inflorescences; III—flowering; IV—fruit formation; V—ripening of fruits.

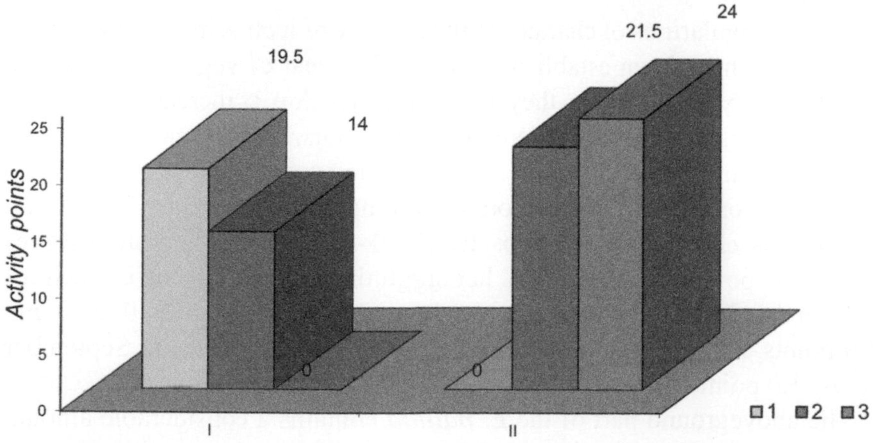

FIGURE 20.13 (See color insert.) Dynamics of activity of lectins in inflorescences of *E. pallida* of the second year of vegetation. I—date of inflorescences forming; II—blossoming inflorescences Sampling time: 1 June; 2 July: 3 August.

The study of rhizomes with roots of *E. pallida* testifies to the absence of lectin activity in samples taken in May, June, and July (Fig. 20.13). The maximum activity was registered by us during in August (21.0 points) the smaller in September (20.0 points).

20.7 CONCLUSION

As a result of the studies, a new technique for conducting mass analysis for determining hemagglutination activity of *Echinacea* extracts is proposed.

The raw material should be extracted with physiological solution and further evaluation should be carried out with using a phosphate-citrate buffer mixture (pH = 4.4) prepared on the basis of physiological solution with the help of human red blood cells, and the activity should be determined visually in points.

As a result of the studies, the activity of *E. purpurea* lectins during different periods of ontogenesis was studied. The results of many years of the research allow us to conclude that they accumulate most of all in roots with rhizomes (6.0–9.0 units), stems (5.5–7.0 units), inflorescences (2.0–6.0 units).

It is established that the basal leaves blade a major role in the formation of the lectin pool of the plant. The peculiarities of accumulation of lectins in stems and root system lead to a thought that there is a lectin-polysaccharide complex, which ensures the necessary functioning of hemagglutinins in the plant.

Certain regularities of changes in the activity of lectins in the ontogenesis of *E. pallida* have been established. In the first year of vegetation in young plants, activity was low, as they grow and develop it increased in leaves to 16.0 points, in generative stems to 14.0 points. In rhizomes with roots, phytolectins are found at the end of the growing season.

In the second year of vegetation, beginning with flowering, high activity of lectins is characteristic for rosette (21.0–24.0 points) and stem leaves (18.0–24.0 points). The peak of hemagglutinating activity of extracts of stems and inflorescences occurred at the end of vegetation (20.0–21.0 and 24.0 points, respectively), and rhizomes with roots in August to September (20.0–21.0 points).

The aboveground part of the *E. pallida* contains a considerable amount of lectins and can be a source of raw materials of these unique protein compounds, which opens the possibility of bioconversion of wastes that are formed on seed crops and after the plantation is eliminated.

KEYWORDS

- **lectins**
- **hemagglutination**
- **purple coneflower**
- **pale purple coneflower**
- ***Echinacea purpurea* (L.) Moench**
- ***Echinacea pallida* (Nutt.) Nutt.**

REFERENCES

Antonjuk, V. O.; Rybak, O. V. Study of Carbohydrate Specificity of Lectins of Underground Organs of *Echinacea purpurea* and *Rudbeckia laciniata. Farmakom.* **2002,** *3,* 153–158. (in Ukr.).

Bauer, R.; Wagner, H. *Echinacea: handbuch für erzte, apotheker und andere naturwissenschaftler;* Wissenschaftliche Verlagsgesellschaft. GmbH: Stuttgart, 1990; p 182.

Dreval. N. V.; Schegoleva, T. Y.; Kolesnikov, V. G. Comparative Analysis of Molecular Mechanisms *Echinacea purpurea* (L.) Moench on Blood Cell for New Biotechnology Making/With *Echinacea* in the Third Millennium. Materials of the International Scientific Conference, Poltava. Terra, 2003, pp 168–172 (in Russ.).

Dubinska, G. M. Pespectives of Use of a Water-Alcohol Extract of *Echinacea purpurea* as a Means of Treatment and Prevention of Homeostasis Disorders in the Liquidators of the Consequences of the Chernobyl Accident/Learning and Using *Echinacea.* Proceedings of the International Conference. -Poltava, Verstka, 1998, pp 118–121 (in Ukr.).

Golynskaya, Y. L.; Pospelov, S. V.; Samorodov, V. N. Patent 276 (USSR). A method for evaluating the physiological activity of lectins to sugars. G 01 N 33/53. 1992. (in. Russ.). **1732**.

Hardman, J. T.; Beck, M. L.; Owensby, C. E. Range Forb Lectins. *Transfusion* **1983,** *23,* 519–522.

Ignatov, V. V. Carbohydrate Recognizing Proteins—Lectins. *Sorosovskii obrazovatel'nyi zhurnal.* **1997,** *2,* 14–20. (in Russ.).

Kondrotas, A.; Janulis, V.; Jurkstiene, V.; Simoniene, G. In *Hemoagglutinative properties of Desmodium Caradense and Echinacea purpurea (phytoimmunostimulators)*, Abstracts of International Scientific Conference "Laboratory and Clinical Immunology," September 19–21, Vilnius, Lithuania, 1996. p. 121.

Kondrotas, A.; Jurkstiene, V.; Janulis, V. Changes in the Activity of Some Indicators of Non-specific Reactivity of the Organism under the Influence of *Echlnacea moench. Immunology, allergology, infektology*. Leningrad, **1999,** *1,* pp 84–85 (in Russ.).

Lutsik, M. D.; Panasjuk, E. N.; Lutsik, A. D. Lectins. *L'vov* **1981,** p 156. (in Russ.).

Miller, S. C. Two Immunoenhancers are Not Better than One. In *Echinacea: The Genus Echinacea;* Miller, S. C., Ed.; CRC Press: Boca Raton, 2004; p 276.

Pohorila, N. F.; Menshova, V. O.; Brajon, O. V. Lectins are Biologically Active Substances of *Echinacea purpurea*. *Farmacevtychnyj zhurnal.* **1997,** *4,* 80–83. (in Ukr.).
Pospelov, S. V. Lectins of *Echinacea purpurea*—Search, Properties and Evaluation of Activity/Learning and using *Echinacea.* Proceedings of the International Conference, Poltava. Verstka. 1998, pp 90–92. (in Russ.).
Pospelov, S. V. Lectins of Representatives of the *Echinacea genus* (*Echinacea* Moench). 1. Some Methodological Aspects of Activity Evaluation. *Khimija Rastitel'nogo Syr'ja.* **2012,** *3,* 143–148. (in Russ.).
Pospelov, S. V. Lectins of Representatives of the *Echinacea* Genus (*Echinacea* Moench.). 2. Features of Activity in the Ontogenesis of *Echinacea pallida* (Nutt.) Nutt. *Khimija Rastitel'nogo Syr'ja.* **2013,** *1,* 128–135. (in Russ.).
Pospelov, S. V. Evaluation of the Activity of Lectin-Containing Extracts of *Echinacea* purpurea. *Visnyk Poltavs'kogo derzhavnogo sil's'kogospodars'kogo instytutu.* **1998**, *1,* 15–17. (in Russ.).
Pospelov, S. V.; Pospelova, A. D. Lectins of representatives of the *Echinacea* genus (*Echinacea* Moench.). 2. Features of activity in the ontogenesis of *Echinacea purpurea* (L.) Moench.). *Khimija Rastitel'nogo Syr'ja.* **2012,** *3,* 149–156 (in Russ.).
Pospelov, S. V.; Samorodov, V. N. *Echinacea purpurea*: from Indian Prairies to Ukrainian Steppes. *Zerno.* **2009,** *6,* 64–68. (in Russ.).
Pospelov, S. V.; Samorodov, V. N. Search and Properties of Lectins of *Echinacea purpurea.* Problems Medicinal Plant. Proceedings of the International Scientific Conference on the Occasion of the 80th Anniversary of the Institute of Medicinal Plant Biochemistry. Poltava, 1996, pp 239–240. (in Ukr.).
Pospelov, S. V.; Samorodov, V. N.; Pospielova, G. D. Main directions and Results of Research of Biology of Lectins in Poltava State Agricultural Institute. *Visnyk Poltavs'koho derzhavnoho sil's'kohospodars'koho instytutu.* **2001,** *4,* 42–47 (in Ukr.).
Samorodov, V. N.; Pospelov, S. V. *Echinacea in Ukraine: The Fifty-Year Experience of the Introduction and Cultivation;* Poltava, Verstka, 1999, p 52. (in Russ.).
Samorodov, V. N.; Pospelov, S. V.; Moiseeva, G. F.; Sereda, A. V. Phytochemical Composition and Pharmacological Properties of Various Species of the Echinacea Moench. Genus (A Review). *Pharm. Chem. J.* **1996,** *4,* 245–251.
Showalter, A. M. Arabinogalactan-Proteins: Structure, Expression and Function. *Cell Mol. Life Sci.* **2001,** *58*(10), 1399–1417.
Vasfilova, E. S.; Bagautdinova, R. A. Features of the Growth and Development of *Echinacea pallida* Variety Prairie Beauty in the Conditions of the Middle Urals. *Visnyk Poltavs'koi' derzhavnoi' agrarnoi' akademii'.* **2011,** *1,* 31–35. (in Russ.).

INDEX

B

C

D

E

F

G

H

I

J

K

L

N

O

Q

R

T

U

V

W

X

Printed and bound by CPI Group (UK) Ltd, Croydon, CR0 4YY
23/10/2024
01777703-0018